Oxford Textbook of
Anaesthesia for Oral and
Maxillofacial Surgery

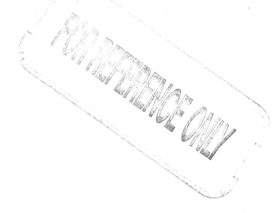

Oxford Textbook of Anaesthesia for Oral and Maxillofacial Surgery

Edited by

Ian Shaw

Consultant Anaesthetist
Royal Victoria Infirmary, Newcastle upon Tyne,
and Honorary Clinical Lecturer
University of Newcastle upon Tyne Medical School

Chandra Kumar

Consultant Anaesthetist and Professor of Anaesthesia
James Cook University Hospital, Middlesbrough

and

Chris Dodds

Consultant Anaesthetist and Professor of Anaesthesia
James Cook University Hospital, Middlesbrough

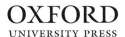

OXFORD
UNIVERSITY PRESS

OXFORD

UNIVERSITY PRESS

Great Clarendon Street, Oxford OX2 6DP

Oxford University Press is a department of the University of Oxford.
It furthers the University's objective of excellence in research, scholarship,
and education by publishing worldwide in

Oxford New York

Auckland Cape Town Dar es Salaam Hong Kong Karachi
Kuala Lumpur Madrid Melbourne Mexico City Nairobi
New Delhi Shanghai Taipei Toronto

With offices in

Argentina Austria Brazil Chile Czech Republic France Greece
Guatemala Hungary Italy Japan Poland Portugal Singapore
South Korea Switzerland Thailand Turkey Ukraine Vietnam

Oxford is a registered trade mark of Oxford University Press
in the UK and in certain other countries

Published in the United States
by Oxford University Press Inc., New York

© Oxford University Press, 2010

British Library Cataloguing in Publication Data
Data available

Library of Congress Cataloging in Publication Data
Data available

Typeset by MPS Limited, A Macmillan Company
Printed in Great Britain
on acid-free paper by
CPI Antony Rowe

ISBN 978–0–19–956421–7

10 9 8 7 6 5 4 3 2

Dedication

Hilary, Catriona, and Susannah Shaw
Suchitra Kumar
Ann Dodds

Foreword

I have always been nervous about anaesthesia for oral and maxillofacial surgery. It could all go so wrong, so quickly. Perhaps I was not helped by a maxillofacial surgeon who remarked that "no patient is so bad that we can't make them worse", when I was a first year anaesthetist. Even if one can avoid the problems of cyanosis ("I *really* should *not* have taken that tube out") or bleeding, or bleeding and cyanosis, one is intimidated by the difficult anatomy, physiology and pathology involved in the head and neck. It is an area that few of us can claim to understand well, and most of us approach with apprehension. One of the reasons for my discomfort has been ignorance, and that has been partly due to the lack of a textbook devoted to maxillofacial anaesthesia. It is curious that no one has had the initiative to bring together the issues of relevance to anaesthetists before.

There is a huge amount of information in this volume, which the specialist will find fascinating, but the book will be welcomed particularly by the occasional oral and maxillofacial anaesthetist and their assistants, thrust into that specialist world, probably when "on call". A survey of the members of the United Kingdom Difficult Airway Society revealed that anaesthesia for maxillofacial surgery was regarded as the source of their greatest anxieties concerning airway matters. The correct timing and conduct of anaesthesia for urgent cases are particularly worrying issues for the inexperienced.

There is pleasure and satisfaction to be had in the practice of anaesthesia, but there is also anxiety and doubt. Much of our apprehension arises from the suspicion that there is a better way of doing something. Finding a source of knowledge and experience is a pleasure recognised by all of us who have felt that we don't know enough, and worse, that others can see that we don't.

Samuel Johnson remarked that "*Knowledge is of two kinds. We know a subject ourselves, or we know where we can find information upon it*". Ian Shaw and his co-editors have persuaded a distinguished list of experts to provide us with the first textbook devoted to oral and maxillofacial anaesthesia, so now we know where to look. I wish it had been available earlier in my career.

Dr Ian Calder MB ChB, DRCOG, FRCA
Consultant Anaesthetist
Department of Neuroanaesthesia and Critical Care
The National Hospital for Neurology and Neurosurgery
Queen Square
London
WC1N 3BG

Preface

Oral and maxillofacial surgery is the surgical specialty concerned with the diagnosis and treatment of diseases affecting the teeth, mouth, jaws, face, and neck and represents one of the commonest indications for anaesthesia worldwide. The anaesthetic care of oral and maxillofacial patients requires specific knowledge and skills on the part of the anaesthetist. An understanding of the subject matter is fundamental to the safe practice of anaesthesia.

This textbook is intended to go some way to address this need. The anaesthetist can be called upon to provide anaesthesia for patients presenting with impacted or carious teeth, infections of the mucosa and adjacent structures, complex facial injuries, head and neck cancers, salivary gland disease, facial disproportion, temporomandibular joint disorders, cysts, and tumours of the jaws. Anaesthetists may also be involved in managing patients experiencing chronic and intractable facial pain and provide anaesthesia for multiple trauma involving the face.

Although primarily written for anaesthetists, this textbook will also be of interest to maxillofacial surgeons, anaesthetic practitioners, anaesthetic nurses, and Operating Department Practitioners involved in providing anaesthesia for dental, oral, and maxillofacial surgery. We would also expect the work to be of interest to those anaesthetists currently in training and studying for their professional examinations.

Ian Shaw
Chandra Kumar
Chris Dodds

Acknowledgements

We would like to acknowledge the patience, assistance, and helpful advice shown by members of the Oxford University Press Production Team throughout the project.

Contents

List of contributors *xv*

Abbreviations *xvii*

Chapter 1 **The history of dental anaesthesia** *1*
Gary Enever

Chapter 2 **Preassessment and optimization of oral and maxillofacial patients** *11*
Diane Monkhouse and Sanjiv Sharma

Chapter 3 **Medicolegal aspects of anaesthesia for oral and maxillofacial surgery** *27*
Christopher Heneghan

Chapter 4 **Recognition and management of the difficult airway** *35*
Charles H. Kates and Steven Gayer

Chapter 5 **The surgical airway** *49*
Kaye Cantlay

Chapter 6 **The innervation of the head and neck** *65*
Bernard J. Moxham and Barry K.B. Berkovitz

Chapter 7 **Regional anaesthetic techniques in oral and maxillofacial surgery** *91*
John Gerard Meechan

Chapter 8 **Conscious sedation** *103*
David Craig

Chapter 9 **Anaesthesia for dental surgery** *119*
Sean Williamson

Chapter 10 **Anaesthesia for aesthetic surgery** *131*
Sandip Pal and Chandra Kumar

Chapter 11 **Infection and oral and maxillofacial surgery: implications for anaesthesia** *143*
Ian D. Clement

Chapter 12 **Oral and maxillofacial related injuries and hazards during anaesthesia** *151*
Hilary Turner and Ian Shaw

Chapter 13 **Oral and maxillofacial imaging for the anaesthetist** *165*
Neil Heath and Iain Macleod

Chapter 14 **Anaesthesia for maxillofacial trauma** *177*
Joy Curran

Chapter 15 **Facial, oral, and airway thermal injuries and anaesthesia** *189*
Tim Vorster

Chapter 16 **Anaesthesia for oral and maxillofacial malignancy** *207*
Anjum Ahmed-Nusrath, Seema Pathare, and Stephen Bonner

Chapter 17 **Adjuvant therapy for head and neck malignancy** *225*
Charles G. Kelly

Chapter 18 Anaesthesia for orthognathic surgery *241*
Viki Mitchell

Chapter 19 Anaesthesia for paediatric maxillofacial surgery *253*
Ann Black and Senthil Nadarajan

Chapter 20 Hypotensive anaesthesia *269*
Andrew Jones

Chapter 21 Anaesthesia for nasal and antral surgery *275*
Sanjiv Sharma and Judith C. Wright

Chapter 22 Orofacial pain *283*
Tara Renton and Joanna Zakrzewska

Chapter 23 Sleep apnoea *299*
Chris Dodds

Chapter 24 Postoperative nursing considerations for the maxillofacial surgical patient *311*
Lindsay Garcia

Index *327*

List of contributors

Dr Anjum Ahmed-Nusrath MB BS DA FRCA
Consultant Anaesthetist
James Cook University Hospital, Middlesbrough

Dr Barry K.B. Berkovitz BDS MSc PhD FDS (Eng)
Emeritus Reader
Anatomy and Human Sciences, King's College London

Dr Ann E. Black MB BS DRCOG DA FRCA
Consultant Anaesthetist
Great Ormond Street Hospital for Children NHS
  Trust, London

Dr Stephen Bonner MB BS MRCP FRCA
Consultant in Anaesthesia and Intensive Care
James Cook University Hospital, Middlesbrough

Dr Kaye Cantlay BA MB ChB MRCP FRCA EDIC
Consultant in Anaesthesia and Critical Care
Royal Victoria Infirmary, Newcastle upon Tyne

Dr Ian Clement BM BCh MA DPhil MRCP FRCA
Consultant Anaesthetist
Royal Victoria Infirmary, Newcastle upon Tyne

Dr David Craig BA BDS MMedSci MFGDP (UK)
Consultant, Sedation and Special Care Dentistry
Guy's and St. Thomas's NHS Foundation Trust, London

Dr Joy Curran MB BS FRCA
Consultant Anaesthetist
Queen Victoria Hospital, East Grinstead

Professor Chris Dodds MB BS MRCGP FRCA
Consultant Anaesthetist and Professor of Anaesthesia
James Cook University Hospital, Middlesbrough

Dr Gary Enever MB BS MA FRCA
Consultant Anaesthetist
Royal Victoria Infirmary, Newcastle upon Tyne

Mrs Lindsay Garcia RGN BSc
Divisional Manager of Intensive Care and Medicine
James Cook University Hospital, Middlesbrough

Dr Steven Gayer MD MBA
Associate Professor of Clinical Anaesthesia
  and Opthalmology and Director of Anaesthesia
  Services, Bascolm Palmer Eye Institute
University of Miami Millar School of Medicine
Miami, Florida, USA

Dr Neil Heath DCR(R) BDS MSc MFDSRCS DDRRCR
Consultant in Oral and Maxillofacial Radiology
Glasgow Dental Hospital, Glasgow

Dr Christopher P.H. Heneghan BA BM BCh FRCA
Consultant Anaesthetist and Barrister
Nevill Hall Hospital, Abergavenny

Dr Andrew Jones BSc LMSSA DGMRCP FRCA
Consultant Anaesthetist
Royal Liverpool Hospital, Liverpool

Dr Charles H. Kates DDS
Associate Professor of Anaesthesia and Surgery,
  Director of Anaesthesia and Pain Control,
  Division of Oral/Maxillofacial Surgery
University of Miami Miller School of Medicine
Miami, Florida, USA

Dr Charles G. Kelly MB ChB MSc FRCP
  FRCR DMRT
Consultant Oncologist
Freeman Hospital, Newcastle upon Tyne

Professor Chandra Kumar MB BS DTCD DA
  FFARCS FRCA MSc
Consultant Anaesthetist and Professor of Anaesthesia
James Cook University Hospital, Middlesbrough

Dr Iain Macleod PhD BDS FDSRCS(Ed) DDRRCR
Consultant in Oral and Maxillofacial Radiology
Newcastle upon Tyne Dental Hospital, Newcastle
  upon Tyne

Dr John Gerard Meechan BSc BDS PhD FDSRCS
  (Edin) FDSRCPS (Glas)
Consultant and Senior Lecturer in Oral and
  Maxillofacial Surgery
School of Dental Sciences, Newcastle University
  Newcastle upon Tyne

Dr Viki Mitchell MB BS FRCA
Consultant Anaesthetist
University College Hospital, London

Dr Diane Monkhouse MB BS MRCP FRCA
Consultant in Anaesthesia and Intensive Care
James Cook University Hospital, Middlesbrough

Professor Bernard J. Moxham BSc BDS PhD
Professor of Anatomy and Deputy Director and Head
  of Teaching at the Cardiff School of Biosciences,
  Cardiff University, Cardiff

Dr Senthil Nadarajan MB BS FRCA
Consultant Anaesthetist
Ipswich Hospital, Ipswich

Professor Sandip K. Pal MB BS FFARCSI MD
Consultant Anaesthetist and Director of Research &
  Development
Mid Essex Hospitals NHS Trust, Broomfield Hospital,
  Chelmsford

Dr Seema Pathare MB BS FRCA
Specialist Registrar in Anaesthesia, Northern Deanery.
James Cook University Hospital, Middlesbrough

Professor Tara Renton BDS MDSc (OS) PhD
  FDSRCS FRACDS FRACDS(OMS)
Professor in Oral Surgery
Kings College Hospital, London

Dr Sanjiv Sharma MB BS FRCA
Specialist Registrar, Northern Deanery
James Cook University Hospital,
  Middlesbrough

Dr Ian Shaw BSc PhD MB BChir DA FRCA
Consultant Anaesthetist
Royal Victoria Infirmary, Newcastle upon Tyne

Dr Hilary Turner MB BS FRCA
Specialist Registrar, Northern Deanery
Royal Victoria Infirmary, Newcastle upon Tyne

Dr Tim Vorster, MB BS BSc FRCA
Consultant in Burns Intensive Care and Anaesthetics,
  McIndoe Burns Centre,
Queen Victoria Hospital, East Grinstead

Dr Sean Williamson MB BChir FRCA
Consultant Anaesthetist
James Cook University Hospital, Middlesbrough

Dr Judith Wright MB ChB FRCA
Consultant Anaesthetist
James Cook University Hospital, Middlesbrough

Professor Joanna M. Zakrzewska BDS MB BChir MD
  FDSRCS FFDRCSI FHEA FFPM RCA
Consultant and Honorary Professor in Oral Medicine
  and Facial Pain Lead,
Eastman Dental Hospital, University College London
  Hospitals

Abbreviations

AAOP	American Academy of Orofacial Pain	DDAVP	1-desamino-8-D-arginine vasopressin
ABA	American Burn Association	DJD	degenerative joint disease
ABG	alveolar bone graft	DMFT	decayed, missing, or filled teeth
ACC	American College of Cardiologists	DPT	dental panoramic tomogram
ACE	angiotensin-converting enzyme	DVT	deep vein thrombosis
AD	advance decision		
AHA	American Heart Association	EBRT	external beam radiotherapy
AO	atypical odontalgia	ECG	electrocardiogram
APA	Association of Paediatric Anaesthetists	EEG	electroencephalography
APTT	activated partial thromboplastin time	EGFR	epidermal growth factor receptor
ARDS	acute respiratory distress syndrome	EMG	electromyography
ASA	American Society of Anesthesiologists	ENT	ear, nose, and throat
ATLS	Advanced Trauma Life Support	ESR	erythrocyte sedimentation rate
		ETT	endotracheal tube
BiPAP	bilevel positive airway pressure	ETTH	episodic tension-type headache
BMI	body mass index		
BMS	burning mouth syndrome	FBC	full blood count
BP	blood pressure	FDA	Federation Dentate International
BSSO	bilateral sagittal split mandibular ramus osteotomy	FEES	fibreoptic endoscopic evaluation of swallowing
		FESS	functional endoscopic sinus surgery
CBS	carotid blowout syndrome	FEV$_1$	forced expiratory volume in 1 second
CCF	congestive cardiac failure	FFP	fresh frozen plasma
CDH	chronic daily headache	FiO$_2$	fraction of inspired oxygen
CH	cluster headache		
CHEOPS	Children's Hospital of Eastern Ontario Pain Scale	POI	fibreoptic intubation
COPD	chronic obstructive pulmonary disease	FVC	forced vital capacity
CPAP	continuous positive airway pressure		
CPEX	cardiopulmonary exercise test	GA	general anaesthetic
CSF	cerebrospinal fluid	GDP	general dental practitioner
CT	computed tomography	GKI	glucose, potassium, and insulin
CTTH	chronic tension-type headache	GMC	General Medical Council
CVA	cerebrovascular accident		
CVP	central venous pressure	HDU	high dependency unit
CVVH	continuous venovenous haemofiltration	HIV	human immunodeficiency virus

IASP	International Association for the Study of Pain		PE	pulmonary embolism
ICU	intensive care unit		PEEP	positive end-expiratory pressure
ID	internal diameter		PEFR	peak expiratory flow rate
ILMA	intubating laryngeal mask airway		PEG	percutaneous endoscopic gastrostomy
IMCA	independent mental capacity advocates		PIFP	persistent idiopathic facial pain
IMF	intermaxillary fixation		POISE	perioperative ischaemic evaluation trial
IMRT	intensity modulated radiotherapy		PONV	postoperative nausea and vomiting
INR	international normalized ratio		PRF	pulse repetition frequency
IPPV	intermittent positive pressure ventilation		PSG	polysomnography
ISS	injury severity scores		PT	prothrombin time
ITU	Intensive Therapy Unit		RA	regional anaesthesia *or* relative analgesia
JVP	jugular venous pressure		RAE	Ring–Adair–Elwyn
			RCRI	revised cardiac risk index
Kg	kilogram/s		RCT	randomized controlled trials
KTP	potassium titanyl phosphate		RDCTMD	Research Diagnostic Criteria for Temporomandibular Disorders
LA	local anaesthetic		REM	rapid eye movement
LMA	laryngeal mask airway		RSI	rapid sequence induction
LPA	lasting power of attorney		RTA	road traffic accident
LST	life-sustaining treatment		SIRS	systemic inflammatory response syndrome
MAC	minimum alveolar concentration		SMV	submentovertex
MAD	mucosal atomization device		SSRI	selective serotonin reuptake inhibitors
mcg	microgram/s		ST	surgical tracheostomy
MHRA	Medicines and Healthcare products Regulatory Agency		SUNCT	short-lasting unilateral neuralgia from conjunctival irritation and tearing
ml	millilitre/s		SWS	slow wave sleep
MMPI	Minnesota multiple personality inventory		TBSA	total body surface area
MRI	magnetic resonance imaging		TCA	tricyclic antidepressants
MS	multiple sclerosis		TCI	target-controlled infusion
			TED	thromboembolus deterrent
NHS	National Health Service		TIA	transient ischaemic attack
NICE	National Institute for Health and Clinical Excellence		TIVA	total intravenous anaesthesia
			TMD	temporomandibular disease
NSAIDS	non-steroidal anti-inflammatory drugs		TMJ	temporomandibular joint
			TNM	tumour, node, and metastases
OAR	organs at risk		TTE	transthoracic echocardiogram
OD	outer diameter		TTH	tension-type headache
OHIP	Oral Health Impact		UK	United Kingdom
OMF	oral and maxillofacial		US	United States
OPG	orthopantomogram			
OSA	obstructive sleep apnoea		VPI	velopharyngeal insufficiency
PCA	patient-controlled analgesia		VTE	Venous thromboembolism
PCI	patient-controlled infusion			
PDT	percutaneous dilatational tracheostomy		WHO	World Health Organization

1

The history of dental anaesthesia

Gary Enever

Introduction

There has been very little published about anaesthesia for oral and maxillofacial surgery in recent years. That is why this book has been written. In the past, however, dental anaesthesia was a hugely important subject, with many books in circulation, and there were prominent sections in the general textbooks on anaesthesia. The history of dental anaesthesia can almost be regarded as the history of anaesthesia itself and, in this chapter, I hope to show why.

A small, scruffy black and white dog picks its way over the cobbles, between the horses hooves and piles of rubbish. It stops at a doorway and sniffs, hopefully, and begins to sidle in. Then it leaps back into the road, barking frantically as a scream from within rends the air. A young man in blue stockings and brown frock coat rushes out, clutching his hand over a copiously bleeding mouth. He is followed into the daylight by a muscular man in a bloodstained apron, clutching a large blackened tooth in a pair of pincers. The 'dentist' leans against his red and white striped pole and shakes his head sadly, then steps back into his shop with a shout of 'next'.

Painful teeth have existed since the dawn of human existence, and the desire to avoid this pain has no doubt existed for a similar length of time. Unfortunately, until relatively recently, life for most people was brutal, painful, and short. Bad teeth were a part of life, and pulling them out without any form of analgesia or anaesthesia was normal. The alternative was to keep them, and suffer continuous agony, or worse. Forceps for extracting teeth are some of the earliest surgical instruments discovered.

From our enlightened age, it is easy to look back at history and assume that man has always striven to conquer pain. The means to alleviate pain over the centuries have been scant and poisonous, and surgery excruciating and dangerous. Alcohol, hemp, poppy, henbane, and mandrake (or all of them mixed together) were used, with minor degrees of success[1]. However, over the past 200 years, scientific advances, allied with innovation and enterprising thinking, have changed attitudes. Driven by increasing demands from society, the search for pain relief accelerated. Techniques such as using cold, pressure, and hypnotism became popular, and are still used by some today. But it is the discovery of general, and then local, anaesthesia that changed the world.

It is easy to believe that anaesthesia as we know it started on 16 October 1846 in Boston, with a young dentist giving ether for the first successful public demonstration of 'painless' surgery[1]. His success, however, was only the culmination of a long series of events stretching back over hundreds of years. The idea of inhaling soporific substances went back at least as far as the Islamic physicians of a thousand years ago. Ether was known from the middle ages, and was described in the sixteenth century by Paracelsus, in the heyday of alchemy. He noted that feeding ether to chickens put them to sleep[1]. Eighteenth century scientists such as Joseph Priestley explored the chemical nature of gases, following the work of Hooke, Boyle, and Newton.

Humphry Davy

By the end of the eighteenth century, a number of gases had been identified and could be produced relatively reliably. Priestley had identified nitrous oxide in 1773. The rapidly expanding British Empire had made many people rich, and the rich were able to indulge themselves in new fads and cures. Bristol had been an extremely rich port, England's second city, with trading in slaves, sugar, rum, and tobacco. Although losing the American colonies had been a blow to Bristol's status, the rich and famous of the West Country still gravitated there. So it was to Bristol that Thomas Beddoes brought these new gases in his 'Pneumatic Institute'[2,3]. To help him in his enterprise, he employed a brilliant young surgeon's apprentice from Penzance by the name of Humphry Davy. Davy prepared gases, supervised treatments, and also observed the effects of gases on both patients and himself. He was particularly interested in nitrous oxide and eventually wrote a scholarly volume on the subject, published in 1800. Interestingly, Davy came into contact with celebrities, notably the romantic poets such as Coleridge, Southey, and Wordsworth. It is well known that they were extremely interested in mind-altering experiences. Nitrous oxide became a favourite recreational drug of the time. The Pneumatic Institute was lampooned in contemporary cartoons, but inhalational therapy was established.

Davy, unfortunately, failed to publicize the truly beneficial qualities of his gas. He had noted that nitrous oxide had a beneficial effect on his own toothache, and reduced his pain. Unfortunately, he had not pursued the observation and a great chance was lost. The fame of Humphry Davy is related to his later work—his lectures at the Royal Society and, in particular, his safe miner's lamp.

For the next 40 years, nitrous oxide, and also ether, was used for frolics and public entertainment. Their anaesthetic qualities went unnoticed, leaving serious investigators experimenting with such agents as carbon dioxide. Henry Hill Hickman, a physician in Shropshire, rendered a number of animals insensible to the pain of surgery, but did not try carbon dioxide on human patients. Had he known that the unconsciousness he saw was probably due to asphyxiation, a concept little understood at the time, perhaps he would not have persisted. Asphyxiation anaesthesia was, however, used in the nineteenth century. It was popular to throttle lunatics in asylums with a stocking around the neck, to make them more amenable to washing and dressing, and, of course, it became an important part of nitrous oxide anaesthesia, but more of that later[4,5].

The dawn of modern anaesthesia

By the 1840s, the time was ripe for 'modern' anaesthesia. Chemistry had progressed; agents were available, if not appreciated. Surgeons and dentists could progress little further as they were limited by the endurance of their patients. It just needed the right spark to start the fire. The blaze could have started in America in 1842, with a family doctor called Crawford Williamson Long. Ether frolics were popular in America, and the young physician had attended them. He had noted that inhaling the vapour had rendered him insensible to an injury. He tried ether inhalation for minor surgery and was successful, but did not advertise his discovery. He had primacy, but not the publicity.

With increasingly refined diets and the use of copious amounts of sugar, tooth decay and so dentistry were on the increase. The need for extractions spiralled, but they were still very painful. Horace Wells, a dentist of Hartford, Connecticut, first tried nitrous oxide successfully on 12 December 1844 for the extraction of one of his teeth. The gas was administered by Gardner Quincy Colton, and the tooth pulled by John Riggs. As with Long, Wells had noted that those under the influence seemed insensible to injury. He had seen nitrous oxide displayed the night before by the travelling chemist and showman, Colton, a purveyor of 'laughing gas'. So, he inhaled nitrous oxide himself and had one of his teeth painlessly extracted. Excited by the wonderful discovery, he repeated his experiments on a number of patients, with equal success. Unfortunately, there followed a very public and very unsuccessful demonstration in the Massachusetts General Hospital. Surgery was attempted before adequate gas had been inhaled, and the patient howled with pain. This failure eventually left Wells a broken man. He had a volatile temperament, falling into depression and then mental illness. He took his own life in prison in 1848 with a combination of chloroform and opening his femoral artery with a razor. Nitrous oxide was not to be taken seriously for another 20 years, although Colton carried on with his laughing gas shows.

On 16 October 1846, William Morton, another dentist, successfully demonstrated the use of ether for the removal of a tumour from a young man's neck in Boston, Massachusetts. He had worked with Horace Wells and knew of his failed attempt with nitrous oxide and had sought something more effective. He experimented, with the help of the chemist Dr Jackson, with sulphuric ether, trying it on his spaniel and then a young man, Eben Frost, again for tooth extraction. Ether rendered the subjects insensible to the pain inflicted. Morton was on the road to fame[1].

It is unlikely that Morton's discovery was purely intended for the alleviation of human suffering. Being able to operate painlessly gave him a huge advantage over his dental competition, and thus potentially increased his income. The successful demonstration was very good publicity. So were comments and papers from those assembled, the senior surgeons from one of America's greatest hospitals. Less noble is the fact that Morton subsequently tried to keep ether secret by calling it 'Letheon' and applying for a patent. He hoped that anaesthesia would be controlled, and tried to sell licences. He also tried to control the supply of his miracle agent but, because of the smell, people soon recognized it for what it was—sulphuric ether. His secret was out. Sadly, the discovery of anaesthesia was subsequently sullied by a number of arguments as to 'who was first'. Wells, Jackson, Morton, Long, and others vied acrimoniously, but in the end history remembers Morton[6].

Following the successful public demonstration, the press and assembled dignitaries in Boston made sure that news of this wonderful breakthrough spread around the world as quickly as ships could carry it. Dr Henry J. Bigelow, present at Morton's demonstration, prophetically stated 'I have seen something today which will go round the world'. The fact that the world was ready is supported by the readiness to try the new wonder. Wherever the news arrived, bottles of ether were procured and patients rendered insensible. That these patients submitted themselves so readily indicated how unpleasant was the alternative.

The term 'anaesthesia' was suggested by another Boston physician, Oliver Wendell Holmes, in a letter to Morton on 21 November 1846, and the name was adopted. The anaesthetic age had begun.

The first anaesthetic in England was almost certainly given in London. On Saturday 19 December 1846, a dentist by the name of James Robinson extracted a tooth from a Miss Lonsdale using ether for the extraction. She was the niece of a Dr Boott, who had just received a letter from Henry Bigelow. Two days later, Robert Liston, after communication from Boott, performed a painless and successful leg amputation. The realization that anaesthesia was a serious proposition, and not 'humbug', started a revolution. Anaesthetics were tried in most parts of Britain by early 1847. Interestingly, the first anaesthetic in Scotland also occurred on 19 December 1846. Dr Frazer had travelled from America on the *Arcadia*, the ship carrying Bigelow's letter. He gave ether at the hospital in

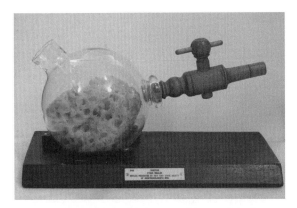

Figure 1.1 Morton's ether inhaler, as used in one of the first successful demonstrations of general anaesthesia in October 1846. See also Plate 1. (Photograph reproduced with the kind permission of the Association of Anaesthetists of Great Britain and Ireland.)

Dumfries, his ship having stopped in Scotland on the way to England.

Early anaesthesia was unpleasant and unpredictable for the patient. The alternative was terrible pain, so many accepted the risks. Ether was dripped onto sponges held inside glass vessels held to the face (Figure 1.1). As the ether evaporated, the glass became extremely cold and sometimes an inadequate amount of vapour was produced. The vapour was noxious, causing coughing and vomiting, and could make the skin so cold that it burned. As most anaesthetics were delivered by untrained assistants, under the direction of untrained operators, quality control was non-existent. Many surgeons, including Liston, were disappointed by the lack of reliability, and abandoned anaesthesia briefly. It needed someone to apply intelligence and science to the problem.

John Snow

John Snow (Figure 1.2) was a physician working in London at the time of Robinson and Boott's first use of ether, and was inspired by what he learned. Snow had an interesting but frustrating career up until 1846. He was born to a poor family in York, but thanks to a well connected uncle, his intelligence was not wasted. As a young surgeon's apprentice in Newcastle, he became acquainted with George and Robert Stephenson of engineering and railway fame. He joined the local Literary and Philosophical Society, and listened to lectures on Victorian engineering, steam, evaporation, condensation, gases, and pressures. When anaesthesia

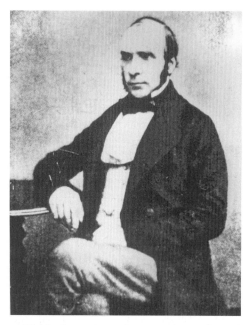

Figure 1.2 John Snow, nineteenth-century pioneer of anaesthesia.

first appeared, Snow probably understood the physics of gases better than any doctor in the country and immediately began his own investigations. He was possibly prompted to action by the untrained and unscientific individuals he met. It is said he was inspired by a pharmacist hurrying along the street with his glass ether vaporizer under his arm, busy developing his 'etherizing' practice. So, in 1847, Snow became Britain's, and the world's, first true dedicated physician/anaesthetist. He created the first proper anaesthetic vaporizers and did extensive animal research. For the next 10 years he gave thousands of anaesthetics, first with ether and then with chloroform and other agents[7]. Ether was difficult and unpleasant for induction, even in Snow's hands, and so in 1848 he switched to chloroform.

Where had chloroform come from? An obstetric surgeon in Edinburgh, James Young Simpson, had used ether in childbirth early in 1847. Because ether was unpleasant, Simpson experimented with other chemicals and at the end of 1847 used chloroform for the first time with great success. Chloroform was much easier to use but was later shown to be much more dangerous in overdose than ether. It was being used widely and indiscriminately, and inevitably soon became incriminated in a number of anaesthetic deaths. But, used carefully in skilled hands, it continued as an anaesthetic almost up to the present day.

In 1853, Snow gave chloroform to Queen Victoria for the birth of Prince Leopold. She called it 'that blessed chloroform', and took it again for her next delivery in 1857.

Reading John Snow's case books revealed that he had a thriving dental anaesthetic practice. He spent his days visiting hospitals, dentists, and surgeon's homes, as well as the homes of more well-to-do patients. Snow gave anaesthetics for about 25 dentists who were working within a mile of his house in Piccadilly. They were the leading practitioners of the capitol, many of them becoming leaders of professional dentistry in Britain.

Unfortunately, Snow suffered from increasing ill health. He had long been teetotal and vegetarian, not easy in Victorian England, and many of his colleagues felt that his habits were a major contributing factor to his frailty. He died on 16 June 1858 at the early age of 46, a few days after a massive stroke. It is interesting to note that, in his last week of work, in early June, he gave six chloroform anaesthetics for the removal of teeth, including one to the Duke of Bedford[8].

Snow is remembered not only by anaesthetists, but also epidemiologists, as he was the first to identify cholera as a waterborne disease. He removed a pump handle in Soho, and stopped an outbreak. To celebrate

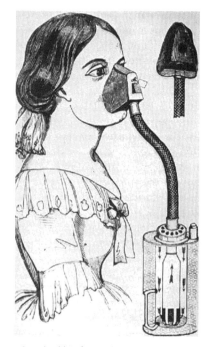

Figure 1.3 Snow's chloroform inhaler. Drawing from an original illustration in Snow's book.

the success, he has a pub named after him—ironic, considering his own drinking habits.

Joseph Clover

At the time of Snow's demise, the Dental Hospital had been founded in Soho, London, later to become the Royal Dental Hospital and School. Joseph Clover was a contemporary of Snow's, developing a career as a 'chloroformist'. He was the second great physician/anaesthetist to work in London, and he was appointed to the staff. Clover consolidated the great work of Snow, and was a prolific and inventive man, despite his poor health as a result of tuberculosis. He worked on safer ways to deliver chloroform, including using a large bag of air with a known percentage of chloroform vapour within.

Clover was also important in popularizing the introduction of nitrous oxide to Britain. After Wells had failed in 1844, Colton continued to tour with his laughing gas show. In 1862, he began to give nitrous oxide successfully for a number of dentists. He moved to Europe, and in Paris found a dentist very willing to use nitrous anaesthesia. Ironically, he was an American, T. W. Evans. Evans and Colton gave many thousands of successful anaesthetics, and Evans came to England on a demonstration tour in 1868. Clover observed Evans' success and began to use nitrous oxide, especially for dental anaesthetics[9]. By 1869, both Clover and a dentist called Alfred Coleman had independently devised masks and equipment to deliver gas nasally. Clover also developed the use of nitrous oxide as an induction agent to smooth ether anaesthesia. This can be indicated by the stopcock on later versions of his ether inhaler, for the introduction of nitrous oxide. If the patient needed oxygen, the mask was lifted slightly to let a little air in! Thus, thanks to dental anaesthesia, the use of ether was repopularized in Britain.

With the introduction of nitrous oxide to Britain, we now enter a time of rapid expansion. Ether and chloroform were not easy to use and carried known risks. They were usually given under the direction of a surgeon, or by one of the few physicians that specialized in anaesthesia. Nitrous oxide, however, appeared to be easy to use and safe. Dentists and their assistants began to give large numbers of anaesthetics. It is probably this fact that popularized the use of anaesthesia more than any other. Initially, nitrous oxide was generated from a special apparatus by the dentist. Soon, however, it could be purchased in rubber bags from chemist shops, and then in the first compressed gas cylinders from companies such as Barth and Coxeter.

Fatalities in dental practice were thankfully few. An early report in the Lancet of 1873 described the demise of a large lady called Miss Wyndham following unsuccessful nitrous oxide for dental extraction[10]. Colton engaged the Lancet in correspondence to defend 'his' anaesthetic, and his writings showed his lack of scientific understanding. Notably, he felt that, as nitrous oxide was made up of one part oxygen to two parts nitrogen, the patient was getting more oxygen than if they were breathing room air. It is amazing that, with this lack of knowledge, he gave over 100 000 anaesthetics without a death.

By the end of the 1860s, simple surgery and dentistry could be rendered relatively painless and less stressful for both operator and patient. Unfortunately, it was still not particularly safe to have an operation. Many who had surgery and survived the anaesthetic and immediate postoperative period died soon after. They had become infected by the myriad of bacteria that infested Victorian operating theatres. Dentistry, in contrast, took place in the homes of patients or dentists and, even with dirty instruments, the risks of sepsis from dental extractions were small. In many cases, removing infected teeth and pus improved the patient's condition.

Following the innovations of Florence Nightingale and Joseph Lister, infection rates finally came under

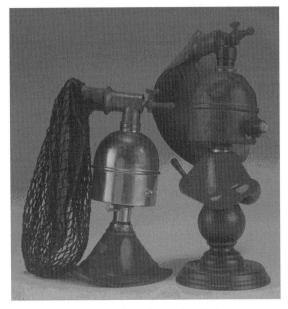

Figure 1.4 Clover's portable regulating ether inhaler.

some control. Surgeons became more ambitious and patients less reluctant. Operation rates increased as new operations were introduced, and hospitals needed more staff to work in the operating theatres. It is of interest to note that even at this time operations were usually brief, with continuous anaesthesia of over 15 minutes rare. The 'house staff', invariably senior medical students, acted as the anaesthetists under the direction of senior surgeons. They had little true training in anaesthesia, and mishaps often occurred, especially in patients with medical illnesses or more complex surgery. For this reason, by later in the nineteenth century, specialist physicians were often appointed to act as consulting anaesthetists. They were still rare, and often held appointments at a number of hospitals. It was these men who started to move anaesthesia forward.

Sir Frederic Hewitt

Sir Frederic Hewitt, born in 1857, had his first paper on anaesthesia published in 1885. He had taken up the specialty as his poor eyesight prevented anything more conventional. As with Clover, he was intelligent and inventive, and was soon a consulting anaesthetist to several London hospitals, including St George's, the London, the King Edward VII, as well as Charing Cross, the Royal Dental, the Royal Hospital for Children and Women, and the National Orthopaedic Hospital. He was the author of one of the first dedicated British textbooks, intended for 'medical and dental practitioners and students'[11]. The book was so popular that it was still being published after Hewitt's death in 1916, the text having been revised many times. Anaesthetists that he instructed, such as Bellamy Gardiner and Blumfeld, also become prominent, publishing their own textbooks[12,13].

Although famous for anaesthetizing royalty and being knighted, Hewitt gave thousands of dental anaesthetics, and was particularly interested in nitrous oxide. He was one of the first to consider the inherent asphyxia caused by pure nitrous oxide seriously, and he developed equipment to allow the entrance of air and later oxygen during continuous anaesthesia. He is certainly credited with being the force behind the use of oxygen with nitrous oxide. He devised many other pieces of equipment, including mouth props, gags, and an improved version of Clover's inhaler with a wider bore.

Because anaesthesia had become an integral part of their working lives, dentists were trained in anaesthesia

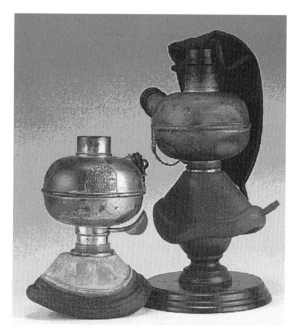

Figure 1.5 Hewitt's wide-bore modification of Clover's portable regulating ether inhaler.

as students, receiving better exposure to the specialty than most medical students. They were particularly trained in the use of nitrous oxide. Dentists were also taught to use ether, but many were dissuaded from the

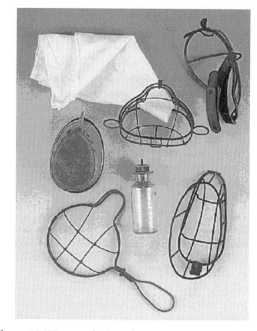

Figure 1.6 Wire anaesthetic masks.

use of chloroform[14–17]. They were also warned of the dangers of ethyl chloride, which made its appearance at about this time. It was not used, as we do today, topically, but as a highly potent induction agent.

With the introduction of specialist anaesthetists came textbooks, new inventions and equipment, and skills and understanding increased. Although new anaesthetic apparatus appeared, many anaesthetics still involved a novice dropping ether or chloroform onto a gauze mask or folded towel.

The dawn of local anaesthesia

It is now an appropriate time to look at other developments that occurred at the end of the nineteenth century. Cocaine had been identified and named by Gaedicke and then Niemann[1] in 1855. It was used topically by a number of physicians, but it was the use on the eye by Carl Koller in 1884 that first stimulated widespread interest. It is perhaps a comment on the quality and safety of general anaesthesia that new methods of achieving painless surgery were still vigorously sought. Experiments were attempted, injecting cocaine into a variety of places. But dosage was not well controlled, solutions were not sterile, and cocaine was toxic. Deaths occurred not infrequently, even when dilute solutions were used. New agents were devised, with Stovaine and procaine appearing after the turn of the century. Cinchocaine was introduced in 1931, and finally lignocaine (xylocaine) in 1943.

Local anaesthesia for dental work was reported by Sauvez, of L'Dentaire in Paris, in 1908, but it was not immediately popular in America or Britain. As stated in one textbook of the time[14], 'Best of all suited for local anaesthetics are the stolid, phlegmatic persons' and that 'Americans are by temperament in no way likely to be good subjects for local anaesthetics, and that the same may be said of the large majority of the Anglo-Saxon race'! Alderson's textbook of 1911 described techniques to manage cocaine toxicity, including forcing a mixture of black coffee and brandy into the patient (presumably via the mouth), and flicking the chest with wet towels[15]. Local anaesthesia was used for dental work by enthusiasts, but was far less popular than general anaesthesia for the next 70 years, in Britain at least.

The early twentieth century

The First World War saw casualties on a vast scale but, even so, anaesthesia was still mostly rudimentary and given by non-specialists. When America joined the conflict in 1917, they brought with them an apparatus credited to Gwathemy that allowed a constant flow of oxygen and nitrous oxide to pass through a vaporizer and then to the patient. The idea was taken up by Boyle of the Royal Army Medical Corp (RAMC), and the Boyle's machine came to Britain. Before then, anaesthesia was either open, using a 'rag and bottle' technique, or an inhaler with to-and-fro rebreathing. Nitrous oxide was given via a bag that was filled from a cylinder and then rebreathed.

Huge numbers of men were injured in the trenches of the First World War and, not surprisingly, many were wounded when they exposed their heads above the trench to enemy fire. This gave a disproportionate number of head and neck wounds, and a specialist unit was set up under the New Zealand surgeon Gillies. He was given two young RAMC doctors, Magill and Rowbotham, to act as his anaesthetists. Ivan Magill, later knighted, is credited for introducing endotracheal intubation and the laryngoscope into everyday anaesthesia. The new technique allowed free access to the face and mouth during surgery, revolutionizing head and neck surgery. Magill also designed his forceps, still used today, an anaesthetic machine, and a circuit (now classified as the Mapleson 'A').

Endotracheal intubation was soon being performed more frequently, which allowed the development of

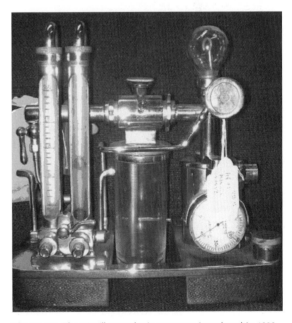

Figure 1.7 The Magill anaesthetic apparatus introduced in 1932.

more complex surgery such as thoracic and abdominal procedures. By the 1930s, reliable intravenous anaesthesia appeared, with the introduction of the barbiturate thiopentone. However, most dental anaesthetics were still 'gas', nitrous oxide, and were often delivered by dentists. By now, dentists were using different anaesthetic equipment from the hospital anaesthetists with their Boyle's machines. Dental surgeries increasingly used demand flow machines, introduced first in 1910 by an American from Toledo, E. I. McKesson[18]. Anaesthesia was delivered continuously via a nasal mask, rather than inducing and removing the mask as had been the case previously. A number of McKesson machines (Figure 1.8) came to Britain, where a similar locally made machine known as the Walton series became popular.

During this period, many famous anaesthetists 'cut their teeth', giving thousands of dental anaesthetics. A group of young men, collectively known as the 'Mayfair Gas, Fight and Choke Company', were driven around the West End of London in expensive cars to provide anaesthesia for surgeries and hospitals. The Mayfair Gas Company was a partnership in anaesthetics founded in 1933 by Robert Macintosh, later to become Professor Sir R. R. Macintosh, William McConnell, and Bernard Johnson. They worked from

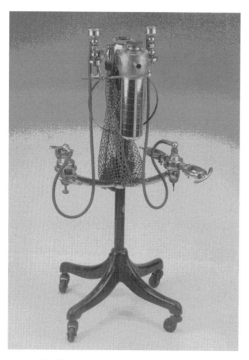

Figure 1.8 The McKesson anaesthesia apparatus.

Macintosh's home at 9a Upper Brook Street, Mayfair, London. Each anaesthetist working for the Mayfair Gas Company was expected to buy their own car as they had to bring their equipment with them. The car was maintained by the company and a driver was employed to help carry the equipment and also to help move patients.

More doctors specializing in anaesthesia began to appear. They were employed to do routine daytime work, while emergencies were still left for the house staff. Soon, further house surgeons were appointed solely for this dedicated task. When they started, they received no training, and were expected to pick up the tricks of the trade quickly. There were, however, many new techniques to learn. Macintosh was made the first professor of anaesthesia in Britain, and academic training of anaesthetists began. His textbook, published in 1940, was entitled *Essentials of General Anaesthesia, with special reference to dentistry*, perhaps reflecting his own experience and the prominence of dental anaesthetics at the time[19].

The period of the Second World War was an important one for anaesthesia. Many doctors were given training and exposure to large numbers of cases, resulting in an expansion of the specialty after the war. New equipment and drugs appeared, including the Macintosh laryngoscope that we still use today, and the first muscle relaxant, curare. Better understanding of the dangers of drugs and techniques developed, such as the practice of intubation under large doses of thiopentone. It is said that American anaesthesiologists unfortunately killed many injured service personnel after the attack on Pearl Harbour by not realizing how dangerous thiopentone was in shock.

After the Second World War, and the introduction of the National Health Service (NHS) in the UK, anaesthesia grew and developed very quickly. A Faculty was founded in the Royal College of Surgeons in London, and a fellowship examination introduced. Senior anaesthetists were given consultant status, and this improved the recruitment of new anaesthetists immensely.

With increased numbers of staff came an expansion of academic anaesthesia, with chairs being established in most large teaching hospitals. The science of anaesthesia was studied, and new drugs and techniques were adopted. Muscle relaxants, lignocaine, and new inhalational agents appeared. Physiology and pharmacology, physics, and clinical measurement appeared in the anaesthetic examinations. The increasing intellectual demands of the specialty engendered a new breed of anaesthetists. They were no longer working for surgeons, but with them, to offer new levels of care to patients. Mortality and morbidity rates improved, as the problems so long ignored were identified and tackled. It was perhaps the 'Golden Age' of anaesthesia. It was also an era of increased interest and use of local anaesthesia, at least in the USA and Europe, following the introduction of lignocaine[20].

Victor Goldman

Dental anaesthesia was still being taught to dental students, and many of the new drugs and techniques appeared attractive[21–23]. Because of the way the UK NHS funded dental procedures, there was great pressure to see large numbers of patients as quickly as possible. This was especially true of paediatric patients. The numbers of children having teeth extracted under anaesthesia soared to millions. But the use of potent new drugs such as halothane[24] and methohexitone started to increase the death rate insidiously. Halothane had first appeared in 1956, and soon Victor Goldman, a consultant at the Royal Free and Eastman Hospitals, introduced a new halothane vaporizer. It was very simple, using the glass bowl from an AC Delco fuel pump, and was intended to fit to a demand flow machine such as a McKesson or Walton. Goldman was one of the most important dental anaesthetists of the twentieth century, not only for his inventions, which included improved nasal masks and other vaporizers, but for his investigations into the risks of dental anaesthesia[25].

As the safety of anaesthesia improved, unexpected deaths during dental anaesthesia came under the spotlight. Cardiovascular collapse in the upright position of the dental chair was soon investigated, and Bourne suggested the concept of fainting while sitting[26]. There were also an increasing number of dentists giving intravenous methohexitone, a short-acting barbiturate, usually from a needle in the antecubital fossa, then proceeding to perform an operation. Although it was called sedation, the boundary into anaesthesia was easily and not infrequently crossed. Not only did patients collapse from hypotension or respiratory obstruction, there was often no training or equipment for resuscitation. Following further widely reported deaths and in consequence increasing public pressure, there was a call for a reduction in the number of dental general anaesthetics, and an increase in safety. This culminated in the report published under

the chairmanship of Sir David Poswillo, *The Report of an Expert Working Party on General Anaesthesia, Sedation and Resuscitation in Dentistry in 1990*. It made recommendations in four areas. It stated that general anaesthesia should be avoided wherever possible. It suggested that Health Authorities took steps to improve the provision of properly funded dental anaesthetic sessions, undertaken only by those with sufficient expertise to do it safely. It did not stop dentists from giving general anaesthetics. Finally, the Poswillo report recommended that standards of equipment, monitoring, and personnel should be the same as for any anaesthetic[27].

Despite declining numbers of dental anaesthetics[28], whether because of increased use of local and sedation techniques or reduced levels of tooth decay, deaths still happened. This resulted in further reports and recommendations. In 1998, the General Dental Council of the UK, after consulting the Royal College of Anaesthetists, issued guidance that in practical terms stopped dentists giving general anaesthetics. In 1999, further guidelines were issued to limit dental anaesthesia to the minimum, and, at the end of 2001, general anaesthesia for dentistry ceased outside of hospitals[29].

Conclusion

This brings us to the present day. Dental anaesthesia is strictly controlled, and is delivered by experienced anaesthetists in hospitals with full access to equipment, monitoring, and resuscitation. Methohexitone and halothane have gone, to be replaced by sevoflurane and propofol. Nitrous oxide is much less popular and is often avoided altogether. The nasal mask is giving way to the laryngeal mask. Demand flow anaesthetic machines have been relegated to museums. Dentists are now no longer trained to remove teeth under general anaesthesia, while there is a huge expansion of sedation and relative analgesia techniques.

References

1. Armstrong Davison MH. (1965) *The Evolution of Anaesthesia*. Altrincham: Sherratt and Son.
2. Davy H. (1800) *Researches Chemical and Philosophical chiefly concerning Nitrous Oxide…and its respiration*. Bristol: Biggs and Cottle.
3. Cartwright FF. (1952) *The English Pioneers of Anaesthesia (Beddoes: Davy: Hickman)*. Bristol: John Wright and Sons.
4. *Souvenir of the Henry Hill Hickman Centenary Exhibition* (1930). London: The Wellcome Foundation.
5. Bellamy Gardiner H. (1901) *The Asphyxial Factor in Anaesthesia*. London: Bailliere, Tindall and Cox.

6. Keys TE. (1945) *The History of Surgical Anesthesia*. New York: Shuman's.

7. Snow J. (1858) *On Narcotism by the Inhalation of Vapours*, facsimile edition. London: Royal Society of Medicine, 1991.

8. Ellis RH. (1994) *The Case Books of Dr. John Snow. Medical History Supplement No 14*. London: Wellcome Institute for the History of Medicine.

9. Duncum B. (1947) *The Development of Inhalation Anaesthesia*. (Reprinted 1994, Royal Society of Medicine.) London: Oxford University Press.

10. Sykes WS. (1961) *Essays on the First Hundred Years of Anaesthesia*, Vols 1 and 2. Edinburgh: E and S Livingstone.

11. Hewitt FW. (1907) *Anaesthetics and their Administration. A text-book for medical and dental practitioners and students*, 3rd edn. London: Macmillan and Co.

12. Bellamy Gardiner H. (1909) *Surgical Anaesthesia*. London: Bailliere, Tindall and Cox.

13. Blumfeld J. (1912) *Anaesthetics*. London: Bailliere, Tindall and Cox.

14. Luke TD, Stuart Ross J. (1919) *Anaesthesia in Dental Surgery*, 4th edn. London: Heinemann.

15. Alderson WE. (1911) *Dental Anaesthetics*. Bristol: John Wright and Sons.

16. Rawdon Smith GF. (1926) *Outlines of Dental Science—Dental anaesthesia*. Edinburgh: E and S Livingstone.

17. Levy AG. (1922) *Chloroform Anaesthesia*. London: John Bale, Sons and Danielson.

18. McKesson EI. (1935) *Nitrous Oxide and Oxygen Anaesthesia in Dentistry*, 3rd edn. Toledo: The McKesson Appliance Co.

19. Macintosh RR, Pratt FB. (1940) *Essentials of General Anaesthesia, with special reference to dentistry*. Oxford: Blackwell Scientific Publications.

20. Seldin HM. (1947) *Practical Anesthesia for Dental and Oral Surgery*, 3rd edn. London: Henry Kimpton.

21. McNaught Inglis J, Campkin V. (1960) *General Anaesthesia for Dentistry*. London: Edward Arnold.

22. Walsh RS. (1960) *General Anaesthesia for Dental Surgery*. London: Longmans.

23. Jorgensen NB, Hayden J. (1967) *Premedication, Local and General Anesthesia in Dentistry*. Philadelphia: Lea and Febiger.

24. Goldman V. (1960) Halothane in the dental surgery. *Br Dent J*, **109**, 259–63.

25. Goldman V. (1958) Deaths under anaesthesia in the dental surgery. *Br Dent J*, **105**, 160–3.

26. Lee JA, Atkinson RS. (1968) *A Synopsis of Anaesthesia*, 6th edn. Bristol: John Wright and Sons.

27. Blayney MR, Malins AF. (2001) Chair dental anaesthesia. *CPD Anaesthesia*, **3**(3), 91–6.

28. Padfield A. (2002) A brief history of British "chair" dental anaesthesia. *International Congress Series*, **1242**, 405–8.

29. Landes DP. (2002) The provision of general anaesthesia in dental practice, an end which had to come? *Br Dent J*, **192**, 129–31.

2

Preassessment and optimization of oral and maxillofacial patients

Diane Monkhouse and Sanjiv Sharma

Introduction

Oral and maxillofacial surgery encompasses a vast array of surgical procedures involving a diverse patient population. At one extreme is surgery for infants with congenital craniofacial malformations while at the other is cancer surgery with microvascular reconstruction for elderly patients with multiple comorbidities. Similarly, there is variability in acuity. Management of the polytrauma victim requiring timely surgical intervention contrasts with elective day case dental surgery for children with learning disabilities. This variety plus the need for a shared airway frequently provides an anaesthetic challenge.

This chapter will deal with the systematic assessment and optimization of the patient listed for oral and maxillofacial surgery. Assessment of the airway is dealt with in detail in Chapter 4. Emphasis will be placed upon some of the difficult issues the anaesthetist may encounter.

Preoperative assessment is the clinical investigation that precedes anaesthesia for surgical procedures[1]. Fundamental aims are to identify potential anaesthetic difficulties, investigate and optimize existing medical conditions, improve safety by assessing and quantifying risk, and facilitate planning of perioperative care[2]. In addition, it should provide an opportunity to obtain informed consent and explain in detail the scheduled perioperative management. Assessment should take place early in the patient's journey so that the patient can be reassured and have his anxieties allayed whilst all essential requirements can be anticipated before the day of surgery, reducing the risk of cancellation for clinical reasons. This may be more difficult in the case of emergency surgery[3].

The Australian Incident Monitoring Study (AIMS)[4] suggested that one in ten of perioperative incidents reported identified inadequate preoperative assessment or preparation. Poor airway assessment, communication problems, and failure to modify the anaesthetic plan based on preoperative evaluations were the most common contributing factors. Respondents suggested that 57% problems were preventable.

The guidelines of the American Society of Anesthesiologists (ASA)[5] recommend that the preanaesthesia visit should include an interview with the patient or guardian to review medical history, previous anaesthetic exposure and recent drug therapy, an appropriate physical examination, a review of investigations, and assignment of ASA physical status score.

The ASA classification (Table 2.1) highlights patient risk only and is based on subjective physician assessment. It does not take into account surgical complexity and environmental factors.

Surgical risk is often categorized on the basis of the invasive nature of the planned surgery and the anticipated blood loss (Table 2.2). The site of surgery is another important predictor of postoperative pulmonary complications[6].

There is no comprehensive risk stratification system that takes into account both the patient's comorbidity combined with the specific surgical risk. Although this is undoubtedly the most effective way of risk-stratifying patients in the preoperative period, it can become a very complex procedure.

Table 2.1 American Society of Anesthesiologists' physical status classification

ASA1	Healthy patient without medical problems
ASA2	Mild, well controlled systemic disease with no impact on daily activity
ASA3	Significant or severe systemic disease that limits normal activity
ASA4	Severe systemic disease that is a constant threat to life
ASA5	Moribund patient who is equally likely to die in the next 24 hours with or without surgery
ASA6	Brain dead organ donor

Suffix E to the classification indicates emergency surgery.

Preoperative investigations

Preoperative investigations can be used to provide additional diagnostic and prognostic information to supplement the clinical history, assess the risk of anaesthesia and surgery, guide therapeutic interventions to lower risk, and provide baseline results to help direct intraoperative and postoperative management[7]. Abnormal investigation results may prompt delay in the surgical procedure whilst the problem is addressed. Input from another specialty, prescription of new medication or correction of physiological abnormalities

Table 2.2 Grading system for surgical procedures

Grade of surgery	Example
Grade 1 (minor)	Excision of skin lesions Drainage of abscess Dental extractions
Grade 2 (intermediate)	Primary repair of inguinal hernia Tonsillectomy/ adenotonsillectomy Knee arthroscopy Haemorrhoids
Grade 3 (major)	Total abdominal hysterectomy Endoscopic resection of prostate Lumbar discectomy Thyroidectomy Laparoscopic cholecystectomy
Grade 4 (major+)—body cavity surgery or major resection	Radical neck dissection Joint replacement Lung operations Colonic resection Upper GI surgery All intracranial surgery Vascular surgery

such as anaemia, hypertension, or hypokalaemia may be required. Modification of the anaesthetic technique, surgical procedure or postoperative destination may be considered. However, there is little evidence to support routine investigation of the asymptomatic patient as it does not significantly contribute to anaesthetic management[8]. An appropriate strategy for rational, cost-effective testing is therefore essential. In the UK, the National Institute for Clinical Excellence (NICE) has published recommendations for pre-operative investigation (Table 2.3) based on the ASA grade of the patient and the grade of the proposed surgery[9].

Drug therapy—continue or stop?

Decisions regarding continuing or stopping regular medication should be based on the patient's comorbidities and the nature of the proposed surgery. Several drugs have beneficial effects during surgery, some are deleterious, and others have significant problems with abrupt cessation. Careful consideration should be given to each medication and clear instructions given to the patient and ward staff at the preoperative visit.

Antihypertensive drugs should be continued on the day of surgery except for angiotensin-converting enzyme inhibitors and angiotensin receptor antagonists, which may contribute to significant intraoperative hypotension.

Aspirin should be continued unless the risk of bleeding outweighs the risk of thrombosis. A meta-analysis evaluating cardiovascular risk of discontinuing aspirin versus the risk of perioperative bleeding complications from its continuation suggested cardiovascular events occurred in 10.2% patients where aspirin had been stopped. Bleeding complications increased by a factor of 1.5 in those continuing aspirin therapy[10].

Antiplatelet agents (e.g. clopidogrel) should be continued if the risk of thrombosis outweighs the risk of bleeding. This needs to be considered on an individual patient basis and may require input from surgical and cardiology colleagues to assess the risks and benefits fully. For patients with bare metal or drug-eluting coronary stents, the risk of stopping clopidogrel must be discussed with the cardiologist. If reversal of antiplatelet effect is required, clopidogrel must be discontinued for at least 7 days before surgery. In emergency situations, platelet transfusions may be required.

Statins are effective cardioprotective agents in the perioperative period. The risk of rhabdomyolysis in patients continuing therapy is very small while the risk

Table 2.3 Summary of recommended preoperative investigations based on NICE guidelines[9]

Investigations required	Patient groups
Full blood count Urea and electrolytes Liver function tests Electrocardiogram	All ASA3 or 4 patients All grade 3 or 4 surgery Any cardiovascular disease—hypertension, ischaemic heart disease, cardiac failure, CVA, TIA, peripheral vascular regardless of grade of surgery All diabetics Respiratory disease that limits exercise Connective tissue and multisystem diseases Patient with impaired renal function Concurrent malignancy Chronic liver disease or jaundice Severe nutritional deficiency Obese patients (BMI >35)
Full blood count	Recent/ongoing history of anaemia History of menorrhagia Surgery for investigation of bleeding All grade 2, 3 or 4 surgery if patient >60 years Pregnant patients having non-obstetric surgery Sickle cell disease or patient requiring sickle cell screen
Coagulation screen	Consider in patients taking anticoagulants depending on admission date Bleeding disorders or history of bleeding tendency Chronic liver disease, jaundice or gallbladder surgery Chronic renal failure All grade 4 surgery Cancer surgery if suspicion of metastases
Random blood glucose	All diabetic patients Obese patients (BMI >35) Patients taking oral steroids All patients undergoing grade 3 or 4 surgery
Electrocardiogram	Patients >60 years
Respiratory function tests	ASA4 respiratory disease Poorly controlled asthma Unexplained poor exercise tolerance Only need PEFR in patients with exercise-limiting chest disease
Sickle cell testing	If status is unknown, Sickledex test required in patients of Afro-Caribbean, Eastern Mediterranean, Middle-Eastern, and Asian descent
Chest X-ray	Children for cardiac surgery Elderly ASA3 or 4 patients with respiratory disease requiring grade 3 or 4 surgery

of acute withdrawal is higher. The current American College of Cardiologists/American Heart Association (ACC/AHA) guidelines recommend continuation of statins as a class 1 recommendation[11].

Diuretics should be discontinued on the day of surgery except for thiazides taken for hypertension.

For advice on insulin and oral hypoglycaemics, see the section on diabetes mellitus.

Warfarin should be discontinued for 4–5 days before surgery and international normalized ratio (INR) should be less than 1.5. The decision regarding introduction of

heparin depends on the initial indication for warfarin therapy and should be discussed in the outpatient department at the time of booking surgery. In emergency situations, vitamin K reverses the effect of warfarin but takes several hours. More rapid reversal can be achieved by administration of fresh frozen plasma or prothrombin complex concentrate.

Antiarrhythmics, antiepileptics, antidepressants, asthma medications, hormone replacement therapy, thyroxine, steroids, and antacids should all be continued on the day of surgery.

Respiratory disorders

A detailed history and thorough physical examination is required to identify patients with a high risk of perioperative pulmonary complications. Common complications include atelectasis, pneumonia, hypoxaemia, pulmonary embolism, acute lung injury, and respiratory failure. This can prolong hospital stay by 1–2 weeks. Perioperative management will include identification of respiratory disease, assessment of severity, and pre-optimization[12,13]. Modification of risk factors such as stopping smoking is of vital importance. Other important steps include incentive spirometry and medical optimization of pulmonary and cardiac function.

Patient-related risk factors include advanced age, obesity, smoking, obstructive sleep apnoea, functional status, asthma, and chronic obstructive pulmonary disease (COPD)[14,15].

Advanced age is an independent risk factor for postoperative pulmonary complications. This is related to loss of elastic recoil, impaired airway protective reflexes, decreased capacity for generating maximal expiratory flow, and functional airway closure. Obesity can contribute to decreased functional residual capacity, intrapulmonary shunting, and hypoxaemia.

Patients who smoke more than ten pack-years are at increased risk of perioperative pulmonary complications. Current smokers have higher risk of pulmonary complications. Stopping smoking even 1 or 2 days prior to the surgical procedure leads to a decrease in carboxyhaemoglobin levels and minimizes the cardiovascular effects of nicotine. However, it takes 6–8 weeks of abstinence to improve lung function[16].

A diagnosis of obstructive sleep apnoea is important as it increases morbidity and mortality (see Chapter 23). The presence of pulmonary hypertension and right heart failure should be recognized during preoperative assessment. ASA status is useful to determine the general health status of a patient. Decreased exercise capacity signifies poor respiratory and cardiac reserve, and increases the risk of perioperative complications.

Asthma is an inflammatory respiratory disease with hypersensitivity of airways to a variety of stimuli, resulting in airway obstruction and limitation of airflow. Accurate history-taking is important to identify the asthmatic patient and the severity of the disease, precipitating factors, current medications (including systemic steroid use), past hospital admissions for acute asthma attacks, and any previous history of admission to the intensive care unit. The commonest risk is bronchospasm during general anaesthesia because of a hyperreactive airway. The role of preoptimization is to identify any reversible element of airflow limitation and treat it with beta$_2$ agonists and steroids preoperatively. Measurement of peak expiratory flow rate is useful. The aim is to achieve the best personal peak expiratory flow rate before scheduled surgery[13,14].

COPD is a chronic lung disease with irreversible and progressive obstruction of airflow. It includes chronic bronchitis and emphysema as two disease entities, but patients usually present with overlapping symptoms. COPD is an independent risk factor for perioperative pulmonary complications. Optimization in the preoperative period includes treatment of associated infection and any reversible element of bronchospasm. Patients with chronic hypoxaemia and pulmonary hypertension should be identified at preoperative assessment. Spirometry shows an obstructive pattern with decreased forced expiratory volume in 1 second (FEV_1) to forced vital capacity (FVC) ratio[17,18].

Cardiac disorders

The goal of evaluation of patients with cardiac disease is to identify high risk patients (Table 2.4), stratify the risk, and develop strategies for risk reduction. In most cases a detailed and accurate history with focused physical examination will be sufficient to identify cardiac disease and relevant risk factors. Specialized tests may be required to stratify risk and determine need for preoperative intervention (Table 2.5). However, unnecessary specialized investigations may contribute to surgical delay, patient harm, and increased cost.

Table 2.4 Important points on history-taking and physical examination

History-taking	Physical examination
Chest pain	Irregularity of pulse
Palpitations	Raised JVP
Irregular heartbeat	Peripheral oedema
Dyspnoea	Displaced apex beat
Orthopnoea	S3 gallop
Paroxysmal nocturnal dyspnoea	S4 heart sound
Haemoptysis	Presence of murmurs
Syncope	
Claudication	
Medications	
Previous history of coronary artery disease	

Table 2.5 Non-invasive tests of cardiac function

Investigation	Information
Electrocardiograph (ECG)	Shows ischaemic changes, arrhythmias, and left ventricular hypertrophy
Transthoracic echocardiogram (TTE)	Demonstrates left ventricular function, regional wall abnormalities, and severity of valvular disease
Exercise stress test	Used to demonstrate exercise-induced ischaemia. Patients with severe ST segment depression at low workload or heart rate <70% of predicted maximum have severe disease
Stress echocardiography	Performed during exercise to show exercise-induced wall motion abnormalities. Dobutamine stress echocardiography can be performed in patients unable to exercise
Cardiopulmonary exercise test (CPEX)	Used to evaluate both cardiac and respiratory function. Cardiac function is evaluated in terms of anaerobic threshold and VO_2 max
Myocardial perfusion scintigraphy	Thallium-201 or technetium-99m sestamibi radionuclide is used. Uptake of radionuclide is proportional to bloodflow. Exercise or intravenous vasodilator can determine reversible ischaemia

Ischaemic heart disease

Patients undergoing oral and maxillofacial surgery may be at risk of cardiac events, not only intraoperatively but also during their recovery period. The risk applies particularly to those with known coronary heart disease but may also apply to asymptomatic individuals. Recognized risk factors for ischaemic heart disease include advanced age, positive family history, smoking, hypercholesterolaemia, diabetes mellitus, and hypertension.

There are multiple risk stratification indices available:

* The ASA index is used for assessment of the patient's physical status and to predict morbidity and mortality (Table 2.1)
* The Goldman cardiac risk index identifies nine independent variables which are weighted based on their ability to predict cardiac morbidity and mortality in patients undergoing non-cardiac surgery[19,20]
* Detsky's modified Goldman cardiac risk index takes into account the severity of angina and differentiates recent from previous myocardial infarction[21,22]

* The revised cardiac risk index (RCRI) assigns one point for six independent predictors of adverse cardiac outcome in patients undergoing non-cardiac surgery[23]
* ACC/AHA guidelines provide a framework for screening and identifying patients during pre-operative assessment who are at high risk for perioperative cardiac events[24–26]. Three major parameters help to determine the risk of cardiac morbidity and mortality for patients undergoing non-cardiac surgery and help determine the need for additional testing or specific pharmacology therapy[27,28]. These are the clinical characteristics of the patient, the inherent cardiac risk of the planned surgical procedure, and the patient's functional capacity.

ACC/AHA stepwise approach to perioperative evaluation of cardiac risk

Step 1: Is there a clinical need for emergency non-cardiac surgery?

In the case of a life-threatening situation, non-cardiac surgery should proceed without extensive cardiac assessment. Recommendations for perioperative surveillance and management are appropriate in patients identified as having substantial pre-existing cardiac conditions.

Step 2: Are there active cardiac conditions?

Active cardiac conditions include unstable coronary syndromes, decompensated heart failure, significant arrhythmias, severe mitral or aortic stenosis[26,27]. The presence of such conditions makes further cardiac evaluation essential prior to elective non-cardiac surgery.

Step 3: Does the planned surgery have low cardiac risk?

The assessment of cardiac risk associated with specific surgical procedure is related to the type and duration of surgery plus physiological stress associated with the procedure. Patients scheduled for low risk surgical procedures do not require extensive preoperative testing. Cardiac risk associated with high risk surgery (aortic or major vascular surgery) is more than 5%, intermediate risk surgery (head and neck surgery) is 1–5% and is less than 1% for low risk surgery (superficial or endoscopic procedures)[28].

Step 4: Does the patient have good functional capacity without symptoms?

Functional status is an important determinant of perioperative risk. It is evaluated by the estimated energy requirement metabolic equivalents (METS) for various activities. The Duke Activity Status Index provides the physician with a set of questions to determine a patient's functional capacity.

Examples include:

♦ 1–4 METS   Ability to eat, dress, walk around the house
♦ 4–6 METS   Ability to climb stairs or play golf
♦ >10 METS   Ability to swim or play tennis.

Patients with functional capacity of 4–5 METS do not require further testing prior to non-cardiac surgery.

Step 5: Does the patient have clinical risk factors?

The following six independent predictors were identified in the RCRI: stable ischaemic heart, compensated heart failure, cerebrovascular disease, diabetes mellitus requiring preoperative insulin therapy, preoperative creatinine level of >177μmol/l, and high risk surgery[23]. Patients without clinical risk factors but poor functional capacity do not require further investigation prior to surgery. However, the presence of clinical risk factors will require more extensive cardiac evaluation.

Medical management

It is essential to optimize medical management prior to surgery. All prescribed antianginal medications should be continued perioperatively. Statins should be continued as they have a cardioprotective effect[29]. Continuation of antiplatelet therapy has to be assessed on a risk–benefit basis.

Beta blockers are used in the treatment of myocardial ischaemia, hypertension, and arrhythmias. They decrease myocardial contractility and sympathetic tone and are negatively chronotropic. The beneficial effects of beta blockade include improvement of myocardial oxygen supply/demand balance. Numerous investigators have found a reduction in ischaemic events and death with use of beta blockers in the perioperative period[30,31]. Interruptions to beta blockade may lead to rebound hypertension and arrhythmias. Based on evidence from existing studies, the target resting heart rate should be less than 65 beats/min[26,27]. Patients who are judged to benefit from beta blockade at preoperative assessment should have careful titration of dose and control of heart rate. The recently published perioperative ischaemic evaluation trial (POISE) demonstrated significant reduction in the rate of non-fatal myocardial infarction with metoprolol therapy compared with placebo[32].

However, the incidence of symptomatic hypotension, significant bradycardia, and stroke was greater with metoprolol therapy.

Coronary revascularization

If the non-invasive stress test result is abnormal, then the patient should be referred for angiography in an attempt to modify the risk[28]. Non-cardiac surgery, such as elective maxillofacial surgery, should be delayed for a minimum or 4–6 weeks after coronary artery bypass graft. In the case of coronary stenting, the decision is based on the type of stent placed. Non-cardiac surgery should be delayed for 4–6 weeks after insertion of bare metal stents and for 6 months after insertion of drug-eluting stents[26]. Dual platelet therapy (aspirin and clopidogrel) should be continued for 4 weeks after bare metal stent insertion and for 1 year after drug-eluting stent insertion.

Congestive cardiac failure

Congestive cardiac failure (CCF) is a common, debilitating condition which may be problematic in the perioperative period. It affects 1% of people between 50 and 59 years, and more than 10% of people over the age of 80. The most common causes of heart failure are ischaemic heart disease and hypertension.

Characteristic findings are of fatigue and impaired exercise tolerance secondary to impaired ventricular performance. It is essential that patients with CCF are identified preoperatively. Those with recent or current decompensation pose the highest operative risk. Concurrent associated diseases such as ischaemic heart disease, diabetes, and hypertension should also be addressed.

Essential investigations should include urea and electrolytes, haemoglobin, ECG, and chest radiograph. Patients treated with diuretics should have correction of any electrolyte disturbance. Anaemia should also be corrected. A transthoracic echocardiogram gives additional information about left ventricular function and valvular pathology. According to the ACC guidelines, the greatest risk of perioperative ischaemic events is seen in patients with an ejection fraction of less than 35%[26]. B-type natriuretic peptide levels can be used to distinguish dyspnoea secondary to pulmonary dysfunction from CCF[33]. Cardiac catheterization should be performed if significant coronary heart disease or valvular dysfunction is suspected as the cause of heart failure.

Medical therapy should be instituted to optimize patients with CCF in the preoperative period.

A combination of diuretics, beta blockers, and ACE inhibitors is used to reduce myocardial work, control heart rate, and reduce afterload[34]. Tachycardia is poorly tolerated because of shortened diastolic perfusion time. Atrial fibrillation with rapid ventricular response and loss of atrial kick can cause significant haemodynamic compromise. This should be urgently addressed and rate control achieved prior to surgery. Patients with low cardiac output states leading to hypotension and deteriorating renal function may require inotropic agents like dobutamine or milrinone.

Elective surgery should be deferred until medical management is optimized. Provision of appropriate level of care in the postoperative period should also be considered. If high risk surgery or emergency surgery is anticipated, critical care support should be arranged.

Hypertension

The goals of preoperative assessment are to identify patients with undiagnosed hypertension or inadequately controlled blood pressure with evidence of end-organ damage.

The Joint National Committee on Prevention, Detection, Evaluation and Treatment of hypertension has classified hypertension (Table 2.6)[35].

The goal of treatment is a blood pressure (BP) of less than 140/90 mmHg; however, for patients with diabetes mellitus or chronic kidney disease, the target is a BP of less than 130/80 mmHg[36,37].

Hypertension is an important risk for coronary heart disease so it is important to identify untreated or suboptimally treated patients. The presence of left ventricular hypertrophy or ST segment abnormalities on preoperative ECG signify increased risk of perioperative cardiac events. Further cardiac testing is indicated in the perioperative management.

Lifestyle modification is important and recommended modifications are weight reduction for overweight patients[38,39], dietary sodium reduction[40,41],

Table 2.6 Classification of hypertension[35]

Class	Systolic (mmHg)	Diastolic (mmHg)
Normal	<120	<80
Prehypertension	120–139	80–89
Stage 1 hypertension	140–159	90–99
Stage 2 hypertension	>160	>100

appropriate physical activity[42], and reduction in consumption of alcohol[43].

Patients on treatment with beta blockers should continue treatment in the perioperative period. Many researchers recommend discontinuation of ACE inhibitors on the morning of surgery in patients with well controlled hypertension to prevent intraoperative hypotension. Parenteral antihypertensive agents should be used in the intraoperative period.

The patients with well controlled hypertension with no evidence of end-organ damage should safely proceed to non-cardiac surgery. Treatment with beta blockers should be initiated in patients diagnosed with hypertension and coronary artery disease for the first time at preoperative evaluation. Patients with known hypertension but inadequate control should have their doses of antihypertensives titrated. The ACC/AHA guidelines do not recommend further cardiac testing or delaying surgery in patients without end-organ damage.

Valvular heart disease

Valvular heart defects have serious implications for non-cardiac surgery. Aortic stenosis is an independent risk factor. Preoperative evaluation should assess the clinical extent of valvular insufficiency, the cross-sectional area of the valve, and the pressure gradient across the stenotic valve.

A degree of aortic stenosis is present in approximately 25% of patients over 65 years of age. The classic symptoms are angina, syncope, and left ventricular failure. A low volume and slowly rising carotid pulse is typical. An ejection systolic murmur is heard at the aortic area with conduction to neck and apex. The normal valve area is 3–4 cm^2. Critical stenosis occurs when the valve area is <0.7cm^2. Patients with aortic stenosis have a fixed cardiac output state because of left ventricular outflow obstruction. Sudden vasodilatation will lead to a profound drop in blood pressure. Patients are dependent on an adequate preload. The ACC/AHA guidelines recommend delaying non-cardiac surgery in patients with severe aortic stenosis[26]. Percutaneous valvuloplasty may be useful in younger patients. Aortic valve replacement is required in symptomatic critical aortic valve stenosis prior to non-cardiac surgery. Patients with a mechanical valve require long-term anticoagulation.

Mitral stenosis usually occurs as a consequence of rheumatic heart disease and is commonly associated with mitral regurgitation. The normal mitral valve area is 4–6 cm^2. Mitral stenosis is critical when the area is less than 1 cm^2 and the patient is symptomatic. Exertional dyspnoea, orthopnoea, and paroxysmal nocturnal dyspnoea are typical complaints. Atrial fibrillation is common. Physical examination findings include an opening snap following S2 and a low-pitched diastolic murmur at the apex. Left atrial pressure is increased, leading to dilatation of the left atrium, pulmonary hypertension, and compromised right ventricular function. The cardiac output is reduced. There is increased risk of thrombus formation with dilated atrium and presence of atrial fibrillation.

A sudden increase in heart rate can precipitate pulmonary oedema. The heart rate should be controlled with digoxin, beta blockers or calcium channel blockers. Adequate control of volume status and heart rate is required in patients prior to non-cardiac surgery. Anticoagulation therapy should be considered to prevent thrombus formation and risk of systemic emboli.

Perioperative infective endocarditis prophylaxis is indicated in all patients with cardiac structural defects undergoing surgical procedures with risk of bacteraemia. Common organisms involved are *Streptococcus viridians* and *Enterococcus*. The recently published NICE guidelines suggest the following patients are at increased risk of developing infective endocarditis[44]:

- Those with acquired valvular heart disease with stenosis or regurgitation
- Those with valve replacement
- Those with structural congenital heart disease, including surgically corrected or palliated structural conditions (exclusions are isolated atrial septal defect, fully repaired ventricular septal defect or fully repaired patent ductus arteriosus, closure devices that are judged to be endothelialized)
- Those with previous infective endocarditis
- Those with hypertrophic cardiomyopathy.

Antibiotic prophylaxis against infective endocarditis is not recommended for people undergoing dental procedures or surgery to the gastrointestinal, genitourinary or respiratory tracts.

Gastrointestinal disorders

Common problems which affect patients requiring oral maxillofacial surgery include aspiration during anaesthesia, peptic ulceration with the risk of bleeding, and postoperative nausea and vomiting. These risks must be thoroughly assessed in the preoperative period[45].

Conditions which predispose to aspiration include a recent meal, morbid obesity, intoxication with alcohol, pregnancy, hiatus hernia, diabetes, the use of opiate analgesia, trauma, and altered conscious level.

Aspiration of gastric contents can result in a broad spectrum of lung injuries, from aspiration pneumonitis to acute respiratory distress syndrome. Prevention of aspiration by identifying patients at risk and ensuring adequate fasting times is fundamental to safe anaesthetic practice. Ingestion of clear fluids until 2 hours before anaesthesia is permitted. Guidelines for the paediatric patient allow healthy infants to consume breast milk up to 4 hours before induction of anaesthesia. This fasting time is extended to 6 hours for formula milk, non-human milk or solids. In adults, the minimum fasting time for solids is 6 hours[46].

Peptic ulcer disease is a common disorder which may be problematic in the perioperative period. Common causative agents include *Helicobacter pylori* infection of the gastric mucosa, ingestion of non-steroidal anti-inflammatory drugs (NSAIDs) or steroids, the stress response to surgery, and shock causing gut mucosal hypoperfusion. Preoperative assessment should identify patients with active peptic ulcer disease and those who may develop symptoms after surgery. Eradication of *H. pylori* and avoidance of NSAIDs and corticosteroids in high risk patients is recommended. Treatment with proton pump inhibitors, H$_2$ antagonists or mucosal protectants should also be considered in high risk groups.

Despite improved anaesthetic techniques and administration of shorter-acting agents, one-third of patients will experience postoperative nausea and vomiting (PONV). This can prolong recovery, increase the duration of hospital stay, and increase costs. Approximately 1% of day case patients require overnight stay because of protracted vomiting[47]. Groups with a high risk of PONV include females, non-smokers, young patients, and those who suffer motion sickness. Pain, anxiety, and dehydration may increase the incidence of PONV. Identification of such risk factors allows modification of the anaesthetic technique and the administration of combination antiemetics to minimize postoperative problems.

Haematological disorders
Anaemia

Anaemia is the most common haematological disorder detected in the preoperative period. The gender-based World Health Organization (WHO) definition is a haemoglobin concentration of less than 13.0 g/dl for men and 12.0 g/dl for women. The aetiology of anaemia is multifactorial, being dietary, autoimmune, secondary to chronic disease such as renal failure, drug-related, and inherited.

Identifying the correct aetiology of anaemia is necessary before appropriate therapy can be instituted. Anaemia is important in the pathogenesis, prognosis, and complications of perioperative cardiovascular events[48,49]. A low haemoglobin is a significant predictor of mortality for patients with chronic cardiac failure and it is recognized as a risk factor for left ventricular hypertrophy in patients with end-stage renal disease. It has been shown to be independently associated with postoperative mortality. In one study, patients with preoperative anaemia had a more than twofold increased risk of death within 90 days of surgery[50].

Treatment with iron or B$_{12}$ and folate are relatively safe but may necessitate delays in surgery. This may be acceptable for elective surgery but is clearly not an option in cancer surgery or more emergent operations. Erythropoietin is commonly used to treat anaemia secondary to chronic kidney disease but is relatively contraindicated in malignancy. Preoperative blood transfusion may be indicated as a means of correcting anaemia in a timely manner, particularly when significant intraoperative blood loss is anticipated. However, this carries inherent risk.

Bleeding disorders

The vast majority of minor oral and maxillofacial procedures involve minimal blood loss. Epistaxis following nasal intubation during dental anaesthesia is not uncommon. In more major maxillofacial cases, the risk of significant blood loss is increased. This may be confounded by underlying bleeding disorders or anticoagulant therapy. A detailed history and focused physical examination is of vital importance in identifying the bleeding disorder.

History-taking should cover the following points:

- Prolonged bleeding after minor cuts and injuries
- Previous history of excessive bleeding after dental extractions, childbirth, and surgery
- Severe and prolonged menstrual periods
- Excessive bruising
- Bleeding more than 3 minutes after brushing teeth
- Frequent nose bleeds

- History of occult or frank blood loss from gastrointestinal or genitourinary tract
- History of bleeding disorders or inherited familial haematological disorders
  - Haemophilia (deficiency of factor VIII)
  - Christmas disease (deficiency of factor IX)
  - Von Willebrand's disease (deficiency of von Willebrand factor)
  - Leukaemia
  - Thrombocytopenia
  - Liver disease
  - Renal failure
  - Malnutrition
  - Malabsorption
  - Collagen vascular disease
- Medications which can alter coagulation profile.

The nature of the defect and therefore the most appropriate initial investigations (Table 2.7) may be suggested by the history and examination.

Vascular and platelet bleeding is suggested by bruising of the skin and bleeding from mucosal membranes. Inherited coagulation disorders are associated with haemarthrosis and muscle haematomas. Thrombocytopenia is the most common cause of abnormal bleeding.

Patients without evidence of risk factors suggestive of bleeding disorder on history-taking and physical

Table 2.7 Investigation of bleeding disorders

Assay	Comments
Platelet count and blood film	Initial investigation
Coagulation screen	
Prothrombin time (PT)	Prolonged with deficiency of factors I, II, V, VII and X or warfarin therapy
Activated partial thromboplastin time (APTT)	Prolonged with deficiency of all coagulation factors except VII or heparin therapy
Thrombin time (TT)	Prolonged with fibrinogen deficiency, dysfibrinogenaemia, disseminated intravascular coagulation
Bleeding time	Abnormal with von Willebrand's disease, blood vessel defects, platelet dysfunction

examination have a low risk for perioperative hae-morrhage, and routine preoperative coagulation test-ing is not recommended.

Haemophilia is an inherited coagulation disorder with factor VIII deficiency. The severity of bleeding depends on levels of factor VIII. Haemophilia is severe when the level is less than 1%. Activated partial thromboplastin time (APTT) is prolonged but pro-thrombin time (PT) is normal. Treatment includes 1-desamino-8-D-arginine vasopressin (DDAVP), pur-ified factor or recombinant factor VIII administration.

Patients with diabetes mellitus

Diabetes mellitus is a progressive endocrinopathy associated with carbohydrate intolerance and insulin dysregulation. Diabetic patients are more susceptible to gingival and dental disease. With the increasing prevalence of diabetic patients undergoing surgery and the increased risk of associated complications, appro-priate perioperative assessment and management are imperative. Mortality rates in diabetic patients have been estimated to be up to five times greater than in non-diabetic patients, often related to the end-organ damage caused by the disease. Chronic complications resulting in retinopathy, nephropathy, neuropathy, and atherosclerosis can increase the likelihood of sur-gical complications due to infections and vasculo-pathies. Diabetes mellitus is an independent predictor of postoperative myocardial ischaemia among patients undergoing cardiac and non-cardiac surgery[51].

During preoperative assessment, details regarding current diabetes management should be explored. Duration of treatment, specific medication regimen, insulin resistance, and hypersensitivity should be documented. Evaluation of the patient's diabetes diary is often helpful, as is a review of the most recent gly-cosylated haemoglobin (HbA$_{1c}$). HbA$_{1c}$ is an indicator of glycaemic control over the preceding 3 months. If HbA$_{1c}$ is greater than 9%, diabetic control is poor and input from the diabetes team is advisable. If HbA$_{1c}$ is above 12%, consideration should be given to improv-ing control before elective surgery is undertaken.

It is important to check for the presence of cardiac, renal, and neurological sequelae of diabetes, as the presence of these may complicate the perioperative management and increase patient risk. In addition, a comprehensive cardiac assessment should be under-taken in diabetic patients requiring intermediate or major non-cardiac surgery.

The general management principle is to minimize the risk of hypoglycaemia and to limit the incidence of hyperglycaemia. For patients who are diet-controlled or who use oral hypoglycaemics, perioperative man-agement depends on the nature of surgery. For minor dental and oral surgery, body surface or endoscopic procedures, oral hypoglycaemic agents should be omitted on the day of surgery. Ideally, the diabetic patient should be first on the list and encouraged to eat as soon as able postoperatively. Oral hypoglycaemic agents should be administered with the first post-operative meal. Caution must be exercised with the use of metformin. Renal function should be satisfactory prior to reintroduction of this agent. For diet- or tablet-controlled diabetics requiring major oral or maxillofacial surgery, an intravenous insulin regimen will be required. This tends to be in the form of a glucose, potassium, and insulin infusion (GKI). This is commenced when the patient is fasted and should continue through the perioperative period.

Patients who are treated with insulin should be ade-quately controlled preoperatively. Long-acting insulin preparations should be continued until the evening of surgery. The patient should then not receive any sub-cutaneous rapid-acting or premixed insulin on the day of surgery. On the morning of the operation, the blood glucose should be checked and a GKI infusion com-menced. Hourly blood glucose monitoring is manda-tory in the perioperative period.

Renal disorders

Acute renal failure is defined as an abrupt and sus-tained decrease in kidney function resulting in inability to maintain fluid and electrolyte balance and to excrete nitrogenous waste products[52]. The causes can be grouped into prerenal, intrinsic, and postrenal. The National Kidney Foundation guidelines[53] classify *chronic* renal disease into five stages based on the esti-mated value of glomerular filtration rate and presence of kidney damage.

The aim of preoperative evaluation should be to assess the cause and severity of any renal abnormality and optimize the patient's condition to minimize perioperative risk. The evaluation should include an estimation of disease duration, urine analysis, and assessment of glomerular filtration rate. The main causes of morbidity and mortality in patients with renal disease are cardiovascular events, haemorrhage, hyperkalaemia, infection, and multiorgan failure[54,55].

Patients with chronic renal failure have a high inci-dence of cardiac disease and are at increased risk of perioperative cardiac events. Hypertension is also common owing to salt and water retention. This should be treated with salt restriction and antihypertensive agent therapy. Poor control of BP can accelerate the progression of renal failure. Antihypertensive agents should be continued during the perioperative period. Atherosclerosis, fluid overload, and anaemia can lead to left ventricular hypertrophy and failure. ACE inhibitors and angiotensin receptor blockers have been proven to slow the progression of renal failure.

There is an increased risk of developing uraemic pericarditis in non-dialysis patients if urea levels exceed 25 mmol/l. Acute coronary syndrome can be more complex to diagnose as troponin levels will be elevated secondary to renal dysfunction.

Hyperkalaemia is common and can be life-threatening. If ECG changes are present, prompt treatment with calcium chloride or gluconate is required. In addition, administration of dextrose and insulin will effect a temporary reduction in potassium levels. Other treatment modalities include bicarbonate and polystyrene ion exchange resin. Dialysis is required to treat uncontrolled hyperkalaemia. In contrast, hypokalaemia is less common, and cautious correction is advised. Hyponatraemia occurs in acute renal failure because of proximal tubular dysfunction and failure to reabsorb sodium. Other electrolyte abnormalities include hyperphosphataemia and hypocalcaemia.

Metabolic acidosis occurs because of the accumulation of acids, decreased buffering of hydrogen ions, and decreased reabsorption of bicarbonate. Profound acidosis can reduce cardiac contractility and depress the response to inotropic agents. Sodium bicarbonate can be used to correct metabolic acidosis but patients with severe acidosis need dialysis.

Platelet dysfunction is the most common bleeding diathesis in patients with renal impairment. Platelet aggregation is abnormal and bleeding time is prolonged. Platelet adhesiveness is reduced owing to impaired activation of glycoprotein IIb–IIIa complex[56,57]. A platelet count and clotting screen should routinely be checked in all patients with renal dysfunction. Administration of cryoprecipitate or DDAVP can reduce the risk of intraoperative bleeding.

Anaemia is common in renal failure patients. It can be caused by decreased erythropoietin production, inhibition of red cell synthesis, and vitamin B_{12} deficiency. Regular treatment with recombinant erythropoietin is often required. Patients with low iron stores need iron supplementation.

Patients on haemodialysis should receive dialysis in the 24-hour period prior to surgery to optimize volume, electrolyte, and acid–base status.

Liver disorders

The identification of liver disease during preoperative assessment is important as it can influence postoperative morbidity and mortality. The liver is vital for protein synthesis, glucose homeostasis, bilirubin excretion, drug metabolism, and toxin removal. Because of its dual blood supply, it has a substantial functional reserve. Consequently, clinical manifestations of hepatic dysfunction tend to occur only after extensive injury. Liver disease is a heterogeneous collection of disorders ranging from asymptomatic transaminitis to end-stage liver disease. The most common causes of advanced liver disease are alcohol-related cirrhosis, hepatitis B and C, autoimmune disease, drugs, toxins, disorders of the biliary tree, and metabolic disorders such as haemochromatosis, alpha-1 antitrypsin deficiency, and Wilson's disease.

Prediction of perioperative risk is based on the degree of liver dysfunction, the clinical status of the patient, and the nature of the proposed surgery. Patients with alcoholic liver disease have an increased risk of postoperative complications if they have hepatitis or cirrhosis compared with fatty liver alone[58]. Poor wound healing, bleeding, infections, and withdrawal delirium are all recognized problems. Alcohol withdrawal occurs when illness interrupts alcohol intake. Tremors, irritability, and nausea characterize minor alcohol withdrawal. Symptoms usually appear within a few hours of reduction or cessation of alcohol consumption and resolve within 48 hours.

Coexisting problems need to be identified and addressed prior to surgery. Correction of any coagulopathy, restoration of intravascular volume, optimization of cardiac function, correction of electrolyte disturbances, and provision of nutrition should be seen as priorities prior to planned surgery[59].

Coagulopathy is a predominant feature of hepatic dysfunction because the liver is responsible for production of the majority of clotting factors. Associated portal hypertension can cause hypersplenism and thrombocytopenia. Administration of vitamin K, fresh frozen plasma, and platelets may be required to optimize coagulation prior to surgery. Ideally, a target INR of less than 1.5 and a platelet count of more than 80×10^3/l should be achieved. However, this may vary depending on the nature and urgency of proposed surgery[60,61].

Ascites can compromise respiratory function in the postoperative period. It should be treated aggressively with diuretics or paracentesis. Similarly, patients with cirrhosis are at increased risk of encephalopathy. This can be exacerbated by hypoxia, CNS depressants, infection, and gastrointestinal bleeding. These risks should be identified preoperatively and postoperative care modified appropriately. Often patients with alcoholic liver disease are malnourished because of poor dietary intake. Correction of nutritional deficiencies should be addressed preoperatively, particularly in patients undergoing major risk surgery.

Patients with oral and maxillofacial malignancy

Squamous cell carcinoma of the head and neck can affect the oral cavity, oropharynx, hypopharynx, and larynx. Patients with these cancers are typically older, with serious coexisting cardiovascular and respiratory disease reflecting the risk factors for development. Any comorbid conditions should be recognized and addressed in preoperative planning. These patients may require extensive surgery, surgical airways, mechanical ventilation, haemodynamic support, and prolonged inpatient care. The accepted complication rate associated with major head and neck surgery is approximately 20–25%, with pulmonary, cardiovascular, and infectious complications being most common[62].

Recognition of risks and aggressive preoperative management is essential.

Symptoms may vary depending upon the primary site but can include sore throat, dysphagia, and odynophagia. Poor oral intake, weight loss, and malnutrition are well recognized sequelae. Nutritional factors have been shown to have a significant impact on survival of patients with oral cancer[63]. In patients with stage III/IV head and neck cancer treated with multiple modalities, the strongest independent predictor of survival is pretreatment weight loss[64]. Malnutrition is associated with an increased risk of postoperative complications such as wound dehiscence, anastomotic breakdown, infection, abscess formation, respiratory failure, and death[65]. Malnourished patients have depressed immune systems, particularly cell-mediated immunity. Consequently, nutritional preoptimization of the patient with head and neck cancer for major surgery requires careful consideration. A multidisciplinary approach to management is preferable. Involvement of a dietician in the presurgical assessment of nutritional status is imperative. Anthropomorphic measurements (triceps skin fold, upper arm diameter) and weight as a percentage of baseline weight have been used to assess nutritional status. Laboratory values include albumen, prealbumin, transferrin, and retinol-binding protein [is/are] also used but have significant limitations. Albumin is handicapped by a long half-life (20 days), whereas the prealbumin, retinol-binding protein, and transferrin are more indicative of the present nutritional state (half-life of 8 days).

The enteral route should be used preferentially. A soft fine bore nasogastric feeding tube can be used for short-term feeding. However, a percutaneous endoscopic gastrostomy (PEG) is superior if longer term feeding is required. A PEG tube is also beneficial in the postoperative period during radiotherapy when swallowing may be impaired owing to reduced salivation and inflamed oropharyngeal mucosa[66].

Patients at the extremes of age
Paediatric patients

Preoperative evaluation of the paediatric patient allows an opportunity to gather information regarding the child's medical and anaesthetic history, as well as the chance to establish rapport with the child and parents[67]. A detailed history dating back to the neonatal period should be sought. In particular, children with craniofacial deformities may have associated conditions, with major anaesthetic implications (see Chapter 19). For example, patients with Pierre Robin syndrome have mandibular hypoplasia, micrognathia, glossoptosis, and cleft palate, with the potential for difficult intubation. Similarly, cleft lip and palate can be associated with congenital syndromes, especially velocardiofacial syndromes and chromosomal abnormalities. Systemic disorders are more common with cleft palate than with cleft lip alone and include skeletal, cardiac, renal, and central nervous system defects[68]. They may have major implications for anaesthesia, particularly associated cardiac problems.

Many children with learning disabilities require general anaesthesia to treat periodontal disease. Preoperative visiting allows an opportunity to organize carers, prescribe sedative premedications to facilitate a smooth transfer to theatre and anticipate intraoperative difficulties and postoperative needs.

Elderly patients

Ageing is associated with a constellation of physiological changes and an increased susceptibility to disease. These factors render the older patient more vulnerable to the complications of anaesthesia and surgery.

The elderly progressively lose physiological reserves because of ageing and cannot mount the necessary prolonged response to injury. This may then lead to single or multiple organ failure. Therefore, when reserves are needed to meet the increased demands of acute illness or surgical stress but are no longer present, organ system failure may result[69]. A team of senior surgeons, anaesthetists, and physicians should be closely involved in the care of elderly patients who have poor physical status and high operative risk. The decision to operate on a high-risk patient should prompt the provision of a higher level of care in the postoperative period. Emergency surgery should not be deferred once the patient is deemed medically fit. Early involvement of specialists in an attempt to optimize existing medical conditions should be encouraged. Optimal fluid balance should be a high priority in the preoperative period to minimize the risk of intraoperative hypotension[70].

Patients requiring solid organ transplantation

The survival rate of patients after solid organ transplantation has improved owing to recent advances in perioperative management and immunosuppression. Systemic infections and rejection dramatically decrease the survival rate in transplant recipients. Since odontogenic inflammation may favour transplant rejection, increase the risk of bacterial endocarditis or lead to life-threatening postoperative infections, all existing or potential sources of dental infection should be eliminated before transplantation surgery[71].

General anaesthesia is best avoided but may be required if extensive dental work is required. Anaesthesia should be conducted by experienced personnel with due consideration to abnormal bleeding tendency, altered drug metabolism, and infectious complications. Optimization of the underlying condition is often extremely limited. The patient with end-stage renal failure requiring regular renal replacement therapy should have surgery arranged within 24 hours of dialysis to ensure control of hyperkalaemia and volume status. Particular attention should be paid to the site of the arteriovenous fistula or graft to prevent inadvertent injury in the perioperative period.

Post-transplantation, elective dental care should be deferred for at least 3 months to reduce the risk of infectious complications during the early period of immunosuppression.

Maxillofacial trauma

Trauma to the maxillofacial area is of great importance to the anaesthetist given the potential for airway compromise and is discussed in detail in Chapter 14. Injuries may be isolated or multiple. A thorough preoperative evaluation requires the luxury of time which may not be available in the polytrauma victim. Under such circumstances, effective teamwork and structured clinical assessment is vital.

Conclusion

Postoperative morbidity and mortality after oral and maxillofacial surgery depends, in part, on the preoperative physiological status of the patient. Thorough preoperative assessment and optimization are essential before assigning the patient to a particular therapeutic option. Early communication between the surgical and anaesthetic team is essential to identify problems and ensure comprehensive preanaesthetic investigation and preparation.

References

1. The Association of Anaesthetists of Great Britain and Ireland. (2009) Pre-operative assessment. The role of the anaesthetist. November 2001. Available online at http://www.aagbi.org (accessed 30 March 2009).
2. Garcia-Miguel FJ, Serrano-Aguilar PG, Lopez-Bastida J. (2003) Preoperative assessment. Lancet, 362, 1749–57.
3. Royal College of Anaesthetists. (2004) Guidance on the provision of anaesthetic services for pre-operative care. Available online at http://www.rcoa.ac.uk (accessed 30 March 2009).
4. Inadequate pre-operative evaluation and preparation: a review of 197 reports from the Australian Incident Monitoring Study. Anaesthesia, 2000; 55, 1173–8.
5. Kluger MT, Tham EJ, Coleman NA, et al. (2002) American Society of Anesthesiologists task force on preanesthesia evaluation. Practice advisory for preanesthesia evaluation: a report by the American Society of Anesthesiologists Task Force. Anesthesiology, 96, 485–96.
6. Brooks-Brunn JA. (1997) Predictors of postoperative pulmonary complications following abdominal surgery. Chest, 111, 564–7.
7. Sweitzer B-J. (ed.) (2008) Overview of preoperative evaluation and testing. In: Sweitzer B-J. (ed.) Preoperative Assessment and Management, pp. 14–47. Lippincott Williams and Wilkins, Philadelphia, USA.
8. American Society of Anesthesiologists. (2002) Practice advisory for preanesthesia evaluation: a report by the American Society of Anesthesiologists task force on preanesthesia evaluation. Anesthesiology, 96(2), 485–96.
9. NICE guidelines (2003). Preoperative tests. The use of routine preoperative tests for elective surgery. Available

online at http://www.nice.org.uk/Guidance/CG3 (accessed 30 March 2009).

10. Burger W, Chemnitius JM, Kneissel GD, *et al.* (2005) Low-dose aspirin for secondary cardiovascular prevention—cardiovascular risks after its withdrawal versus bleeding risks with its continuation—review and meta-analysis. *J Intern Med*, **257**, 399–414.

11. Fleisher LA, Beckman JA, Brown KA, *et al.* (2006) ACC/AHA 2006 guideline update on perioperative cardiovascular evaluation for non-cardiac surgery. *Circulation*, **113**, 2662–74.

12. Smetana G. (1999) Preoperative pulmonary evaluation. *N Engl J Med*, **340**, 937–44.

13. Qaseem A, Snow V, Fitterman N, *et al.* (2006) Risk assessment for and strategies to reduce perioperative pulmonary complications for patients undergoing non-cardiothoracic surgery: a guideline from the American College of Physicians. *Ann Intern Med*, **144**, 575–80.

14. Warner D. (1996) Perioperative respiratory complications in patient with asthma. *Anesthesiology*, **85**, 455–66.

15. Smetana GW, Lawrence VA, Cornell JE. (2006) Preoperative pulmonary risk stratification for non-cardiothoracic surgery: systematic review for the American College of Physicians. *Ann Intern Med*, **144**, 581–95.

16. Barrera R, Shi W, Amar D, *et al.* (2005) Smoking and timing of cessation: impact on pulmonary complications after thoracotomy. *Chest*, **127**, 1977–83.

17. Celli BR, MacNee W, Agusti A, *et al.* (2004) Standards for the diagnosis and treatment of patients with COPD: a summary of the ATS/ERS position paper. *Eur Respir J*, **23**, 932–46.

18. Srinivas RB, Julia FW, Tara S, Eugene SC, Richard KA. (2007) Preoperative evaluation of the patient with pulmonary disease. *Chest*, **132**, 1637–45.

19. Mangano DT, Goldman L. (1995) Preoperative assessment of patients with known or suspected coronary disease. *N Engl J Med*, **333**, 1750–56.

20. Goldman L, Caldera DL, Nussbaum SR, *et al.* (1977) Multifactorial index of cardiac risk in noncardiac surgical procedures. *N Engl J Med*, **297**, 845–50.

21. Palda VA, Detsky AS. (1997) Perioperative assessment and management of risk from coronary artery disease. *Ann Intern Med*, **127**, 313–28.

22. Detsky AS, Abrams HB, Forbath N, *et al.* (1986) Cardiac assessment for patients undergoing noncardiac surgery. A multifactorial clinical risk index. *Arch Intern Med*, **146**, 2131–4.

23. Lee TH, Marcantonio ER, Mangione CM, *et al.* (1999) Derivation and prospective validation of a simple index for prediction of cardiac risk of major noncardiac surgery. *Circulation*, **100**, 1043–9.

24. Eagle KA, Brundage BH, Chaitman BR, *et al.* (1996) Guidelines for perioperative cardiovascular evaluation for noncardiac surgery: report of the American College of Cardiology/American Heart Association Task Force on Practice Guidelines (Committee on Perioperative Cardiovascular Evaluation for Noncardiac Surgery). *J Am Coll Cardiol*, **27(4)**, 910–48.

25. Eagle KA, Berger PB, Calkins H, *et al.* (2002) ACC/AHA guideline update for perioperative cardiovascular evaluation for noncardiac surgery—executive summary: a report of the American College of Cardiology/American Heart Association Task Force on Practice Guidelines (Committee to Update the 1996 Guidelines on Perioperative Cardiovascular Evaluation for Noncardiac Surgery). *Circulation*, **105**, 1257–67.

26. Fleisher LA, Beckman JA, Brown KA, *et al.* (2007) ACC/AHA 2007 guidelines on perioperative cardiovascular evaluation and care for noncardiac surgery: executive summary: a report of the American College of Cardiology/American Heart Association Task Force on Practice Guidelines (Writing Committee to revise the 2002 guidelines on perioperative cardiovascular evaluation for noncardiac surgery). *J Am Coll Cardiol*, **50(17)**, 1707–32.

27. Eagle KA, Berger PB, Calkins H, *et al.* (2002) ACC/AHA guideline update for perioperative cardiovascular evaluation for non cardiac surgery. *J Am Coll Cardiol*, **39**, 542–53.

28. Freeman WK, Gibbons RJ. (2009) Perioperative cardiovascular assessment of patients undergoing noncardiac surgery. *Mayo Clinic Proceedings*, **84(1)**, 79–90.

29. Hindler K, Shaw AD, Samuels J, *et al.* (2006) Improved postoperative outcomes associated with preoperative statin therapy. *Anesthesiology*, **105(6)**, 1260–72.

30. Devereaux PJ, Beattie WS, Choi PT-L, *et al.* (2005) How strong is the evidence for the use of perioperative beta blockers in non cardiac surgery? Systematic review and meta-analysis of randomised control trials. *BMJ*, **6**, 313–21.

31. Auerbach AD, Goldman L. (2002) Beta blockers and reduction of cardiac events after non cardiac surgery. *JAMA*, **287**, 1435–44.

32. POISE Study Group. (2008) Effects of extended release metoprolol succinate in patients undergoing noncardiac surgery (POISE Trial): a randomised trial. *Lancet*, **371**, 1839–47.

33. McCullogh PA, Nowak RM, McCord J, *et al.* (2002) B-type natriuretic peptide and clinical judgement in emergency diagnosis of heart failure: analysis from Breathing Not Properly (BNP) Multinational Study. *Circulation*, **106**, 416–22.

34. Hunt SA, ACC/AHA Task Force on Practice guidelines. (2005) ACC/AHA 2005 guideline update for the diagnosis and management of chronic heart failure in the adult: a report on the American College of Cardiology/American Heart Association Task Force on Practice Guidelines. *J Am Coll Cardiol*, **46**, 1–82.

35. Herman WW, Konzelman JL, Prisant LM. (2004) New national guidelines on hypertension. A summary for dentistry. *J Am Dent Assoc*, **135(5)**, 576–84.

36. Mitka M. (2000) Hypertension experts recommend new focus on the systolic reading. *JAMA*, **284**, 1638–9.

37. Arauz-Pacheco C, Parrott MA, Raskin P. (2003) American Diabetes Association. Treatment of hypertension in adults with diabetes. *Diabetes Care*, **26** (Suppl. 1), S80–2.

38. The Trials of Hypertension Prevention Collaborative Research Group. (1997) Effects of weight loss and sodium

reduction intervention on blood pressure and hypertension incidence in overweight people with high-normal blood pressure. The Trials of Hypertension Prevention, phase II. *Arch Intern Med*, **157**, 657–67.

39. He J, Whelton PK, Appel LJ, *et al.* (2000) Long-term effects of weight loss and dietary sodium reduction on incidence of hypertension. *Hypertension*, **35**, 544–9.

40. Sacks FM, Svetkey LP, Vollmer WM, *et al.* (2001) DASH-Sodium Collaborative Research Group. Effects on blood pressure of reduced dietary sodium and the Dietary Approaches to Stop Hypertension (DASH) diet. DASH-Sodium Collaborative Research Group. *N Engl J Med*, **344**, 3–10.

41. Vollmer WM, Sacks FM, Ard J, *et al.* (2001) DASH-Sodium Trial Collaborative Research Group. Effects of diet and sodium intake on blood pressure: subgroup analysis of the DASH-sodium trial. *Ann Intern Med*, **135**, 1019–28.

42. Kelley GA, Kelley KS. (2000) Progressive resistance exercise and resting blood pressure: a meta-analysis of randomized controlled trials. *Hypertension*, **35**, 838–43.

43. Xin X, He J, Frontini MG, Ogden LG, Motsamai OI, Whelton PK. (2001) Effects of alcohol reduction on blood pressure: a meta-analysis of randomized controlled trials. *Hypertension*, **38**, 1112–17.

44. NICE guidelines on prophylaxis for endocarditis (March 2008). Available online at http://www.nice.org.uk/Guidance/CG64 (accessed 30 March 2009).

45. Ogle OE. (2006) Gastrointestinal diseases and considerations in the perioperative management of oral surgical patients. *Oral Maxillofacial Surg Clin N Am*, **18**, 241–54.

46. Practice guidelines for preoperative fasting and the use of pharmacological agents to reduce the risk of pulmonary aspiration: application to healthy patients undergoing elective procedures: a report by the American Society of Anaesthesiologists Task Force on Preoperative Fasting. *Anesthesiology*, 1999; **90**, 896–905.

47. Tramer MR. (2001) A rational approach to the control of postoperative nausea and vomiting: evidence from systematic reviews. Part 1. Efficacy and harm of antiemetic interventions and methodological issues. *Acta Anaesthesiol Scand*, **45**, 4–13.

48. Shander A, Knight K, Turner R, *et al.* (2004) Prevalence and outcomes of anaemia in surgery: a systematic review of the literature. *Am J Med*, **116**, 58S–69S.

49. Carson JL, Duff A, Poses RM, *et al.* (1996) Effect of anaemia and cardiovascular disease on surgical morbidity and mortality. *Lancet*, **348**, 1055–60.

50. Scott BW, Karkouti K, Wijeysunders DN, *et al.* (2009) Risk associated with preoperative anemia in non-cardiac surgery: a single-center cohort study. *Anesthesiology*, **110**, 574–581.

51. Coursin DB, Connery LE, Ketzler JT. (2004) Perioperative diabetic and hyperglycemic management issues. *Crit Care Med*, **32(4)**, S116–124.

52. Mcphee SJ, Papadakis MA. (2008) *Current Medical Diagnosis and Treatment*, 47th edn. Lange, USA.

53. National Kidney Foundation. (2002) K/DOQI clinical practice guidelines for chronic kidney disease: evaluation, classification and stratification. *Am J Kidney Dis*, **39** (2 Suppl. 1), S19.

54. Kellerman PS. (1994) Perioperative care of the renal patient. *Arch Intern Med*, **154**, 1674–88.

55. Shiplak MG, Fried LF, Crump C, *et al.* (2002) Cardiovascular disease risk status in elderly patients with renal insufficiency. *Kidney Int*, **62**, 997–1004.

56. Kaw D, Malhotra D. (2006) Platelet dysfunction and end-stage renal disease. *Semin Dial*, **19**, 317–22.

57. Eberst ME, Berkowitz LR.(1994) Haemostasis in renal disease. *Am J Med*, **96**, 168–79.

58. Rizvon MK, Chou CL. (2003) Surgery in the patient with liver disease. *Med Clin North Am*, **87(1)**, 211–27.

59. Ziser A, Plevak DJ, Wiesner RH, *et al.* (1999) Morbidity and mortality in cirrhotic patients undergoing anesthesia and surgery. *Anesthesiology*, **90(1)**, 42–53.

60. Clarkson E, Bhatia SJ. (2006) Perioperative management of the patient with liver disease and management of the chronic alcoholic. *Oral Maxillofacial Surg Clin N Am*, **18**, 213–25.

61. Friedman LS. (1999) The risk of surgery in patients with liver disease. *Hepatology*, **29(6)**, 1617–23.

62. Harris CM, Nierzwicki BL, Blanchaert RH. (2006) Perioperative management of maxillofacial tumour and reconstruction patients. *Oral Maxillofacial Surg Clin N Am*, **18**, 227–39.

63. Liu S-A, Tai W-C, Wong Y-K, *et al.* (2006) Nutritional factors and survival of patients with oral cancer. *Head and Neck*, **28**, 998–1007.

64. Mick R *et al.* (1991) Prognostic factors in advanced head and neck cancer patients undergoing multimodality therapy. *Otolaryngology Head & Neck Surgery*, **105**, 62–73.

65. Bozetti F, Gavazzi C, Miceli R. (2000) Perioperative total parenteral nutrition in malnourished, gastrointestinal cancer patients: a randomized, clinical trial. *J Parenter Enteral Nutr*, **24(1)**, 7–14.

66. Brown AE, Prein J. (1999) The team approach in the management of oral cancer. In: Ward Booth P, Schendel SA, Hausamen JE (eds) *Maxillofacial Surgery*, Vol. 1. Churchill Livingstone, pp. 325–30. London, UK.

67. Evans L, Prosser DP. (2006) Preoperative assessment and preparation for anaesthesia in children. *Anaesthesia and Intensive Care Medicine*, **7**, 375–9.

68. Disability. In: Scully C, Cawson RA (eds). *Medical Problems in Dentistry*. Elsevier Churchill Livingstone, pp. 427–30. London, UK.

69. Rosenthal RA, Kavic SM. (2004) Assessment and management of the geriatric patient. *Crit Care Med*, **32**, S92–S105.

70. *Extremes of age. The 1999 report of The National Enquiry into Perioperative Deaths.* November 1999. NCEPOD, London. See www.ncepod.org.uk/pdf/1999/99full.pdf for further details.

71. Meyer U, Weingart D, Deng MC, *et al.* (1999) Heart transplants—assessment of dental procedures. *Clin Oral Invest*, **3**, 79–83.

3

Medicolegal aspects of anaesthesia for oral and maxillofacial surgery

Christopher Heneghan

Introduction

The law relating to anaesthesia for oral and maxillofacial surgery is the law that governs all medical practice, and in this respect anaesthetists are no different from other doctors. The range of patients encountered will include those aged from under 5 to those over 100 years, the mentally incompetent and the all too competent, the litigious, and the obstinate. The involvement of other doctors (surgeons) in decision-making, while from time to time putting extra difficulties in our way, does not change the need to work to the correct standard.

Some of the law governing medical practice is common law, the judicial response to a legal vacuum; some is statute (including statutory instrument), which ranges from laws codifying the common law to wholly new departures. Law is a function of government, and differs between jurisdictions. This chapter will address the law of England and Wales, and, where appropriate, may include comments about other jurisdictions. These writings should not be seen as a substitute for legal advice, though they may of course help understand such advice, and where comments are included regarding the law of other jurisdictions, they should be seen as illustrative rather than instructive.

Structure of law

Detailed knowledge of the structure of the law is not the remit of this chapter. It will suffice to understand that criminal law addresses divergence from accepted forms of behaviour so serious that the state regards them as requiring control, while civil law addresses differences between persons reaching to lower levels of seriousness.

There is some overlap, as for example where negligence causes death, where sufficiently serious negligence may reach the level of crime and initiate manslaughter charges. Both civil and criminal law are adversarial, designed to answer a question, be it of guilt or blame, and issue orders based on those answers: sentences, damages, injunctions, and so on. Medical law has the added dimension of the Coroner's court, the sole court that merely seeks information and has no powers beyond announcing the results of its inquiry: if it seeks to take matters further, it must send its information to the criminal authorities.

Most of what we do is covered by the law of negligence, one of the civil wrongs ('torts') developed by judges over centuries in the process known as the common law. Statute law covers those matters to which the sovereign in parliament has directed his attention and passed a law. Common law covers all the rest, where parliament has been silent and judges must decide, governed by precedent and sometimes common sense. The law defining murder is still common law, though parliament has decided on the proper sentence. Parliament can adjust common law as it wishes, and has recently done so by codifying the law with regard to consent and capacity in the Mental Capacity Act 2005[17].

Negligent acts or omissions

Negligence may be by action or failure to act—omission. The law here has been fairly stable for some years now. The authoritative reference is to Lord Atkin's judgment in Donoghue v Stevenson[1]:

> The liability for negligence...is no doubt based upon a general public sentiment of moral wrongdoing for

which the offender must pay. But acts or omissions which any moral code would censure cannot in a practical world be treated so as to give a right to every person injured by them to demand relief. In this way rules of law arise which limit the range of complaints and the extent of their remedy. The rule that you are to love your neighbour becomes in law, you must not injure your neighbour; and the lawyer's question, 'Who is my neighbour?' receives a restricted reply. You must take reasonable care to avoid the acts or omissions which you can reasonably foresee would be likely to injure your neighbour. Who, then, in law is my neighbour? The answer seems to be, persons who are so closely and directly affected by my act that I ought reasonably to have them in contemplation as being so affected when I am directing my mind to the acts or omissions which are called into question.

Once someone is our patient, they always fall within the definition of the foreseeable neighbour mentioned in the judgment. The next question to be considered is: could we reasonably foresee that our acts or omissions would injure that patient? Here the usually quoted judgment is that of McNair J in Bolam[2]:

> …I must tell you what I mean in law by 'negligence'. In the ordinary case which does not involve any special skill, negligence in law means a failure to do some act which a reasonable man in the circumstances would do, or the doing of some act which a reasonable man in the circumstances would not do; and if that failure or the doing of the act results in injury, then there is a cause of action. How do you test whether this act or failure is negligent? In the ordinary case it is said you judge it by the action of the man in the street. He is the ordinary man. In one case it has been said you judge it by the man on the top of the Clapham omnibus. He is the ordinary man. But where you get a situation which involves the use of some special skill or competence, then the test as to whether there has been negligence or not is not the test of the man on the top of a Clapham omnibus, because he has not got this special skill. The test is the test of the ordinary skilled man exercising and professing to have that special skill. A man need not possess the highest expert skill: it is well established law that it is sufficient if he exercises the ordinary skill of the ordinary competent man exercising that particular art…

Incorporated in that judgment are two concepts that are crucial to medical negligence: first, the test, whether we exercise the ordinary skill of the ordinary competent anaesthetist. This has come to mean that our actions would be acceptable to a responsible (or reputable or respectable) body of practitioners in the field, and the term the 'responsible minority defence' is often used to encapsulate the idea. Thus, it does not matter whether some practitioners might criticize your

actions, when there is another group who regard it as acceptable. This allows for differences of opinion, and for development of the specialty.

The second concept is that our failing, act or omission, must result in an injury for liability to arise. A 2005 case[3] has thrown that into doubt, and it will be addressed under the section on consent, but the rule that will be applied except in very rare circumstances is: if the patient is not damaged in some way, there is no tort, and no right to sue*.

The law has decided what is a body of opinion: how many or how few doctors must regard something as acceptable to be regarded as a 'body of opinion'. A 'body of opinion' suggests quite a few, but it can in fact be as few as 12 (a spinal surgery case)[4], and, by implication at least, only one[5]. This case actually turned on whether the unique practice of one individual anaesthetist was negligent: no consideration was given to whether one individual could be a body of opinion, so he must have been.

The case mainly went to the next question-was he a responsible body of opinion? He had been dropping systolic blood pressure during middle ear surgery to 35–40 mmHg, and had done so for years. Then, in 1979, a patient suffered damage. It was decided that the doctor was not responsible on the basis that he failed to follow up these cases himself, and that he did not conduct animal research. He had started a patient-based research project that came to nothing[†], but he did publish a series of 700 cases in the British Journal of Anaesthesia[6]: this was not regarded as sufficient to be called responsible.

What is responsible was considered and modified further in Bolitho[7]. This case said that, for the opinion of doctors to be responsible, it must be reasonable and/or logical (depending which judgment you read): if it is not, the court may reject it. This judgment initially raised concerns that judges might regularly reject medical evidence on acceptable practice. As well as allowing the opinions of someone only sketchily versed in medicine to over-rule those of experts, this would have had the further disadvantage of making the law unpredictable. In fact, Bolitho has not been applied much: it has been referred to in only 12 cases in 10 years

---

* This is not relevant to clinical governance issues: employers are not limited by the rule that damage must result from negligence before right of action arises, as their rights and duties derive from employment law, and the duties of the doctors to the GMC.

† Those who feel this was an unfair application of 1995 standards to 1979 events, or that reputation was more important than responsibility, will not find me disagreeing.

of medical law reports (*Lloyd's Rep Med*)—in only four of these was expert evidence not followed, with three of these regarding doctors (the fourth was a midwife). Thus the effect of Bolitho is not to over-rule medical opinion much, more to reserve the right to do so, so that doctors are only advising the court, not deciding cases.

Causation

Damage done to a patient must be caused by the act or omission that constituted negligence. Whilst that seems obvious, for a period the law relied on a more robust approach to causation that derived from employment law: where there is failure to perform an act which is specifically designed to prevent a certain outcome, and that outcome occurs, then it is reasonable to blame the outcome on the failure[8]. This was reversed in Wilshire[9], so that where there are several possible causes of damage, some of which are non-negligent, the claimant must show on the balance of probabilities that negligence did cause the damage.

In passing, this highlights an interesting divergence between medical and legal language: doctors will often talk of a probable cause of an event, meaning a cause more likely than any one of the other possibilities. Lawyers use the same phrase to mean the possibility which is more likely than all the others put together. We should be clear when advising lawyers that they have the same understanding of such language.

Consent

Consent from the patient has always been required before treatment can be given: only in certain prescribed circumstances can treatment be imposed without consent, and that is almost invariably where there is no capacity to consent (see below).

Two matters must be dealt with under this heading. The first is that a consent form is not a requirement *in law*. Local protocols and common practices have made them indispensable in certain parts of medical practice, such as surgery, and never used at all in others, such as general practice or, curiously, anaesthesia. In any debate about the desirability or otherwise of consent forms, it should be realized that a consent form is merely evidence of consent at the time the form was signed[10]. It is not a contract, and consent may be withdrawn or modified at any time the patient has capacity. Consent may be verbal, or by action or acquiescence, and may be evidenced by a signed form, a note in the records or statements from witnesses.

The other point of interest is that we call it 'consent', which implies that the doctor is asking the patient to be allowed to treat him/her, in turn implying our desire to treat may be greater than the patient's to be treated. While we, who work with them regularly, realize that such an analysis of the interaction may apply with surgeons, it is a rather curious way of viewing most doctor-patient interactions, and 'request for treatment' might be a more appropriate formulation. 'Consent', however, is here to stay.

Information and consent

How much or what information a patient should receive before consenting came into English law with Sidaway[11], a decision on whether a patient who was paralysed following neck surgery should have been warned of the risk of paralysis. This 1985 judgment is interesting insofar as it illustrates the changes since then. It is long and detailed (and contradictory), but basically states that what needs to be told to a patient should be decided by doctors, and the Bolam test of negligence decides whether enough information has been given. However, the judgment goes on with many extra comments, some of which are summarized as follows:

- Informed consent forms no part of English law
- A patient should have enough information to make an informed decision
- If a doctor judges that to give full information might frighten a patient off accepting really necessary treatment, he should withhold that information
- If a patient asks, we must answer truthfully
- We should not withhold information of a substantial risk of grave adverse consequences—the example, from a Canadian case[12] was a 10% risk of a stroke
- If the court thought we had blundered, it would be entitled to say so.

Interestingly, when stating what in general judges thought we really must tell patients, as well as setting a two-part test in (1) substantial risk of (2) grave adverse consequences, the examples for how that test may be fulfilled were (1) 10% risk of (2) stroke. Today we are told, for example by trust legal advisors, that we should advise of a greater than 1% risk, with no consideration as to the gravity of consequence. There is no case law to support this, and if it is the correct level, that is because so many doctors have become convinced of it that there is no longer a responsible body of opinion that would not advise of a 1% risk. In practice, many doctors are advising of *all* risks (or trying to), and advice is being given of risks estimated at less than 0.01% (e.g. infection after spinal anaesthesia). Do we have to do this? There is no law on these precise percentages because Sidaway still applies, so what is the correct information to give will be tested on expert evidence, but this is also covered by Bolitho, that it must be reasonable/logical, and further, in Pearce[12], that we should advise patients of '...a significant risk which would affect the judgement of a reasonable patient... so that the patient can determine for him or herself as to what course he or she should adopt...' This reinforces the patient-based aspects of Sidaway, and perhaps we would have no major difficulty with it, apart from the unpredictability of what a judge might think a reasonable patient might think.

Of course, when we move to the practical application of the law, if doctors agree on a certain standard, that effectively becomes the legal standard. The General Medical Council (GMC) has pronounced on what the standard should be[13], using a patient-centred approach, and, for example, stating that we '...must tell patients if an investigation or treatment might result in a serious adverse outcome, even if the likelihood is very small...,' with *adverse outcome* defined as '...resulting in death, permanent or long-term physical disability or disfigurement, medium- or long-term pain or admission to hospital; or other outcomes with a long-term or permanent effect on a patient's employment, social or personal life.' The guidance in this document is there for all to read. I would be surprised if any medical expert was prepared to support a different standard in court.

It used to be that it hardly mattered what information you gave to patients, as it was very difficult to demonstrate that the outcome would have been different had the information been given (thus completing the necessary step in proving negligence, proving damage was caused by the negligence). This is because it will usually be the case that treatment offered will be accepted, as it is intended to address life- or limb-threatening, or painful, conditions, and on average the benefits will far outweigh the risks. Whilst there are areas where this may not apply, for example areas such as cosmetic surgery where patient choice is a vital issue, it has proved difficult to convince a court that a different outcome would have ensued, and therefore that damage was caused by failure to inform.

Chester (Chester v Afshar)[14] is another spinal surgery/damage case, where the patient was not told of risks, had the operation, the risks materialized, and she said she would not have consented. The defence argued that she would have had the operation anyway, but not that day. Whilst there was some discussion of the question of whether, had she had the operation another day, the 2% risk of damage would have materialized, seeming to take the view that it is a random risk rather than one based on factors present whenever she had the operation, the majority (three of five) of judgments supporting the patient's claim were based on the following logic, quoting Lord Steyn (at para 24):

> Standing back from the detailed arguments, I have come to the conclusion that, as a result of the surgeon's failure to inform the patient, she cannot be said to have given informed consent* to the surgery in the full legal sense. Her right of autonomy and dignity ought to be vindicated by a narrow and modest departure from the traditional causation principles.

Lord Walker (at para 101) also said

> I agree ... that the patient ought not to be without a remedy, even if it involves some extension of existing principle...

This is a real break with precedent, as it amounts to giving the patient a remedy even when she was not physically or mentally damaged by the negligence, or where the only damage was to her autonomy! This amounts, in my opinion, to punishing the surgeon for not advising of risks, even though that lack of advice did not cause injury. This logic could be extended to permit doctors to be sued for any damage that follows negligence, whether caused by it or not!

However, this does not look likely to be going to happen[15]. There is no reported case that follows the precedent of *Chester*, and there are reported remarks suggesting disagreement by other senior members of the judiciary[16]. Nevertheless, the current law seems to be that, in consent cases, if we fail to advise of a significant risk and the risk materializes, the patient may win against the doctor even without being able to prove a causative link. Doctors should be well advised, therefore, to advise of significant, serious risks.

Competence and consent

The long string of case law in this area has recently been codified in the Mental Capacity Act 2005 ('the Act')[17]. The Act has introduced a number of new principles, while leaving unaltered most of the existing law. To date, there have been no judgments regarding

---

* A concept that "forms no part of English Law"—see Sidaway second bullet point above.

consent to medical treatment since this act came into force, so speculation as to the precise meaning of the Act is inevitable.

The Mental Capacity Act 2005 can be found and read in detail at http://www.opsi.gov.uk/ACTS/ acts2005/pdf/ukpga_20050009_en.pdf, with codes of practice available at http://www.dca.gov.uk/menincap/ legis.htm, and a helpful, easy-to-read summary at http://www.dca.gov.uk/menincap/mca-act-easyread. pdf. Worth noting as unchanged in the Act are the following (s1–2):

♦ Capacity is assumed, which means lack of capacity has to be proved

♦ Patients should not be treated as incompetent unless all practicable steps to help them make decisions have failed

♦ Patients are not to be 'deemed incompetent' merely because they make an unwise decision

♦ Any act or decision taken on behalf of an incompetent person must be in his or her best interests*[18]

♦ Before an act is done or a decision made, the decision-maker must consider whether its purpose can be as effectively achieved less restrictively of a patient's rights and freedom of action, i.e. do the minimum

♦ When considering whether a patient has capacity we:

a. Must not go by age/appearance alone

b. Must consider whether the patient will regain capacity soon enough to decide

c. Must encourage participation by the patient

d. Must not be motivated by a desire to bring about death

It is a little surprising that a legislator evidently thought there is a need for a statement that doctors must not be motivated by a desire to bring about death, but there it is: it was against the law before this, and it is still against the law.

---

* Best interests in medicine is not redefined by the Act, nor is there yet a judgment on it. However, regarding appointment of a Deputy, a recent case[19] emphasizes that capacity is not all or nothing but is decision-specific; and notes that while the protected person's wishes are not paramount in deciding best interests, if he or she expresses a wish that is not irrational, not impractical, and not irresponsible, it should be followed unless strongly outweighed.

Emphasized in this act (s2(1)) is the point that 'a person lacks capacity in relation to a matter if *at the material time* he is unable to make a decision for himself *in relation to the matter ...*' Capacity relates to a particular decision, and is not a general phenomenon. A banal illustration might be that a patient knows very well whether he or she wants tea or coffee, but may not have capacity to decide which operation to have (if any). The consequence for doctors, therefore, seems to be that the practitioner who seeks the decision has to assess capacity, and this is not a function that might be delegated, for example, to a psychiatrist.

Modest changes to the law include an extension of the test of capacity, to read (s3):

♦ A person [lacks capacity] if he is unable to

○ Understand information relevant to the decision

○ Retain that information

○ Use or weigh that information as part of a decision-making process

♦ or

○ Communicate the decision (talking, sign language, other means).

We should note that the conjunction between the parts is 'or', which means that you lack capacity if you fail any part of the test. New to this test compared to the old common law formulation[18] is that there is no longer a requirement for the patient to believe the information he has been told, and in addition there is a requirement to be able to communicate the decision. Those of us frequently working with patients with Alzheimer's will recognize failure to understand, to retain, and to use the information, one or all of which may cause lack of capacity.

If we conclude (which should be on balance of probabilities) that a patient lacks capacity, normally we should take that decision based on their best interests, but we should also:

♦ Consider, and so far as reasonably ascertainable, the patient's past or present wishes, values, and feelings (and any relevant written statement made when they had capacity)

♦ Take into account, if it is practicable and appropriate to consult them, the views of:

○ Anyone named by the person as someone to be consulted on the matter in question or on matters of that kind

○ Anyone engaged in caring for the person or interested in his welfare

○ Any donee of a lasting power of attorney granted by the person

♦ And

○ Any deputy appointed for the person by the court.

It should be noted that there is no reference to next of kin. We know of course that next of kin never had the power to make decisions on behalf of their relative in English law, but there have often been protocols regarding contacting them, and not infrequently they have not actually seen the patient for years: an estranged spouse, for example, can be the legal next of kin to someone who has been living with someone else for decades. The law now requires taking into account the views of those listed above. Thus anyone known to the patient may be consulted, including a carer, friend, next door neighbour, even the milkman, if they are interested in the patient's welfare.

It should also be noted that the requirement is to 'take into account'. This does not mean the person consulted is a decision-maker, but that they should be consulted to find out what the patient would have wanted (if known), and such information does not absolve the deciding doctor from the need to decide. 'Taking into account' means including with all the other factors for consideration, not following slavishly.

The Act also identifies (S3(9)) that there is sufficient compliance with it if a deciding doctor *reasonably believes* what he does or decides is in the best interests of the patient, and that where there is reference to 'relevant circumstances', it means circumstances of which the deciding doctor is aware, and which it would be reasonable to regard as relevant. The tenor of the Act (apart from the remark about not being motivated by a desire to bring about death) is generally trusting of doctors to behave properly rather than a tough restrictive code, which, as previously mentioned, follows the old common law. That is not to say we will not be subject to criticism, or will get away with things, but in large part if we carry on as before we will not be far wrong.

New concepts in the act

In England and Wales, doctors have always made decisions for the incapacitated, acting in their best interests. This has worried some, perhaps concerned that power corrupts, and wondering *Quis custodiet ipsos custodes?** Other jurisdictions have addressed this by using substitute decision-making, whether by next of kin or other nominated individuals to decide on behalf of the incapacitated, or by 'living wills'. The Act has attempted to introduce these ideas into English law, with what success remains to be seen.

There are four new parts of the Act.

♦ Lasting power of attorney

♦ Advance decisions

♦ Independent mental capacity advocates (IMCAs)

♦ Court of protection and public guardian.

Lasting power of attorney (LPA)

This amounts to a variation on the old 'enduring power of attorney', which allowed appointment of someone to manage your financial affairs if you lose capacity. Someone given LPA may take medical decisions as well. The appointment is strictly regulated. The LPA is subject to the same rules about acting in the patient's best interests as are doctors' decisions. The appointing document has to be in the correct form and registered with the public guardian to be effective. It is specifically set out (s11(7)(c)) that the terms of the LPA may extend to giving or refusing consent to the carrying out or continuation of a treatment, and (S11(8)(a)) 'does not authorize the giving or refusing of consent to the carrying out or continuation of life-sustaining treatment, *unless the instrument contains express provision to that effect*', the 'instrument' being the document appointing the LPA.

As far as can be understood from the Act, the intention is to create a powerful, but tightly restricted, position, so that, if properly done, just about any medical decision can be made on behalf of a patient, in their best interests. It is supervised and governed by the court of protection, and the Office of the public guardian's website* provides forms for setting up an LPA that seem absolutely explicit and clear. Litigation on what constitutes life-sustaining treatment is to be expected, as for example much of what we do on intensive care might come under that heading, but if it is part of a treatment package that is intended to bring about recovery, the edges start blurring.

---

* Latin tag = who will keep watch over the watchers, who will protect us from our protectors?

* http://www.publicguardian.gov.uk.

Advance decisions

For some years competent patients have attempted to exercise personal control of medical care that might be offered when they are no longer competent. 'Living will' and 'advance directive' were the terms for the documents used to attempt this, wherein patients set out their desires. There was never a problem accepting such documents as evidence of a patient's wishes, though there was no litigation on whether they are binding in circumstances where we might not think the decision to be in the patient's best interests.

The Act (Ss 24–29) has introduced the concept into English law, calling it, presumably for avoidance of confusion, the advance decision (AD). Patients can now *refuse* (but not insist on) specified treatment in specified circumstances. This can include life-sustaining treatment (LST), though it must then include a statement that it applies to LST even if the patient's life is at risk. Such documents must be written, signed, and witnessed to be effective, but can be completely withdrawn verbally at any time by a patient who still has (or regains) capacity. An amendment to the AD will need to be in writing if it covers LST. Acts by the patient that are inconsistent with the terms of the AD may invalidate it, as may subsequent appointment of an LPA (see above) with powers covering the same treatment. Unforeseen circumstances may also invalidate an AD.

The AD does not have to be registered; indeed, there are no provisions for registration. A central registry for easy access by treating emergency doctors has been suggested, but not implemented. It is expected that these decision will be made known to patients' general practitioners, and potentially stored on computerized records when they are fully operational: there are, of course, difficulties with being sure that such records and registers are up to date, especially when we consider that the AD may be withdrawn verbally without notice. No doubt practices will develop.

If we are unhappy that the AD is valid, or that it covers treatment we believe to be indicated, we are allowed to continue the treatment until uncertainties are clarified, if necessary by the court. To date, there appears to have been no litigation on ADs.

Independent mental capacity advocates (IMCAs)

If you do not have anyone you wish to nominate as your LPA (or cannot afford the fees), have not thought of an advance decision (or not in time), have no one caring for you or interested in your welfare-in short, you are one of the many in the modern age living alone and isolated-none of the changes we have discussed can help you, or doctors trying to discover your wishes, and work out your best interests. The Act has tried to address this with the new IMCA.

This is intended to work as follows: if serious medical* treatment is proposed for someone who lacks capacity, and there is no one** to consult regarding the patient's best interests, before we start the treatment, we *must* appoint an IMCA. The IMCA is paid to:

- Provide support, so the patient may participate as fully as possible in a decision
- Obtain and evaluate relevant information, ascertaining what the patient's wishes and feelings would be likely to be, and the beliefs and values that would be likely to influence the patient, if he had capacity
- Ascertain alternative courses of action available in relation to the patient
- Obtaining further medical opinion where the IMCA thinks necessary
- Report his or her findings in writing.

Much of this seems a bit vague, but in part this is because it is meant to cover decision-making for the long-term incapacitated, perhaps regarding accommodation, as well as medical treatment, both acute and chronic.

There are provisos. For example, for urgent treatment we need not wait (perhaps days) for the IMCA to be instructed and report-though we should record why we did not wait. When the IMCA has reported, we must take the content into account; as before, this does not mean that the IMCA tells us what to do, but that we weigh that information in the balance when deciding.

It should be noted that we are *required* to instruct an IMCA as set out. This is not an option, to be ignored if inconvenient.

It should also be noted that the requirement operates when we are proposing 'serious medical treatment': we need to know what the law thinks is serious under this heading, and it can be summarized as where there is a fine balance between risk and benefit, and where there may be serious consequences. Examples include cancer treatments, sterilization and termination, cardiac surgery or neurosurgery, and amputations. If in doubt

---

* Not mental.   ** Excluding paid professionals.

about the need for an IMCA, we are advised to consult our colleagues. If still in doubt, one should get one.

Experience so far has been that IMCAs, who range from solicitors to registered nurses, have been unwilling to challenge decisions regarding serious medical treatment. It is early days yet, of course.

Court of protection and the public guardian

This is a new court which is a superior court of record, i.e. equal in status to the High Court. Its functions include to:

- Decide whether a person has capacity
- Make declarations, etc. on financial/welfare regarding people who lack capacity
- Appoint deputies to make decisions for people who lack capacity
- Make decisions regarding enduring and lasting powers of attorney.

It is to this court we will be applying for orders and declarations regarding difficult contested decisions in our patients who lack capacity.

The final new concept in the Act is the office of public guardian. This is an official, overseen by a board, who essentially deals with the administration of some of the other new concepts of the Act, looking after the paperwork, keeping the registers, and so on. A fuller discussion of the public guardian's role is beyond the remit of this chapter. For those seeking further information, the public guardian's website* gives a wealth of detail.

Children and consent

The Mental Capacity Act does not apply to those under 16 years of age (s2(3)), only amending some transitional arrangements. The way this is phrased implies that the law on consent to treatment of children is unchanged. In England and Wales, this is that a parent or guardian, the care authority for children in care, and the courts may consent for medical treatment on behalf of a child. If a child is over 16 but under 18, he or she may also consent for his or her own medical treatment[19], and is assumed to have capacity. If under 16, the law is as set out in the Gillick case[20], which decided that a child under 16 may consent to his or her own treatment provided he or she has sufficient

* http://www.publicguardian.gov.uk

intelligence and understanding to appreciate fully what is proposed. In the decided case, this applied to contraception, and is limited by consideration of best interests, set out by Lord Fraser in the House of Lords' judgment. This is of limited applicability to anaesthesia for oral and maxillofacial surgery and will not be discussed further. Authoritative professional guidance can be found in the relevant GMC publication[21].

Note that in English and Welsh law, if one of those with the right to consent does so, refusal of consent by another with that right does not invalidate the consent already given: this applies even if the child refuses, and is over 16 and refuses consent[22]. In Scotland the law allows any child who may give consent also to withhold it.

Please note

Law changes: This chapter was contemporary at the time of writing and obviously cannot address any subsequent changes to the law should they have arisen.

References

1. Donoghue v Stevenson. [1932] AC 562 (HL).
2. Bolam v Friern HMC. [1957] 1WLR 582.
3. Chester v Afshar. [2005] *Lloyd's Rep Med*, 109 (HL).
4. De Freitas v O'Brien & Connolly. [1995] *Med LR*, 108 (CA).
5. Hepworth v Kerr. [1995] *Med LR*, 139 (QBD).
6. Kerr AR. (1977) Anaesthesia without profound hypotension for middle ear surgery. *Br J Anaesth*, **49(5)**, 447–52.
7. Bolitho v City & Hackney HA. [1998] AC 232 (HL).
8. McGhee v NCB. [1973] 1WLR 1.
9. Wilshire v Essex AHA. [1988] 1AC 1074 (HL).
10. Chatterton v Gerson. [1981] 1All ER 257.
11. Sidaway v Board of Governors of Bethlehem Royal Hospital. [1985] AC 871 (HL).
12. Pearce v United Bristol Healthcare NHST. [1999] PIQR 53.
13. Consent: patients and doctors making decisions together. GMC 2008.
14. Chester v Afshar. [2005] *Lloyd's Rep Med*, 109 (HL).
15. See commentary following Chester v Ashfar. [2005] *Lloyd's Rep Med*, 128 (HL).
16. Gregg v Scott. [2005] *Lloyd's Rep Med*, 130 para 217 (HL).
17. Mental Capacity Act, C 9 of 2005.
18. Re C (Refusal of Medical Treatment). [1994] 1FLR 31.
19. Family Law Reform Act, 1969, s8.
20. Gillick v Norfolk & W Wisbech AHA. [1986] AC112.
21. *0–18 years: guidance for all doctors* (2007) General Medical Council UK.
22. Re W (a minor) (medical treatment). [1992] 4All ER 627.

4

Recognition and management of the difficult airway

Charles H. Kates and Steven Gayer

Introduction

Anaesthesia for oral and maxillofacial surgery presents a number of complex problems not shared with most other specialties. These procedures demand special attention in the establishment and maintenance of a patent, functional airway. Anaesthetists must conduct a meticulous evaluation of the upper respiratory tract, understand the unique nature of certain pathologies, and establish ventilatory access that does not interfere with the planned procedure. A great deal of skill in airway manipulation is requisite.

The amount of upper respiratory tract variations and issues coincident with oral surgery are too numerous to tabulate and provide comprehensive answers to, but the provider with adequate background and an armamentarium of knowledge and expertise can deal with these problems as they arise. A recurrent theme of this chapter is that the foremost challenge in the delivery of anaesthesia for oral and maxillofacial surgery relates to airway management. Our discussion is limited to means of evaluating and recognizing the difficult oral surgery patient airway, but also includes management and maintenance of that airway, such that once successfully acquired, its patency is not compromised.

The majority of the chapter's discussion applies to general anaesthesia for maxillofacial surgery in the hospital setting; however, many of the same principles and techniques are applicable to day case outpatient practice as well. The airway management of patients undergoing monitored intravenous sedation (Chapter 8) is an additional special challenge that will also be addressed.

Assessing the airway

There are four elements to consider in the airway assessment:

◆ Will mask ventilation be possible after the patient has been anaesthetized?

◆ Will it be feasible to introduce a supraglottic device if needed?

◆ Is endotracheal intubation achievable with direct laryngoscopy?

◆ Is it possible to create a surgical airway if needed?

The main elements of assessing the degree of anticipated ease or difficulty of direct laryngoscopy include evaluation of the mobility of the laryngeal structures, the laryngeal angle, the temporomandibular joint (TMJ) and its function, and more. The anaesthetist must examine the anatomical relationships of structures and inspect for congenital or acquired abnormalities.

The angle of the larynx is often underappreciated when evaluating the ease of direct laryngoscopy (Figure 4.1). The so-called 'anterior larynx' is usually a change in angle of the larynx in relation to the anaesthetist's view of it through the mouth [1].

As the larynx tilts or flattens, the opportunity for visualization decreases substantially.

This can be assessed externally by noting the angle of the laryngeal protuberance in the neck. It cannot always be seen easily, but can be appreciated in lateral radiographic examination. This is not to suggest that all patients having anaesthesia for oral or maxillofacial surgery have a lateral radiographic neck evaluation,

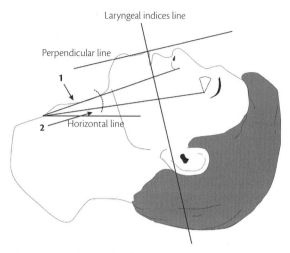

Figure 4.1 The laryngeal angle.

however, if there is any question preoperatively, it can certainly be worthwhile.

The TMJ presentation may be the most important determinant of ease of visualization. Because direct laryngoscopy depends, for the most part, on the mobility of the mandible, opening the mouth while protruding the mandible may allow the anaesthetist to obtain a direct view of the larynx. The best way to diagnose TMJ mobility is by palpation of the mandibular condyles during mouth opening. Having the patient protrude his/her mandible in a closed position is inadequate because it does not evaluate the three-dimensional movements of the condyles in the glenoid fossae. The vector movement is forward and downward when the mouth opens and closes. These combined movements of the TMJ exist so that an elliptical motion is developed with coordination of the tongue, allowing for proper formation of the food bolus in preparation for swallowing.

There are essentially six movements of the mandible. These are unique to primates and are especially well developed in humans. The motions are: opening and closing, protrusion and retrusion, and the 'Bennett shift', which is the lateral motion of the condyle in the glenoid fossae. As the mandible opens, the condyle translates forward in the glenoid fossae and also moves laterally, depending on the angle at which it meets the joint. This vector movement is positioned approximately 18–20 cm inferior to the chin. If the mouth opens without forward translation of the condyle, there will be a hinge-axis rotation which will make visualization impossible. There are few things in airway management which are absolute but the hinge-axis vector rotation of the TMJ is one of the best predictors of unattainable direct visualization using conventional laryngoscopic techniques.

Evaluation is conducted by palpation of the TMJ on both sides while the patient opens his/her mouth. One should feel the condyles rotate and slide forward beneath the tips of the palpating fingers. There should be full forward and downward translation of the condyles in the sigmoid fossae (Figure 4.2). Simultaneously, one should note the distance between the occlusal edges of the incisor teeth. Anywhere from 32 mm to 45 mm is within normal limits. Less than 20 mm will cause difficulty with insertion of standard laryngoscope blades, and may also interfere with tongue compression during laryngoscopy [2].

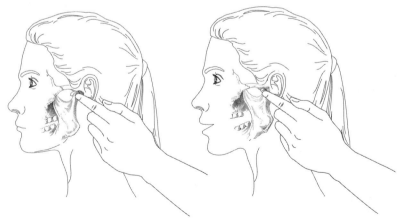

Figure 4.2 Evaluation of temporomandibular joint (TMJ) mobility. Palpation of the TMJ should be with one finger on each of the two sides.

A simple and rapid method to assess the inter-incisive distance, as well as the relationship between the mentis and the larynx is to apply the '3–3–2 Fit' rule:

- 3 of the patient's fingers should fit between the mandibular and maxillary incisors
- 3 fingers should fit between the mentis and the thyroid cartilage
- 2 fingers should fit between the thyroid and hyoid cartilages.

The Mallampati classification has been a staple of airway evaluation for prediction of ease of intubation for many decades[3]. Scoring is derived by examination of the oral cavity, specifically inspecting the visibility of the uvula, the faucial pillars, and the soft palate. The tonsils, uvula, and soft palate are fully evident in class 1 airways; one may only perceive the upper portion of the tonsils and uvula in class 2; in class 3, only the base of the uvula is readily apparent; while in class 4 the uvula is not discernable. A higher score has traditionally been thought to correlate with increased difficulty of direct laryngoscopy. However, it is the authors' opinion that the Mallampati taxonomy is flawed because it is a soft tissue-dependent diagnostic system that does not take into consideration other, more pertinent variables, particularly for the oral and maxillofacial surgery patient[4]. Additionally, it is often incorrectly applied. There are too many variables, such as altering results with phonation, which would suggest that it is not a reliable predictor of direct laryngoscopic success[5]. Oral and maxillofacial surgery patients frequently have restricted mouth openings, trauma, or other intraoral abnormalities, which often limits the utility of airway evaluation using the Mallampati classification.

Prediction of the difficult airway beyond Mallampati

- Ask the patient to swallow and note the mobility of the larynx. If the larynx does not shift vertically during normal deglutition, there may be restriction of laryngeal movement from scarring or other abnormality. Also, notice the symmetry of the laryngeal movement. If there is rotation of the larynx, or if there seems to be a lag on one side or the other, there may be tumour, impingement, encroachment, or other protrusions at that level. A patient with this particular abnormality should have fibreoptic laryngeal evaluation prior to surgery to determine if there are problems that might lead to difficulty with direct laryngoscopy

- The thyromental distance should be measured to help determine whether or not the larynx is higher than expected—the so-called 'anterior larynx' (Figure 4.3)[6].

- Thorough examination of the oral cavity may reveal evidence of potential difficulty with direct laryngoscopy (Figure 4.4). One of these is the high arched palate. This can be associated with a reduced distance between the upper teeth because of a v-shaped, elongated and enlarged maxilla. An interincisive distance of less than 20 mm will reduce oral access. Additionally, bulging of the tongue can interfere with the use of the laryngoscope because the traditional laryngoscope requires that the tongue be compressed or moved to the left. Macroglossia can be a function of long-time edentulism, as the tongue grows to fill in the space created by missing teeth so that speaking and swallowing are normalized. Swallowing and speaking require tongue and lip seal. Mandibular or maxillary torri can hinder direct laryngoscopy even though the interincisive distance is greater than 40 mm. Some outsized maxillary torri can occupy the entire palatal space.

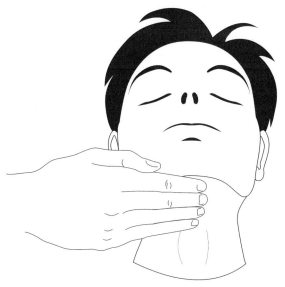

Figure 4.3 Thyromental distance. Also assess the thyrohyoid distance (see text).

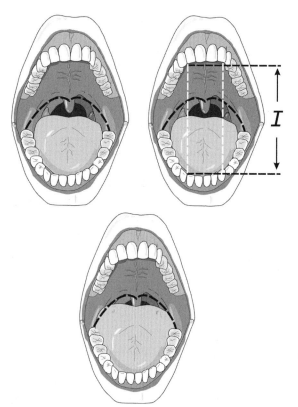

Figure 4.4 Examination of the oral cavity. Palatal morphology, mandibulo/maxillary, anteroposterior relationships, size and shape of the tongue, and interincisive distance are all important prognosticators of successful direct laryngoscopy.

Mandibular torri can cause tongue protrusion on a scale that precludes insertion of a laryngoscope

♦ Obesity or pregnancy may limit or prevent insertion of the laryngoscope by the sheer size of the patient's chest[7]. Obese patients often have fat lobules protruding from lateral borders of the oropharynx that can block the view of the larynx. Patients who are in cervical traction or protective collar are prevented from flexion/extension movements which are important for direct laryngoscopy. A short or immobile neck can sometimes make direct laryngoscopy virtually impossible. Congenital deformities, including but not limited to facial dystocias, macroglossia, and subglottic stenosis, are a problem for the same reason (Chapter 19)

♦ Gross infections or haematomata may cause potential airway encroachment. Soiling and contamination of the upper airway can occur if the patient has an expanding posterior pharyngeal abscess or haematoma, which might easily be lacerated during intubation with a conventional laryngoscope. Patients with dental infection can be especially difficult because of trismus and elevation of the tongue and floor of the mouth (Chapter 11). When evaluating the mouth of the oral surgery patient, it is essential that the tongue be pulled aside and its floor be examined in order to determine if there is a submandibular or submaxillary abscess which might rupture during attempted direct laryngoscopy. Additionally, mass effect can distort the view of the airway

♦ Prior tracheostomy can cause constriction of the airway below the chords, scarring of supraglottic tissues, and flattening of the trachea

♦ Vocal cord paralysis is a common finding in the traumatized victim who has received neck and laryngeal trauma. Neuromuscular blocking agents to facilitate intubation may diminish or erase ability to achieve visualization by direct laryngoscopy

♦ Thyroid goitre may cause compression and sometimes fixation of the laryngeal apparatus, such that direct visualization of the vocal cords is hindered or absent

♦ Regurgitation and/or bleeding can obliterate the field of vision during indirect as well as direct laryngoscopy.

Airway management for oral and maxillofacial surgery

Since the twentieth century, the sine qua non of airway management under general anaesthesia has been direct pharyngeal laryngoscopy and oral intubation. Nasal intubation is often preferred for oral and maxillofacial surgery in order to allow the surgeon unrestricted access to the mouth and pharynx. A McGill's forceps placed through the oral inlet can clasp and guide the endotracheal tube through the vocal chords. In many circumstances, congenital malformations, disease pathology, or trauma render direct laryngoscopy and oral/nasal intubation demanding and problematic. In these instances, the endotracheal tube may be placed via indirect laryngoscopy or without visualizing the glottic opening at all ('blindly'). One may elect to induce anaesthesia first or obtain the airway with the patient awake and breathing spontaneously. This is often a critical decision, since the 'can't ventilate, can't intubate' situation is a real possibility during airway management for oral and maxillofacial surgery. Blind nasal intubation is a classical technique which has largely been supplanted by intubation with a flexible fibreoptic bronchoscope. Although not commonly used, all anaesthetists should master this technique since the added skill of being adept with a blind nasal technique, requiring no extraneous apparatus, may help secure an airway when other techniques have failed. Finally, in appropriate situations, the anaesthetist may opt for maintaining ventilation with a supraglottic device. It is apparent, therefore, that for oral and maxillofacial surgery, the anaesthetist should possess a large armamentarium of airway access tools, methods, and skills to safely secure ventilation.

Awake intubation and sedation

Awake intubation, whether it is 'blind' or fibreoptic-guided, requires two key elements—sedation and topical anaesthesia. A small dose of glycopyrrolate may diminish secretions and improve view should a fibreoptic bronchoscope be utilized. This should be given to the patient 20 minutes prior to the anticipated airway management in order to achieve maximum desiccation of the airway. Sedation can be accomplished in many ways. Continuous titrated infusion of propofol and/or a small amount of narcotic or benzodiazepine are common strategies. The titrated infusion of dexmeditomodine is enjoying a surge in popularity just now.[8] Whatever practice is chosen, the goal should be a patient who is able to cooperate and be comfortable during this potentially stressful situation.

Topical local anaesthesia for awake intubation

Airway local anaesthesia to provide pain management can be accomplished using a topical or spray inhalation technique, or a combination of the above with nerve blocks. The following is the authors' preferred technique:

- The nostril to be intubated is chosen based on its patency and size. Since the choice will ultimately depend on physical evaluation, both nostrils are initially prepared with the least noxious topical agent

- One ml of warm 4% lidocaine is carefully dropped into each nostril and the patient instructed to simultaneously sniff. Because topical lidocaine is very benign, the patient does not suffer nasal irritation; the patient then accepts the initial topicalization much more readily. Once this is accomplished, a more aggressive topical anaesthetic technique can proceed

- Cotton swabs are prepared with 4% lidocaine and a vasoconstrictor, such as phenylephrine or oxymetazoline. The cotton swabs are passed into the chosen nostril in the following manner:

  ○ The first cotton swab is passed all the way in until the tip rests against the posterior pharyngeal wall

  ○ Pressure is applied to the handle end of the cotton swab. This pressure anaesthesia will produce a reasonable field block of the glossopharyngeal nerve

  ○ Following this, additional cotton swabs are stacked in the nostril in such a way that the majority of the nasal mucosa comes in contact with the topical anaesthetic. Particular attention should be paid to the area of Kiesselbach's plexus. This area can bleed severely if accidentally lacerated during the insertion of the endotracheal tube

  ○ Once the cotton swabs have been placed, additional liquid anaesthetic with vasoconstrictor is added through the nostril to increase the contact of the anaesthetic with the nasal mucosa

- A transtracheal block is then accomplished utilizing 1.5 ml of 4% lidocaine in a 2–3-ml syringe. The injection is made with a 20-G 1-inch needle. This needle size has been chosen because it allows for very rapid injection. Should the patient cough violently, there is little danger of needle fracture. Some practitioners use a catheter rather than a needle to avoid the possibility of needle breakage. This manoeuvre, while seemingly safe, has its own hazard as during the cough it is possible that the catheter might kink and not be easily removed from the cricothyroid membrane. Having correctly sited the needle the:

  ○ Patient is told to take a 'deep breath and hold it'

  ○ Injection is made, and the needle quickly withdrawn

  ○ The patient usually coughs moderately, spreading and spraying the topical anaesthetic throughout the posterior pharynx, the upper and lower larynx, and the epiglottis

- Following the transtracheal block, the cotton swabs are removed from the nose, and the nostril is then sprayed for 1 second with benzocaine or its equivalent. This is very effective, but can be somewhat caustic. However, the prior topicalization provides sufficient analgesia to prevent discomfort. Beware of methaemoglobinemia if employing benzocaine

- The last drug to be instilled in the nostril is 1 ml of 2% viscous lidocaine. The patient is encouraged to inhale, gargle, and then swallow. This will usually anaesthetize any areas that have been neglected in the prior orchestrations. Some practitioners prefer inhalation of finely sprayed liquid lidocaine delivered via a mucosal atomizing device; however, we find the atomizing technique unreliable and patchy

- The nostril, oropharynx, nasopharynx, and mouth, are suctioned with a 16F catheter. This tactic has the dual purpose of clearing excess material and testing the level of analgesia. The patient should have no sensation during the use of the suction catheter. If there is discomfort, additional topicalization is necessary. Although it may seem that this volume of topical anaesthetic may cause overdose, this has not been a problem, and patients generally are able to tolerate the 'awake' manoeuvres that follow, comfortably

- Once sedation and analgesia has been accomplished, the anaesthetist may proceed with intubation. This can be blind awake; awake fibreoptic; or even direct intubation. If direct intubation is employed, additional analgesia will be required to obtund the gag reflex and anesthetize the tongue. This can be quickly accomplished with 5% lidocaine paste applied to the back of the tongue with a tongue depressor. The paste will melt and spread itself across the back of the tongue and the valeculae which will substantially reduce or eliminate gagging. With patient cooperation and relative comfort at this point, even retrograde intubation, provided that skin and subcutaneous tissues above the cricothyroid ligament have been anaesthetized, can be well tolerated.

Nerve blocks for awake intubation

Direct nerve block is also an effective method to augment analgesia of the upper airway. Recurrent laryngeal nerve blocks are accomplished by instilling a few millilitres of local anaesthetic 1 cm inferior to the greater horn of the hyoid bones. Be wary of potential phrenic nerve block occurring simultaneously. Regional anaesthesia techniques in oral and maxillofacial surgery are discussed in Chapter 7.

Flexible fibreoptic bronchoscopy

The flexible fibreoptic bronchoscope consists of bundled fibreoptic lights that illuminate the airway and transmit an image back to the anaesthetist. It is the gold standard solution for management of the difficult airway. An endotracheal tube, softened by having been placed in warm water, is placed through the selected nostril and advanced into the upper pharynx as far as is comfortable. Silicone tubes are not thermoplastic, so will readily adapt to passage through the nares without prior warming.

If the oral route is chosen, a guiding oral airway such as the Ovassapian Airway (Hudson RCI, North Carolina, USA) or Williams Airway Intubator (Anaesthesia Associates, San Marcos, California, USA) allow passage of the bronchoscope between the closed upper and lower teeth. The technique involves inserting the fibreoptic device through the endotracheal tube until it reaches beyond the tube's tip. Oxygen is connected to the suction port on the airway to provide an enriched FiO_2 environment and to propel secretions away from the field of vision. There have, however, been case reports of barotrauma, so carefully consider the use of oxygen in this setting in this manner[9]. Facilitatory manoeuvres include lifting the chin, applying cricoid pressure, and, provided there is no contraindication, turning the head slightly to optimize the field of vision. Neck extension, jaw thrust, tongue traction, lifting the tongue and epiglottis with a laryngoscope, or attempting fibreoptic bronchoscopy through a supraglottic airway may also be beneficial. The combination of using the smallest diameter endotracheal tube with the largest fibreoptic bronchoscope improves likelihood of success.

Blind nasal intubation

Correct patient positioning is the key to successful blind nasal intubation, whether the patient is awake and breathing, asleep with spontaneous ventilation, or asleep and paralysed. The technique involves hyperextension of the neck, rotation of the head towards the side of the intubated nostril, then guiding the tube either with breath sounds or by feel and visibility (Figure 4.5). The endotracheal tube is introduced until it reaches the posterior nasopharynx, where it then curves downward and enters the oropharynx. In the awake patient this is done as quickly as possible to reduce distress. Warming of the first few centimetres of the distal end of the endotracheal tube prior to intubation can be of assistance in reducing discomfort when using a standard thermoplastic tube. It is inadvisable to warm the entire tube since its preformed curve will be compromised.

The authors prefer silicone rubber non-thermoplastic endotracheal tubes as they are pliable and cause minimal trauma upon insertion. The device is lubricated and passed gently through the nose into the nasopharynx and then onward to the oropharynx. At this point the

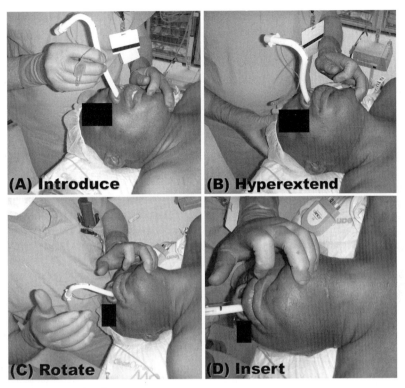

Figure 4.5 Blind nasal intubation. See also Plate 2.

contralateral nostril is sealed by the anaesthetist's left thumb. The left index finger seals the lips, the chin is elevated with the remaining fingers of the left hand, and the tube is advanced into the trachea during inhalation. Peak inspiratory flow can be as high as 50 litres per minute. If the tube is advanced during the inspiratory phase of respiration, the patient will, quite literally, inhale it. Provided there is excellent topical anaesthesia and adequate sedation, intubation can thus be painlessly and easily accomplished. Use of a gum elastic bougie may allow the anaesthetist to receive tactile confirmation of the tracheal rings.

The same technique is used during blind asleep intubation. In this case the patient is unable to cooperate, so the vortex of air guiding the tube is simply a normal but depressed breath. Although this increases the difficulty of the technique, with practice it is still possible to accomplish the desired goal.

Blind nasal intubation can be achieved in the paralysed non-breathing patient, without breath sounds to guide the positioning of the endotracheal tube. The operator stands at the head of the operating table, the head of the patient is positioned as in the previous technique, but this time the guidance is

through the tactile and visual senses of the anaesthetist. Once the tube is in the pharynx, there may be obstruction to its movement. This generally means that the endotracheal tube has lodged in the vallecula and external bulging of tissue may be noted. The tube is withdrawn slightly, rotated either to the left or right, advanced again past the obstruction, and then swivelled back toward the centre. The endotracheal tube may appear to be seen sliding or 'crawling' under the skin as it passes between the vocal cords. The position of the airway is then confirmed by the usual manoeuvres: chest rise, auscultation, and end-tidal CO_2.

Transillumination

A transtracheal light wand such as the TrachLight (Laerdal Medical AS, Toronto, Ontario, Canada) can expedite blind intubation via transillumination of the glottic airway[10]. It is particularly useful when direct intubation is not possible. The device is usually inserted in the unconscious patient, but awake intubation is possible if the patient is properly sedated. Placement requires reduced ambient light such that cervical transillumination is possible. The technique for its use is quite simple. The light wand is slipped onto the track of the light handle which protrudes through the endotracheal tube lock. The endotracheal tube is then slid over the light wand and secured onto the slide. The stylet is then advanced to an appropriate position so the measurement marker on the light wand corresponds with the corresponding marker on the endotracheal tube. There is a label approximately 4 cm from the tip of the tube for a right-angle bend of the endotracheal and light wand complex. This curvature is a key element for success with this device. Once the tube is properly mounted, the mandible is pulled forward with the left hand, and the endotracheal tube and light wand are passed gently through the mouth and blindly into the oropharynx. The apparatus is manipulated until transillumination through the neck can be appreciated below the cricothyroid membrane (Figure 4.6). The wire stylet is then pulled back approximately 3 cm, allowing the tip of the endotracheal tube and light wand to feed forward and slide further into the trachea. Once this has occurred, the endotracheal tube is released from the tracheal tube lock and the device is removed, leaving the endotracheal tube in the trachea. This appliance is easily and rapidly employed and is quite inexpensive. It is a useful airway adjunct for difficult intubations where other techniques have failed. One should be wary, however, that its use may be relatively contraindicated in the presence of significant oropharyngeal trauma or disease.

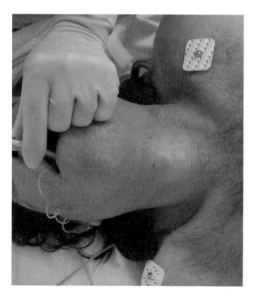

Figure 4.6 Transillumination. See also Plate 3.

Nasal airway with endotracheal connector

In some circumstances, such as oral trauma or subluxated teeth, a mask or oral airway may be inadvisable. A nasopharyngeal airway attached to a 60° endotracheal connector may be a suitable solution for airway management (Figure 4.7). It is then connected to the breathing circuit, and forms an insufflation system which can be useful for anaesthetic delivery or oxygen supplementation during deep sedation. The contralateral nostril is obturated with a dental roll to facilitate leak-proof ventilation. This airway modality is commonly used in day-care anaesthesia for oral surgery and dentistry.

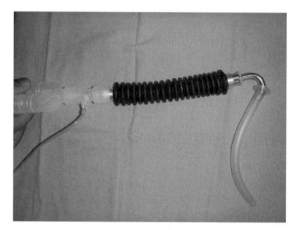

Figure 4.7 Nasal airway with endotracheal connector.

Flexible laryngeal mask airway

Supraglottic devices such as the laryngeal mask airway (LMA) have become popular in recent years as a substitute for mask anaesthesia, ventilation via nasal airway, or endotracheal intubation[11]. A modified, flexible wire re-enforced tube rather than the traditional rigid curved cylinder can be useful for oral surgery (Figure 4.8)[12]. The technique for placement is similar to that of a classic LMA [12], but it is usually inserted from the front rather than from the head of the patient in order to maintain control of the longer, more pliant shaft. One of the problems with this device for oral surgery is that it can obstruct surgical access, particularly to the more posterior teeth. It is not a definitive airway, can rotate *in situ*, and does not prevent aspiration. If the patient requires ventilation above 20 cm of water, the

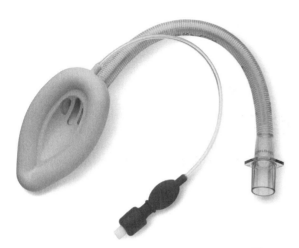

Figure 4.8 Flexible laryngeal mask airway. (LMA Flexible™ courtesy of LMA North America, Inc.).

device may leak and the aspiration risk increases. One must remember that this device is not a definitive airway.

Nevertheless, from a practical standpoint, the LMA is useful for day case outpatient oral surgery anaesthesia.

Supraglottic airway assisted intubation

For those patients who are not at risk of aspiration of blood or gastric contents, intubation may be accomplished via a traditional supraglottic device such as the Air-Q Intubating Laryngeal Airway (Cookgas LLC, Saint Louis, Missouri, USA). Other intubating airways such as the FasTrach or CTrach (LMA North America Inc., La Jolla, California, USA) are rigid, curved appliances with a formed inflatable seal for the glottic outlet. These devices act to secure ventilation and provide a guided path for blind or flexible fibreoptic-assisted introduction of an endotracheal tube. Patients with suspected cervical spine injury may experience less neck extension compared to use of traditional direct laryngoscopy[13]. Success may be limited by gross anatomic abnormality, TMJ stenosis, or small oral inlet.

Video-assisted laryngoscopes

Video-assisted laryngoscopes such as the Glidescope (Verathon Inc., Bothell, Washington, USA), and McGrath (LMA North America Inc., La Jolla, California, USA) are relatively new airway adjuncts which are particularly valuable in those situations where direct laryngoscopy and/or fibreoptic intubation have not been successful[14]. These are modified laryngoscopes that have an additional non-pliable bend, enabling the operator to see around the curve of the upper airway. They contain a fibreoptic bundle, a light source, and a high-definition camera (Figure 4.9). A liquid crystal display panel allows vivid indirect clear visualization of the airway.

These instruments are used in the same manner as a traditional laryngoscope. They can be especially useful in patients with suspected cervical spine injury where any movement of the cervical spine could be disastrous. They are also useful in patients with limited mouth opening, grossly distorted upper airway anatomy, or as a means for endotracheal tube exchange. Nasotracheal intubation guided by oral placement of a video laryngoscope may be quicker than direct laryngoscopy and use of Magill's forcep[15]. Contraindications to their use include inadequate operator experience, a small oral inlet, traumatic injury, or deformity of the larynx and posterior pharynx. The McGrath is self-contained and thus highly portable and conveniently uses common household batteries. The screen view is small and it requires costly disposable blade attachments. The Glidescope has a rechargeable battery, a larger view screen, and needs no disposable parts.

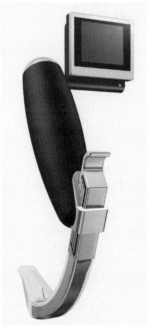

Figure 4.9 McGrath® video-assisted laryngoscope. (Courtesy of LMA North America, Inc).

A particularly useful application for video-assisted laryngoscopes is the elective tube exchange from oral to nasal (or even nasal to oral). The entire process can be visualized without danger of airway loss. In extreme cases, a tube exchanger or fibreoptic laryngoscope can still be left in place while the second tube is passed behind it. The tube exchanger or fibreoptic laryngoscope remain during the tube replacement and can be used as a visual guide or as a backup for re-intubation should problems be encountered.

Retrograde intubation

This is an invasive technique indicated for patients who have severely limited mouth opening, and in whom traditional laryngoscopic, fibreoptic, or blind techniques have been unsuccessful. It is also useful for patients with restricted neck mobility, grossly distorted upper airway anatomy, and can be the last airway adjunct attempted before the establishment of a surgical airway. Translaryngeal-guided intubation is contraindicated when less invasive methods are available or when there is evidence of trauma or deformity of the larynx.

The patient is prepared for awake intubation as described above. The neck is prepped, and a small amount of 1% lidocaine solution is injected in the area of the cricothyroid space. A 22-G needle attached to a 5-ml syringe, with the bevel facing upwards, (or a catheter over needle) is passed through the cricothyroid membrane in a cephalad direction. Aspiration of air confirms correct positioning. A dedicated guidewire is passed through the needle and directed between the vocal cords onward to the oropharynx. One method to accomplish this is to align the number 1 on the 5-ml syringe with the bevel of the needle. This allows for visual monitoring of the position of the bevel. The guidewire is then passed through the needle and into the oropharynx or nasopharynx. If the patient's head is hyperextended and rotated either to the right or to the left, the wire will usually emerge through the corresponding nostril.

Once the wire has protruded from the nostril, it is gently withdrawn whilst simultaneously pushing it in through the cricothyroid membrane until the marker at the cervical end of the wire is visible near the skin and clamped. The wire is withdrawn through the nose, at which time the plastic tube exchanger is passed over the wire and into the nasopharynx. The tube exchanger continues down until the wire protrudes from the proximal end. A fibreoptic laryngoscope can be substituted for the tube exchanger, by feeding the wire through the suction port of the bronchoscope, thereby allowing direct visualization during the process. If the fibreoptic guidance technique is chosen, it is important to cut the pliant part of the wire before inserting it into the bronchoscope. Failure to do this may result in a 'jam' of the wire in the suction port. The wire is then grasped and the tube exchanger continues to pass until it has entered the larynx. A mark on the proximal end of the wire then appears, indicating that the tube exchanger has entered and is at the anterior wall of the larynx. Since the tube exchanger length is the same length as the distance between the two markings on the guidewire, this ensures that it is well within the larynx. At this point the tube exchanger is held firmly in position and the clamp is released from the distal end of the guidewire. The wire is then pulled gently until it just drops below the skin, at which point it is passed further into the tube exchanger and larynx. The tube exchanger is then advanced into the trachea. This last manoeuvre is necessary to prevent the coupled lines from dislodging from the larynx due to head movement or other accident. Once the tube exchanger is well within the trachea, the endotracheal tube is passed over it, through the nose, and into the trachea, at which point, the tube exchanger and wire are pulled out of the endotracheal tube. Should the guidewire emerge through the mouth rather than through the nose, the technique for nasal intubation still applies, except that the wire tube exchanger and endotracheal tube are passed through the mouth rather than the nose.

Surgical airway

Failing the use of the above airway adjuncts, it may be necessary to execute a surgical airway. This might include a cricothyrotomy, a traditional tracheostomy, or a percutaneous tracheostomy utilizing a dilator and are described in Chapter 5.

Maintaining a secure airway

Frequently, once anaesthesia has been induced and the airway secured, the surgeon may request that the patient be repositioned. This means that most surgeries are performed with the patient's head at some distance from the anaesthetist, placing the anaesthetist at a disadvantage. The anaesthetist must assure that once successfully acquired, the difficult airway's patency is not compromised. Maxillofacial surgeons prefer to operate 180° around the head of the patient in order to achieve the best possible visibility and access to the operative site.

The key to success and safety is preplanning. The use of extendable breathing tubes is a handy adjunct. These are disposable breathing tubes that can be lengthened from 1.5 to as much as 3 metres by simply pulling on them. The breathing circuit can remain in place or be disconnected from the anaesthesia machine during table rotation. One should be aware that the sampling lines for end-tidal CO_2 and anaesthetic agent analysis are often fairly short. Temporarily disconnecting these lines from the anaesthesia machine can prevent accidental extubation. The only monitor that must remain in place during the rotation is the pulse oximeter, so that there is an audible indication of pulse rate and oxygen saturation during the process. It is essential that the lines, monitoring wires, and airway be protected during the rotation of the operating table.

When properly executed, table turning should take no more than 30 seconds. It is essential that following this rotation or any other major repositioning of the patient, the airway be re-evaluated to be sure there has been no change, i.e. endobronchial intubation or disconnection. If the patient is rotated 90° or 180° and been nasally intubated, maintaining a secure airway is especially important (Figure 4.10).

The endotracheal tube or supraglottic airway must be positioned in such a way that the surgeon is able to operate effectively and efficiently without compromising the ability of the anaesthetist to gain rapid access to the airway should it become necessary (Figure 4.10(1)). Competition for the same valuable space is often at a premium. The endotracheal tube or supraglottic airway must be secured in such fashion as to maximize retention and stability of the endotracheal tube and prevent the surgeon or the assistants from inadvertently dislodging, disabling, occluding, or kinking the airway.

For nasally intubated patients the authors prefer to use an endotracheal tube tree, placing it upside down under the patient's head cushion prior to securing the breathing tube to the tree (Figure 4.10(2)). This stabilizes the hoses such that manipulation of the head during the procedure will not cause disconnection. A flat profile is essential for satisfactory operating conditions. For oral intubation, the tubes are brought along the chest, off to the patient's side, and the patient's skin is protected with foam tape and padding to prevent any pressure damage. A nasotracheal tube can be secured to the patient's forehead, padding it

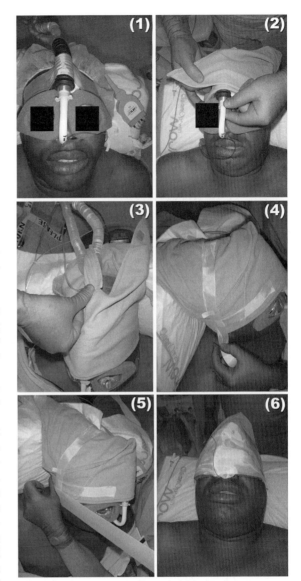

Figure 4.10 Head wrap. The nasal endotracheal tube, connection, and hoses are secured in such a fashion as to avoid the operative field, have a low profile, yet remain secure throughout the procedure. **1** Protect the eyes and tape the tube extender to the forehead; **2** wrap the head with a towel, pulling the extender forward to avoid pressure on the nares; **3** pull the towel through the breathing circuit Y-piece to prevent accidental dislodgement of the endotracheal tube from traction on the hoses; **4** secure with thick tape; **5** tape the towel over the face; **6** complete by taping across the angle of the tube as it enters the nose.

minimally to avoid a high profile. The head is then wrapped with a towel which is taped to the face (Figure 4.10.(3–5)). This method should be implemented in such a way that it avoids encroachment of the operating field (Figure 4.10(6)). If an oral tube is used, it should be taped to one side or the other of the patient's mouth, so that if the surgeon needs to work intraorally, the tube is not in the way and will not accidentally become dislodged during surgery.

Outpatient versus inpatient airway management

As a general rule of thumb, simple intraoral operations tend to be outpatient day case-based procedures, in contrast to major facial reconstruction, cancer management, and traumatic injuries, which necessitate a level of care that can only be provided in a hospital setting. Typically maxillofacial procedures that are performed in the dental surgery involve either infiltration of local anaesthesia alone (Chapter 7) or monitored light sedation and local anaesthetic infiltration. Deep sedation and local anaesthetic infiltration and general anaesthesia can safely and efficiently be accomplished in the dental surgery when proper equipment, well trained staff, and proper supervision are in place: USA, Canada, Japan, Australia, New Zealand, etc. The use of conscious or light sedation, as well as deep sedation techniques, are covered in Chapter 8 and will not be addressed here.

Anaesthetic delivery for short outpatient oral procedures such as dental extractions, creates certain airway challenges. Most anaesthetics are accomplished without the benefit of an endotracheal tube. The classical method is to position the patient in a semi-sitting position. A nasal hood is applied and a bite block or mouth gag is used to hold the mouth open. The anaesthetic proceeds with the anaesthetist supporting the chin to maintain the airway, and to provide counter pressure for the surgical procedures. The airway is protected with an oropharyngeal partition made of a folded gauze. It is very lightly moistened, tucked under the tongue at the posterior of the side being operated upon and carefully molded across the back of the tongue between the vibrating line of the palate and circumvallate papilla of the tongue. This provides a barrier to particulate matter, but does not prevent mouth breathing or liquid intrusion. The surgical assistant must be expert at evacuating fluid and debris with a high-speed dental evacuator. The use of this classical device has certain obvious hazards; however, the technique has been employed for numerous years and has had an excellent safety record. The effectiveness of

this method can be enhanced by the placement of a nasopharyngeal airway.

A further refinement of this technique is to avoid the nasal hood altogether, and place a dental cotton roll in the contralateral nostril. The nasopharyngeal airway is connected to a 60° endotracheal connector which is then attached to the anaesthetic breathing circuit. End-tidal CO_2 monitoring in the non-intubated patient is usually accomplished with a modified nasal prong device. These are now available with a gas sampling port, allowing for breath-by-breath analysis of end-tidal CO_2 and anaesthetic gasses. While quantitative measurement is invalid, qualitative measurement indicates the presence of ventilation.

As discussed above, the flexible LMA has gained popularity and can be used instead of a nasal mask or nasopharyngeal connected airway[16]. Where the airway is questionable or if there is a high risk of significant airway soiling, then endotracheal or nasotracheal intubation should be adopted.

Trauma, major facial reconstruction, and cancer

The establishment of an airway in patients who suffer from traumatic injuries, extensive cancer, or require major facial reconstruction is a major challenge in oral and maxillofacial surgery (Chapter 14). The use of flexible fibreoptic laryngoscopy, usually the gold standard for these cases, may often not be suitable due to contamination of the lens during insertion. Secretions and bleeding in the posterior pharynx, oropharynx, and nasal passages can quickly obliterate either the light source and/or the lens of the bronchoscope, rendering it useless for establishing an airway. However, many of the alternative airway acquisition techniques described above may be apropos.

Awareness of the type of facial injury is extremely important. Attempting to ventilate a patient by mask with intraoral injuries, loose teeth, or other debris is fraught with danger. It is therefore essential that a high-quality preoperative evaluation, including detailed inspection of the mouth and pharynx, be accomplished prior to deciding whether the patient should be intubated awake or while under general anaesthesia.

There are occasions when a surgical airway is prudent and necessary (Chapter 5) and there should be no hesitation to opt for that alternative if indicated. The attempt at other modalities can be life threatening, and therefore it is essential to have a surgical team at the ready should there arise a need for an emergency tracheostomy or cricothyrotomy.

Voice, tone, hoarseness, stridor, and dyspnoea are all indicators of potential hidden laryngeal trauma. Patients who exhibit these particular signs should be evaluated radiographically and, if possible, with fibreoptics prior to attempting airway intervention. There may be a tear in the upper airway which can lead to subcutaneous emphysema and/or pneumothorax should mask ventilation be attempted. A partially transected trachea can become fully transected by the inadvertent blind intersection of an endotracheal tube without fibreoptic visual guidance.

Haemorrhage and haematoma are always possible with the traumatized mid-face, mandible, and oral structures. Concealed bleeding can be posterior to the pharyngeal wall. The pharynx may slowly expand forward due to transection of the greater palatine arteries in Le Fort-type fractures. This insidious enlargement can cause obliteration of the airway. Soiling of the airway can occur should a laryngoscope inadvertently puncture the mucosa. Subcutaneous emphysema can cause a dangerous elevation of the tongue, rendering visualization of the vocal cords and even positive pressure ventilation exceedingly difficult.

Facial fractures include Le Fort I, II, III, and panfacial fractures. Bilateral mandible fractures in the region of the body and/or mandibular condyles can prevent the patient from protruding his/her tongue, thereby causing anatomical airway obstruction. These are often best treated with immediate surgical airway rather than intubation. Cervical spine and soft tissue injuries also can be a problem because of restriction of head and neck positioning to facilitate intubation.

Laryngotracheal damage is sometimes not obvious until the patient has been observed for several hours. Burns can create difficulties including swelling, permanent damage to the tracheobronchial tree, and pulmonary oedema (Chapter 15). Penetrating injuries involving the neck and the trachea can cause partial or complete transection of the trachea, severe haemorrhage, and nerve damage. Crush injuries usually require immediate surgical airway intervention.

As we can see, the status of the cervical spine is a key consideration in many maxillofacial trauma procedures. This presents an especially difficult challenge for establishment of the airway where no cervical movement, hyperextension, hypo-extension, or lateral movement of the head is advisable[18].

In these cases, use of fibreoptic equipment, a lighted stylet, or retrograde intubation may be best suited for establishment of the airway. Patients should remain awake, but well sedated. Good topical local anaesthesia to keep them comfortable, prevent inadvertent movement, and minimize possible cervical spine damage is essential.

The anaesthetist should be familiar with facial nerve (cranial nerve VII) issues associated with mandibular surgery. To gain access to the mandible, the surgeon must carefully dissect down to the bone, avoiding incising the marginal mandibularis. In order to test for its presence the surgeon will often use an electrical nerve stimulator. The effectiveness of this device is markedly reduced if the patient has profound neuromuscular blockade. The use of longer-acting neuromuscular blocking drugs is frequently avoided for induction of anaesthesia of those oral surgery patients with potential difficult airway; however, in some circumstances the anaesthetist may elect to utilize such paralytics. In these instances, prior to induction of anaesthesia a conference with the surgeon is necessary to find out at what point the critical incision will be accomplished. For example, there are times when a mandibular fracture or mandibular surgery involves the placement of arch bars on the teeth and wiring of the teeth prior to the incision. Should this be the case, a non-depolarizer for intubation is not a problem since it will probably have run its course within 20 minutes. The average time required placing arch bars and wiring of teeth is about 45 minutes; the currently used non-depolarizing muscle relaxants can be reversed after 20–30 minutes if necessary.

Postoperative considerations are similar to those of orthognathic surgery procedures and involve judgement as to whether or not a patient may be safely extubated in the operating room or in the recovery room, or if the patient should be allowed to have some time in the intensive care unit before considering the removal of the endotracheal tube. In any event, these patients should not be extubated without the bedside availability of skilled operators and emergency equipment should it be deemed necessary to re-establish the airway. This might include the facility to carry out an emergency cricothyrotomy or tracheostomy if necessary.

Conclusion

Recognition, acquisition, management, and maintenance of the airway for oral and maxillofacial surgery patients requires careful preoperative assessment, thorough evaluation of circumstances unique to the surgical specialty, familiarity with multiple airway tools and techniques, and an expertise in airway manipulation.

References

1. Roberts JT, Abouleish AE, Curlin FJ, *et al.* (1994) The failed intubation: maximizing successful management of the patient with a compromised or potentially compromised airway. In: Roberts JT (ed). *Clinical Management of the Airway.* Philadelphia, PA: Saunders Company, pp. 187–213.

2. Aiello G, Metcalf I. (1992)Anaesthetic implications of temporomandibular joint disease. *Can J Anesth,* **39,** 610–16.

3. Mallampati SR, Gatt SP, Gugino LD, *et al.* (1985) A clinical sign to predict difficult tracheal intubation: a prospective study. *Can Anaesth Soc J,* **32,** 429–34.

4. Lee A, Fan LTY, Gin T, *et al.* (2006) A systematic review (meta-analysis) of the accuracy of the Mallampati tests to predict the difficult airway. *Anesth Analg,* **102,** 1867–78.

5. Oates JDL, Oates PD, Pearsall FJ, *et al.* (1990) Phonation affects Mallampati classification. *Anaesthesia,* **45,** 984.

6. Frerk CM, Till CBW, Bradley AJ. (1996) Difficult intubation: thyromental distance and the atlanto-occipital gap. *Anaesthesia,* **51**(8), 738–40.

7. Cormack RS, Lehane J. (1984). Difficult tracheal intubation in obstetrics. *Anaesthesia,* **39,** 1105–11.

8. Grant SA, Breslin DS, MacLeod DB, *et al.* (2004) Dexmedetomidine infusion for sedation during fiberoptic intubation: a report of three cases. *J Clin Anesth,* **16**(2), 124–6.

9. Ovassapian A, Mesnick PS. (1997) Oxygen insufflation through the fiberscope to assist intubation is not recommended. *Anesthesiology,* **87**(1), 183.

10. Davis L, Cook-Sather SD, Schreiner MS. (2000) Lighted stylet tracheal intubation: A review. *Anesth Analg,* **90,** 745–56.

11. Todd D. (2002) A comparison of endotracheal intubation and use of the laryngeal mask airway for ambulatory oral surgery patients. *J Oral Maxillofac Surg,* **60**(1), 2–4.

12. Wat LI. (2003) The laryngeal mask airway for oral and maxillofacial surgery. *Int Anesthesiol Clin,* **41**(3), 29–56.

13. Waltl B, Melischek M, Schuschnig C, *et al.* (2001) Tracheal intubation and cervical spine excursion: direct laryngoscopy vs. intubating laryngeal mask. *Anaesthesia,* **56**(3), 221–6.

14. Jones PM, Armstrong KP, Armstrong PM, *et al.* (2008) A comparison of GlideScope videolaryngoscopy to direct laryngoscopy for nasotracheal intubation. *Anesth Analg,* **107,** 144–8.

15. Dupanovic M. (2009) Nasotracheal intubation, direct laryngoscopy, and the Glidescope. *Anesth Analg,* **108** (2), 674.

16. Bennett J, Petito A, Zandsberg S. (1996) Use of laryngeal mask airway in oral and maxillofacial surgery. *J Oral Maxillofac Surg,* **54,** 1346–51.

17. Dibiase AT, Samuels RHA, Ozdiler E, *et al.* (2000) Hazards of orthodontics appliances and the oropharynx. *J Orthod,* **27**(4), 295–302.

18. Fuchs G, Schwarz G, Baumgartner A, *et al.* (1999) Fiberoptic intubation in 327 neurosurgical patients with lesions of the cervical spine. *J Neurosurg Anesthesiol,* **11,** 11–16.

5

The surgical airway

Kaye Cantlay

Introduction

A surgical airway is an airway created by an invasive technique, as opposed to an airway maintained via an anatomical route such as the oropharynx or nasopharynx. The circumstances prompting the use of a surgical airway are extremely varied, ranging from the desperate emergency where oxygenation cannot be achieved by any other means, to the airway fashioned in a controlled manner as part of an elective surgical procedure or to facilitate weaning from ventilatory support. A number of surgical approaches to the airway exist, including needle cricothyroid puncture and cricothyroidotomy, surgical and percutaneous dilatational tracheostomy, and the submental airway. Each of these will be discussed in turn, focusing on technique, indications, contraindications, and complications.

Needle cricothyroid puncture and surgical cricothyroidotomy

Needle cricothyroid puncture and surgical cricothyroidotomy are emergency surgical airway procedures that are most commonly performed in the situation in which oxygenation cannot be achieved by any other means. Both procedures gain access to the airway via the cricothyroid membrane. One of the most difficult aspects of these techniques is recognizing that they need to be performed, and that further attempts to either intubate or ventilate by conventional means may be potentially catastrophic.

Indications

Indications are fortunately rare, but include the patient who is impossible to both intubate and ventilate and the patient with impending or actual complete airway obstruction.

An inability to intubate and ventilate a patient may ensue following a failed intubation, where the priority is to maintain oxygenation until such time as the patient regains spontaneous ventilation and consciousness. If it becomes impossible to maintain a patent airway to enable either spontaneous ventilation or hand ventilation by ordinary means, then an emergency airway must be created.

Needle cricothyroid puncture or surgical cricothyroidotomy may be necessary in patients with impending or actual complete airway obstruction in whom there is no time to reverse the underlying problem, or to attempt either conventional intubation or time-consuming surgical procedures such as a tracheostomy. The underlying problems might include severe maxillofacial trauma, epiglottitis, anaphylaxis, and laryngeal pathology such as tumour.

Contraindications

Needle cricothyroid puncture and surgical cricothyroidotomy would not usually be performed in anything other than the absolute emergency. If time allows, then an airway should be achieved by other means where possible. This may be via the conventional orotracheal or nasotracheal route, or if this is found to be, or is likely to be, impossible then via a surgical tracheostomy.

A surgical cricothyroidotomy is contraindicated in the paediatric patient under the age of about 12 years of age. These patients have extremely small, pliable, and mobile laryngeal and cricoid cartilages, making the procedure extremely difficult in this age group. In these patients a needle cricothyroidotomy should be performed or, if time allows, a surgical tracheostomy under direct vision.

In a situation in which there is complete upper airway obstruction, a needle cricothyroid puncture should not be performed, as this relies on exhalation of gases through the upper airway. In complete obstruction, air trapping and barotrauma will ensue on attempted insufflation of gas, as discussed below. In

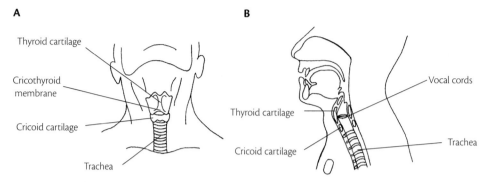

Figure 5.1 Anatomy of the airway illustrating the relative positions of the thyroid cartilage, cricothyroid membrane, cricoid cartilage, and the trachea. **A** Anterior view; **B** sagittal view.

such a situation, a surgical cricothyroidotomy would be the emergency technique of choice.

As these techniques are generally performed in a desperate emergency where other means to create an airway have failed, most other contraindications are relative. These include situations which might make the procedure more difficult such as previous neck surgery or scarring, obesity, haematoma, coagulopathy, overlying infection, and neck trauma.

Practical aspects

Both techniques access the cricothyroid membrane. This membrane has the advantage over the trachea in the emergency setting in that it is more anterior than the trachea with less overlying tissue, easier to fix to facilitate puncture or incision, and generally a less vascular area and there is therefore less danger of significant bleeding.

Of the two techniques, needle cricothyroid puncture is simpler, quicker, and associated with less bleeding. The needle cricothyroid puncture is a more temporary solution, however, and simply buys time during which a more definitive airway must be achieved.

Needle cricothyroid puncture

- If possible, extend the neck of the patient as the landmarks will be easier to identify. The cricothyroid membrane must then be identified as the soft depression between the thyroid cartilage above and the cricoid cartilage below (Figure 5.1). Note that this membrane is proportionally smaller in children under the age of 12 owing to greater overlap of the two cartilages
- If time allows, although commonly it will not, prepare the skin with an antiseptic solution such as 2%

chlorhexidine in alcohol, and anaesthetize the skin with a solution of lidocaine and adrenaline

- The thyroid and cricoid cartilages should then be immobilized, and overlying skin tautened, by placing the thumb and middle finger of the non-dominant hand on either side. The index finger of the same hand confirms the location of the cricothyroid membrane
- A 10-ml syringe attached to a wide bore cannula (14–16G) is held in the dominant hand. The needle and cannula are then used to puncture the skin and cricothyroid membrane whilst aspirating with the syringe. The cannula should be directed caudally, in the midline, at approximately 30° to the skin. Free aspiration of air confirms entry into the trachea (Figure 5.2a)
- The cannula is then advanced over the needle into the tracheal lumen, and the needle removed (Figure 5.2b). Air should be aspirated from the cannula to confirm correct placement within the trachea. The cannula should now be securely taped into place
- The cannula must now be connected to an oxygen source. Various methods have been used, including the following:
  - High-flow oxygen at 15 l/min from the pipeline supply or a cylinder via oxygen tubing. This may be connected either directly to the cannula or via an open three-way tap connected to the cannula. If oxygen tubing alone is used, a small hole the size of a fingertip should be cut in the tubing just before it connects to the cannula. Insufflation of oxygen into the trachea is achieved by placing a fingertip over either the hole in the oxygen tubing or the open side port of the three-way tap for 1 second.

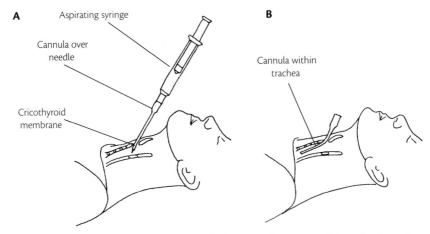

Figure 5.2 Emergency needle cricothyroidotomy. **A** A syringe attached to a cannula over a needle is used to locate the trachea as described in the text. **B** The cannula is then railroaded over the needle into the trachea and the needle removed. The cannula should now be secured and an oxygen source such as a Sanders injector connected to it.

Exhalation is then achieved by removing the fingertip occlusion for at least 3 seconds. It must be noted that exhalation does not occur through the cannula. Gases must be allowed to escape passively from the lungs through the upper airway. Application of airway opening manoeuvres and insertion of airway adjuncts may assist with this. If complete obstruction to the upper airway has occurred, expiration will be impossible, resulting in gas trapping and barotrauma

○ A Sanders injector connected to an oxygen supply may be attached via a Luer lock system to the cannula. This is used in a similar manner to the oxygen source described above, but, owing to the much higher pressures generated (45–50 pounds per square inch (psi)), will achieve greater insufflation through the high resistance of the cannula. A ratio of 1 second's insufflation to 3 seconds' exhalation should still be observed and attention paid to optimizing upper airway patency.

It should be noted that, with this technique, although oxygenation may be achieved, ventilation will be poor. This is particularly the case when using high-flow oxygen, and the patient will become rapidly and progressively hypercapnic. Jet ventilation using the Sanders injector will usually achieve better ventilation, but may perform less well in situations of increasing upper airway obstruction[1,2]. In addition, the needle cricothyroidotomy offers no airway protection. This manoeuvre is therefore only a temporary solution

which buys about 30–40 minutes, during which a more definitive airway which will facilitate both oxygenation and ventilation must be achieved.

Complications of needle cricothyroidectomy

Complications of needle cricothyroidectomy are included in Table 5.1.

Technique of surgical cricothyroidotomy

Compared to needle cricothyroidotomy, surgical cricothyroidotomy is the method of choice in adults if

Table 5.1 Complications of needle cricothyroidotomy

- Misplacement of the cannula with development of subcutaneous emphysema or pneumothorax on attempted insufflation
- Kinking and obstruction of the cannula
- Trauma to structures other than the trachea with the needle
- Bleeding
- Barotrauma owing to failure of adequate expiration or excessive pressures from the Sanders injector
- Progressive hypercapnia
- Reflex coughing on insufflation, which may be ameliorated by an injection of lidocaine down the cannula

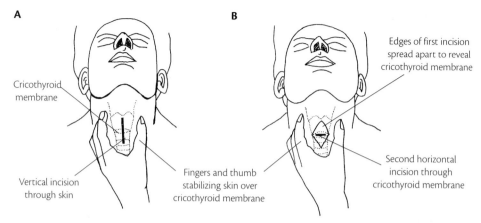

Figure 5.3 Emergency surgical cricothyroidotomy. **A** The skin on either side of the airway is stabilized using the non-dominant hand. A vertical incision overlying the cricothyroid membrane is made using a scalpel held in the dominant hand. **B** The edges of the skin incision are spread to reveal the cricothyroid membrane. A second horizontal incision is made through the membrane. An endotracheal tube should now be passed through the second incision into the trachea.

skills allow as it will facilitate both oxygenation and ventilation[2]

- The patient is positioned as for a needle cricothyroid puncture, and the cricothyroid membrane identified. If time allows, the skin should be prepared with antiseptic solution and then injected with a mixture of lidocaine with adrenaline

- The larynx should be immobilized using the thumb and middle finger of the non-dominant hand placed on either side of the thyroid and cricoid cartilages, as for the needle cricothyroidotomy

- A vertical midline skin incision approximately 1.5 cm in length is then made with a scalpel using the dominant hand (Figure 5.3a)

- The skin on either side of the incision is then retracted laterally either using the thumb and middle finger of the non-dominant hand, or a retractor if available, to expose the cricothyroid membrane

- A horizontal incision through the inferior part of the cricothyroid membrane is now made using the scalpel (Figure 5.3b). This avoids the superior cricothyroid vessels which run horizontally near the upper border of the membrane. The blade should be directed inferiorly to avoid trauma to the true vocal cords

- The incision should now be opened up to facilitate the passage of a tracheal tube though it. This may be achieved either by using a pair of forceps passed into the incision to dilate the incision in the vertical

plane, or a tracheal hook to apply downward traction to the lower border of the incision and the cricoid cartilage; if such instruments are not immediately available, however, the handle of the scalpel may be placed through the incision and rotated by 90° to open up the hole in the vertical plane

- An endotracheal tube is now passed through the opening into the trachea. The tube may be by necessity a small diameter tube such as a size 6.0 mm, but should ideally be a cuffed tube. Either a conventional translaryngeal tube or a tracheostomy tube may be used. The cuff should now be inflated and correct placement established with capnography and clinically

- The patient may now be ventilated with an appropriate circuit.

Commonly, the emergency surgical cricothyroidotomy will be revised within the first 24 hours to a surgical tracheostomy, as this has traditionally been thought to be associated with lower longer term airway morbidity. This is controversial, however, and some would argue that continued ventilation via the cricothyroidotomy is not associated with an increased incidence of complications[3,4].

Complications of surgical cricothyroidectomy

The complications associated with surgical cricothyroidotomy are given in Table 5.2.

Table 5.2 Complications of surgical cricothyroidotomy

- Procedural complications such as bleeding, subcutaneous emphysema, pneumothorax, failure to locate the trachea, creation of a false passage, trauma to the trachea and surrounding structures
- Intermediate complications such as infection or bleeding
- Late complications such as subglottic stenosis

Cricothyroidotomy kits

A number of complete commercial cricothyroidotomy kits are available for use in the emergency setting. These are useful if both immediately available and familiar to the user. Examples of these kits include the following:

CricKit®

CricKit® is marketed by North American Rescue Incorporated and contains sachets of antiseptic solution, a scalpel, a tracheal hook, a size 6.0 mm cuffed cricothyroidotomy tube, a syringe with which to inflate the cuff, and a tie to secure the tube after insertion.

Mini-Trac® II

Mini-Trac® II is manufactured by Portex and contains a scalpel, a size 4.0 mm uncuffed cannula loaded onto a curved introducer to aid insertion, a neck tape, and a suction catheter.

The PCK®

The PCK® kit is manufactured by Portex and contains a scalpel, a size 6.0 mm cuffed cricothyroidotomy tube mounted on a Veress needle designed to reduce the chances of injury to the posterior wall of the trachea, a tube tie, a suture, and a heat and moisture exchanger.

Tracheostomy

Tracheostomy refers to the creation of a surgical airway through the wall of the trachea. The indications for a tracheostomy range from the emergency to the elective. There are two principal techniques, namely surgical and percutaneous dilatational. The surgical tracheostomy (ST) may be done as an emergency or as a more elective procedure, whilst the percutaneous dilatational tracheostomy (PDT) is usually performed in an elective manner, and is usually to facilitate longer term intubation and/or ventilation in the critically ill patient. These techniques will be discussed in turn below.

Indications

Tracheostomy may be indicated to relieve impending or anticipated upper airway obstruction due to pathology such as airway tumour, infection, oedema, trauma, or congenital malformation. A tracheostomy may also be part of an elective surgical procedure to ensure a patent airway. This may be permanent in the case of laryngectomy, or temporary following other major maxillofacial procedures where transient airway swelling is anticipated.

In critical care patients requiring protracted intubation and ventilation, tracheostomy is an alternative to orotracheal or nasotracheal intubation. A surgical airway facilitates weaning from mechanical ventilation in the patient with reversible respiratory failure and allows tracheobronchial toilet in the patient with insufficient ability to clear respiratory secretions. Patients on long-term ventilation, such as those with irreversible respiratory failure owing to a high cervical spinal injury or neuromuscular disease, benefit from a tracheostomy. It may also provide airway protection in the patient with impaired airway reflexes because of reduced conscious level or bulbar disorders.

Advantages

The advantages of a tracheostomy over endotracheal intubation are most apparent in the critically ill population. These include the following: patient comfort, reduction in sedation requirements, reduced resistance to breathing through a shorter tracheal tube, possibly more rapid weaning from mechanical ventilation, improved tracheal toilet, better oropharyngeal hygiene, and an ability to eat and speak.

Contraindications

There are few contraindications to a ST although certain conditions such as morbid obesity, limited neck extension or severe kyphoscoliosis, large thyroid goitres, or overlying infection may make the procedure technically more difficult.

There are few absolute contraindications to percutaneous dilatational tracheostomy, and many of the contraindications that have previously been felt to have been absolute have been challenged[5]. The need for emergency airway access is generally considered an absolute contraindication to PDT. In such a situation cricothyroidotomy or ST are usually the techniques of choice, depending on the time and skills available. The technique is also considered to be contraindicated in children below the age of 12 years, in whom an open ST would be the technique of choice in the more controlled setting, or needle cricothyroidotomy in the emergency situation.

Relative contraindications to PDT include morbid obesity, anterior neck masses such as goitres, previous neck surgery, limited neck extension or unstable neck injury, coagulopathies, high ventilatory requirements such as high positive end expiratory pressure (PEEP) dependency or high inspired oxygen concentration. In such patients, if a tracheostomy were considered to be indicated, an open ST might be favoured over a PDT.

Surgical versus percutaneous dilatational tracheostomy in critical care

Although there are definite logistical advantages to PDT at the bedside in critical care patients, the short- and long-term advantages and disadvantages of per-cutaneous versus ST are less clearcut. There have been many studies performed, including a number of ran-domized controlled trials attempting to address this question. There have also been several published meta-analyses, the two largest of which have looked at around 1000 patients each. The conclusions drawn include that PDT is associated with a lower incidence of wound infection and unfavourable scarring, and that there is no difference in terms of bleeding, late stenosis or mortality. PDT may have a cost benefit and is faster to perform[6,7].

Surgical tracheostomy

A surgical or open tracheostomy (ST) is most com-monly performed in the operating theatre, although may less commonly be undertaken at the bedside in the intensive care unit.

Technique of surgical tracheostomy

♦ Ideally the patient is positioned supine with the shoulders elevated and the neck extended. This position will maximally expose the trachea, and may be facilitated by placing a shoulder roll between the scapulae, or a pillow behind the patient's shoulders. Although neck extension facilitates the procedure, overextension should be avoided, as it firstly tends

to narrow the airway, and secondly may encourage the operator to place the stoma in too caudal a position, particularly in the paediatric patient with a very small and mobile trachea. A low position may result in a tube encroaching on the carina, or very close to the innominate artery[8]. In the patient with a cervical spine injury, however, neck extension may be precluded, and inline immobili-zation should be maintained. In the more unusual situation where such a procedure is being performed in the awake patient under local anaesthesia, posi-tioning may have to be compromised to minimize patient distress, and, for example, it may be neces-sary to have the patient almost sitting or semi-recumbent

♦ A wide area from the chin to below the clavicles should be cleaned with an antiseptic solution such as 2% chlorhexidine, and then draped with sterile drapes. The skin overlying the second tracheal ring is then identified and infiltrated with a mixture of lidocaine and a vasoconstrictor such as adrenaline

♦ A vertical skin incision is now made in the midline approximately 2–3 cm in length. Some would advocate a horizontal incision which may provide a better long-term cosmetic outcome, but may trap more secretions

♦ Sharp dissection is used to divide the platysma muscle. Any vessels such as aberrant anterior jugular veins are cauterized or ligated. Haemostasis should be meticulous

♦ Midline blunt dissection is then used to divide the strap muscle tissues. These are then retracted lat-erally to expose the thyroid isthmus. If the isthmus lies superior to the third tracheal cartilage, it may simply be mobilized superiorly to gain access to the trachea. More commonly, however, the isthmus overlies the second and third rings, and must be incised or even completely divided to gain greatest access to the trachea

♦ Access to the tracheal lumen is often associated with inadvertent puncture of the underlying endotracheal tube cuff, resulting in a ventilatory leak. The oro-pharynx should therefore be aspirated of all secretions prior to surgical incision of the trachea. Tracheal lumen access can be achieved in one of three ways:

  ○ Ring removal—the anterior portion of one or more of the tracheal rings is removed to create a rectan-gular stoma. Stay sutures are placed in the tracheal wall at either side of the stoma and left uncut. These

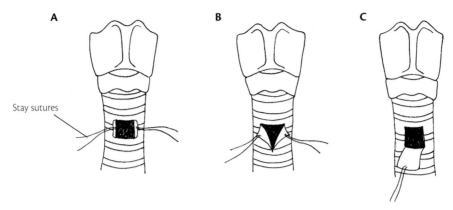

Figure 5.4 Approaches to surgical tracheostomy. **A** Ring removal; **B** 'T' shaped incision; **C** inverted U-shaped incision.

sutures are used to provide countertraction during the insertion of the tracheostomy tube, but are also usually left *in situ* following the procedure to facilitate reinsertion of an accidentally displaced tube (Figure 5.4a)

○ T-shaped opening – a 2-cm incision is made horizontally through the tracheal wall between the second and third tracheal rings, or the third and fourth rings. A vertical incision is then made perpendicular to the first incision in the midline through the distal one or two tracheal rings using heavy scissors. Stay sutures are then inserted into each flap and taped to either side of the neck or upper chest (Figure 5.4b)

○ U-shaped flap – this method, described by Björk[9], involves the creation of an inverted U-shaped tracheal wall flap. In this technique, the flap is made at the level of the second to fourth tracheal rings, and reflected downwards, with its upper border sutured to the skin, creating a bridge of tracheal tissue that assists with tube placement (Figure 5.4c). In the emergency replacement of the displaced tube, the flap will not only assist in guiding the tracheal tube into the trachea lumen, but will also help to prevent the creation of a false passage through pretracheal tissues. A modification of this method involves the creation of an H-shaped flap in which the tracheal flaps are reflected and secured to skin both superiorly and inferiorly

○ Once the tracheal stoma has been created, the endotracheal tube (if one is *in situ*) should be withdrawn, such that the tip lies proximal to the upper border of the stoma. Any secretions or blood within the trachea should be suctioned. The tracheostomy tube is then inserted through the stoma under direct vision, usually with an obturator *in situ* to guide it into place

○ Once tracheal tube placement has been confirmed as satisfactory, for example with adequate ventilation and capnography, the endotracheal tube may be removed.

Percutaneous dilatational tracheostomy (PDT)

Tracheostomy is commonly used in critical care as an alternative to translaryngeal endotracheal intubation in the patient expected to require protracted periods of mechanical ventilation.

Although in the past the majority of tracheostomies were performed surgically in the operating theatre, over time the technique of PDT has become increasingly popular. This latter technique may be performed quickly and simply at the bedside, without the need to transport the patient, and by non-surgical doctors.

The earliest dilatational tracheostomies were performed by a serial dilatational method developed by Ciaglia[10]. A number of other dilatational techniques have also been described, including a modification of the Ciaglia method employing a single dilator (e.g. Blue Rhino, Cook)[11], dilatational forceps (e.g. Griggs)[12], a screw-action dilator (PercuTwist)[13], and a translaryngeal method of placement (Fantoni)[14]. The technique currently most commonly used in the UK is that using a single dilator and this will be described in detail below.

Technique of percutaneous tracheostomy using a single tapered dilator

- The patient should be adequately anaesthetized and paralysed with an appropriate muscle relaxant of intermediate duration

- The patient should be ventilated with 100% oxygen. A volume-controlled mode of ventilation may be preferable to pressure-controlled as there will be a variable leakage of inspired gases during the procedure

- The patient's endotracheal tube should now be repositioned such that there is no danger of either the tube or, perhaps more importantly, its cuff being punctured as the trachea is located with a needle. This will entail deflating the cuff of the tube and withdrawing it under direct vision using a laryngoscope, until the cuff lies across the cords. The cuff is then reinflated to provide a seal, and the tube resecured. A throat pack may usefully be placed if a leak is still apparent, but this must not be forgotten, and must be removed at the conclusion of the procedure. An alternative to this manoeuvre that may be useful, in the patient who is not on high levels of ventilatory support, is the substitution of the endotracheal tube with a laryngeal mask

- The patient should now be positioned as for an open tracheostomy with the neck extended such that the larynx is elevated and the trachea more accessible. This may be achieved by placing a pillow behind the patient's shoulders

- The operator should now scrub and put on a gown, sterile gloves, hat, and a mask with a visor

- All equipment should be checked and a suitable size of tracheostomy tube selected. The tracheostomy tube cuff should be checked, and the tube loaded onto an appropriately sized dilator. Both the dilator and the tracheostomy cuff should be lubricated well with water-soluble gel

- A wide area of skin should be cleaned with an antiseptic solution such as 2% chlorhexidine in alcohol and sterile drapes placed

- The landmarks should be defined and the skin overlying the second to fourth tracheal rings identified

- The skin should be infiltrated with up to 10 ml of 1% lidocaine containing adrenaline, the latter providing vasoconstriction to reduce the risk of bleeding during the procedure

- A horizontal skin incision should be made, approximately the length of the outer diameter of the intended tracheostomy tube

- The subcutaneous tissues are now bluntly dissected down to the trachea

- A second operator should now pass a bronchoscope into the trachea via the patient's endotracheal tube or laryngeal mask airway to observe the subsequent stages of the procedure directly

- The trachea is now located using a cannula-over-needle attached to a syringe (Figure 5.5a). The operator should aim to puncture the trachea as close to the midline as possible, between either the second and third, or the third and fourth tracheal rings. Aspiration of air confirms that the trachea has been entered. The cannula is then advanced over the needle into the trachea and the syringe and needle are removed

- A guidewire is now passed through the cannula (Figure 5.5b). This wire should pass freely and should be observed by the bronchoscopist to advance towards the carina. The cannula is now removed, leaving the wire within the trachea

- A small dilator is now passed over the wire into the trachea. A distinct 'give' is appreciated as the dilator passes through the tracheal wall. The dilator is then removed, leaving the wire within the trachea

- The large tapered dilator has a hydrophilic coating. By dipping the dilator in water prior to use, this coating will form a lubricant that will reduce tissue drag and thereby reduce the potential for tissue damage

- The large dilator loaded over a guiding catheter is now passed over the guidewire in one movement into the trachea. The dilator should be advanced until the bold black marker is at the skin (Figure 5.5c). This dilator is then left *in situ* for a few seconds to facilitate tissue stretch. The dilator is then removed, leaving both the guidewire and the guide catheter in the trachea

- The tracheostomy tube preloaded onto its dilator is now passed over the wire and guiding catheter into the trachea (Figure 5.5d). The wire, guiding catheter, and dilator are now removed, leaving only the tracheostomy tube in the trachea

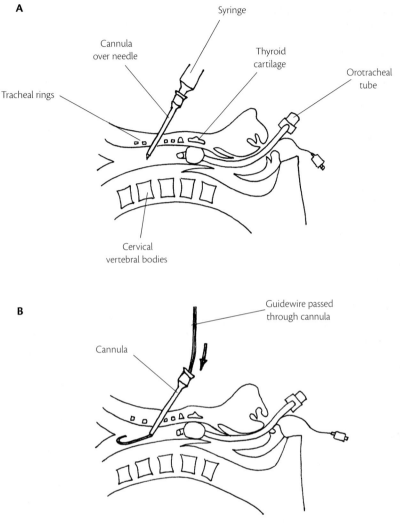

Figure 5.5 Percutaneous dilatational tracheostomy using a single tapered dilator. **A** The trachea is located using a syringe attached to a cannula over a needle. This should be guided by a bronchoscope passed via the endotracheal tube, but this has been omitted from the figures for clarity. **B** The cannula is passed over the needle into the trachea and the needle removed. A guidewire is passed through the cannula into the trachea. **C** The large tapered dilator loaded onto the guiding catheter is passed over the guidewire into the trachea until the black line is at the skin incision. **D** The tracheostomy tube loaded onto an appropriately sized dilator is passed over the guiding catheter and guidewire into position in the trachea.

- The bronchoscope is used to ascertain that the tracheostomy tube has entered the trachea and that the entire cuff is within the tracheal lumen. By passing the bronchoscope through the tracheostomy tube itself, tracheal placement may be double checked and the distance from the carina measured

- The cuff should now be inflated and ventilation transferred to the tracheostomy tube. The tube should be secured with either sutures or tapes

- A chest radiograph is commonly performed following the procedure to rule out complications such as pneumothorax.

Alternative techniques for percutaneous tracheostomy

Serial dilator technique

This was described by Ciaglia in 1985[10]. It is a technique broadly similar to that outlined above, but using a series of dilators of gradually increasing gauge to create

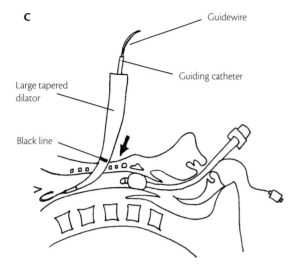

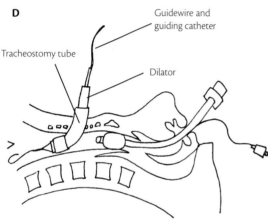

Figure 5.5 Continued

the stoma. In comparison to single dilator techniques, this method is slower, with greater potential for deterioration in oxygenation.

Dilatational forceps technique

One version of this was developed by Griggs in 1990 [12]. A Seldinger technique is used to locate and pass a guidewire into the trachea as in the tapered dilator technique. A pair of customized forceps is then threaded over the wire, firstly through the skin and subcutaneous tissue. The forceps are then opened up to stretch up these tissues. The forceps are advanced further along the wire into the trachea itself, and opened up a second time to stretch up a hole in the

tracheal wall. A tracheostomy tube is then passed over the wire through the passage created.

Screw-action dilatation

A technique developed by Rusch known as PercuTwist[13] involves a single-step dilatation of the tracheal wall. In this case the dilator is a screw-like device that actually lifts the anterior wall of the trachea during its use. This is in contrast to the posterior displacement of the anterior tracheal wall commonly observed with the use of the Blue Rhino dilator. This has the advantage of ensuring an unobstructed bronchoscopic view of the procedure, and may potentially be associated with a lower incidence of tracheal ring fractures and posterior tracheal wall injury.

Translaryngeal technique

This was developed by Fantoni in 1993[14]. In this method, the guidewire placed in the trachea is directed superiorly through the larynx. A specially designed tracheostomy tube is then threaded over the guidewire and passed through first the larynx and then through the anterior tracheal wall. This technique may theoretically reduce the risk of damage to the posterior tracheal wall, but is possibly more complicated than other techniques with a high incidence of technical difficulties[15].

Complications of surgical and percutaneous tracheostomy

There are many potential complications associated with both surgical and percutaneous tracheostomy (Table 5.3), and so the risk:benefit ratio must be carefully considered in every patient before proceeding, particularly in the critical care setting. The complications may be divided into immediate (procedural), early, and late. Any complications more specific to PDT or ST are indicated.

Choice of tracheostomy tube
Size

The size of a tracheostomy tube is expressed in millimetres, and generally corresponds to its internal diameter (ID). The actual internal and outer diameter (OD) of the tube will usually be displayed on the packaging or on the tube itself and will vary depending on the design and manufacturer of the tube. When selecting a tube, both internal and external diameters must be considered. A tube with too small an internal diameter will provide an increased resistance to

Table 5.3 Complications of surgical and percutaneous tracheostomy

Immediate

Bleeding

Pneumothorax

Surgical emphysema

Damage to tissues during puncture with needle (PDT)

    Eccentric puncture

    Puncture of structures other than the trachea

    Damage to the posterior tracheal wall and oesophagus

    Cartilage fracture

Misplacement of tracheostomy tube

    Pretracheal

    Endobronchial

    Passage through posterior tracheal wall

Hypoxia and de-recruitment of alveolae

Hypercapnea owing to inadequate ventilation

Early

Infection of the tracheostomy site

Blockage of the tracheostomy tube with secretions

Displacement of the tracheostomy tube

Erosion of tissue due to pressure from the tracheostomy tube or cuff

    Mucosal ulceration

    Erosion of innominate artery

    Tracheo-oesophageal fistula

Late

Tracheal granulomas

Tracheal stenosis

Tracheomalacia

Persistent sinus at the tracheostomy site

respiration and may be difficult to clear secretions through. If it is a cuffed tube, a smaller tube will require an increased pressure to create a seal within the trachea. A tube with too large an OD will be difficult to pass into the trachea, and may hinder the ability of the patient to breathe around the tube through the upper airway with the cuff deflated.

A tube with an OD that is approximately three-quarters of the diameter of the patient's trachea should be selected. A size 8.0 mm ID tube (11 mm OD) will usually be appropriate for the average adult male, and a 7.0 mm tube (10 mm OD) for the average adult female.

Length

Many tubes are preformed to fit the average adult patient, such that the outer flange will lie comfortably and flush with the anterior neck wall, whilst the distal end of the tube sits within the trachea parallel to the tracheal walls. Preformed tubes may create problems, however, particularly in the obese patient or patient with more extensive pretracheal tissues. In these patients, the tube may be too short, such that the end of the tube abuts the posterior tracheal wall. This may lead to ulceration, formation of granulation tissue on the posterior wall of the trachea, and obstruction of the tube. In the very large patient, the tube cuff may not sit completely within the tracheal lumen. In larger patients a tube with a variable flange position may therefore be suitable. Conversely, in the very small patient, a preformed tube may be too long, and the tube may curve forward and ulcerate or even erode through the anterior tracheal wall.

Material

Metal tubes are usually only used in patients with permanent tracheostomies. These are silver-coated which is bactericidal and non-irritant. Metal tubes are uncuffed, and do not have a standard 15 mm connector and so are unsuitable for providing positive pressure ventilation. They are also extremely rigid. Plastic tubes are more flexible and may be made from polyvinyl chloride (PVC) or silicone. PVC tubes tend to soften at body temperature, conforming to patient anatomy. Silicone tubes are the most flexible and naturally soft regardless of temperature.

Cuffed versus uncuffed tracheostomy tubes

Tubes may be cuffed or uncuffed. The uncuffed tube is useful for clearance of secretions but provides no airway protection. Although an uncuffed tube may be used to provide a degree of mechanical ventilation, positive pressure ventilation is much more effectively provided with a cuffed tube, particularly with incompliant lungs. A large volume low pressure cuff is desirable as this will dissipate pressure over a wider surface area. This will reduce the incidence of tracheal wall erosion and ulceration, and longer term stenosis.

Fenestrated versus non-fenestrated

The fenestrated tube is similar in construction to the standard tracheostomy, but has one or more holes in the posterior wall, above the level of the cuff. With the cuff deflated and the tracheal tube occluded at its outer end, the patient may breathe via the upper airway. This will allow phonation, and may also be a useful step in the assessment of a patient prior to decannulation, as discussed below.

Inner tubes

Some tracheostomy tubes are designed to be used with a coaxial inner tube. Occasionally the 15 mm universal connector is part of the inner tube, and so a ventilator circuit may not be attached without the inner tube in place. The advantage of an inner tube is that it may be removed for cleaning or replaced at intervals. A non-fenestrated inner tube placed within a fenestrated outer tube may convert a fenestrated tube to one which is effectively non-fenestrated.

Decannulation

Decannulation decision-making will depend on the reason for which the tracheostomy was performed. In the case of a tracheostomy performed for upper airway obstruction, the tracheostomy may be removed if and when the underlying airway obstruction has sufficiently resolved and a patent upper airway is restored. Endoscopic examination of the upper airway may assist in confirming this. Prior to decannulation, the cuff of the tracheostomy may be deflated and, on occlusion of the tracheostomy tube, the patient should be observed to breathe comfortably, without respiratory distress through their upper airway and around the tracheostomy tube.

In the case of a tracheostomy tube performed to facilitate prolonged mechanical ventilation, decannulation is usually considered once the patient has successfully weaned from mechanical ventilation, including PEEP. The patient will usually have demonstrated stable gas exchange on no mechanical support for at least 24 hours.

The patient should also be able to demonstrate an effective cough such that he or she will be able to expectorate secretions adequately. Occasionally, where the secretion load is still very high, or the patient's cough strength borderline, a mini-tracheostomy may be placed as an interim measure to assist with secretion clearance.

Prior to formal decannulation, a 'physiological decannulation' is sometimes performed by occluding the tracheostomy tube with a tracheostomy button and deflating the cuff. This will allow additional time to assess the patient for respiratory distress, stable gas exchange, and cough effectiveness prior to actually removing the tube. To reduce the resistance to breathing around a large tracheostomy tube during such a trial, some physicians would advocate first exchanging the tube for a fenestrated tube, or a smaller diameter tube.

Tracheostomy in critical care

When a tracheostomy is performed in the critical care setting, the procedure is generally carried out in a planned and controlled manner, and the patient will usually already be intubated. If the patient is not already anaesthetized, anaesthesia should be induced and maintained with an appropriate agent. In the critical care setting this would usually involve an intravenous induction and maintenance with a short-acting agent such as propofol. If the procedure is to be carried out in the operating theatre, the option of a volatile anaesthetic will be available. A short-acting opiate administered either as an infusion or in the form of boluses will be useful to obtund the sympathetic response to airway manipulation. The patient should be paralysed with a muscle relaxant of intermediate duration to prevent coughing during the procedure.

Tracheostomy for airway obstruction

The urgent tracheostomy performed for airway obstruction will require more careful consideration and preparation. The patient will not uncommonly present with a variable, sometimes severe, degree of respiratory distress and stridor. They may be extremely frightened and uncooperative, agitated, using their accessory muscles of respiration, and will often adopt a position in which airflow is maximized such as sitting upright. Depending on the pathology, the patient may also be unable to swallow, and may be drooling and have pooled secretions in the airway. In the emergency setting, the patient may also have a full stomach.

In addition to the usual assessment, the anaesthetist must focus in particular on the airway to formulate an appropriate management plan (Chapter 4).

Anaesthesia for emergency tracheostomy

In broad terms the choice lies firstly between performing the procedure under either local or general anaesthesia. If the procedure is performed under general anaesthesia, then the anaesthetist must decide how best to secure the airway, and how to induce anaesthesia.

Local anaesthesia

Only very rarely will it be necessary to undertake a tracheostomy under local anaesthesia. This will usually only be required in the situation where it is felt that attempting to secure an airway via the oral or nasal route will either be impossible or unduly hazardous, and that the safest option is to have a patient who is conscious and maintaining his or her own airway until a surgical airway has been created.

Performing a tracheostomy under local anaesthesia will avoid the risk of losing the airway completely under general anaesthesia with potentially catastrophic consequences. It will also avoid the need for a potentially difficult awake fibreoptic intubation. The disadvantages of performing the procedure under local anaesthesia are that it may prove to be extremely distressing for the patient, particularly in the patient with severe respiratory embarrassment. In the patient with a critically obstructed airway the patient may be unable to lie flat with the neck extended, and the surgeon may have to attempt the procedure with the patient sitting or semi-recumbent. The patient's respiratory rate may be high, and the excursion of the trachea may be increased as the patient attempts to overcome the obstruction. This will clearly add to surgical difficulty.

Local anaesthesia per se will usually be achieved by simple infiltration of the tissues with a mixture of lidocaine and adrenaline. An injection of lidocaine into the trachea itself injected via the cricothyroid membrane may help to reduce coughing during airway manipulation.

General anaesthesia

In the majority of cases the tracheostomy will take place under general anaesthesia with the airway having been first secured via the oral or nasal route. General anaesthesia offers the advantage of greater control over the surgical field, and removes the risk of patient distress or lack of cooperation during the procedure itself. However, securing the airway and administering anaesthesia may prove hazardous and technically challenging. For this reason, an experienced anaesthetist should always be involved in the planning and management of such a case.

A number of options will be available to the anaesthetist, and these will depend on the individual patient's circumstances and pathology. A detailed description of all potential techniques that may be employed is beyond the scope of this chapter, but the basic principles will be discussed below.

Factors influencing the decision are multiple. If the patient's mouth opening is severely restricted and unlikely to improve under anaesthesia (Chapter 11), then direct laryngoscopy will not be an option. Local pathology can distort the normal anatomy and obscure an adequate view of the vocal cords. A nasendoscopy performed by the ENT surgeon may give valuable information in this regard. The patient may not be able to cooperate with an awake fibreoptic intubation and in some circumstances an awake fibreoptic intubation may actually precipitate complete airway obstruction or the size of the scope may be too large to traverse a narrowed larynx. The patency of the nostrils or presence of a base of skull fracture may influence whether the nasal route may be used. Other factors to consider are the patient's fasting status and the skills of the anaesthetic team and the equipment available to them.

A decision must first be made as to whether or not it is necessary to secure the airway prior to induction of anaesthesia; in other words, whether or not an awake fibreoptic intubation is indicated. An awake fibreoptic intubation might be appropriate in the patient in whom direct laryngoscopy is unlikely to provide a view of the larynx, for example due to pathology such as tumour or swelling in the supraglottic region. In addition, the patient might either be unfasted, or there may be concern about the ability to maintain an airway following induction of anaesthesia, such that asleep fibreoptic intubation is precluded.

A fasted patient in whom direct laryngoscopy is unlikely to be successful, but is not expected to present undue difficulties in maintaining an airway following induction of anaesthesia, can be managed with an asleep fibreoptic intubation. Induction of anaesthesia may be achieved by the intravenous or inhalational route. However, an intravenous induction will run the risk of rendering the patient apnoeic with the potential for the situation of not being able to ventilate an unintubatable patient. A gaseous induction with a non-irritant volatile agent such as sevoflurane will facilitate the induction of deep anaesthesia in the spontaneously breathing patient. If the airway becomes impossible to maintain adequately at any stage, then the volatile may be turned off and the patient allowed to regain consciousness, and an alternative plan followed. Once the patient is deeply anaesthetized, an assessment of the ability to hand-ventilate may be made. If this is easy, a muscle relaxant may be administered, but if there is any doubt as to the adequacy and ease of hand-ventilation, then spontaneous respiration should continue. A fibreoptic intubation may then be undertaken via either the nasal or oral route as clinically indicated.

In the patient in whom direct laryngoscopy is likely to provide a view of the larynx, albeit a distorted one, and there is no major concern over the ability to maintain an airway following induction of anaesthesia, the inhalational induction of anaesthesia is an acceptable technique. With the patient breathing spontaneously under deep inhalational anaesthesia, laryngoscopy may be attempted, and the patient intubated if possible. The anaesthetist should have a range of endotracheal tubes available, and be prepared to use one of a very small diameter if necessary.

Submental approach to intubation

Submental intubation is an alternative to tracheostomy where both nasal and oral intubation is contraindicated, and protracted intubation and ventilation not anticipated. Such an airway was first described by Hernandez Altmir in 1986[16], and has proved useful in areas such as complex craniomaxillofacial trauma, and oncological cranial base surgery[17,18]. The submental airway facilitates surgical access to the base of skull, facial bones, and oropharynx, and allows control over dental occlusion. It has the potential advantage of avoiding breach of the tracheal wall, and the complications of tracheostomy.

Technique of submental tracheal intubation

- The establishment of a submental airway requires first that a conventional oropharyngeal intubation is performed, usually with a reinforced endotracheal tube (Figure 5.6a)

- A 2-cm skin incision is then made in the submental area adjacent to the lower border of the mandible

- Blunt dissection with Kelly forceps is then used to divide the muscular layers of the floor of the mouth. The mucosa of the floor of the mouth is then incised over the tip of the forceps, and the forceps then opened to create a tunnel

- The pilot balloon of the endotracheal tube is then brought through this tunnel. The patient is then

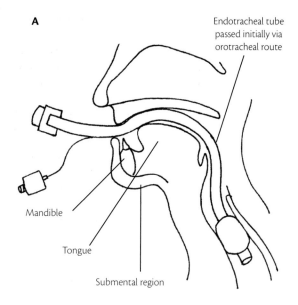

A   Endotracheal tube passed initially via orotracheal route

Mandible

Tongue

Submental region

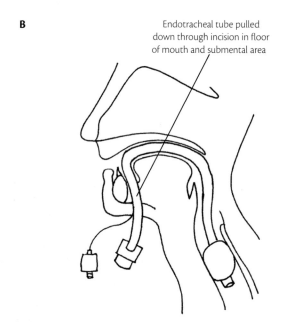

B   Endotracheal tube pulled down through incision in floor of mouth and submental area

Figure 5.6 The submandibular airway. **A** The patient is first intubated via the orotracheal route. **B** The proximal end of the tube is then pulled through an incision created through the floor of the mouth and submental region.

disconnected from the ventilator, the universal connector removed from the endotracheal tube, and the proximal end of the tube drawn through the tunnel to emerge through the skin of the submental region (Figure 5.6b and Plate 14)

- The universal connector is reconnected and the patient attached once more to the breathing circuit and ventilator

- After checking that the position of the tube is satisfactory, it is then sutured into place

- At the end of the surgical procedure, the tube is replaced into the mouth and the patient extubated in the conventional manner.

Complications

There are few complications of submental intubation reported in the literature. However, potential complications include haemorrhage, injury to the sublingual glands, Wharton's duct or lingual nerve, fistulas, infection, and submental or oral scarring.

Conclusion

Securing a surgical airway is a potentially hazardous procedure. It is important for the anaesthetist to understand the dangers and pitfalls associated with the various surgical approaches and the complications that can arise.

References

1. Craven RM, Vanner RG. (2004) Ventilation of a model lung using various cricothyrotomy devices. *Anaesthesia*, **59** (6), 595–9.
2. Scrase I, Woollard M. (2006) Needle vs surgical cricothyroidotomy: a short cut to effective ventilation. *Anaesthesia*, **61(10)**, 962–74.
3. DeLaurier GA, Hawkins ML, Treat RC, Mansberger AR Jr. (1990) Acute airway management. Role of cricothyroidotomy. *Am Surg*, **56**, 12–5.
4. Gillespie MB, Eisele DW. (1999) Outcomes of emergency surgical airway procedures in a hospital-wide setting. *Laryngoscope*, **109(11)**, 1766–9.
5. Bardell T, Drover JW. (2005) Recent developments in percutaneous tracheostomy: improving techniques and expanding roles. *Current Opin Crit Care*, **11(4)**, 326–32.
6. Delaney A, Bagshaw SM, Nalos M. (2006) Percutaneous dilatational tracheostomy versus surgical tracheostomy in critically ill patients: a systematic review and meta-analysis. *Crit Care*, **10(2)**, R55.
7. Higgins KM, Punthakee X. (2007) Meta-analysis comparison of open versus percutaneous tracheostomy. *Laryngoscope*, **117(3)**, 447–54.
8. Grant CA, Dempsey G, Harrison J, Jones T. (2006) Tracheo-innominate artery fistula after percutaneous tracheostomy: three case reports and a clinical review. *Br J Anaesth*, **96(1)**, 127–31.
9. Björk VO. (1960) Partial resection of the only remaining lung with the aid of respirator treatment. *J Thorac Cardiovasc Surg*, **39**, 179–88.
10. Ciaglia P, Firsching R, Syniec C. (1985) Elective percutaneous dilatational tracheostomy: a new simple bedside procedure; preliminary report. *Chest*, **87(6)**, 715–19.
11. Byhahn C, Lischke V, Halbig S, Schiefler G, Westphal K. (2000) Ciaglia blue rhino: a modified technique for percutaneous dilatation tracheostomy. Technique and early clinical results. *Anaesthetist*, **49(3)**, 202–6.
12. Griggs WM, Worthley LI, Gilligan JE, Thomas PD, Myburg JA. (1990) A simple percutaneous tracheostomy technique. *Surg Gynaecol Obstety*, **170(6)**, 543–45.
13. Westphal K, Maeser D, Scheifler G, Lischke V, Byhahn C. (2003) PercuTwist: a new single-dilator technique for percutaneous tracheostomy. *Anaesth Analg*, **96(1)**, 229–32.
14. Fantoni A, Ripamonti D. (1997) A non-derivative, non-surgical tracheostomy: the translaryngeal method. *Intensive Care Med*, **23(4)**, 386–92.
15. Cantais E, Kaiser E, Le-Goff Y, Palmier B. (2002) Percutaneous tracheostomy: prospective comparison of the translaryngeal technique versus the forceps-dilational technique in 100 critically ill adults. *Crit Care Med*, **30(4)**, 815–19.
16. Altemir FH. (1986) The submental route for endotracheal intubation. *J Maxillofac Surg*, **14**, 64–5.
17. Biglioli F, Mortini P, Goisis M, Bardazzi A, Boari N. (2003) Submental orotracheal intubation: an alternative to tracheotomy in transfacial cranial base surgery. *Skull Base*, **13(4)**, 189–95.
18. Caubi AF, Vasconcelos BC, Vasconcellos RJ, Araújo de Morais HH, Rocha NS. (2008) Submental intubation in oral maxillofacial surgery: Review of the literature and analysis of 13 cases. *Med Oral Patol Oral Cir Bucal*, **13(3)**, E197–200.

6

The innervation of the head and neck

Bernard J. Moxham and Barry K.B. Berkovitz

Introduction

The distinguished anatomist and zoologist, J.Z. Young, in his account of the evolution of the vertebrate head and neck (cephalization), suggested that the initial location of the head from a creature with repeated body segments (e.g. an earthworm-like animal) was merely related to the opening of the gut, the mouth, at one end of the creature as it moved forward. At about the same time, organs of special sense would evolve around the mouth so that the animal could better find, and select, its food and consequently the front end of the neural tube would evolve into a brain in order to 'analyse' the information received from these organs of special sense. In evolutionary terms, therefore, the mouth is the primary organ of the head; the special senses are secondary and the brain tertiary. This is all reflected in understanding the functions of the human head and neck. The primary function is metabolic, being concerned with the selection and ingestion of food and with respiration through the nose (a derivative of the foregut) and mouth. The head, having a very complex array of special senses and peripheral nerves, also functions overall as an 'analyser' of the external environment and as a means of recognizing other creatures (both friend and foe). Given these functions it is therefore not surprising that the mouth is so important biologically and physiologically, that it is associated with a complex sensory and motor innervation, and that clinically the treatment of the face, jaws, and mouth requires a thorough-going knowledge of the complex innervation.

This chapter serves as an 'introduction' to the peripheral nervous system of the head and neck in order to provide essentially background information preparatory to a more detailed perspective in relation to

clinical situations in subsequent chapters. Specialist reference texts should be consulted if further detail is required[1-7].

The innervation of the face

The face is bordered by the pinnae of the ears laterally, by the chin inferiorly, and by the hairline superiorly. This region is known to anatomists as the 'superficial face'. This region continues superiorly into the scalp. The 'deep face' is the temporal fossa, the parotid region, and the infratemporal fossa. There are two major nerves innervating the superficial face. The fifth cranial nerve, the trigeminal nerve, for all three of its divisions is the 'great sensory nerve' of the head (only the mandibular division has a motor component primarily supplying the muscles of mastication). The seventh cranial nerve, the facial nerve, is the 'great motor nerve' of the head, supplying primarily the muscles of facial expression (only the nervus intermedius component has a major sensory element, associated with taste).

The cutaneous innervation of the face

Three large areas of the face can be mapped out to indicate the peripheral nerve fields associated with the three divisions of the trigeminal nerve (Figure 6.1). Embryologically, each division of the trigeminal nerve is associated with a developing facial process which gives rise in the adult to a particular area of the face. The mandibular nerve is associated with the mandibular process of the first pharyngeal (branchial) arch, the maxillary nerve with the maxillary process from the first arch, and the ophthalmic nerve with the frontonasal process overlying the developing prosencephalon.

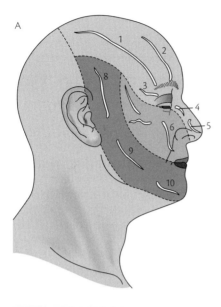

1 Supraorbital nerve – V1
2 Supratrochlear nerve – V1
3 Lacrimal nerve – V1
4 Infratrochlear nerve – V1
5 External nasal nerve – V1
6 Infraorbital nerve – V2
7 Zygomaticofacial and zygomaticotemporal nerves – V2
8 Auriculotemporal nerve – V3
9 Buccal nerve – V3
10 Mental nerve – V3

1. Supraorbital nerve and artery
2. Supratrochlear nerve and artery
3. External nasal nerve
4. Branch of lacrimal nerve
5. Infraorbital nerve
6. Mental nerve

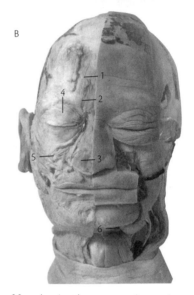

Figure 6.1 A The cutaneous innervation of the face **B** Frontal view of face showing the cutaneous innervation

The cutaneous branches of the mandibular nerve

The area supplied by the mandibular nerve includes the skin overlying the mandible, the lower lip, the fleshy part of the cheek, part of the auricle, and part of the temple. It has three cutaneous branches:

* The *mental nerve* is a branch of the inferior alveolar nerve. It emerges onto the face through the mental foramen of the mandible. It supplies the skin of the lower lip and the skin overlying the mandible (except around the angle of the mandible)

* The *buccal branch of the mandibular nerve* is sometimes referred to as the long buccal nerve to distinguish it from the buccal branch of the facial nerve. It emerges onto the face from behind the ramus of the mandible to supply the skin overlying the fleshy part of the cheek

* The *auriculotemporal nerve* appears on the face behind the temporomandibular joint, and ascends over the zygomatic arch. It supplies the tragus, concha, external acoustic meatus and tympanic membrane of the ear, and the posterior part of the temple (beard part of the temple).

The cutaneous branches of the maxillary nerve

The maxillary nerve supplies the skin of the lower eyelid, the prominence of the cheek, the ala part of the nose, part of the temple, and the upper lip. It has three cutaneous branches:

* The *infraorbital nerve*, the largest cutaneous branch of the maxillary nerve, emerges onto the face through the infraorbital foramen. As well as supplying skin overlying the maxilla, it gives off

palpebral branches to the lower eyelid, nasal branches to the ala of the nose, and labial branches to the
upper lip

- The *zygomaticofacial nerve* is one of the two branches
of the zygomatic nerve. It emerges from the orbit
onto the face at the zygomaticofacial foramen. It
supplies skin overlying the prominence of the cheek

- The *zygomaticotemporal nerve* is the remaining
branch of the zygomatic nerve. It enters the temporal fossa via the zygomaticotemporal foramen on
the deep surface of the zygomatic bone. It supplies
skin over the anterior part of the temple (non-beard
part of temple).

The cutaneous branches of the ophthalmic nerve

This nerve has three branches (frontal, nasociliary, and
lacrimal) which are distributed to the face. The area
supplied is extensive, including the forehead, the upper
eyelid, and much of the external surface of the nose. Five
nerves are concerned with the cutaneous innervation:

- The *supraorbital nerve* is the largest ophthalmic
branch on the face. It is one of the two terminal
branches of the frontal nerve. It emerges from the
orbit through the supraorbital notch (or foramen)
and supplies much of the forehead and most of the
upper eyelid

- The *supratrochlear nerve* supplies a small area of skin
over the medial part of the forehead and over the
medial part of the upper eyelid. It is also a terminal
branch of the frontal nerve and emerges from the
orbit medial to the supraorbital nerve. Its name
indicates that it runs above the trochlea associated
with the superior oblique muscle of the eye

- The *infratrochlear nerve* is one of the two terminal
branches of the nasociliary nerve (the other being
the anterior ethmoidal nerve). It supplies skin over
the bridge of the nose and at the medial corner of
the upper eyelid. As its name suggests, it leaves the
orbit below the trochlea associated with the superior
oblique muscle

- The *external nasal nerve* is the terminal part of the
anterior ethmoidal nerve. It supplies the skin of the
nose below the nasal bones (excluding the ala portion around the external nares)

- The *lacrimal nerve* is the smallest branch of the
ophthalmic nerve. It emerges from the upper lateral
margin of the orbit to supply the lateral part of the
upper eyelid.

The great auricular nerve

One part of the face which does not receive its cutaneous innervation from the trigeminal nerve is the
angle of the mandible. The skin in this region is supplied by the great auricular nerve. This nerve is derived
from the cervical plexus (anterior primary rami of the
second and third cervical nerves). Appearing at the
posterior border of the sternocleidomastoid muscle, it
passes forwards and upwards across the muscle to
reach the angle of the mandible.

The mandibular nerve

The mandibular nerve (Figure 6.2) is the largest division of the trigeminal nerve and is the only one which
contains motor as well as sensory fibres. Developmentally, it is the nerve of the first pharyngeal
(branchial) arch and is thus responsible for supplying
structures derived from it. Its sensory fibres supply the
mandibular teeth and their supporting structures, the
mucosa of the anterior two-thirds of the tongue and
the floor of the mouth, and the skin of the lower part
of the face (including the lower lip and parts of the
temporal region and auricle). Its motor fibres supply
the four muscles of mastication and the mylohyoid,
anterior belly of digastric, tensor veli palatini, and
tensor tympani muscles.

The mandibular nerve is formed in the infratemporal fossa by the union of the sensory and motor
roots immediately after they leave the skull at the
foramen ovale. Within the foramen ovale, the motor
root (or roots) lie posteromedially to the sensory root
and these roots are accompanied by emissary veins, the
lesser petrosal nerve (from the glossopharyngeal nerve)
going to the otic ganglion, and by the accessory
meningeal artery. As the mandibular nerve leaves the
foramen ovale, it lies on the tensor veli palatini muscle
and is covered laterally by the upper head of the lateral
pterygoid muscle (slightly anterior to the neck of the
mandible). After a short course, the nerve divides into
a smaller anterior trunk and a larger posterior trunk.
Before this division, the main trunk gives off two
branches—the meningeal branch and the nerve to
medial pterygoid. The anterior trunk of the mandibular nerve is mainly motor, the posterior trunk
mainly sensory.

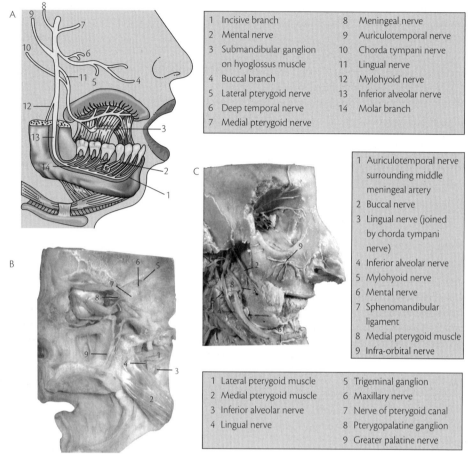

1	Incisive branch	8	Meningeal nerve
2	Mental nerve	9	Auriculotemporal nerve
3	Submandibular ganglion on hyoglossus muscle	10	Chorda tympani nerve
4	Buccal branch	11	Lingual nerve
5	Lateral pterygoid nerve	12	Mylohyoid nerve
6	Deep temporal nerve	13	Inferior alveolar nerve
7	Medial pterygoid nerve	14	Molar branch

1	Auriculotemporal nerve surrounding middle meningeal artery
2	Buccal nerve
3	Lingual nerve (joined by chorda tympani nerve)
4	Inferior alveolar nerve
5	Mylohyoid nerve
6	Mental nerve
7	Sphenomandibular ligament
8	Medial pterygoid muscle
9	Infra-orbital nerve

1	Lateral pterygoid muscle	5	Trigeminal ganglion
2	Medial pterygoid muscle	6	Maxillary nerve
3	Inferior alveolar nerve	7	Nerve of pterygoid canal
4	Lingual nerve	8	Pterygopalatine ganglion
		9	Greater palatine nerve

Figure 6.2 A The mandibular nerve. **B** Medial view of infratemporal fossa showing the medial pterygoid muscle and the mandibular nerve **C** Infratemporal fossa of left side viewed posteriorly showing pterygoid muscles

Branches of the mandibular nerve

- Meningeal branch (nervus spinosus)

- Nerve to medial pterygoid

- Anterior trunk: masseteric nerve, deep temporal nerves, nerve to lateral pterygoid and buccal nerve

- Posterior trunk: auriculotemporal nerve, lingual nerve and inferior alveolar nerve (and nerve to mylohyoid).

The *meningeal branch of the mandibular nerve (nervus spinosus)* arises from the main trunk of the mandibular nerve. It is a 'recurrent nerve' as it runs back into the middle cranial fossa through the foramen spinosum. It supplies the dura mater lining the middle and anterior cranial fossae and the mucosa of the mastoid antrum and mastoid air cells.

The *nerve to the medial pterygoid muscle* enters the deep surface of the muscle and also gives slender branches that pass uninterrupted through the otic ganglion to supply the tensor tympani and tensor veli palatini muscles.

The *masseteric nerve* is usually the first branch of the anterior trunk of the mandibular nerve. It passes above the upper border of the lateral pterygoid muscle (accompanying the posterior deep temporal nerve) and then crosses the mandibular notch (between the condylar and coronoid processes) to be distributed into the masseter muscle. It also gives an articular branch to the temporomandibular joint. The nerve enters the masseter muscle as two branches. The upper branch is smaller and runs to the deeper layers of the muscle. The larger, lower trunk innervates the more superficial layers of the masseter muscle.

The *deep temporal nerves* also pass above the lateral pterygoid muscle. Anatomists have provided varying descriptions for them. Anterior, middle, and posterior deep temporal nerves may be recognized.

The *nerve to the lateral pterygoid muscle* may arise separately or may run with the buccal nerve before entering the deep surface of the lateral pterygoid muscle.

The *buccal branch of the mandibular nerve* is the only sensory branch of the anterior trunk of the mandibular nerve. On emerging between the upper and lower heads of the lateral pterygoid muscle, it passes downwards and forwards across the lower head to contact the medial surface of the temporalis muscle as it inserts onto the coronoid process of the mandible. It then clears the ramus of the mandible to lie on the lateral surface of the buccinator muscle in the cheek. At this point, it is close to the retromolar fossa of the mandible. It now gives branches to the skin of the cheek (see Figure 6.1) before piercing the buccinator to supply its lining mucosa, the buccal sulcus, and the buccal gingiva related to the mandibular molar and premolar teeth. It may also carry secretomotor fibres to minor salivary glands in the buccal mucosa, these being post-ganglionic fibres from the otic ganglion. The buccal branch of the mandibular nerve may be seen to 'anastomose' with the buccal branches of the facial nerve.

The *auriculotemporal nerve* is the first branch of the posterior trunk of the mandibular nerve. It is essentially sensory but it also distributes autonomic fibres to the parotid gland derived from the otic ganglion. It usually arises as two roots (approximately 75% of cases) that encircle the middle meningeal artery and unite behind the artery. The nerve then runs backwards under the lateral pterygoid muscle to lie beneath the mandibular condyle (between the condyle and the sphenomandibular ligament). On entering the parotid region, it turns to emerge superficially between the temporomandibular joint and the external acoustic meatus. From the upper surface of the parotid gland, the auriculotemporal nerve ascends on the side of the head with the superficial temporal vessels, passing over the posterior part of the zygomatic arch. It gives several branches along its course:

◆ *Ganglionic branches* which communicate with the otic ganglion

◆ *Articular branches* which enter the posterior part of the temporomandibular joint; these carry proprioceptive information important in mastication

◆ *Parotid branches* which convey parasympathetic secretomotor fibres and sympathetic fibres to the parotid gland; these fibres are related to the otic ganglion. Sensory fibres from the auriculotemporal nerve supply the gland (with the exception of the capsule, which is innervated by the great auricular nerve)

◆ *Auricular branches* (usually two) which supply the tragus and crus of the helix of the auricle, part of the external acoustic meatus, and the outer (lateral) surface of the tympanic membrane

◆ *Superficial temporal branches* which are cutaneous nerves supplying part of the skin of the temple (see Figure 6.1).

The *lingual nerve* is the second branch of the posterior trunk of the mandibular nerve. It is essentially a sensory nerve but, following union with the chorda tympani branch of the facial nerve, it also contains parasympathetic fibres. Initially, the nerve lies on the tensor veli palatini muscle deep to the lateral pterygoid muscle. Here, the chorda tympani nerve (which has entered the infratemporal fossa via the petrotympanic fissure and passed over the spine of the sphenoid bone) joins the posterior surface of the lingual nerve. After emerging from the inferior border of the lateral pterygoid muscle, the lingual nerve curves downwards and forwards in the space between the ramus of the mandible and the medial pterygoid muscle (pterygomandibular space). At this level, it lies anterior to, and slightly deeper than, the inferior alveolar nerve. The lingual nerve then leaves the infratemporal fossa, passing downwards and forwards to lie close to the lingual alveolar plate of the mandibular third molar. Before curving forwards into the tongue, the nerve is found above the origin of the mylohyoid muscle and lateral to the hyoglossus muscle.

The close relationship of the lingual nerve to the third molar tooth makes the nerve susceptible to damage during removal of the tooth. In addition, in about one in seven cases, the lingual nerve is actually located above the lingual bony plate in the third molar region and is liable to damage during surgery.

The lingual nerve supplies the mucosa covering the anterior two-thirds of the dorsum of the tongue, the ventral surface of the tongue, the floor of the mouth, and the lingual gingivae of the mandibular teeth. The chorda tympani fibres travelling with the lingual nerve are of two types: sensory and parasympathetic. The sensory fibres are associated with taste for the anterior two-thirds of the dorsum of the tongue. The parasympathetic fibres are preganglionic fibres that pass to the submandibular ganglion. Postganglionic fibres are distributed to the submandibular and sublingual salivary glands.

The *chorda tympani branch* of the facial nerve is distributed through the lingual nerve and has two types of fibres. Sensory fibres are associated with taste to the anterior two-thirds of the tongue. Parasympathetic fibres are preganglionic to the submandibular ganglion. Postganglionic fibres are secretomotor to the submandibular and sublingual glands.

The *inferior alveolar nerve* is the largest branch of the mandibular division of the trigeminal nerve. It is the third branch of the posterior trunk of the mandibular nerve. Although it is essentially a sensory nerve, it also carries motor fibres which are given off as the mylohyoid nerve. Indeed, the mylohyoid nerve contains all the motor fibres of the posterior trunk of the mandibular nerve. The inferior alveolar nerve descends deep to the lateral pterygoid muscle, posterior to the lingual nerve in the pterygoid hiatus. Here, it is crossed by the maxillary artery. On emerging at the inferior border of the muscle, it passes between the sphenomandibular ligament and the ramus of the mandible to enter the mandibular foramen. It is accompanied in its course by inferior alveolar blood vessels.

The *mylohyoid nerve* is given off just before the mandibular foramen. It pierces the sphenomandibular ligament and runs in a groove (the mylohyoid groove) which lies immediately below the mandibular foramen. The mylohyoid nerve supplies the mylohyoid muscle and the anterior belly of the digastric. The mylohyoid nerve may also contain sensory fibres that supply the skin of the chin and medial parts of the submandibular triangle in the suprahyoid region.

The main distribution of the inferior alveolar nerve is to the mandibular teeth and their supporting structures, there being molar and incisive branches. The mental nerve is a cutaneous branch that supplies the skin of the chin and the lower lip. It arises within the mandible in the premolar region, but soon exits onto the face via the mental foramen (see Figure 6.1).

The trigeminal nerve, although not specifically having parasympathetic fibres, is associated with the parasympathetic ganglia of the head and indeed conveys postganglionic parasympathetic fibres to target organs. The mandibular nerve in this context is associated with the otic ganglion in the infratemporal fossa and the submandibular ganglion in the floor of the mouth.

The otic ganglion

This parasympathetic ganglion lies immediately below the foramen ovale on the medial surface of the main trunk of the mandibular nerve. It is concerned primarily with supplying the parotid gland. Like other parasympathetic ganglia in the head, three types of fibres are associated with it: parasympathetic, sympathetic, and sensory fibres. However, only the parasympathetic fibres synapse in the ganglion. The preganglionic parasympathetic fibres originate from the inferior salivatory nucleus in the brainstem. The fibres pass out in the glossopharyngeal nerve, appearing as the lesser (superficial) petrosal nerve from the tympanic plexus in the middle ear cavity. The lesser petrosal nerve reaches the otic ganglion by a complex course. Passing through the petrous part of the temporal bone, the lesser petrosal nerve comes to lie in the floor of the middle cranial fossa. Here, it is lateral to the greater (superficial) petrosal branch of the facial nerve. The lesser petrosal nerve usually enters the infratemporal fossa through the foramen ovale to join the otic ganglion. On occasion, the lesser petrosal nerve passes through the sphenopetrosal fissure. The sympathetic root of the otic ganglion is derived from postganglionic fibres from the superior cervical ganglion. They are said to reach the otic ganglion from the plexus on the middle meningeal artery. Other descriptions have it that the sympathetic root arises from the deep petrosal nerve or directly from the internal carotid plexus. The sensory root is derived from the auriculotemporal nerve. The postganglionic parasympathetic fibres (with sympathetic and sensory components) reach the parotid gland by way of the auriculotemporal nerve. Parasympathetic fibres may also innervate the minor salivary glands in the cheek, passing with the buccal branch of the mandibular nerve.

The submandibular ganglion

This parasympathetic ganglion is found in the floor of the mouth, on the superficial surface of the hyoglossus muscle and under cover of the mylohyoid muscle. The ganglion lies between the lingual nerve and the deep part of the submandibular gland. Indeed, it is suspended by two roots from the lingual nerve. The prime function of the submandibular ganglion is to supply the submandibular and sublingual salivary glands.

In common with the other parasympathetic ganglia in the head, the submandibular ganglion has a parasympathetic, a sympathetic, and a sensory supply. Only the parasympathetic fibres synapse within the ganglion. Preganglionic parasympathetic fibres originate from the superior salivatory nucleus in the brain stem. The fibres pass with the nervus intermedius of the facial nerve into the internal acoustic meatus and exit the skull with the chorda tympani nerve at the petrotympanic fissure. The chorda tympani nerve joins the lingual nerve in the infratemporal fossa and by this route the parasympathetic fibres reach the submandibular ganglion. It is claimed that the preganglionic parasympathetic fibres pass via the posterior root linking the ganglion to the lingual nerve. The sympathetic supply to the ganglion is derived from the superior cervical ganglion. It reaches the submandibular ganglion via the sympathetic nerve plexus surrounding the facial artery. The sensory supply arises from the adjacent lingual nerve.

Branches from the ganglion pass directly to the submandibular gland. The sublingual gland, however, is supplied by fibres which re-enter the lingual nerve by the anterior connecting root.

The innervation of the temporomandibular joint

The temporomandibular joint is richly innervated, particularly its upper aspect. Of special significance are the encapsulated proprioceptive nerve endings important in the reflex control of mastication. Free nerve endings associated with nociception are also present. Innervation for the joint is provided by the auriculotemporal, masseteric, and deep temporal nerves. The auriculotemporal branch of the mandibular division of the trigeminal nerve winds around the back of the temporomandibular joint, between it and the external acoustic meatus, before ascending in front of the tragus of the auricle to the temporal region. It provides multiple branches supplying the temporomandibular joint. The masseteric branch of the mandibular division of the trigeminal nerve passes through the mandibular notch to enter the posterior surface of the masseter muscle and, during its course, also gives multiple branches supplying the temporomandibular joint. The (posterior) deep temporal branch of the mandibular division of the trigeminal nerve arises in the infratemporal fossa and, passing up to supply the temporalis muscle, provides a branch to the temporomandibular joint. Additional sources of supply for the temporomandibular joint have been reported to be provided by the facial nerve and the otic ganglion.

The maxillary nerve

This division of the trigeminal nerve (the fifth cranial nerve) contains only sensory fibres. Functionally, it supplies the maxillary teeth and their supporting structures, the hard and soft palate, the maxillary air sinus, much of the nasal cavity, and skin overlying the middle part of the face.

The maxillary nerve (Figure 6.3) arises from the trigeminal ganglion on the floor of the middle cranial fossa. It passes along the lateral dural wall of the cavernous sinus to exit the cranial cavity at the foramen rotundum. It emerges from the foramen rotundum in the upper part of the pterygopalatine fossa, where most of the branches are derived. These branches can be classified into those which come directly from the maxillary nerve and those which are associated with the pterygopalatine parasympathetic ganglion.

Branches from the main maxillary nerve trunk

- ◆ Meningeal nerve
- ◆ Ganglionic branches
- ◆ Zygomatic nerve, zygomaticotemporal nerve, zygomaticofacial nerve
- ◆ Posterior superior alveolar nerve
- ◆ Infraorbital nerve, middle superior alveolar nerve, anterior superior alveolar nerve.

Branches from the pterygopalatine ganglion

- ◆ Orbital nerve
- ◆ Nasopalatine nerve
- ◆ Posterior superior nasal nerve
- ◆ Posterior inferior nasal nerve
- ◆ Greater (anterior) palatine nerve
- ◆ Lesser (posterior) palatine nerve
- ◆ Pharyngeal branch.

The meningeal nerve is the only branch from the main trunk of the maxillary nerve that does not originate in the pterygopalatine fossa; it arises within the middle cranial fossa, before the foramen rotundum. It runs with the middle meningeal artery and innervates the dura mater lining the middle cranial fossa.

The ganglionic branches are usually two in number and connect the maxillary nerve to the pterygopalatine ganglion.

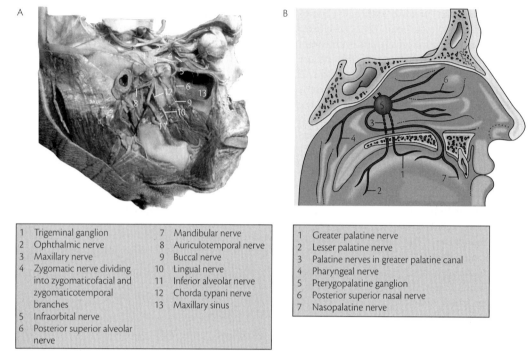

1	Trigeminal ganglion	7	Mandibular nerve
2	Ophthalmic nerve	8	Auriculotemporal nerve
3	Maxillary nerve	9	Buccal nerve
4	Zygomatic nerve dividing into zygomaticofacial and zygomaticotemporal branches	10	Lingual nerve
		11	Inferior alveolar nerve
		12	Chorda typani nerve
		13	Maxillary sinus
5	Infraorbital nerve		
6	Posterior superior alveolar nerve		

1	Greater palatine nerve
2	Lesser palatine nerve
3	Palatine nerves in greater palatine canal
4	Pharyngeal nerve
5	Pterygopalatine ganglion
6	Posterior superior nasal nerve
7	Nasopalatine nerve

Figure 6.3 A The course of the maxillary nerve **B** Branches of the pterygopalatine ganglion

The zygomatic nerve leaves the pterygopalatine fossa through the inferior orbital fissure. It passes along the lateral wall of the orbit before dividing into zygomaticotemporal and zygomaticofacial branches. These pass through the zygomatic bone to supply overlying skin (see Figure 6.1). The zygomaticotemporal nerve exits the zygomatic bone at its temporal (medial) surface. It pierces the temporal fascia to supply skin over the temple. The zygomaticotemporal nerve also gives a branch to the lacrimal nerve, which carries autonomic fibres to the lacrimal gland. The zygomaticofacial nerve leaves the zygomatic bone on its lateral surface to supply skin overlying the prominence of the cheek.

The posterior superior alveolar nerve(s) is one of three superior alveolar nerves that supply the maxillary teeth. The middle and anterior superior alveolar nerves are branches of the infraorbital nerve (see below). The posterior superior alveolar nerve(s) leaves the pterygopalatine fossa through the pterygomaxillary fissure. Thence, it runs onto the tuberosity of the maxilla and eventually pierces the bone to supply the maxillary molar teeth and the maxillary sinus. Before entering the maxilla, the nerve provides a gingival branch which innervates the buccal gingivae around the maxillary molars. The extra-bony course of the posterior superior alveolar nerve is variable. The nerve can subdivide into several branches just before, and just after, it enters the maxilla. Alternatively, it may arise as several distinct branches at the main trunk of the maxillary nerve.

The infraorbital nerve can be regarded as the terminal branch of the maxillary nerve proper. It leaves the pterygopalatine fossa to enter the orbit at the inferior orbital fissure. Initially lying in a groove in the floor of the orbit (the infraorbital groove), the infraorbital nerve runs into a canal (the infraorbital canal) and passes onto the face at the infraorbital foramen (see Figure 6.1 for the cutaneous distribution of the nerve). The middle and anterior superior alveolar nerves arise from the infraorbital nerve in the orbit.

The infraorbital nerve supplies the conjunctiva and skin of the lower eyelid. It also innervates the skin over the upper jaw (see Figure 6.1).

The branches of the maxillary nerve that arise with the pterygopalatine ganglion contain not only sensory fibres from the maxillary nerve, but also autonomic fibres from the ganglion, which are mainly distributed to glands and blood vessels.

The orbital nerve passes from the pterygopalatine ganglion into the orbit through the inferior orbital fissure. It supplies periosteum and, via sympathetic fibres, the orbitalis muscle. The orbital nerve can also supply part of the maxillary sinus and may pass through the posterior ethmoidal foramen to innervate posterior ethmoidal air cells and the sphenoid air sinus. It may also connect with the ciliary ganglion.

The nasopalatine nerve runs medially from the pterygopalatine ganglion into the nasal cavity through the sphenopalatine foramen. It passes across the roof of the nasal cavity to reach the back of the nasal septum. The nasopalatine nerve then passes downwards and forwards within a groove on the vomer to supply the posteroinferior part of the nasal septum. It passes through the incisive canal, where it usually forms a single nerve with its fellow of the opposite side, and emerges on the hard palate at the incisive fossa to supply the oral mucosa around the incisive papilla and palatal gingiva of the anterior teeth.

The posterior superior nasal nerve enters the back of the nasal cavity through the sphenopalatine foramen. It divides into lateral and medial branches. The lateral branches supply the posterosuperior part of the lateral wall of the nasal fossa. The medial branches cross the roof of the nasal cavity to supply the nasal septum overlying the posterior part of the perpendicular plate of the ethmoid.

The posterior inferior nasal nerve supplies the inferior part of the lateral wall of the nose in the region of the inferior nasal concha. It may arise directly from the pterygopalatine ganglion or appear as a branch from the anterior palatine nerve.

The greater (anterior) palatine nerve passes downwards from the pterygopalatine ganglion, through the palatine canal, and onto the hard palate at the palatine foramen. Within the greater palatine canal, it can give off nasal branches that innervate the posteroinferior part of the lateral wall of the nasal fossa. On the palate, it runs forwards at the interface between the palatine process and the alveolar process of the maxilla to supply much of the mucosa of the hard palate and palatal gingivae (except around the incisive papilla).

The lesser (posterior) palatine nerve(s) passes downwards from the pterygopalatine ganglion initially through the palatine canal. It then passes through the lesser palatine canal in the pyramidal process of the palatine bone and onto the palate at the lesser palatine foramen (or foramina). It runs backwards to supply the soft palate.

The pharyngeal branch originates from the pterygopalatine ganglion and passes through the palatovaginal canal to supply the mucosa of the nasopharynx.

The palatovaginal canal is formed when the groove on the undersurface of the vaginal process of the sphenoid bone articulates with the upper surface of the sphenoid process of the palatine bone. The pharyngeal branch has also been reported to pass through the vomerovaginal canal, which generally transmits the pharyngeal branch of the sphenopalatine artery. The vomerovaginal canal lies between the upper surface of the vaginal process of the sphenoid bone and the ala of the vomer and is often continuous with the pterygoid canal.

The parasympathetic ganglion associated with the maxillary nerve is the pterygopalatine ganglion that is located within the pterygopalatine fossa.

The pterygopalatine ganglion

This parasympathetic ganglion is situated below the maxillary nerve in the pterygopalatine fossa, connected by two ganglionic branches. It is concerned primarily with supplying the nose, palate, and lacrimal gland.

As with other parasympathetic ganglia in the head, three types of fibres enter the pterygopalatine ganglion: parasympathetic, sympathetic, and sensory fibres. However, only the parasympathetic fibres synapse in the ganglion. The preganglionic parasympathetic fibres originate from the superior salivatory nucleus in the brainstem. The fibres pass with the nervus intermedius of the facial nerve. They subsequently emerge as the greater (superficial) petrosal nerve. This occurs within the facial canal of the temporal bone, close to the geniculate ganglion of the facial nerve. The greater petrosal nerve then passes through the bone to appear on the floor of the middle cranial fossa. It then runs medially in a shallow groove towards the foramen lacerum. Passing within the foramen lacerum, the greater petrosal nerve enters the pterygoid canal which lies at the base of the pterygoid process. After passing along the pterygoid canal, the nerve emerges into the pterygopalatine fossa and joins the pterygopalatine ganglion. Postganglionic sympathetic fibres run to the pterygopalatine ganglion by a complex course. From the superior cervical ganglion, sympathetic fibres run to the internal carotid plexus surrounding the internal carotid artery. From this plexus, a branch called the deep petrosal nerve is given off that enters the pterygoid canal to reach the pterygopalatine ganglion. The greater petrosal nerve and the deep petrosal nerve join within the pterygoid canal to become the nerve of the pterygoid canal. The sensory fibres to the ganglion run in the ganglionic branches of the maxillary nerve.

The nerves leaving the pterygopalatine ganglion are the orbital nerve, the nasopalatine nerve, the greater and lesser palatine nerves, the posterior superior and inferior nasal nerves, and the pharyngeal nerve. These nerves are described above with the maxillary nerve. The parasympathetic component will be distributed within these nerves to supply the minor salivary glands. The parasympathetic component of the pterygopalatine ganglion is also responsible for supplying the lacrimal gland. The fibres first pass from the ganglion in one of the ganglionic branches to the maxillary nerve. They then travel with the zygomatic and zygomatico-temporal branches. Within the orbit, they pass from the zygomaticotemporal nerve to the lacrimal nerve (of the ophthalmic nerve) to reach the lacrimal gland.

The ophthalmic nerve

The ophthalmic nerve (Figure 6.4) is a division of the trigeminal nerve (the fifth cranial nerve) and is a sensory nerve that travels through the orbit to supply primarily the upper part of the face. Developmentally, it is the nerve of the frontonasal process.

The trigeminal ganglion in the floor of the middle cranial fossa is the site where the ophthalmic nerve arises. The nerve passes along the lateral dural wall of the cavernous sinus and gives off three main branches just before the superior orbital fissure.

Branches of the ophthalmic nerve

- Lacrimal nerve
- Frontal nerve: supraorbital nerve, supratrochlear nerve
- Nasociliary nerve: sensory branches to the ciliary ganglion, long ciliary nerves, posterior ethmoidal nerve, anterior ethmoidal nerve (and external nasal nerve), infratrochlear nerve.

The *lacrimal nerve* enters the orbit through the superior orbital fissure, above the common tendinous ring of the recti muscles. Here, it is situated lateral to the frontal and trochlear nerves. The lacrimal nerve passes forwards along the lateral wall of the orbit on the superior border of the lateral rectus muscle. It passes through the lacrimal gland and the orbital septum to

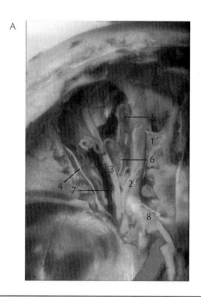

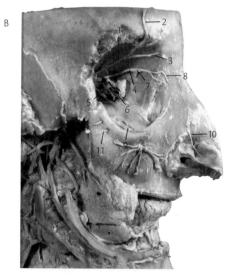

1	Superior oblique muscle	4	Lacrimal nerve
2	Trochlear nerve	5	Ophthalmic artery
3	Frontal nerve dividing into	6	Nasociliary nerve
	supraorbital and	7	Superior ophthalmic vein
	supratrochlear nerves	8	Optic nerve

1	Frontal nerve	7	Anterior ethmoidal nerve
2	Supra-orbital nerve	8	Infratrochlear nerve
3	Supratrochlear nerve	9	Infra-orbital nerve
4	Nasociliary nerve	10	External nasal nerve
5	Ciliary ganglion	11	Zygomaticofacial nerve
6	Short ciliary nerves		

Figure 6.4 A Orbit viewed from above showing distribution of nerves **B** View of medial wall of orbit showing distribution of nerves. See also Plate 4.

supply conjunctiva and skin covering the lateral part of the upper eyelid (see Figure 6.1). The lacrimal nerve communicates with the zygomatic branch of the maxillary nerve. By this means, parasympathetic fibres associated with the pterygopalatine ganglion are conveyed to the lacrimal gland.

The *frontal nerve* is the largest branch of the ophthalmic nerve. It enters the orbit through the superior orbital fissure, above the common tendinous ring of the recti muscles, and lies between the lacrimal nerve laterally and the trochlear nerve medially. The frontal nerve passes forwards on the levator palpebrae superioris muscle, towards the rim of the orbit. About halfway along this course, it divides into the supraorbital and supratrochlear nerves.

The *supraorbital nerve* is the larger of the terminal branches of the frontal nerve. It continues forwards along the levator palpebrae superioris muscle and leaves the orbit through the supraorbital notch (or foramen) to emerge onto the forehead. The supraorbital nerve supplies mucous membrane lining the frontal sinus, skin and conjunctiva covering the upper eyelid, and skin over the forehead and scalp (see Figure 6.1).

The *supratrochlear nerve* runs medially above the pulley for the superior oblique muscle. It gives a descending branch to the infratrochlear nerve and ascends onto the forehead through the frontal notch. It supplies skin and conjunctiva covering the upper eyelid, and skin over the forehead (see Figure 6.1).

The *nasociliary nerve* passes into the orbit through the superior orbital fissure, within the common tendinous ring of the recti muscles. Initially, the nerve lies lateral to the optic nerve. It then runs forwards and medially across the optic nerve and, coursing between the superior oblique and medial rectus muscles, comes to lie close to the medial wall of the orbit. Near the anterior ethmoidal foramen, the nasociliary nerve divides into its terminal branches: the anterior ethmoidal and infratrochlear nerves.

The first branches of the nasociliary nerve are sensory branches to the ciliary ganglion. They leave the ganglion in the short ciliary nerves, running to the eyeball to supply the cornea, the ciliary body, and the iris.

Two or three long ciliary branches arise from the nasociliary nerve as it crosses the optic nerve. These ciliary nerves pierce the sclera at the back of the eye and pass forwards to provide sensory innervation to the cornea and iris. They also distribute sympathetic fibres to the dilator pupillae muscle. The sympathetic fibres originate from the superior cervical ganglion.

They are postganglionic fibres which travel in the plexus surrounding the internal carotid artery. They join the ophthalmic nerve in the cavernous sinus.

The posterior ethmoidal nerve passes beneath the superior oblique muscle and leaves the orbit through the posterior ethmoidal foramen to enter the nose. It supplies the sphenoidal sinus and the posterior ethmoidal air cells.

The anterior ethmoidal nerve exits the orbit through the anterior ethmoidal foramen. It enters the anterior cranial fossa where the cribriform plate of the ethmoid bone meets the orbital part of the frontal bone. It then runs into the roof of the nose through a small foramen at the side of the crista galli. The anterior ethmoidal nerve supplies the anterior and middle ethmoidal air cells and some of the mucosa covering the nasal septum and the lateral wall of the nose. It terminates on the face as the external nasal nerve (see Figure 6.1).

The infratrochlear nerve passes forwards along the medial wall of the orbit below the pulley of the superior oblique muscle. It passes above the medial palpebral ligament to reach the side of the nose. It supplies the lacrimal sac, the caruncle, the conjunctiva at the medial canthus, and the skin on the medial aspect of the upper eyelid.

The parasympathetic ganglion associated with the ophthalmic nerve is the ciliary ganglion that is located within the orbit and is described in this chapter elsewhere.

The facial nerve

The facial nerve (Figure 6.5), the seventh cranial nerve, consists of two components: the motor facial nerve 'proper' and the nervus intermedius. The facial nerve 'proper' leaves the skull through the stylomastoid foramen. The nerve then passes over the styloid process of the temporal bone and its attached muscles to enter the parotid gland. Before entering the parotid, the facial nerve gives rise to a posterior auricular nerve and a digastric nerve.

The *posterior auricular nerve* supplies the auricular muscles (muscles of facial expression).

The *digastric nerve* supplies the posterior belly of the digastric muscle together with the accompanying stylohyoid muscle.

The facial nerve gives rise to five named branches: temporal, zygomatic, buccal, (marginal) mandibular, and cervical. These branches arise from two main trunks or divisions within the gland, namely the

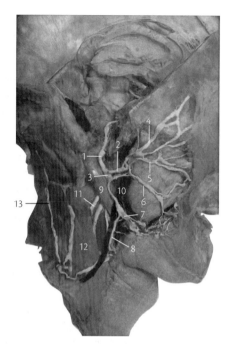

1	Facial nerve at stylomastoid faramen
2	Temporofacial branch of facial nerve
3	Cervicofacial branch of facial nerve
4	Temporal branch of facial nerve
5	Zygomatic branch of facial nerve
6	Buccal branch of facial nerve
7	Mandibular branch of facial nerve
8	Cervical branch of facial nerve
9	Posterior belly of digastic muscle
10	Retromandibular vein and external carotid artery
11	Spinal accessory nerve
12	Sternocleidomastoid muscle
13	Lesser occipital nerve

Figure 6.5 Lateral view of the face showing contents and deep relations of the parotid gland

temporofacial and the cervicofacial divisions. The temporal and zygomatic branches usually arise from the temporofacial division while the mandibular and cervical branches arise from the cervicofacial division. The buccal branch has a variable origin.

Within the parotid gland, the facial nerve divides into the temporofacial and cervicofacial divisions at a point termed the pes anserinus ('goose's foot'). Variations of these two main divisions are common. There are frequently many 'anastomoses' between them, thus forming a 'parotid plexus' within the substance of the gland. Six distinctive patterns can, however, be recognized. For the *Type I* pattern (13%), no 'anastomoses' occur between adjacent branches. For the *Type II* pattern (20%), an arcade of 'anastomoses' exists between the branches of the temporofacial division and usually occurs beyond the anterior border of the parotid. For the *Type III* pattern (28%), a single large 'anastomosis' occurs between the temporofacial and cervicofacial divisions (again beyond the anterior margin of the gland). For the *Type IV* pattern (24%), there are 'anastomotic' loops between the temporal and zygomatic branches, as well as connections within the gland between the cervicofacial division and the buccal and zygomatic branches. For the *Type V* pattern (9%) there

are connections between the cervicofacial division and the temporofacial division arising either from the buccal branch or directly from the point where the facial nerve trunk divides. Finally, for the *Type VI* pattern (6%), there is a marked plexus of 'anastomoses'. This is the only pattern of the facial nerve in which the (marginal) mandibular branch is reinforced by an 'anastomosis' from an adjacent branch.

The *temporal nerve* (three or four branches) crosses the zygomatic arch just anteriorly to the superficial temporal vessels. The nerve supplies the auricular muscles and the muscles of the forehead and orbicularis oculi.

The *zygomatic nerve* (one, two, or three branches) runs below the inferior border of the zygomatic arch. It also innervates the orbicularis oculi muscle and the muscles of the nose and the upper lip.

The *buccal branch of the facial nerve* has a variable origin from the cervicofacial and/or the temporofacial divisions. Usually, there is only one branch, occasionally two. A line drawn from the labial commissure to the tragus indicates the level of the buccal nerve. Where the nerve is single, it is usually found below the origin of the parotid duct. Where there are two branches, one branch passes above and one below the parotid duct. The buccal nerve passes beneath the zygomaticus muscle to supply the buccinator muscle and the muscles of the upper lip.

The *(marginal) mandibular nerve* (usually two branches) has an important surgical relationship with the lower border of the mandible (hence its name), usually running 1–2 cm below the border. The mandibular nerve supplies the muscles of the lower lip and lies deep to the platysma muscle but superficial to the investing layer of deep cervical fascia.

The *cervical nerve* also passes deep to the platysma muscle but superficial to the investing layer of deep cervical fascia. It runs behind the superficial part of the submandibular gland where it divides into several branches that supply the platysma muscle.

The innervation of the orodental tissues

The oral mucosa receives its sensory innervation primarily from the maxillary and mandibular divisions of the trigeminal nerve. The trigeminal nerve also supplies the teeth and their supporting tissues. The salivary glands are supplied by secretomotor, parasympathetic fibres from the facial and glossopharyngeal nerves. The motor innervation of the oral musculature is derived mainly from the mandibular, facial, accessory, and hypoglossal nerves.

The innervation of the teeth and gingivae

The dentition in the lower jaw is innervated by the mandibular nerve. The teeth receive their nerve supply from the molar and incisive branches of the inferior alveolar nerve. The lingual gingivae are supplied mainly by the lingual branch of the mandibular nerve.

The labial gingivae are innervated by the mental branch of the inferior alveolar nerve and the buccal gingivae by the buccal branch of the mandibular nerve.

The innervation of the dentition in the upper jaw is derived almost entirely from the maxillary nerve. The teeth are supplied by the anterior, middle, and posterior superior alveolar branches. The palatal gingivae are innervated by the nasopalatine and greater (anterior) palatine branches via the pterygopalatine ganglion. The labial and buccal gingivae are supplied by the infraorbital and the posterior superior alveolar branches.

Table 6.1 summarizes the nerve supply to the teeth and gingivae.

The inferior alveolar nerve

The inferior alveolar nerve (Figure 6.6) is the terminal branch of the posterior trunk of the mandibular nerve. It arises in the infratemporal fossa, deep to the lower head of the lateral pterygoid muscle. On emerging from beneath this muscle, the inferior alveolar nerve lies within the pterygomandibular space. Here, it gives off a mylohyoid branch which is a motor nerve to the anterior belly of the digastric muscle and the mylohyoid muscle (it may also have sensory fibres which enter the mandible in the mental region to participate in the nerve supply to the lower incisors). The inferior alveolar nerve enters the mandible through the mandibular foramen.

The course of the inferior alveolar nerve through the mandible is variable. The molar branches to the premolar and molar teeth come either directly from the inferior alveolar nerve in the mandibular canal by short or long branches, or indirectly from the nerve outside the mandibular canal by a series of alveolar

Table 6.1 Sensory innervation of teeth and gingivae. The teeth are numbered according to their position along the tooth row

	Nasopalatine nerve	Greater palatine nerve		Palatal gingiva
Maxilla	Anterior superior dental nerve	Middle superior alveolar nerve	Posterior superior alveolar nerve	Teeth
	Infraorbital nerve	Posterior superior alveolar and buccal nerve		Buccal gingiva
	1 2 3	4 5 6 7 8		
Mandible	Mental nerve	Buccal nerve and perforating branches of inferior alveolar nerve		Buccal gingiva
	Incisive nerve	Inferior alveolar nerve		Teeth
	Lingual nerve and perforating branches of inferior alveolar nerve			Lingual gingiva

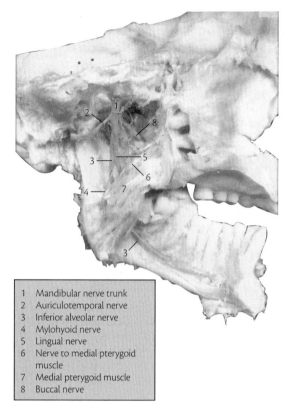

1	Mandibular nerve trunk
2	Auriculotemporal nerve
3	Inferior alveolar nerve
4	Mylohyoid nerve
5	Lingual nerve
6	Nerve to medial pterygoid muscle
7	Medial pterygoid muscle
8	Buccal nerve

Figure 6.6 Medial view of infratemporal fossa showing inferior alveolar nerve

branches. The mandibular canal may be closely related to the roots of the mandibular molars, even to the extent of occasionally perforating a root.

The main trunk of the inferior alveolar nerve divides near the premolars into mental and incisive nerves. The mental nerve runs for a short distance in a mental canal before leaving the body of the mandible at the mental foramen to emerge onto the face. It supplies the skin and mucosa of the lower lip, and the labial gingivae of the mandibular anterior teeth. The incisive nerve runs forwards in an incisive canal. This nerve usually innervates only the incisor and canine teeth, but occasionally it supplies the first premolar.

The superior alveolar nerves

There are usually three superior alveolar nerves (see Figure 6.3) supplying the maxillary dentition: the posterior, middle, and anterior superior alveolar nerves.

The *posterior superior alveolar nerve* arises from the maxillary nerve in the pterygopalatine fossa. It

descends onto the posterior wall of the maxilla, passing through the pterygomaxillary fissure, and divides into dental and gingival branches. The dental branches enter the maxilla and run in narrow canals above the roots of the molar teeth. The gingival branch does not enter the bone but runs along the outer surface of the maxillary tuberosity to supply the buccal gingivae of the maxillary molar teeth.

The *middle superior alveolar nerve* is found in about 70% of individuals. The nerve generally arises in the floor of the orbit from the infraorbital branch of the maxillary nerve. It can also arise directly from the maxillary nerve in the pterygopalatine fossa. The middle superior alveolar nerve runs in the posterior, lateral, or anterior wall of the maxillary air sinus. It terminates above the roots of the premolar teeth.

The *anterior superior alveolar nerve* arises from the infraorbital nerve within the infraorbital canal. It generally appears as a single nerve, occasionally as two or three branches. The nerve runs in the anterior wall of the maxillary sinus and terminates near the anterior nasal spine after giving off a small nasal branch.

The three superior alveolar nerves form a plexus just above the roots of the maxillary teeth. Indeed, it is difficult to trace the precise innervation of the teeth from a specific superior alveolar nerve. As a general rule, however, the incisors and canine are supplied by the anterior nerve, the molars by the posterior nerve, and the premolars by the middle nerve.

The sensory innervation of the lips and cheeks

The mucosa of the upper lip is supplied by the infraorbital branch of the maxillary nerve. The lower lip is innervated by the mental branch of the mandibular nerve. The mucosa of the cheeks is innervated by the buccal branch of the mandibular nerve.

The *buccal nerve* is the terminal branch of the anterior trunk of the mandibular nerve. It arises in the infratemporal fossa, behind the upper head of the lateral pterygoid muscle. The buccal nerve passes between the two heads of the lateral pterygoid muscle and crosses the infratemporal fossa. It runs into the upper part of the retromolar fossa at the anterior border of the ramus of the mandible. The buccal nerve breaks up into several branches within the buccinator muscle. It innervates both the mucosa and the skin of the cheek and the buccal gingivae of the mandibular cheek teeth (perhaps even of the maxillary cheek teeth).

The sensory innervation of the tongue and the floor of the mouth

Concerning general sensation (i.e. excluding taste), three distinct nerve fields can be recognized on the dorsum of the tongue. The anterior part of the tongue, in front of the circumvallate papillae, is supplied by the lingual branches of the mandibular nerves (see Figure 6.2). Behind, and including, the circumvallate papillae, the tongue is innervated primarily by the glossopharyngeal nerves. Small areas on the posterior part of the tongue around the epiglottis are supplied by the superior laryngeal branches (internal branches) of the vagus nerves. Concerning taste, the anterior part of the tongue is innervated by the chorda tympani branches of the facial nerves. These are distributed through the lingual nerves. The posterior part of the tongue, including the circumvallate papillae, has a similar innervation for taste as that for general sensation.

The mucosa on the ventral surface of the tongue and on the floor of the mouth is supplied by the lingual branches of the mandibular nerves.

The *lingual nerve* is derived from the posterior trunk of the mandibular nerve within the infratemporal fossa. It receives the chorda tympani branch of the facial nerve beneath the lateral pterygoid muscle. At the level of the mandibular foramen, the lingual nerve lies on the medial pterygoid muscle and is anterior to the inferior alveolar nerve. The lingual nerve then leaves the infratemporal fossa, passing downwards and forwards to lie close to the lingual alveolar plate of the mandibular third molar tooth. Before curving forwards into the tongue, the nerve is found above the origin of the mylohyoid muscle and lateral to the hyoglossus muscle. On the superficial surface of the hyoglossus muscle, the lingual nerve twists twice around the submandibular salivary duct, first on the lateral side of the duct and then on the medial side. It enters the tongue behind the sublingual salivary gland. Suspended from the lingual nerve as it runs across the hyoglossus muscle is the submandibular parasympathetic ganglion.

The lingual nerve itself supplies the mucosa covering the anterior two-thirds of the dorsum of the tongue, the ventral surface of the tongue, the floor of the mouth, and the lingual gingivae of the mandibular teeth.

The chorda tympani fibres travelling with the lingual nerve are of two types: sensory and parasympathetic. The sensory fibres are associated with taste for the anterior two-thirds of the dorsum of the tongue. The parasympathetic fibres are preganglionic fibres that pass to the submandibular ganglion. Postganglionic fibres are distributed to the submandibular and sublingual salivary glands.

The sensory innervation of the palate

The sensory supply to the palate (Figure 6.3) is derived mainly from branches of the maxillary nerve via the pterygopalatine ganglion. A small area behind the incisor teeth is supplied by the nasopalatine nerves. The remainder of the hard palate is innervated by the greater palatine nerves. The soft palate is supplied by the lesser palatine nerves. There is evidence to suggest that some areas supplied by the lesser palatine nerves may also be innervated from the facial nerves. The posterior part of the soft palate and the uvula may be supplied by the glossopharyngeal nerves.

The *nasopalatine nerve* runs along the nasal septum from the pterygopalatine ganglion and emerges onto the hard palate at the incisive fossa behind the maxillary first incisor teeth. The nasopalatine nerve innervates the gingivae behind the maxillary incisor teeth.

The *greater and lesser palatine nerves* pass from the pterygopalatine ganglion, down the greater palatine canal at the back of the lateral wall of the nose. The greater palatine nerve runs through the greater palatine foramen and onto the back of the hard palate. It passes towards the front of the hard palate at the interface between the palatine and alveolar processes of the maxilla. In addition to supplying the mucosa of the palate, the greater palatine nerve innervates the palatal gingivae for the maxillary cheek teeth. The lesser palatine nerve emerges onto the palate at the lesser palatine foramen. It runs backwards into the soft palate.

The sensory innervation of the oropharyngeal isthmus

The mucosa over the pillars of the fauces is supplied by the glossopharyngeal nerve.

The innervation of the oral musculature

The innervation of the various muscles associated with the mouth is derived from the mandibular division of the trigeminal, the facial, the cranial part of the accessory and the hypoglossal cranial nerves, and the first cervical spinal nerves. The innervation is summarized in Table 6.2.

Table 6.2 Innervation of the oral musculature

Region	Muscle	Nerve
Lips	Orbicularis oculi	Facial
Cheeks	Buccinator	Facial
Tongue (intrinsic musculature)	Transverse Longitudinal Vertical	Hypoglossal
Tongue (extrinsic musculature)	Genioglossus Hyoglossus Styloglossus	Hypoglossal
	Palatoglossus	Accessory (cranial part)
Floor of mouth	Mylohyoid	Mandibular division of trigeminal
	Geniohyoid	First cervical spinal nerve (via hypoglossal)
Palate	Tensor veli palatini	Mandibular division of trigeminal
	Levator veli palatini; Palatoglossus; Palatopharyngeus; Salpingopharyngeus; Musculus uvulae	Accessory (cranial part)

The innervation of the salivary glands

The lesser petrosal branch of the glossopharyngeal nerve supplies the parotid gland via the otic parasympathetic ganglion. Postganglionic fibres pass to the gland through the auriculotemporal branch of the mandibular nerve.

The greater petrosal branch of the facial nerve probably supplies palatal and pharyngeal glands via the pterygopalatine parasympathetic ganglion. Postganglionic fibres reach the palate with the nasopalatine, greater palatine, and lesser palatine branches of the maxillary nerve.

The chorda tympani branch of the facial nerve provides secretomotor fibres parasympathetic to the submandibular and sublingual salivary glands via the submandibular ganglion. It probably also provides the innervation of minor salivary glands in the lips, cheeks and tongue.

The innervation of the nasal cavity

Special sensation related to olfaction is associated with the olfactory nerves (i.e. the first cranial nerves). General sensation to the nasal mucosa is related to branches from the ophthalmic and maxillary divisions of the trigeminal nerves (i.e. the fifth cranial nerves).

The olfactory epithelium is located in the roof of the nasal cavity, extending onto the lateral walls of the nasal fossae (above the superior nasal conchae) and the uppermost part of the nasal septum. Filaments of the olfactory nerves (about 20 on each side) pass upwards through the cribiform plate of the ethmoid bone into the cranial cavity to synapse in the olfactory bulbs. Each filament is ensheathed by the meninges. Thus, a potential pathway exists for the spread of infection from the nose to the cranial cavity.

The anterior ethmoidal nerve is the only branch of the ophthalmic nerve which supplies the nasal mucosa. It arises from the nasociliary nerve and mainly supplies an area in front of the nasal conchae (it also innervates the anterior extremities of the middle and inferior conchae). After leaving the orbit through the anterior ethmoidal foramen, the anterior ethmoidal nerve enters the cranial cavity onto the cribiform plate of the ethmoid. It leaves the cranial cavity through a small slit near the crista galli and enters the roof of the nasal cavity. Here, the nerve runs in a groove on the inner surface of the nasal bone. The anterior ethmoidal nerve passes downwards and forwards and gives rise to lateral and medial internal nasal branches. The lateral internal nasal branches pass to the lateral wall of the nose whereas the medial internal nasal branches run to the nasal septum. When the anterior ethmoidal nerve emerges at the inferior margin of the nasal bone it becomes the external nasal nerve.

The maxillary nerve contributes many branches which supply the nasal mucosa. The infraorbital and the posterior superior alveolar nerves arise directly from the maxillary nerve. The posterior superior nasal, greater palatine and nasopalatine nerves arise indirectly by way of the pterygopalatine ganglion.

The infraorbital nerve is the terminal branch of the maxillary nerve. After passing onto the face at the infraorbital foramen, it provides a nasal branch which supplies the skin of the vestibule and the mobile part of the nasal septum. The anterior superior alveolar branch of the infraorbital nerve also supplies nasal mucosa. Its nasal branch passes through a small canal in the lateral wall of the nose (below the level of the inferior concha) to innervate the anterior part of the inferior meatus and the adjacent part of the floor of the nose and adjoining nasal septum.

The posterior superior nasal nerve originates at the pterygopalatine ganglion. It enters the back of the nasal cavity through the sphenopalatine foramen and gives off lateral and medial branches. The lateral branches supply the posterosuperior part of the lateral wall of the nose around the superior and middle nasal conchae. The medial branches cross the roof of the nasal cavity to supply the septum overlying the posterior part of the perpendicular plate of the ethmoid.

The greater (anterior) palatine nerve also arises from the pterygopalatine ganglion. It descends in the greater palatine canal where it gives off posterior inferior nasal branches. These branches pass through small openings in the perpendicular plate of the palatine bone to supply the posteroinferior portion of the lateral wall of the nose (below, and including, the middle meatus).

The nasopalatine nerve passes from the pterygopalatine ganglion into the nasal cavity through the sphenopalatine foramen. It runs across the roof of the nasal cavity to reach the back of the nasal septum. It then passes downwards and forwards, lying in a groove on the vomer, to supply the posteroinferior part of the septum. The floor of the nose is supplied anteriorly by the nasal branch of the anterior superior alveolar nerve and posteriorly by the nasal branches of the greater (anterior) palatine and by the nasopalatine nerves. Autonomic fibres to glands and vessels in the nose are distributed with the above mentioned branches of the maxillary nerve via the pterygopalatine ganglion. In addition, autonomic fibres are presumed to be distributed with the anterior ethmoidal nerve via the ciliary ganglion.

The nerves within the orbit

Both motor and sensory nerves are found in the orbit (see Figure 6.4). The motor nerves are the oculomotor,

trochlear, and abducent nerves. They supply the extraocular muscles. There are also motor nerves derived from the autonomic nervous system. Parasympathetic fibres from the oculomotor nerve (via the ciliary ganglion) supply the sphincter pupillae and ciliary muscles. Parasympathetic fibres from the facial nerve (via the pterygopalatine ganglion) supply the lacrimal gland. Sympathetic fibres supply the dilator pupillae muscle. The sensory nerves within the orbit are the optic, ophthalmic, and maxillary nerves. The ophthalmic and maxillary nerves are essentially only passing through the orbit to supply the face and jaws.

The oculomotor nerve

This is the third cranial nerve. It is the main source of innervation of the extraocular muscles. The oculomotor nerve also contains parasympathetic fibres which relay in the ciliary ganglion.

The oculomotor nerve emerges at the midbrain, on the medial side of the crus of the cerebral peduncle. It passes along the lateral dural wall of the cavernous sinus. The oculomotor nerve then divides into superior and inferior divisions and runs beneath the trochlear and ophthalmic nerves. The two divisions of the oculomotor nerve enter the orbit through the superior orbital fissure, within the common tendinous ring of the recti muscles. Here, the nasociliary branch of the ophthalmic nerve lies between the divisions of the oculomotor nerve.

The superior division of the oculomotor nerve passes above the optic nerve to enter the inferior surface of the superior rectus muscle. It supplies this muscle and provides a branch which runs to the levator palpebrae superioris muscle.

The inferior division of the oculomotor nerve divides into three branches: medial, central, and lateral. The medial branch passes beneath the optic nerve to enter the lateral surface of the medial rectus muscle. The central branch runs downwards and forwards to enter the superior surface of the inferior rectus muscle. The lateral branch travels forwards on the lateral side of the inferior rectus muscle to enter the superior surface of the inferior oblique muscle. The lateral branch also communicates with the ciliary ganglion to distribute parasympathetic fibres to the sphincter pupillae and ciliary muscles.

The trochlear nerve

This is the fourth cranial nerve. It is the only cranial nerve which emerges from the dorsal surface of the brain. The trochlear nerve passes from the midbrain onto the lateral surface of the crus of the cerebral peduncle. It runs through the lateral dural wall of the cavernous sinus. The nerve then crosses the oculomotor nerve and enters the orbit through the superior orbital fissure, above the common tendinous ring of the recti muscles. Here, it lies above the levator palpebrae superioris muscle and medial to the frontal and lacrimal nerves. The trochlear nerve travels but a short distance to enter the superior surface of the superior oblique muscle. Indeed, the innervation of the superior oblique muscle is the sole function of the trochlear nerve.

The abducent nerve

The abducent nerve is the sixth cranial nerve. It emerges from the brain stem, between the pons and the medulla oblongata. The abducent nerve is related to the cavernous sinus but, unlike the oculomotor, trochlear, ophthalmic, and maxillary nerves which merely invaginate the lateral dural wall, it passes through the sinus itself. The abducent nerve enters the orbit through the superior orbital fissure. It is here situated within the common tendinous ring of the recti muscles, first below and then between the two divisions of the oculomotor nerve and lateral to the nasociliary nerve. The abducent nerve passes forwards to enter the medial surface of the lateral rectus muscle. The innervation of this muscle is the sole function of the abducent nerve.

The *ophthalmic nerve and its branches* are described elsewhere in this chapter.

The *maxillary nerve* gives rise directly to two nerves that pass into the orbit (the zygomatic and infraorbital nerves) and indirectly to an orbital branch from the pterygopalatine ganglion. All three nerves enter the orbit through the inferior orbital fissure.

The optic nerve

The optic nerve is the second cranial nerve. It arises from the optic chiasma on the floor of the diencephalon. It enters the orbit through the optic canal, accompanied by the ophthalmic artery. The shape of the optic nerve changes from being flattened at the chiasma to being rounded as it passes through the optic canal. The optic nerve in the orbit passes forwards, laterally, and downwards. It pierces the sclera at the lamina cribrosa, slightly medial to the posterior pole. The optic nerve has a slightly wavy course which allows for movements of the eye.

Within the orbit, the optic nerve is surrounded by extensions of the three meninges. This reflects the fact that the nerve is really an 'outgrowth' of the brain.

The optic nerve has important relationships with other orbital structures. As the nerve leaves the optic canal, it lies superomedial to the ophthalmic artery. The oculomotor, nasociliary, and abducent nerves (and sometimes the ophthalmic veins) are situated between the optic nerve and the lateral rectus muscle. The optic nerve is also closely related to the origins of the four recti muscles. More anteriorly, however, the muscles diverge and the nerve becomes separated from them by a substantial amount of orbital fat. Just beyond the optic canal, the ophthalmic artery and the nasociliary nerve cross the optic nerve to reach the medial wall of the orbit. The central artery of the retina enters the substance of the optic nerve about halfway along its length. Near the back of the eye, the optic nerve becomes surrounded by long and short ciliary nerves and vessels.

The ciliary ganglion

The ciliary ganglion is a parasympathetic ganglion which is located near the apex of the orbit. It lies in front of the optic canal, between the lateral rectus muscle and the optic nerve, and close to the ophthalmic artery. The ganglion appears as a small swelling connected to the nasociliary nerve. Short ciliary nerves pass from the ganglion to the eyeball. Functionally, the ciliary ganglion is related to the eye, in particular the motor supply of intraocular muscles.

The parasympathetic fibres to the ciliary ganglion arise from the Edinger–Westphal nucleus of the oculomotor nerve. The preganglionic fibres run with the oculomotor nerve into the orbit, leaving in the branch to the inferior oblique muscle. The fibres then pass to the ciliary ganglion where they synapse. Postganglionic fibres travel to the back of the eye in the short ciliary nerves.

The sympathetic fibres to the ciliary ganglion arise from the plexus around the internal carotid artery within the cavernous sinus. These postganglionic fibres form a fine branch which enters the orbit through the superior orbital fissure, inside the common tendinous ring of the recti muscles. This branch then travels through the ganglion (without synapsing) and into the short ciliary nerves.

The sensory fibres to the ciliary ganglion are derived from the nasociliary nerve. They also pass through the ganglion to the short ciliary nerves without synapsing.

The *short ciliary nerves* convey parasympathetic, sympathetic and sensory fibres between the eyeball and the ciliary ganglion. The nerves pierce the sclera at the back of the eye and run forwards between the sclera and the choroid. The parasympathetic fibres are distributed to the sphincter pupillae and ciliary muscles. Contraction of the ciliary muscles is associated with the accommodation reflex. The sympathetic fibres supply arteries within the eye. (The sympathetic fibres supplying the dilator pupillae muscle are thought to run in the long ciliary nerves.) The sensory fibres carry sensation from the cornea, the ciliary body, and the iris.

The innervation of the neck

The neck, being an 'intermediate zone' between the trunk and the head, is innervated from both spinal nerves (anterior and posterior primary rami) and cranial nerves (mainly Cr IX, X, XI, XII). In contrast, the head is primarily innervated by cranial nerves (the back of the head is innervated by posterior primary rami of spinal nerves) and the trunk by spinal nerves (not ignoring the important contributions of Cr X).

The cutaneous innervation of the neck

The skin of the neck is innervated by branches of primary cervical spinal nerves, via both posterior and anterior rami (Figure 6.7). The posterior rami supply skin over the back of the neck and scalp. The anterior rami supply skin covering the lateral and anterior portions of the neck and even extend onto the face over the angle of the mandible.

The posterior primary rami of the first, sixth, seventh, and eighth cervical nerves have no cutaneous distribution. From the medial branch of the posterior ramus of the second cervical nerve comes the greater occipital nerve. This pierces the trapezius muscle close to its attachment onto the superior nuchal line of the occiput and then ascends to supply the skin over the occipital part of the scalp up to the vertex of the skull. The medial branches of the posterior rami of the third, fourth, and fifth cervical nerves also pierce trapezius to supply skin over the back of the neck in a serial manner.

The anterior primary rami of the second, third, and fourth cervical nerves supply cutaneous branches via the cervical plexus. This plexus is located deep to the sternocleidomastoid muscle and supplies both motor and sensory branches to structures in the neck. The cutaneous branches from the plexus are the lesser occipital, the great auricular, the transverse cervical, and the supraclavicular nerves. All four nerves appear from beneath the sternocleidomastoid muscle at its posterior margin.

The *lesser occipital nerve* takes fibres mainly from the second cervical nerve, although fibres from the third cervical nerve may contribute. It ascends along the posterior margin of the sternocleidomastoid muscle to supply the scalp above and behind the ear and a small area on the cranial surface of the auricle.

The *great auricular nerve* receives fibres from the second and third cervical nerves. It runs up the superficial surface of the sternocleidomastoid muscle towards the ear. It supplies the skin overlying the mastoid process (the mastoid branch), much of the auricle (auricular branches), and the parotid region, and the angle of the mandible (facial branches).

The *transverse cervical nerve* also takes fibres from the second and third cervical nerves. It crosses the sternocleidomastoid muscle horizontally to supply

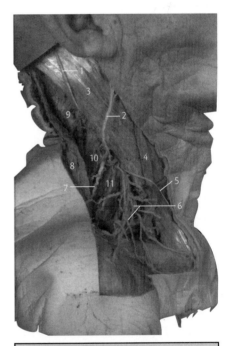

1	Lesser occipital nerve
2	Greater auricular nerve
3	Sternocleidomastoid muscle
4	External jugular vein
5	Transverse cervical nerve
6	Supraclavicular nerves
7	Spinal accessory nerve
8	Trapezius muscle
9	Splenius capitis muscle
10	Levator scapulae muscle
11	Scalenus medius muscle

Figure 6.7 Lateral view of the neck showing the cutaneous innervation from the cervical plexus

skin overlying the anterior part of the neck from the mandible to the sternum.

The *supraclavicular nerves* receive fibres from the third and fourth cervical nerves. Initially, it is a single nerve. This passes downwards towards the clavicle where it divides into three branches (medial, intermediate, and lateral supraclavicular nerves). These nerves supply skin at the root of the neck and over the upper part of the thorax.

The nerves of the neck

Within the carotid sheath runs the vagus nerve. Related to the carotid sheath near the base of the skull are the glossopharyngeal, accessory, and hypoglossal nerves. Lying behind the carotid sheath, and in front of the prevertebral fascia, is the cervical sympathetic trunk. Deep to the internal jugular vein, and in front of the scalenus medius and levator scapulae muscles (at the level of the first four cervical vertebrae), lies the cervical plexus of nerves. Associated with the cervical plexus is the ansa cervicalis. The brachial plexus for the arm lies in the deep part of the posterior triangle in the root of the neck. Both the cervical and brachial plexuses are derived from the anterior primary rami of cervical spinal nerves. The cutaneous contributions of the posterior rami have already been described.

The glossopharyngeal nerve

This is the ninth cranial nerve. It emerges from the medulla oblongata of the brain stem as three or four rootlets. These rootlets are found in a groove between the olive and the inferior cerebellar peduncle. At this site, the glossopharyngeal nerve lies above the rootlets of the vagus nerve. The glossopharyngeal nerve has sensory, motor, and parasympathetic fibres.

The glossopharyngeal nerve leaves the skull through the central part of the jugular foramen. Within the foramen, the nerve shows the superior and inferior ganglia. Below the foramen, the glossopharyngeal nerve is located anterior to the vagus and accessory nerves, passing between the internal jugular vein and the internal carotid artery. It then runs anteriorly between the internal and external carotid arteries and onto the stylopharyngeus muscle. Winding around this muscle, it passes between the superior and middle constrictor muscles of the pharynx to be distributed to the tonsil, pharynx, and tongue. Branches include:

- Tympanic nerve
- Lesser petrosal nerve
- Carotid branch
- Pharyngeal branches
- Stylopharyngeus (muscular) branch
- Tonsillar branches
- Lingual branches.

The *tympanic nerve* arises from the inferior ganglion. It passes upwards through the tympanic canaliculus to reach the middle ear cavity. Here, it contributes to the tympanic plexus, which is found on the promontory of the medial wall of the tympanic cavity. This plexus provides sensory fibres to the mucosa of the tympanic cavity, the auditory tube, and the mastoid air cells. From the plexus arises the lesser petrosal nerve.

The *lesser petrosal nerve* contains preganglionic parasympathetic fibres which relay through the otic ganglion to the parotid salivary gland. The nerve passes from the tympanic plexus, through the anterior wall of the tympanic cavity and onto the floor of the middle cranial fossa. It then emerges through the foramen ovale to join the otic ganglion in the infratemporal fossa.

The *carotid branch(es)* arises just below the skull, as the glossopharyngeal crosses the internal carotid artery. It then passes between the internal and the external carotid arteries to the carotid sinus and the carotid body. During its course it is joined by the carotid branch of the vagus nerve.

The *pharyngeal branches* contribute to the pharyngeal plexus on the middle constrictor muscle (the other components of this plexus being from the sympathetic trunk and the pharyngeal branch of the vagus). The glossopharyngeal contribution to the plexus is sensory to the pharynx.

The *stylopharyngeus branch* supplies the stylopharyngeus muscle (the nerve and muscle being associated embryologically with the third pharyngeal arch).

The *tonsillar branches* supply the palatine tonsil. They form a plexus with the lesser palatine nerve. Branches from the plexus are distributed to the soft palate.

There are two *lingual branches* of the glossopharyngeal nerve. One branch supplies the region around the sulcus terminalis of the tongue, including the circumvallate papillae. The other branch supplies the posterior third of the tongue. The lingual branches are concerned with both taste perception and general sensation.

The vagus nerve

The vagus nerve is the tenth cranial nerve. It has the most extensive distribution of any of the cranial nerves and contains sensory, motor, and para-sympathetic fibres.

The vagus emerges from the brain stem at the medulla oblongata, between the olive and the inferior cerebellar peduncle. It exits the cranium through the jugular foramen with the glossopharyngeal and accessory nerves.

The vagus nerve has two ganglia, the superior and inferior ganglia. The superior ganglion lies within the jugular foramen. The inferior ganglion is situated just below.

Just below the inferior ganglion, the vagus is joined by the cranial part of the accessory nerve. The vagus then passes downwards within the carotid sheath and enters the thorax at the root of the neck.

The vagus nerves in the neck differ in one important respect, namely the origins of the recurrent laryngeal nerves. Branches include:

- Meningeal branch
- Auricular branch
- Pharyngeal branch
- Branches to the carotid body
- Superior laryngeal nerve
- Recurrent laryngeal (right) nerve
- Cardiac branches.

The *meningeal branch(es)* arises from the superior ganglion in the jugular fossa. It supplies dura in the posterior cranial fossa. There is some evidence that this nerve is not truly a branch of the vagus but is derived from upper cervical nerves and/or the superior cervical sympathetic ganglion.

The *auricular branch* also arises from the superior ganglion. It enters the temporal bone via the mastoid canaliculus on the lateral wall of the jugular fossa. It then passes out through the tympanomastoid fissure and divides into two branches. One branch joins the posterior auricular branch of the facial nerve, the other contributes to the innervation of the skin of the auricle, external acoustic meatus, and tympanic membrane.

The *pharyngeal branch* is, in fact, derived from the cranial part of the accessory nerve. It runs from the inferior ganglion of the vagus, between the internal and external carotid arteries, and towards the middle constrictor of the pharynx. There it forms the pharyngeal plexus with branches from the sympathetic trunk, and the glossopharyngeal and external laryngeal

nerves. The pharyngeal nerve is the main motor nerve to the muscles of the pharynx and palate.

Although the carotid body is supplied mainly by the glossopharyngeal nerve, the vagus nerve can also contribute.

The *superior laryngeal nerve* also arises from the inferior ganglion. It then passes deep to both the internal and external carotid arteries on its way to the larynx. It divides into internal and external branches. The internal branch passes between the middle and inferior constrictor muscles to supply sensation to the larynx. The external branch runs down on the inferior constrictor muscle (with the superior thyroid artery) to supply the cricothyroid muscle of the larynx.

The *right recurrent laryngeal nerve* arises in the root of the neck. It leaves the vagus in front of the subclavian artery, loops below, and behind the artery, and then ascends towards the larynx.

The *left recurrent laryngeal nerve* arises in the thorax, as the vagus passes across the arch of the aorta. Both recurrent laryngeal nerves reach the larynx by passing upwards in grooves between the trachea and the oesophagus and they are closely related to the inferior thyroid arteries. They pass beneath the inferior borders of the inferior constrictor muscles to supply the mucosa of the larynx and most of the intrinsic muscles.

Usually two or three *cardiac branches* emanate from the vagus nerve in the neck. They run downwards and medially into the thorax, terminating at the deep part of the cardiac plexus.

The accessory nerve

This is the eleventh cranial nerve. It consists of two distinct parts, the cranial accessory and the spinal accessory nerves.

The *cranial part* of the accessory nerve is a motor nerve which emerges from the medulla oblongata between the olive and the inferior cerebellar peduncle. It joins the spinal part of the accessory at the jugular foramen. Once through the jugular foramen, the cranial and spinal parts again separate. The cranial part then joins the vagus nerve, eventually to be distributed in the pharyngeal branch of the vagus to the pharyngeal and palatine musculature. Some of its fibres also run with the recurrent laryngeal nerve and the cardiac branches of the vagus. Because of its close association with the vagus, some anatomists consider the cranial part of the accessory nerve to be a part of the vagus and not a separate cranial nerve.

The *spinal part* of the accessory nerve is also a motor nerve, although there may be some sensory fibres. It is derived from the upper five segments of the cervical spinal cord. A series of rootlets emerge from the cord between the dorsal and ventral roots of the upper cervical nerves. They join to form the main nerve trunk which passes intracranially through the foramen magnum. At the jugular foramen, the spinal and cranial parts of the accessory nerve unite but soon separate on exiting the cranium. The spinal part of the accessory nerve then crosses the internal jugular vein (usually on its lateral surface) and runs obliquely downwards and backwards to reach the upper part of the sternocleidomastoid muscle. It passes into the substance of this muscle and subsequently enters the posterior triangle of the neck. It crosses the posterior triangle on the levator scapulae muscle before entering the trapezius muscle. The spinal part of the accessory nerve provides the motor supply of the sternocleidomastoid and trapezius muscles.

The hypoglossal nerve

This is the twelfth cranial nerve and is a motor nerve supplying the musculature of the tongue. It originates as a series of rootlets on the medulla oblongata, between the pyramid and the olive.

The hypoglossal nerve runs through the hypoglossal canal of the occipital bone and emerges deep to the carotid sheath. It then passes downwards and, under cover of the posterior belly of the digastric muscle, outwards between the internal jugular vein and the internal carotid artery. Subsequently, it runs forwards across the vagus nerve and the external and internal carotid arteries. Indeed, it loops around the occipital artery near its origin (at its sternocleidomastoid branch). Continuing forwards, it passes below the submandibular salivary gland, onto the hyoglossus muscle to be distributed to the muscles of the tongue.

Like most cranial nerves, the hypoglossal nerve has connecting branches with other cranial and cervical spinal nerves and with the sympathetic system. An important connection is with the anterior primary ramus of the first cervical nerve.

Branches include:

♦ Meningeal branch

♦ Upper root of ansa cervicalis

♦ Muscular branches to thyrohyoid and geniohyoid

♦ Muscular branches to the tongue.

The *meningeal branch* is probably derived from the upper cervical and sympathetic fibres which communicate with the hypoglossal. It appears as the hypoglossal nerve emerges through its canal in the occipital bone. It mainly supplies the dura in the posterior cranial fossa.

The *upper root of the ansa cervicalis* is also derived from the anterior ramus of the first cervical nerve. This branch first appears as the hypoglossal nerve loops around the occipital artery. It passes down on the carotid sheath covering the carotid arteries and is joined by the lower root of the ansa cervicalis from the cervical plexus to form the ansa cervicalis. The upper root of the ansa cervicalis gives a branch to the superior belly of the omohyoid muscle.

The *muscular branches supplying the thyrohyoid* and *geniohyoid* muscles are also derived from the first cervical spinal nerve. The nerve to thyrohyoid arises as the hypoglossal nerve reaches the hyoglossus muscle. The nerve to geniohyoid is given off in the floor of the mouth, above the mylohyoid muscle.

The *branches to the tongue musculature* are the only true branches of the hypoglossal nerve. They are distributed to the intrinsic muscles of the tongue and to the styloglossus, hyoglossus, and genioglossus muscles.

The cervical sympathetic trunk

The sympathetic outflow for all parts of the body is derived principally from the thoracic spinal cord (segments T1 to L2). These preganglionic fibres then pass into the sympathetic trunk via the spinal nerves as white rami communicantes. Here, they may synapse at a ganglion or they pass up or down the sympathetic trunk to a ganglion at a different level. In this manner, the cervical part of the sympathetic trunk receives its preganglionic fibres from the upper thoracic nerves.

The cervical sympathetic trunk exhibits a variable number of ganglia (usually between two and four). The ganglia are designated according to their position (superior, middle, inferior).

The *superior cervical ganglion* lies at the level of the second and third cervical vertebrae. It is situated behind the carotid sheath on the longus capitis muscle (a prevertebral muscle). It is the largest of the cervical sympathetic ganglia and is believed to represent the coalescence of four ganglia which correspond with the upper four cervical spinal nerves.

The branches from the superior cervical ganglion are variable, but can be broadly classified into lateral, medial, and anterior groups.

The lateral branches include the grey rami communicantes to the upper four cervical spinal nerves. In addition, there are branches which communicate with some of the cranial nerves: to the inferior ganglion of the glossopharyngeal nerve, to both ganglia of the vagus nerve, and to the hypoglossal nerve. The nerve which joins the glossopharyngeal and vagus nerves is termed the jugular nerve. The lateral branches of the superior cervical ganglion also include nerves to the superior jugular bulb and to the meninges of the posterior cranial fossa.

There are two medial branches of the superior cervical sympathetic ganglion. There is a laryngopharyngeal branch (which supplies the carotid body and the pharyngeal plexus), and a cardiac branch.

The anterior branches pass onto the common and external carotid arteries to form plexuses. In addition to supplying the blood vessels, the plexus around the facial branch of the external carotid provides the sympathetic supply to the submandibular parasympathetic ganglion. The plexus around the middle meningeal artery (a branch of the maxillary artery from the external carotid) serves the otic parasympathetic ganglion.

Emerging above the superior ganglion is the internal carotid nerve. This nerve may be thought of as the cranial part of the sympathetic system. It passes with the internal carotid artery into the carotid canal. Within the canal, it forms the internal carotid plexus around the internal carotid artery.

The *internal carotid plexus* can be divided into two parts, lateral and medial. The lateral part gives branches which communicate with the trigeminal and abducent cranial nerves. Superior and inferior caroticotympanic nerves traverse the posterior wall of the carotid canal to communicate with the tympanic branch of the glossopharyngeal nerve. An important branch is the deep petrosal nerve. This nerve is destined for the pterygopalatine ganglion. It passes through the foramen lacerum and, joining the greater petrosal branch of the facial nerve, becomes the nerve of the pterygoid canal.

The medial part of the internal carotid plexus supplies the internal carotid artery itself and communicates with the oculomotor, trochlear, ophthalmic division of the trigeminal, and the abducent cranial nerves. Branches also pass through the superior orbital fissure to the ciliary ganglion in the orbit. These branches subsequently run with the short ciliary nerves to be distributed to the blood vessels of the eyeball. The fibres to the dilator pupillae travel by a different course (via the ophthalmic, nasociliary, and then the long ciliary nerves). The terminal branches of the internal carotid plexus form plexuses around the ophthalmic artery and the anterior and middle cerebral arteries of the brain, passing eventually to the pia mater.

The *middle cervical ganglion* is usually situated at the level of the sixth cervical vertebra. It is the smallest cervical ganglion and is occasionally absent. It may fuse with the superior cervical ganglion. The middle ganglion lies close to the inferior thyroid artery just before it enters the gland. Some claim that it represents the coalescence of two ganglia which correspond with the fifth and sixth cervical segments.

Branches from the middle cervical ganglion communicate with the fifth and sixth cervical spinal nerves (also sometimes the fourth and seventh). Two distinct cords pass down to the inferior cervical/cervicothoracic sympathetic ganglion. The anterior cord loops in front and below the subclavian artery as the ansa subclavia. The posterior cord encloses the vertebral artery. The middle cervical ganglion also sends branches to the thyroid gland (along the inferior thyroid artery), to the heart via its cardiac branches, and to the trachea and oesophagus.

An occasional ganglion known as the vertebral ganglion may be found on the front of the vertebral artery. It can be considered as either a low middle cervical ganglion or as a detached part of the inferior ganglion. When present, it gives rise to the ansa subclavia.

The *inferior cervical* often combines with the first thoracic ganglion to form the cervicothoracic ganglion (stellate ganglion). The inferior cervical ganglion (or upper end of the cervicothoracic ganglion) is situated just posterior to the vertebral artery. The lower end of a cervicothoracic ganglion lies behind the subclavian artery on the first thoracic vertebra.

Branches from the inferior cervical ganglion pass to the seventh and eighth cervical nerves and to the first thoracic nerve. There are also cardiac branches and fibres which form plexuses around the subclavian artery and its derivatives. Around the vertebral artery is a plexus which continues up into the skull. This plexus eventually meets the plexus around the internal carotid artery. Some anatomists believe this to be the main intracranial extension of the sympathetic system.

The cervical plexus

This plexus lies deep to the sternocleidomastoid muscle and the internal jugular vein, and in front of the scalenus medius and levator scapulae muscles. It is formed by the anterior primary rami of the upper four cervical spinal nerves (i.e. Cl, C2, C3, C4). The cervical plexus contains both sensory and motor fibres. In addition, grey rami communicantes near the origins of the anterior rami of the cervical nerves supply sympathetic fibres.

Branches from the cervical plexus are distributed to some of the muscles of the neck, to the diaphragm, and to much of the skin of the back of the head, the neck, and the chest around the thoracic inlet. The cutaneous nerves are superficial, the muscular branches deep.

The cutaneous nerves from the cervical plexus are the lesser occipital (C2), great auricular (C2, C3), transverse cervical (C2, C3), and supraclavicular (C3, C4) nerves.

The deep (mainly motor) branches can be subdivided into those which pass medially and those which pass laterally.

The medial branches supply the following muscles:

* Longus capitis (C1, C2, C3)
* Longus colli (C2, C3, C4)
* Rectus capitis anterior (C1, C2)
* Rectus capitis lateralis (C1).

Other medial branches are the inferior root of the ansa cervicalis (C2, C3) and the phrenic nerve (C3, C4, C5). Some branches also communicate with the hypoglossal and vagus nerves, and the sympathetic trunk.

The lateral branches supply the following muscles:

* Levator scapulae (C3, C4)
* Scalenus medius (C3, C4)
* Sternocleidomastoid (C2)
* Trapezius (C3, C4).

There is also a communicating branch to the accessory nerve (C2, C3, C4).

The *phrenic nerve* arises from the cervical plexus and usually takes fibres from the third, fourth, and fifth cervical nerves (mainly from the fourth). It provides the motor nerve supply to the diaphragm.

The phrenic nerve in the neck passes downwards and medially on the superficial surface of the scalenus anterior muscle. Here, it lies under cover of a layer of the prevertebral fascia. As it passes through the thoracic inlet, it runs behind the subclavian vein and in front of the subclavian artery and its internal thoracic branch.

Some of the roots may not join the main nerve trunk until just before leaving the neck. Such roots are called accessory phrenic nerves.

The phrenic nerve contains not only motor fibres but also proprioceptive fibres to the diaphragm and sensory fibres to the pleura and pericardium. Sympathetic fibres may join the phrenic nerve from cervical sympathetic ganglia.

The *branches to the hypoglossal nerve* from the cervical plexus arise mainly from the first cervical spinal nerve. These fibres leave the hypoglossal nerve as four distinct nerves: the meningeal branch of the hypoglossal nerve; the superior root of the ansa cervicalis; and the motor nerves to the thyrohyoid and the geniohyoid muscles. Some Cl fibres also travel with the vagus nerve, and indeed may form its meningeal branch.

The *ansa cervicalis* is a nerve plexus located in front of the common carotid artery. It is formed by the union of two nerve trunks, the superior root of the ansa cervicalis from the hypoglossal nerve (conveying Cl fibres) and the inferior root of the ansa cervicalis from the cervical plexus (conveying C2 and C3 fibres). The superior root is also called the descendens hypoglossi, indicating its path from the hypoglossal nerve as it crosses the external carotid artery. The inferior root may also be termed the descendens cervicalis. It usually appears lateral to the internal jugular vein, crossing the vein to join the superior root. Occasionally, the inferior root may run medial to the internal jugular vein.

The ansa cervicalis supplies all the infrahyoid muscles with the exception of the thyrohyoid muscle. The innervation of the superior belly of the omohyoid muscle is often given off from the superior root just before it reaches the ansa cervicalis.

The brachial plexus

This plexus lies in the deep part of the posterior triangle of the neck, between the clavicle and the lower part of the posterior border of the sternocleidomastoid muscle. It emerges between the scalenus anterior and scalenus medius muscles to pass between the clavicle and first rib, around the axillary artery, and into the upper limb.

The brachial plexus is formed by the anterior primary rami of the fourth to the eighth cervical nerves and by most of the anterior ramus of the first thoracic nerve. The plexus provides the innervation for structures in the upper limb.

The branches arising from the brachial plexus above the clavicle in the neck are:

- Nerves to the scalene and longus colli muscles (C5, C6, C7, C8)
- Communicating branch to the phrenic nerve (C5)
- Dorsal scapular nerve to the rhomboid muscles (C5)
- Long thoracic nerve to serratus anterior muscle (C5, C6, C7)
- Nerve to the subclavius (C5, C6)
- Suprascapular nerve to the supraspinatus and infraspinatus muscles and to the shoulder joint (C5, C6).

Thus, the branches are mainly motor.

The innervation of the pharynx

Most of the pharynx derives its sensory nerve supply from the glossopharyngeal nerve through its pharyngeal and tonsillar branches. The pharyngeal branch arises just before the glossopharyngeal nerve passes onto the posterior surface of the stylopharyngeus muscle. This branch then joins the pharyngeal branch of the vagus to reach the pharyngeal plexus. The tonsillar branch of the glossopharyngeal nerve supplies the region around the oropharyngeal isthmus.

The anterior part of the nasopharynx is not supplied by the glossopharyngeal nerve but by the pharyngeal branch of the maxillary nerve. Furthermore, the soft palate is innervated by the lesser palatine branch of the maxillary nerve. Both the pharyngeal and lesser palatine nerves are branches of the maxillary division of the trigeminal nerve via the pterygopalatine ganglion.

The lower part of the pharynx is innervated by the superior laryngeal branch of the vagus nerve.

The muscles of the pharynx derive their innervation from the nucleus ambiguus in the brain stem. Fibres pass from this nucleus within the glossopharyngeal, vagus, and cranial accessory nerves. The cranial accessory nerve, however, joins the vagus nerve shortly after emerging through the jugular foramen of the skull. These fibres, together with those already in the vagus, reach the pharyngeal plexus via the pharyngeal branch of the vagus to supply most of the muscles of the pharynx. The stylopharyngeus muscle, however, is supplied by fibres from the nucleus ambiguus that run with the glossopharyngeal nerve.

The pharyngeal plexus lies on the external surface of the middle constrictor muscle. It is formed by the pharyngeal branches of the glossopharyngeal and vagus nerves, with contributions from the superior cervical sympathetic ganglion. The glossopharyngeal nerve supplies only sensory fibres to the plexus. The vagus contains motor fibres associated with the cranial part of the accessory nerve which, in addition to supplying the muscles of the pharynx, also supply the muscles of the soft palate.

Conclusion

As can be appreciated from the above description, there is considerable anatomical variation in the innervation of the head and neck. Therefore, the 'standard' anatomy that is outlined in this chapter is inevitably a 'consensus' view of human anatomy and the perceptive, and skilled, clinician will be aware that his, or her, patients may have different anatomies, minor or major.

References

1. Berkovitz BKB, Moxham BJ (eds). (2002) *Head and Neck Anatomy – A Clinical Reference*. London: Martin Dunitz/Taylor Francis.
2. Bernstein L, Nelson RH. (1984) Surgical anatomy of the extra-parotid distribution of the facial nerve. *Arch Otolaryngol*, **110**, 177–83.
3. Hollinshead WH (ed) (1982) *Anatomy for Surgeons: Volume 1 – The Head and Neck*, 3rd edn. New York: Harper & Row.
4. Langdon JD, Berkovitz BKB, Moxham BJ (eds). (2003) *Surgical Anatomy of the Infratemporal Fossa*. London: Martin Dunitz/Taylor Francis.
5. May M. (1986) *The Facial Nerve*. Thieme: Stuttgart.
6. Nortje CT, Farman AG, Grotepass FW. (1977) Variations in the normal anatomy of the inferior dental (mandibular) canal: a retrospective study of panoramic radiographs from 3,612 routine dental patients. *Br J Oral Surg*, **15**, 55–63.
7. Standring S (ed). (2009) *Gray's Anatomy*, 40th edn. Edinburgh: Churchill Livingstone.

Regional anaesthetic techniques in oral and maxillofacial surgery

John Gerard Meechan

Introduction

Many procedures in oral surgery can be performed under local anaesthesia with or without sedation. In addition, local anaesthesia can be used to supplement general anaesthesia. There are advantages of local anaesthesia during general anaesthesia, and these include haemostasis (from the vasoconstrictor in many local anaesthetic solutions), reduced surgical stimulation, and improved postoperative pain control.

Local anaesthetics that are used intraorally are often supplied in prefilled cartridges of varying volumes, ranging from 1.8 to 2.2 ml. The concentration of adrenaline (epinephrine) in some prefilled cartridges for dental use (1:80 000 [12.5 μg/ml]) is greater than that used in other sites. Some syringes that are used by dentists do not permit aspiration when prefilled cartridges are used and these cannot be recommended as the mouth and perioral structures are well vascularized so inadvertent intravascular injection can occur. Positive aspirates may occur in around 20% of intraoral regional blocks[1,2].

This chapter will describe infiltration, regional block, and specialized injections that are used to provide local anaesthesia of the mouth and perioral structures.

Infiltration anaesthesia

Infiltration techniques can be used to anaesthetize the soft tissues and some of the teeth and associated bone. The maxillary teeth and bone are susceptible to infiltration anaesthesia. In the mandible, the anterior teeth and deciduous dentition can be anaesthetized by infiltration; however, this method is not always successful for permanent (adult) mandibular molar teeth and associated bone, so regional block methods are usually employed in this region.

To anaesthetize the maxillary teeth and bone, solution is deposited in the buccal sulcus by piercing the reflected mucosa and advancing towards the apex of the tooth in question. Solution should be deposited in a supraperiosteal location. If bone is contacted, the needle should be withdrawn slightly before aspiration and deposition of the anaesthetic. At least 1.0 ml of a solution such as 2% lidocaine with 1:80 000 adrenaline should be deposited over a period of about 30 seconds. This is the so-called buccal infiltration technique.

The buccal infiltration will anaesthetize the buccal soft tissues, the tooth in question plus the contiguous teeth and associated buccal bone; however, the palatal soft tissues and bone are not affected by this injection. These can be anaesthetized either by infiltration or by one of the regional block methods described below. Injection into the palatal soft tissues is uncomfortable, especially in the anterior hard palate as this soft tissue is not very compliant. A very slow injection technique is needed for anterior palatal infiltrations in the conscious patient.

A similar technique to that described above is used in the anterior mandible for the lower incisors. In this region, infiltration both buccally and lingually significantly improves the success of dental anaesthesia[3].

Regional anaesthetic techniques for the maxillary nerve and its branches

The regional nerve blocks that are used to anaesthetise the branches of the maxillary division of the trigeminal nerve are given in Table 7.1.

Maxillary nerve block

The maxillary nerve may be blocked by extraoral or intraoral approaches. Blockade of this nerve anaesthetizes all the maxillary teeth, and associated buccal and palatal hard and soft tissues, including the skin and mucosa of the upper lip.

Extraoral approach

The landmark for skin penetration is the most concave point of the inferior aspect of the arch of the zygoma. A long needle is used and it is inserted at right angles to both the skin and the sagittal plane. Contact is maintained with the inferior border of the zygomatic arch during advancement of the needle, which progresses until the lateral pterygoid plate is contacted (Figure 7.1). When the bone of the pterygoid plate has been contacted, a note is made of how much needle penetration has occurred. This is an essential part of the procedure as it determines the correct amount of insertion for the final injection. The next stage is to partially withdraw the needle and redirect it towards the pterygopalatine fossa. This is done by pointing the needle 15° more anteriorly and 10° more superiorly compared to the original insertion. It is advanced again at this new orientation until the depth of insertion determined by the initial penetration to the

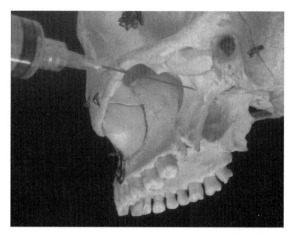

Figure 7.1 The initial approach to the extraoral method of anaesthetizing the maxillary and mandibular nerves. The needle is inserted below the most concave part of the zygomatic arch until the lateral pterygoid plate is contacted (via the sigmoid notch of the mandible, which has been removed in this skull). See text for details of the final needle position.

pterygoid plates is reached. This is the endpoint for injection.

Intraoral approaches

There are two ways of anaesthetizing the maxillary nerve from inside the mouth. These are the tuberosity approach and the greater palatine canal approach.

The tuberosity approach involves inserting a needle in the maxillary buccal sulcus distal to the third molar tooth. A long (35-mm) needle is needed as it is inserted to a depth of around 30 mm. The needle is advanced superiorly, posteriorly, and medially into the pterygomaxillary fissure (Figure 7.2) and 1.5–2.0 ml of solution deposited.

The greater palatine method involves inserting the needle into the greater palatine foramen and then advancing it along the length of the greater palatine canal until it enters the pterygomaxillary fissure (Figure 7.3).

Posterior superior alveolar nerve block

This technique is very similar to that described above for the tuberosity approach to the maxillary nerve block. It follows the technique exactly with the exception of depth of penetration. In this method, the needle is inserted so that it lies at the posterior surface of the maxillary tuberosity and anaesthetizes the posterior superior alveolar nerve as it enters the posterior surface of the maxilla. An injection of 1.5–2.0 ml of solution

Table 7.1 The regional nerve blocks used to anaesthetize the branches of the maxillary division of the trigeminal nerve

Maxillary nerve block
Posterior superior alveolar nerve block
Maxillary molar nerve block
Anterior superior alveolar nerve block
Infraorbital nerve block
Anterior middle superior alveolar nerve block
Palatal anterior superior alveolar nerve block
Greater palatine nerve block
Nasopalatine nerve block

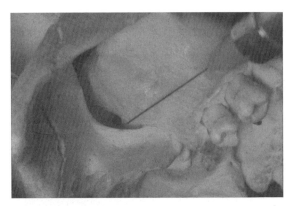

Figure 7.2 The tuberosity approach to the maxillary nerve.

will anaesthetize the maxillary molar teeth and associated buccal bone and soft tissues. Occasionally, the first molar area is not satisfactorily anaesthetized (see below).

A

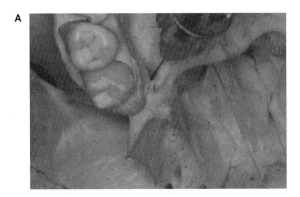

B

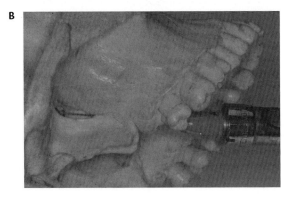

Figure 7.3 The greater palatine canal approach to the maxillary nerve. **A** The needle is inserted into the greater palatine foramen; **B** the tip of the needle in the pterygomaxillary fissure.

Maxillary molar nerve block

This technique anaesthetizes the maxillary molar teeth and associated buccal soft and hard tissues[4]. It was developed to overcome failure of anaesthesia in the first molar region as this area can receive supply from both the posterior and middle superior alveolar nerves. The operator palpates the zygomatic process of the maxilla and then advances the finger distally towards the maxillary tuberosity. The needle penetrates mucosa high in the buccal sulcus between the finger and the distal surface of the zygomatic process and is advanced about a centimetre into the space above the buccinator attachment. A dose of 2.0 ml of solution is injected while maintaining finger pressure. This produces a swelling above the buccinator. At completion of the injection the patient closes the mouth slightly and the solution is massaged superiorly, medially, and distally towards the posterior superior alveolar foramen.

Anterior superior alveolar nerve block

This technique anaesthetizes the anterior teeth and associated hard and buccal soft tissues on one side of the maxilla. It can be achieved by using the infraorbital nerve block described below or by depositing 1.5–2.0 ml of solution in the region of the apex of the maxillary canine tooth.

Infraorbital nerve block

This injection anaesthetizes the incisor, canine, and premolar teeth and associated buccal soft and hard tissues, the soft tissues of the upper lip, and part of the side of the nose. It may be administered via the mouth or extraorally.

The intraoral technique involves inserting a long needle parallel to the roots of the premolar teeth in the zone between the first and second maxillary premolars and advancing toward the infraorbital foramen. About 1.5 ml solution should be injected at the foramen.

The extraoral approach is via skin towards the same target area as described for the intraoral method.

Anterior middle superior alveolar nerve block

This method[5] requires the use of a slow delivery system as provided by computerized syringes (Figure 7.4). The injection point is in the palate halfway between the midline and the gingival margin in the mid premolar point. About 1.0 ml of solution is injected very slowly and solution enters the cancellous space in the maxilla via the multiple foramina that are present on the

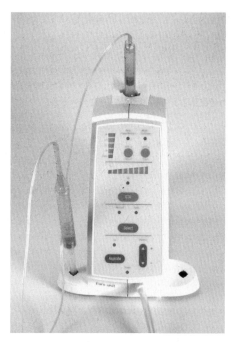

Figure 7.4 Computerized syringes are required for techniques such as anterior middle superior alveolar and palatal anterior superior alveolar nerve block (see text for details).

palatal aspect. This injection can anaesthetize the pulps of the premolar, canine, and incisor teeth on one side together with the associated palatal soft tissues. The buccal soft tissues are not affected.

Palatal anterior superior alveolar nerve block

This injection[6] also relies on the use of computerized delivery systems. In this method the needle is inserted into the incisive papilla palatal to the maxillary central incisors. While injecting slowly, the needle is advanced into the nasopalatine canal, where around 1.0 ml of solution is injected. This anaesthetizes the pulps of the anterior teeth bilaterally and may also provide some anaesthesia to the premolars. The labial soft tissues are not affected by this injection.

Greater palatine nerve block

The greater palatine nerve block will anaesthetize one side of the hard palate as far as the canine region. The injection of 0.2 ml of solution at the greater palatine foramen readily achieves this.

Nasopalatine nerve block

This is the most uncomfortable of the intraoral injections in the conscious patient. The method involves deposition of 0.2 ml of solution on one side of the incisive papilla in the anterior hard palate. Bilateral palatal soft tissue anaesthesia adjacent to the incisor teeth ensues.

Regional anaesthetic techniques for the mandibular nerve and its branches

Regional block techniques are more usually employed in the mandible as infiltration methods are not so successful in the lower jaw. This is a result of the dense cortical plate of bone inhibiting diffusion of solution after deposition supraperiosteally. The blocks employed include the mandibular nerve block, inferior alveolar and lingual nerve block, mental and incisive nerve block, and the long buccal nerve block.

Mandibular nerve block

The mandibular nerve block is given by an extraoral approach. The closest intraoral technique to a true mandibular nerve block is the Gow–Gates method described below.

Extraoral approach to the mandibular nerve

In this method the foramen ovale is approached via the sigmoid notch of the mandible. The landmark for skin penetration and the approach to the lateral pterygoid plate are both identical to those described above for the extraoral approach to the maxillary nerve (Figure 7.1). A long needle is used and it is inserted at right angles to both skin and the sagittal plane. As mentioned with the extraoral approach to the maxillary nerve, the depth of insertion to the pterygoid plate is noted as it determines the correct amount of insertion for the final injection. The next step is to withdraw the needle until the tip is just under the skin. The needle is advanced again but at a different angle. This time the correct angulation is 60° to the sagittal plane. This allows the needle to pass posteriorly to the pterygoid plates. The endpoint for injection is no more than 4 mm deeper than that ascertained at the original penetration to the pterygoid plates.

Inferior alveolar and lingual nerve block

There are many methods described to anaesthetize the inferior alveolar and lingual nerves. Some of these anaesthetize only these two nerves, while others (such as the Gow–Gates method) will affect transmission in other nerves. Several intraoral approaches have been described.

Direct (Halstead) approach

This is probably the most commonly used technique for anaesthesia of the inferior alveolar and lingual nerves within dentistry (Figure 7.5). When successful it provides anaesthesia of the teeth on one side of the jaw and the associated bone, the buccal soft tissues anterior to the mental foramen, the soft tissues of the lip, chin, and anterior two-thirds of tongue. As with all regional block techniques, structures in the midline (such as the central incisor tooth) may not achieve successful anaesthesia unless some other technique is used to counter crossover supply from the contralateral side.

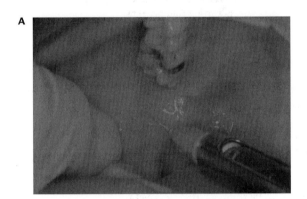

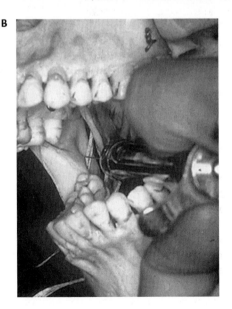

Figure 7.5 The direct approach to the inferior alveolar and lingual nerves. **A** Site of needle penetration; **B** bony endpoint.

The approach is designed to allow deposition of solution close to the mandibular foramen on the medial aspect of the mandibular ramus. The patient has the mouth wide open and a syringe, fitted with a 27-gauge long (35-mm) needle, is advanced across the premolar teeth of the contralateral side to the puncture point, which is half way between the internal oblique ridge of the mandible (which is palpated) and the pterygomandibular raphe (which is visualized). The height of penetration is at the level of halfway up the operator's thumbnail when the thumb is located in the coronoid notch of the mandibular ramus. The needle is advanced 20–25 mm until the medial surface of the ramus is contacted; it is then withdrawn slightly to be supraperiosteal and after aspiration 1.5 ml of solution is deposited. Contact with bone is important prior to injection as it is possible to direct the needle posterior to the ramus and enter the parotid gland. Injecting into this gland can result in hemifacial paresis as transmission in the motor nerves of the facial nerve can be affected. This method will anaesthetize the inferior alveolar nerve and invariably also blocks transmission in the lingual nerve; however, if the lingual nerve needs to be anaesthetized, withdrawing the needle halfway and depositing 0.5 ml at this point is appropriate.

Indirect method

One of the problems that can occur with the direct approach to the inferior alveolar nerve is contacting bone too soon, in the region of the internal or external oblique ridge of the ramus. To circumvent such a possibility, the indirect method may be used. In this technique, the needle is inserted at the same puncture point as described above but the approach is across the teeth on the ipsilateral side. After advancing the needle 10–15 mm, the syringe is swung over towards the premolar teeth of the contralateral side and the method continues as described for the direct technique.

Akinosi–Vazirani method

This technique[7] has two unusual features for an intraoral approach to the mandibular nerve. Firstly, there is no bony endpoint during the approach. Secondly, the patient has the mouth closed during the injection. The landmarks for this method are very simple when a 35-mm needle is used. The patient has the mouth closed and the needle is introduced at the level of and parallel to the maxillary mucogingival junction on the ipsilateral side (Figure 7.6). The needle

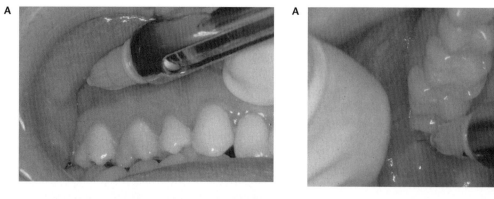

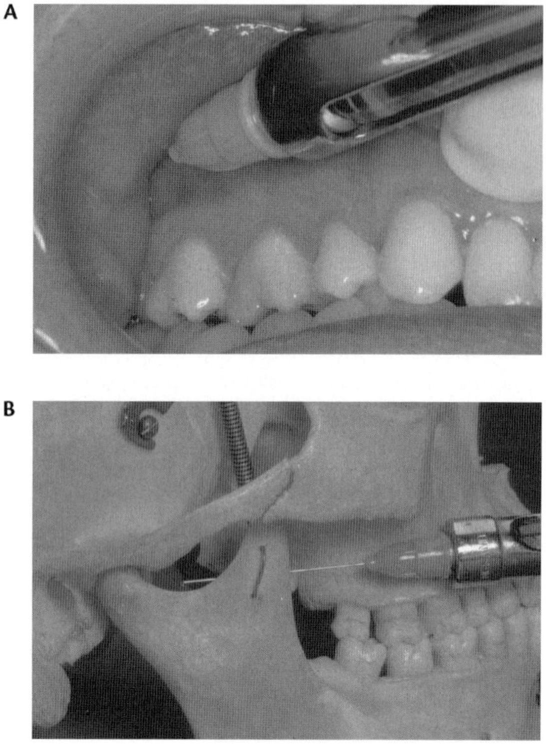

Figure 7.6 The Akinosi-Vazirani technique. **A** The clinical appearance; **B** endpoint of injection.

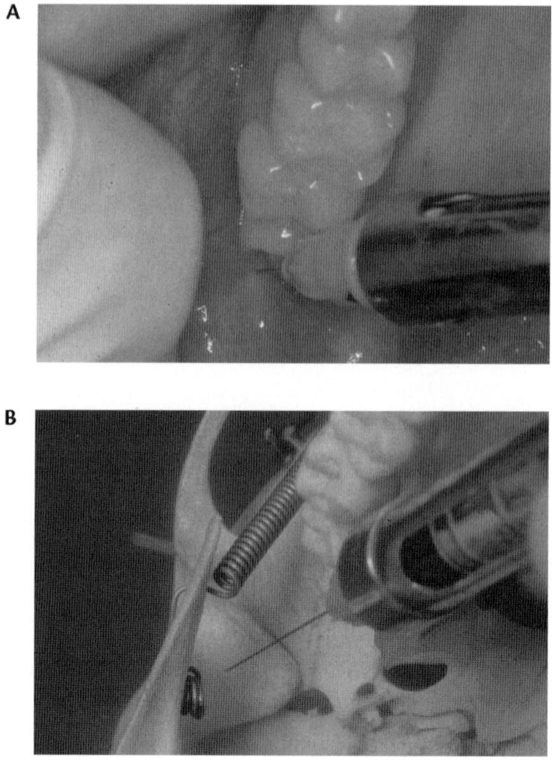

Figure 7.7 The Gow-Gates approach to the mandibular nerve. **A** The point of needle penetration; **B** the endpoint of injection.

penetrates the mucosa in the region of the maxillary tuberosity, and advancement continues until the hub of the needle is parallel to the distal surface of the upper second molar tooth. This is the point of solution delivery and 2.0 ml should be injected following aspiration. This injection will anaesthetize the inferior alveolar, lingual, and mylohyoid nerves.

Gow–Gates method

This technique[8] delivers local anaesthetic solution more superiorly than the other methods described, thus is more likely to anaesthetize fibres leaving the mandibular nerve proximal to the inferior alveolar nerve. In addition to the inferior alveolar, it also anaesthetizes branches of the lingual, mylohyoid, and long buccal nerves. The auriculotemporal nerve may also be affected. To administer this injection, the patient has the mouth wide open and the syringe is advanced from the contralateral maxillary canine across the palatal cusps of the ipsilateral maxillary second molar (Figure 7.7). The syringe is parallel to a line drawn from the angle of the mouth to the intertragal notch. The needle is advanced until bony contact has been made with the mandibular condyle. The needle is then withdrawn slightly and 2.0–3.0 ml injected after aspiration.

Mental and incisive nerve block

This injection provides good soft tissue anaesthesia of the lip and chin. It also anaesthetizes the premolar and anterior teeth, but crossover supply from the midline reduces efficacy for the central incisors. Solution is deposited at the mental foramen via either an intraoral or extraoral approach. The intraoral approach is simpler and the target is the area just below the point halfway between the apices of the mandibular premolar teeth. This is approached via the mandibular buccal sulcus and, following aspiration, 1.5 ml of solution is injected. Massaging the solution through the mental foramen aids the early development of anaesthesia of the teeth.

Long buccal nerve block

This injection anaesthetizes the buccal mucosa and skin in the area opposite the mandibular molar teeth. This can be achieved by infiltration anaesthesia but the true long buccal block is performed by inserting the needle through mucosa in the region of the coronoid notch in the anterior ramus of the mandible and delivering 0.5 ml of solution.

Specialized intraoral techniques

There are some methods[9] that are unique to intraoral anaesthesia; although these may be of limited application in the field of maxillofacial surgery, they merit a mention. They can be especially useful when conventional methods do not provide satisfactory anaesthesia of the teeth. These techniques include intraligamentary or periodontal ligament anaesthesia, intraosseous anaesthesia, and intrapulpal anaesthesia. These techniques have rapid onset but limited duration of anaesthesia. They provide a more localized zone of anaesthesia compared to the other injections described.

Intraligamentary anaesthesia

Intraligamentary anaesthesia (Figure 7.8) is really a subset of intraosseous but as the technique differs it is considered separately. This method relies on deposition of local anaesthetic into the periodontal ligament. From this zone the anaesthetic enters the cancellous bone of the jaws via the cribriform plate of the tooth socket wall. Small doses are used. Only 0.2 ml of solution is deposited into the periodontal ligament on the mesiobuccal aspect of each root of the tooth in question. This technique can be performed with conventional local anaesthetic equipment although

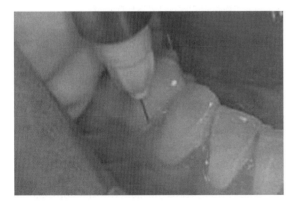

Figure 7.8 The intraligamentary or periodontal ligament injection.

specialized syringes are available that have a mechanical advantage provided by a lever. Narrow (30-gauge) needles are recommended and the injection should be performed slowly as it is possible to extrude teeth from their sockets if excessive force is used.

Intraosseous anaesthesia

Intraosseous anaesthesia (Figure 7.9) is most readily achieved using specialized kit. In this method a hole is made through already anaesthetized buccal attached gingiva distal to the tooth being anaesthetized using a perforator attached to a dental drill. This perforation is carried through the cortical bone until cancellous bone is reached. The perforator is then replaced with a needle of matching diameter and 0.5–1.0 ml of solution injected. Some systems allow perforation and injection with the same needle, thus eliminating the need to change equipment.

The entry of local anaesthetic into the circulation after intraligamentary and intraosseous methods is as rapid as after intravascular injection, and aspiration is not performed during these techniques. Much smaller doses are used than in conventional methods; however, the quick systemic entry must be remembered.

Intrapulpal anaesthesia

Intrapulpal anaesthesia is unique in that no local anaesthetic agent is required. Double-blind studies have shown saline to be as effective as local anaesthetic solutions[10]. In this method, solution is forced into the exposed root canals of teeth and anaesthesia is obtained by ischaemia (Figure 7.10). The method has limited application and can be very unpleasant but has good success. The important feature in governing success is injection against strong back pressure.

Complications of maxillofacial local anaesthesia

Complications resulting from local anaesthetic injections can be localized or generalized. They can be further divided into pharmacological and non-pharmacological. Pharmacological complications may be more common in the maxillofacial region as a result of two factors. Firstly, the area is highly vascularized and inadvertent intravascular injection may occur. Secondly, a higher concentration of the vasoconstrictor adrenaline (1:80 000 or 12.5 μg/ml) is used routinely in this region compared to other regions of the body. The reader is referred to textbooks of

A

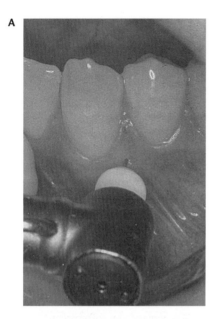

B

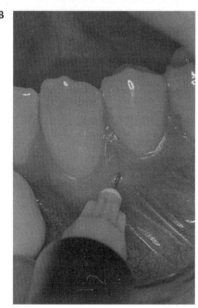

Figure 7.9 The intraosseous injection. **A** Penetration of cancellous. **B** Insertion of needle.

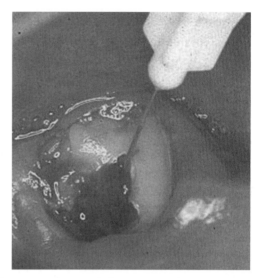

Figure 7.10 The intrapulpal injection.

pharmacology and drug interactions for detailed descriptions of the pharmacological complications of local anaesthesia[11,12].

Localized complications

These can be the result of trauma from the needle or attributable to the injected solution.

Failure of anaesthesia

Failure of anaesthesia is probably the commonest complication. This is more likely after regional block techniques. Failure may be the result of incorrect technique, anatomical variations, presence of inflammation or pharmaceutical problems. The latter can be excluded if the local anaesthetic solution has been properly stored and used before its expiry date.

The correction of poor technique is self-evident. The proper positioning of the needle is important. In addition, the injection of solution at a slow rate (no faster than 30 seconds per ml) increases the efficacy of both infiltration and intraoral regional block techniques[13].

A number of anatomical variations can lead to failure of regional block methods. Alterations of the position of landmarks such as the mandibular foramen can occur[14]. If appropriate radiographs such as panoramic views are available these can be used to locate such landmarks. In addition, collateral supply may decrease the efficacy of regional block injections. This is apparent in midline structures where bilateral nerve supply is common. In the mandible, nerves other than the inferior alveolar nerve may supply the teeth and bone, and these may not always be anaesthetized by the standard inferior alveolar nerve block. The nerves implicated in producing accessory supply to the lower teeth and mandible include the lingual nerve, the long buccal nerve, the nerve to mylohyoid, the auriculotemporal nerve, and the cervical nerves.

These nerves can be countered by using high mandibular blocks such as the extraoral approach, Gow–Gates or Akinosi techniques, or by using supplemental methods such as buccal and lingual infiltrations, periodontal ligament anaesthesia or intraosseous injections.

The presence of inflammation reduces the efficacy of both infiltration and regional block anaesthesia[15]. This reduced efficacy is the result of hyperalgesia caused by activation and sensitization of nociceptors. The presence of inflammation, however, is not a contraindication to the use of local anaesthesia. It is unwise to inject into a site of acute inflammation; however, the use of appropriate regional blocks is possible. As a result of decreased sensitivity of inflamed nerves to local anaesthetics, increased volumes of solution are often necessary, particularly as technique combinations such as intraligamentary, infiltration, and regional block may be employed. This means that knowledge of maximum doses is important to avoid a toxic reaction. This is discussed below. Inflammation is associated with a greater incidence of central effects, and the prophylactic use of systemic anti-inflammatory drugs such as ibuprofen has been shown to increase local anaesthetic efficacy in the maxillofacial region[16].

Injection pain

Some injection pain may occur during delivery of local anaesthesia intraorally and is most apparent during injections in the anterior palate. Using chasing techniques through already anaesthetized buccal interdental papillae to gain access to the palate can decrease this discomfort[17]. The use of topical anaesthetics in the mouth is worthy of discussion. There are very few well controlled trials that have investigated the efficacy of intraoral topical anaesthesia. Those that have appeared show conflicting results. There is evidence that topical anaesthetics do have a pharmacological (in addition to any psychological) effect, as some well designed studies show increased efficacy when topical anaesthetics have been compared to placebo. One study has shown a dose response with topical lidocaine[18]. What is apparent from the literature is that, although topical anaesthetics can reduce the discomfort of needle penetration in the mouth, they have little if any effect on the discomfort of solution deposition. The major factor in reducing the latter is slow injection; this decreases the discomfort of both infiltration and regional block methods.

Severe pain at the time of injection may be the result of subperiosteal deposition. When bone is contacted the needle should be withdrawn a millimetre or so to avoid this complication. Subperiosteal injection may also lead to postinjection pain.

Intravascular injection

Inadvertent intravascular injection may occur in the orofacial region as this area is very well vascularized. As mentioned in the introduction to this chapter, up to 20% of some intraoral regional block techniques show evidence of positive aspirates of blood during injection[1,2]. It is essential that an aspirating syringe system is used when prefilled local anaesthetic cartridges are employed; a variety of such systems are available.

Accidental intravascular injection may occur into the arterial or venous side of the circulation. The latter is more common and may lead to systemic effects attributable to the local anaesthetic or vasoconstrictor; an example would be a tachycardia secondary to increased plasma adrenaline levels.

Unintentional intra-arterial injection can cause localized blanching and, on occasion, tissue necrosis. In addition, injection of local anaesthetic into an artery in the maxillofacial region may interfere with special senses and produce other intracranial effects. These complications and the strategies used to avoid them are described below.

Alteration of special senses and intracranial effects

Diplopia, temporary blindness, and deafness have all been reported after intraoral injection of local anaesthetics[19,20]. These most probably arise as the result of inadvertent intra-arterial injection into a vessel with an intracranial course such as the middle meningeal artery. An alternative route intracranially is the so-called reverse carotid flow[21]. This can occur if solution is injected under force into a branch of the external carotid artery, which results in flow of anaesthetic in a retrograde fashion to the carotid bifurcation, at which point some solution is redirected to the internal carotid artery. This phenomenon has been demonstrated in animal models and accounts for those rare cases of temporary hemiplegia reported after injection in the maxillofacial region. Use of an aspirating syringe system should reduce these temporary complications. In addition, a slow injection rate should eliminate the possibility of reverse carotid flow.

Trismus

Inability to open the mouth may occur after inferior alveolar nerve blocks. This is the result of bleeding into the medial pterygoid muscle, producing muscle spasm. There is nothing that can be done to prevent this.

Recovery to normal function can be slow, taking up to 3 or 4 weeks in some cases.

Hemifacial paresis

A temporary hemiparesis of the face may arise following mandibular block techniques if solution is unintentionally injected into the parotid gland. The thick parotid fascia, which normally prevents diffusion of solution into the gland, retains solution in the gland and a temporary paralysis of the facial nerve may occur. The most important effect is loss of the blink reflex, so the eye must be protected with a patch until normal function returns.

Nerve damage

Regional block in the maxillofacial region can cause damage to nerve trunks[22]. The cause of this damage may be physical trauma from the needle or may be the result of chemical damage from the local anaesthetic solution. This latter is an area of controversy as some believe that the use of more concentrated solutions (such as 4% prilocaine and 4% articaine) produce more non-surgical paraesthesia than 2% lidocaine[23,24]. The nerve most commonly affected is the lingual nerve. The reason for this may be, that as well as being at risk during the approach to the mandibular foramen, the lingual nerve may be damaged during withdrawal of the needle. When the needle is removed, it has developed a fish-hook appearance as a result of tip deformation as it travels through the tissue, whether or not bone is contacted[25]. Another explanation as to why the lingual nerve may be more susceptible to long-term loss of sensation compared to the inferior alveolar nerve, for example, is the result of its structure. The former has fewer fascicles and so recovery may be less forthcoming[26]. Many patients will experience an electric-shock type of feeling during mandibular block injections (again, usually in the lingual nerve); however, not all patients who suffer from post-injection nerve damage will have noticed such an effect. Most cases will recover in less than 2 weeks; however, some remain intransigent. Unfortunately, non-surgical nerve damage is unsuitable for surgical repair and the type of problem produced tends to be a dysaesthesia.

Infection

There are sporadic reports of latent herpes infection being reactivated at the site of intraoral needle penetration. This is a rare complication.

Self-inflicted trauma

As a result of the extensive soft tissue anaesthesia that may occur after regional block techniques in the orofacial region, patients (especially young patients and their parents) must be warned about the dangers of self-inflicted trauma, particularly to the lips and tongue. They should be warned about the dangers of taking excessively hot food and drink whilst the anaesthesia is still effective and not to test anaesthesia by biting the soft tissues. This is a real concern as significant amounts of soft tissue can be lost as a result of self-inflicted trauma[27].

Generalized complications

Syncope

Syncope may occur in the conscious patient prior to intraoral injections. This is prevented by having the patient in a supine position.

Allergy

Allergy to amide local anaesthetics, although possible, is very rare indeed. Ester local anaesthetics were much more likely to cause allergic reactions. These days the only ester anaesthetics in routine use are the topical agents benzocaine and amethocaine. The preservatives contained in some amide solutions (such as para-amino benzoic acid) can trigger allergic reactions as they are structurally related to the ester anaesthetics; however, most modern local anaesthetic formulations are preservative-free. Some local anaesthetic cartridges contain latex and these should be avoided in individuals with severe latex allergies. Most individuals who are tested for allergy to local anaesthetics are found to be non-allergic. Symptoms that patients may mistake for allergy include tachycardia, tiredness, syncope, and localized swelling at the site of injection. Obviously if an individual reports symptoms that are consistent with an allergic reaction such as breathing difficulty, rash or non-localized swelling, then they should be formally tested for allergy. In addition to determining if an allergy exists this will also provide information on an alternative safe anaesthetic.

Toxicity

The subject of toxicity is worth mentioning in relation to injections in the maxillofacial region, particularly intraoral injections. As a result of the highly vascular nature of this region, systemic uptake is more rapid than in other areas of the body, even when adrenaline at a concentration of 12.5 µg/ml is used.

Recommendations for the maximum safe dose of local anaesthetics in this region are inconsistent. Nevertheless, most authorities on this subject suggest lower maximum doses compared to those used elsewhere in the body[28,29]. One recommendation when using prefilled dental local anaesthetic cartridges is to limit the dose to one-tenth of a cartridge per kilogram of body weight. This is a reasonable approximation to the recommended maximum dose for most formulations available in dental cartridges, and, although not absolute, is a reasonable rule of thumb in otherwise healthy patients.

Conclusion

A number of different local anaesthetic techniques are used in the maxillofacial region. Some of these are unique to this location. The highly vascular nature of this part of the body and the use of local anaesthetic solutions with relatively high concentrations of adrenaline mean that systemic effects may be more likely than in other areas.

Distinctive complications can arise from administration of local anaesthetics in the maxillofacial region.

References

1. Rood JP. (1972) Inferior dental nerve block: routine aspiration and a modified technique. *Br Dent J*, **132**, 103–5.
2. Meechan JG, Blair GS. (1989) Clinical experience in oral surgery with two different automatic aspirating syringes. *Int J Oral Maxillofac Surg*, **18**, 87–9.
3. Meechan JG, Ledvinka JIM. (2002) Pulpal anaesthesia for mandibular central incisor teeth: a comparison of infiltration and intraligamentary injections. *Int Endodont J*, **35**, 629–34.
4. Adatia AK. (1976) Regional nerve block for maxillary permanent molars. *Br Dent J*, **140**, 87–9.
5. Friedman MJ, Hochman MN. (1998) The AMSA injection: A new concept for local anesthesia of maxillary teeth using a computer-controlled injection system. *Quintessence International*, **29**, 297–303.
6. Friedman MJ, Hochman MN. (1999) P-ASA block injection: A new palatal technique to anesthetize maxillary anterior teeth. *Journal of Esthetic Dentistry*, **11**, 63–71.
7. Akinosi JO. (1977) A new approach to the mandibular nerve block. *Br J Oral Surg*, **15**, 83–7.
8. Gow-Gates GAE. (1973) Mandibular conduction anaesthesia: a new technique using extraoral landmarks. *Oral Surgery, Oral Medicine, Oral Pathology*, **36**, 321–8.
9. Meechan JG. (2002) Supplementary routes to local anaesthesia. *Int Endodont J*, **35**, 885–96.
10. Birchfield J, Rosenberg PA. (1975) Role of anaesthetic solution in intrapulpal anaesthesia. *J Endodont*, **1**, 26–7.
11. Rang H, Dale M, Ritter J, Flower R. (eds) (2007) *Rang and Dales Pharmacology*, 6th edn. London: Churchill Livingstone.
12. Baxter K (ed.) (2007) *Stockley's Drug Interactions*, 8th edn. London: Pharmaceutical Press.
13. Kanaa MD, Meechan JG, Corbett IP, Whitworth JM. (2006) Efficacy and discomfort associated with slow and rapid inferior alveolar nerve block injection. *J Endodont*, **32**, 919–23.
14. Afsar A, Haas DA, Rossouw PE, Wood RE. (1998) Radiographic localization of mandibular anesthesia landmarks. *Oral Surg, Oral Med, Oral Pathol, Oral Radiol, Endodont*, **86**, 234–41.
15. Hargreaves KM, Keiser K. (2002) Local anesthetic failure in endodontics. *Endodontic Topics*, **1**, 26–39.
16. Modaresi J, Dianat O, Mozayeni MA. (2006) The efficacy comparison of ibuprofen, acetaminophen-codeine, and placebo premedication therapy on the depth of anesthesia during treatment of inflamed teeth. *Oral Surg, Oral Med, Oral Pathol, Oral Radiol, Endodont*, **102**, 399–403.
17. Welbury RR, Duggal MS, Hosie M-T (eds) (2005) *Textbook of Paediatric Dentistry*, 3rd edn. Oxford: Oxford University Press, pp. 97–8.
18. Hersh EV, Houpt MI, Cooper SA *et al.* (1996) Analgesic efficacy and safety of an intra-oral lidocaine patch. *J Am Dent Assoc*, **127**, 1626–34.
19. Rishira B, Epstein JB, Fine D, Nabi S, Wade, NK (2005). Permanent vision loss in one eye following administration of local anesthesia for a dental extraction. *Int J Oral Maxillofac Surg*, **34**, 220–3.
20. Tan TS, Shoeb M, Winter S, Frampton MC. (2007) Acute sensorineural hearing loss immediately following a local anaesthetic dental procedure. *Eur Arch Otorhinolaryngol*, **264**, 99–102.
21. Aldrete JA, Narang R, Sada T, Tan Liem S, Miller GP. (1977) Reverse carotid blood flow—a possible explanation for some reactions to local anesthetics. *J Am Dent Assoc*, **94**, 1142–5.
22. Smith MH, Lung KE. (2006) Nerve injuries after dental injection: a review of the literature. *J Can Dent Assoc*, **72**, 559–64.
23. Haas DA, Lennon D. (1995) A 21 year retrospective study of reports of paresthesia following local anesthetic administration. *J Can Dent Assoc*, **61**, 319–20, 323–6, 329–30.
24. Hillerup S, Jensen R. (2006) Nerve injury caused by mandibular block analgesia. *Int J Oral Maxillofac Surg*, **35**, 437–43.
25. Rout PG, Saksena A, Fisher SE. (2003) An investigation of the effect on 27-gauge needle following a single local anaesthetic injection. *Dent Update*, **30**, 370–4.
26. Pogrel MA, Schmidt BL, Sambajon V, Jordan RCK. (2003) Lingual nerve damage due to inferior alveolar nerve blocks. A possible explanation. *J Am Dent Assoc*, **134**, 195–9.
27. Akram A, Kerr RMF, Mclennan AS. (2008) Amputation of lower left lip following dental local anaesthetic. *Oral Surgery*, **1**, 111–13.
28. Malamed SF (ed.) (2004) *Handbook of Local Anesthesia*, 5th edn. New York: Mosby.
29. Meechan JG. (2002) *Practical Dental Local Anaesthesia*. London: Quintessence.

8

Conscious sedation

David Craig

Introduction

Many patients regard all dental treatment, and especially surgical procedures, as potentially painful and stressful. Reactions range from 'normal' apprehension, through various degrees of anxiety to irrational fear or even phobia. The adverse physiological effects of these psychological responses can increase the risk of treatment and should be controlled. This is particularly important for patients suffering from medical conditions which are made worse by fear.

Conscious sedation is considered by both the United Kingdom (UK) General Dental Council and the UK Department of Health to be an integral element of the control of pain and anxiety[1–3]. In other words, conscious sedation is an important aspect of the modern practice of dentistry.

The UK Department of Health defines conscious sedation as 'A technique in which the use of a drug or drugs produces a state of depression of the central nervous system enabling treatment to be carried out, but during which verbal contact is maintained throughout the period of sedation. The drugs and techniques used to provide conscious sedation should carry a margin of safety wide enough to render loss of consciousness unlikely. The level of consciousness must be such that the patient remains conscious, retains protective reflexes, and is able to understand and respond to verbal commands'[2].

In the UK, the most commonly used dental conscious sedation techniques (titrated intravenous midazolam or titrated inhaled nitrous oxide/oxygen) have an excellent safety record. For many patients, conscious sedation combined with effective local anaesthesia is a very acceptable alternative to general anaesthesia. Explaining the benefits and risks of local anaesthesia, sedation, and general anaesthesia is an important part of the consent process. Despite the safety, efficacy, and cost-benefits of using conscious sedation techniques there are still indications for general anaesthesia for some dental/surgical procedures and certain patient groups.

This chapter provides an introduction to conscious sedation techniques for dental or oral surgery procedures, patient assessment and treatment planning, essential pharmacology, sedation equipment, clinical sedation ('standard' and 'alternative'[4]), sedation for medically compromised patients, and the avoidance/management of sedation-related complications. However, before administering any form of conscious sedation the dental team must have received appropriate training in accordance with contemporary professional guidance[2–8].

Patient assessment and treatment planning

A satisfactory first visit is crucial to the success of subsequent treatment under conscious sedation. There is a great deal of information to be acquired from the patient. At the same time, it should never be forgotten, that the patient is also assessing the dental team. The first meeting should ideally be out of the dental surgery environment and in the nature of an informal 'chat'. The following areas need to be explored:

What is the problem?

It is often helpful to get the patient to complete a questionnaire asking the nature of their fears. This breaks the ice, and other questions may be included which will steer the conversation in the right direction. Remember that for some patients even discussing dentistry can be frightening (Table 8.1).

Medical history

A detailed medical history must be obtained. From the sedation point of view, special note should be made of respiratory and cardiovascular problems, and liver and

Table 8.1 Typical signs and symptoms of anxiety

Signs	Symptoms
Clenched fists/sweaty hands	Fainting
Pallor	Sweating
Distracted appearance	Dry mouth
Not sitting back fully in the dental chair	Need to visit lavatory
Holding handbag/tissue tightly	Nausea
Throat clearing	Tiredness
Looking around	
Not smiling	
Touching/fiddling	
Licking lips	
Very quiet or voluble	
Aggressive behaviour	

kidney disease. Prescribed medication may alert the operator to undisclosed medical conditions and also raise the question of drug interactions. Some medicines potentiate the effect of sedation drugs. It may sometimes be necessary to discuss the patient's medical history with their general medical practitioner or hospital consultant. Baseline recordings of arterial blood pressure, heart rate, and arterial oxygen saturation should be obtained and the results recorded in the clinical notes.

Prescribing sedation can be beneficial in many cases (Table 8.2). The sedation technique may need to be modified to accommodate specific patient risk factors (Table 8.3). Caution should be exercised in the presence of some coexisting medical conditions and expert opinion sought in order to establish the most appropriate environment for conscious sedation (Table 8.4).

Having collected this information it is now possible to assess the operative and/or sedation risk according to the scale of physical fitness devised by the American Society of Anesthesiologists (ASA, see Chapter 2).

Patients classified as ASA 1 or 2 are generally considered suitable for treatment in a primary dental care setting. Those falling into categories 3 and 4 should be referred to a specialist centre such as a teaching hospital or specialist sedation clinic. Some patients oscillate between ASA 3 and 4 according to the severity of their disease and other factors such as the season of the year or a change in medication. Examples of this type of fluctuating condition include: poorly controlled

Table 8.2 Examples where sedation is almost certainly beneficial

Angina: may be provoked by anxiety or stress during the procedure. Sedation reduces the likelihood of angina-related symptoms

Hypertension: the anxiety of treatment can cause an increase in heart rate and an elevation of blood pressure. Sedation modifies these responses and protects the patient

Asthma: sedation is helpful when attacks are known to be provoked by stress

Epilepsy: midazolam is particularly useful in preventing fits when the patient is poorly controlled

Movement disorders: in patients with uncontrolled movements, intravenous sedation will very often suppress the activity

asthma; diabetes mellitus; and epilepsy. It may be preferable to refer such patients or, better still, wait until their condition becomes more stable before providing treatment under sedation. If a patient suffers from two relevant illnesses, or appears to be ASA 2 but with the use of multiple drugs, it is probably sensible to consider the patient to be ASA 3. The ASA scale is a useful 'shorthand' method of recording a patient's medical status but it requires common sense and careful application in order to avoid creating either unnecessary concern or confidence.

When assessing the medical status of an elderly patient, it must be remembered that some physiological functions decline naturally with age and even the apparently healthy patient with no declared medical problems cannot be treated exactly like a young fit adult. Elderly patients with one controlled illness

Table 8.3 Examples of conditions where the technique might require modification

Controlled heart failure: patients might be distressed when supine. Liver perfusion (therefore drug metabolism) is likely to be reduced

Chronic anaemia (diagnosed and managed): be aware of the potential effects of falling oxygen saturation levels and respond promptly

Chronic airways disease(s): interpretation of oxygen saturation levels in smokers and chronic bronchitics may be difficult

Well-controlled diabetes: ensure that the patient is managed appropriately. If possible, have a chairside measure of blood sugar at the beginning of treatment to avoid any later difficulties in assessing levels of consciousness. Avoid unnecessary starvation prior to sedation

Table 8.4 Examples where caution is required—referral should be considered

Severe cardiorespiratory disease: the patient may be breathless at rest or after minimal exertion
Hepatic disease: if there is active liver disease or known impairment of function, drug metabolism may be ineffective (apart from the other problems which could affect treatment)
Severe psychological illness: where antipsychotic or 'major' tranquillizers are used
Drug abuse: opioid dependence or frequent recreational drug use
Alcohol: high levels of alcohol intake or known alcoholism

(e.g. angina) may be suitable for treatment in a primary care setting but the presence of two known conditions (bearing in mind that other disease processes may be present but undiagnosed) should indicate referral.

Dental history

The patient's experiences at the dentist over the years are important; questioning may yield valuable information[9] which will assist during treatment planning (Table 8.5). It must be remembered that non-anxious patients may also be better managed under sedation if the proposed dental procedure is potentially threatening and/or prolonged.

Social factors

The patient's domestic circumstances are very important. An escort will be required for most sedation appointments. In addition, having responsibility for children or elderly relatives may make it difficult for the patient to attend or to be able to recover safely at home.

Table 8.5 Useful dental history questions

Has 'normal' dentistry been possible in the past?
When did dental anxiety start?
What provoked the fear?
When did the patient last visit a dentist?
Has the patient had treatment under general anaesthetic or conscious sedation in the past?
If sedation, what technique was used?
Was this treatment successful?
What concerns the patient most about their teeth?
Are there any current symptoms (particularly pain)?

Dental examination

Whilst some patients will allow a full intraoral examination, the operator may have to be content with a visual examination at this stage. Many phobic patients fear the dental probe and so this should only be used when absolutely necessary, and then with extreme caution. For a very few patients, intraoral radiographs may also be threatening or cause gagging, and so will have to be carried out under sedation.

Discussion and treatment planning

Selection of the most appropriate method of pain and anxiety control requires careful consideration of a number of interlinking factors including the proposed dental treatment, the patient's health and degree of anxiety, the operator's training and experience, and the environment in which the treatment is to be carried out. No matter how fashionable, it is impossible to design a 'care pathway' or 'protocol' which incorporates all the relevant factors. The correct and most successful approach involves a commitment by the whole team (surgeon/sedationist/nursing staff) to careful consideration of a range of options for each individual. A 'one size fits all' approach to pain and anxiety management is rarely successful.

Once a preliminary dental treatment plan has been formulated the treatment options (Table 8.6) may then be considered and discussed with the patient. Advantages and disadvantages of techniques are included in Tables 8.7 and 8.8.

The simplest technique which will enable treatment to be carried out is generally considered to be the most appropriate. However, it is entirely inappropriate to subject patients to a rigid cascade of management options by only being prepared to consider more complex or 'alternative' forms of sedation when all 'simpler' techniques have failed. This is unnecessarily distressing for patients (and the dental team) and may serve to increase anxiety.

Table 8.6 Treatment options

Local anaesthesia (LA) alone
LA with intravenous midazolam
LA with oral or intranasal midazolam
LA with alternative sedation drugs/techniques
LA with inhalational sedation
General anaesthesia

Table 8.7 Advantages and disadvantages of intravenous midazolam sedation

Advantages:
Rapid onset (3–4 minutes or less)
Adequate patient co-operation
Good amnesia
Disadvantages:
No clinically useful analgesia
Respiratory depression
Occasional disinhibition effects
Occurrence of sexual fantasies (rare)
Postoperative supervision for a minimum of 8 hours is required
Older patients are easily over-sedated
Less predictable sedation in young patients

Written consent is required for both the dental procedure and the administration of conscious sedation. Consent for dentistry under conscious sedation should, under all but emergency circumstances, be obtained at the assessment appointment rather then when he/she attends for treatment. If extractions or advanced procedures are required, these must be agreed on a tooth-by-tooth basis; however, this is not usually practical for routine restorative dentistry.

Finally, patients must be given written and verbal pre- and postoperative instructions (Table 8.9) and be

Table 8.8 Advantages and disadvantages of inhalational sedation

Advantages:
No 'needles'
Level of sedation easily altered
Minimal impairment of reflexes
Rapid induction and recovery
Some analgesia
An escort is not mandatory for fit adult patients
Disadvantages:
Sedation depends also on good physiological support
Mask may make oral access difficult
Post-operative amnesia variable
Nitrous oxide atmospheric pollution

Table 8.9 Patient instruction prior to sedation for dental treatment

For your safety, please read and follow these instructions carefully:
Before sedation—on the day of treatment:
Take your routine medicines at the usual times
Have only light meals and non-alcoholic drinks on the day of your appointment
Bring a responsible adult with you. Someone who is able to escort you home and then care for you for the rest of the day. (Not mandatory for adult patients receiving nitrous oxide/oxygen sedation)
After sedation—until the following day:
Do not travel alone—travel home with your escort, by car if possible
Do not drive or ride a bicycle
Do not operate machinery
Do not drink alcohol
Do not return to work or sign legal documents

given the opportunity to ask questions. Some, but not all sedationists, prefer that patients are starved in preparation for treatment under conscious sedation.

Pharmacology

Benzodiazepines

Benzodiazepines act throughout the central nervous system. Specific benzodiazepine receptors are located on neuronal membranes within the brain and spinal cord. All benzodiazepines have a common core shape, which enables them to attach to these receptors. The effect of attaching benzodiazepines to cell membrane receptors is to alter an existing physiological 'filter'.

The normal passage of information through sensory neurons to the brain is damped or filtered by the GABA (gamma-amino-butyric acid) system. GABA is an inhibitory chemical, which is released from sensory nerve endings as electrical nerve stimuli pass from neuron to neuron over synapses. Once released, GABA attaches itself to receptors on the cell membrane of the postsynaptic neuron. The postsynaptic membrane becomes more permeable to chloride ions, which has the effect of stabilizing the neuron and increasing the threshold for firing. During this period, no further electrical stimuli can be transmitted across the synapse. In this way, the number of sensory messages, which travel the whole distance from their origin to the areas of the brain where they are perceived, are reduced or filtered.

Benzodiazepine receptors are located close to GABA receptors. The effect of having a benzodiazepine in place on a receptor is to prolong the time it takes for repolarization after a neuron has been depolarized by an electrical impulse. This further reduces the number of stimuli reaching the higher centres and produces pharmacological sedation, anxiolysis, amnesia, muscle relaxation, and anticonvulsant effects.

All benzodiazepines, which are central nervous system depressants, have a similar shape with a ring structure on the same position of the diazepine part of each molecule. By contrast, flumazenil, the benzodiazepine antagonist, does not have this ring structure and has a neutral effect on the workings of the GABA system. Flumazenil is an effective antagonist, as it has a greater affinity for the benzodiazepine receptor than the active drugs and therefore displaces them. Flumazenil has a shorter half-life than midazolam. When it was first introduced there was a suggestion that administering flumazenil to a sedated patient would result in a short period of reversal followed by re-sedation some 50–60 minutes later. This is not true. The displaced midazolam continues to be redistributed and metabolized independently of the presence of flumazenil. The cessation of action of flumazenil (approximately 50 minutes) coincides with the point at which patients would normally be expected to be fit for discharge after a single dose of midazolam.

The anterograde amnesia produced by midazolam is a desirable effect in terms of reducing the patient's memory of stressful or prolonged treatment. The most profound amnesia occurs immediately after induction but some disturbance to short-term memory may persist for several hours or even until the following day. It is therefore essential to warn both patients and their escorts. It is advisable not to guarantee complete amnesia as this effect varies between patients and in the same patient on different occasions. The effect of anterograde amnesia is often misinterpreted by patients with the result that they believe that they have been unconscious. This may lead to difficulties if the patient returns for further treatment under sedation when they may insist that they are undersedated or more awake than before.

The muscle relaxant effect of benzodiazepines contributes to the difficulty in standing, walking, and maintaining balance experienced by many patients following treatment.

Allergy to the benzodiazepines is fortunately very rare. However, as the common core structure of these drugs is almost identical, a patient who exhibits an allergic reaction to any benzodiazepine must not be managed with flumazenil, which would only worsen the situation.

Metabolism of benzodiazepines takes place in the liver. It has no metabolites which are active once the parent drug has been removed. This is a major advantage of midazolam and is the principal reason for its being considered the drug of choice for outpatient conscious sedation. The water-soluble metabolites of the benzodiazepines are excreted via the kidneys.

All benzodiazepines produce respiratory depression. This is usually mild in healthy patients if the drug is administered intravenously by slow titration. It can, however, be a significant problem in unwell or elderly people. Even in a fit healthy individual, a fast injection or a large quantity of midazolam has the potential to depress respiration to the point of apnoea.

Benzodiazepine-induced respiratory depression affects all patients who are sedated with these drugs by any route of administration. For this reason, respiration must be monitored clinically by observation of the rate and depth of breathing and, since it is not always easy to detect small changes in respiratory function, a pulse oximeter is mandatory. Capnography is considered desirable by some authorities but it is not currently a practical proposition.

Benzodiazepines have few significant cardiovascular effects in healthy people. There is a decrease in mean arterial pressure, cardiac output, stroke volume, and systemic vascular resistance. This may present as a small fall in arterial blood pressure immediately following induction of sedation. However, this is normally compensated by the baroreceptor reflex and is of negligible clinical significance except in people with compromising cardiovascular disease.

Propofol

Propofol (Diprivan 1%) is a synthetic phenol anaesthetic induction agent which has rapid onset, short duration (2–4 minutes) and fast recovery. In lower doses it is a safe and effective sedative agent. However, in order to maintain sedation at a constant level, it is necessary to administer propofol by continuous infusion. The elimination half-life is about 60 minutes in fit patients.

Propofol is sometimes painful on injection particularly when a small vein is used. However, injecting into a large vein and/or adding 1 ml of 1% plain lidocaine (approximately 0.1 mg/kg) to each 20 ml (200 mg) of propofol helps to reduce the pain. Pain on injection is of greater significance for conscious sedation than the induction of anaesthesia.

Propofol's pharmacokinetic properties make it very useful for short procedures when sedation is required for only a few minutes, for example, the extraction of a single tooth. Recovery occurs rapidly after the drug is discontinued. The short redistribution half-life prevents the accumulation of drug in the body and, as a consequence, propofol is also an appropriate agent for much longer cases, for example, maxillofacial or implant surgery. There is no antagonist agent for propofol.

As with midazolam, propofol tends to depress respiration. The frequency of hypersensitivity reaction is similar to that of other anaesthetic induction agents. Propofol is not currently recommended for use in patients with any history of epilepsy.

Opioids

For some patients, midazolam on its own does not provide an adequate degree of sedation. In these cases a combination of agents may make treatment possible, thereby avoiding the need for general anaesthesia. The most frequently used combination of agents is an opioid and midazolam. Individual opioids, like benzodiazepines, act through central nervous system receptors and have either agonist or antagonistic actions. These drugs produce a number of therapeutic effects including analgesia, sedation, and euphoria. Their undesirable effects include cardiorespiratory depression and nausea and vomiting. The most important of these in relation to conscious sedation is respiratory depression. Great care must always be taken when a combination of an opioid and a benzodiazepine is used for sedation.

In dental sedation the most frequently used opioid is fentanyl (and its derivatives). When an opioid/midazolam combination is administered it is imperative that the opioid is given before midazolam is titrated. The incidence of vomiting is about 30% using this technique. It is sometimes necessary to administer an antiemetic. If any opioid is used for sedation, naloxone (Narcan) must be available. Naloxone is an opioid antagonist and reverses respiratory depression, analgesia, and sedation.

Nitrous oxide

Nitrous oxide is an anaesthetic gas. It has a blood/gas solubility coefficient of 0.47 and a MAC (minimum alveolar concentration) of 105%. The blood/gas solubility coefficient determines the rate at which the gas concentration in the lungs equilibrates with that being administered which, in turn, relates to the speed of induction and of recovery. Nitrous oxide is poorly soluble in blood and so induction and recovery are rapid.

MAC value relates to the potency of the gas and determines the concentration needed to induce sedation. Nitrous oxide is not very potent, which means that it is a very safe gas for conscious sedation. In sufficient concentrations (in excess of 100%), the drug will induce light surgical anaesthesia, but only at the expense of adequate oxygenation. In lesser concentrations, it has excellent analgesic and sedative properties. There are very few cardiovascular or respiratory effects and no direct depression of myocardial function or reduction in ventilation. The drug has a central analgesic and anaesthetic effect (the exact mechanism is not clear) and is excreted unchanged via the lungs very rapidly after discontinuing its administration.

Sevoflurane

Sevoflurane is a fluorinated derivative of methyl isopropyl ether which was first synthesized in the early 1970s[10]. It has a MAC of 2% and a blood gas solubility coefficient of 0.6. These physical characteristics make sevoflurane a potent anaesthetic agent with rapid uptake and speedy recovery. It is pleasant to inhale, non-irritant and non-pungent.

The properties that make sevoflurane a useful anaesthetic agent also make it a promising sedation agent. However, a specially calibrated vaporizer is required in order to titrate low concentrations of sevoflurane (up to 1%) in oxygen (or nitrous oxide and oxygen). Sevoflurane is partly metabolized (5%) and so some care is required in people with severe liver or kidney disease.

At present sevoflurane is not widely used for dental sedation because of the practical problems associated with incorporating a vaporizer into any of the currently available dental inhalational sedation machines.

Intravenous sedation using midazolam

Midazolam is the benzodiazepine of choice for intravenous dental sedation[11]. It has a variety of presentations (e.g. 10 mg/5 ml; 10 mg/2 ml; 5 mg/5 ml). The more dilute presentations are easier to administer in small increments whilst observing the patient's response. The National Patient Safety Agency has recently recommended that the 5 mg/5 ml concentration is the most appropriate for sedationists[12]. Whatever concentration is used, a titration technique must always be used in order to reduce the risk of oversedation. It is impossible to determine the correct dosage of midazolam by any form of calculation based on the patient's physical characteristics, for example, age, body weight, body mass index (BMI), or body surface area. Overdosage and/or excessively rapid bolus injections often cause profound respiratory depression or even respiratory arrest. Midazolam produces a period of sedation (acute detachment from the individual's surroundings) for 20–30 minutes followed by a state of relaxation for a further hour or so.

Anxiolysis differs from sedation. Anxiolysis (literally 'dissolving anxiety') may be described as 'dissociating the patient from the perceived threat'. An ideal sedation drug would be anxiolytic rather than merely sedative, as this would leave the patient fully aware, but completely unconcerned about the dental treatment. Unfortunately, no such drug exists. It is important to consider the degree of anxiolysis and not just the depth of sedation when assessing the quality of sedation.

Midazolam produces anterograde amnesia (a reduction in recall following administration of the drug) so most patients have little or no recall of the operative procedure. This effect must, of course, be fully explained to both the patient and their escort before discharge.

Allergy to any benzodiazepine represents an absolute contraindication to intravenous sedation with midazolam. However, benzodiazepine allergy is very rare. A degree of caution is needed when using midazolam during pregnancy and breastfeeding, severe psychiatric disease, alcohol or drug abuse, impaired hepatic function, phobia of needles and injections, poor venous access, and when there are doubts about the ability to provide a suitable escort home.

Equipment

Since the vast majority of adult patients (under 65 years of age) require more than 5 mg midazolam to produce effective sedation, the most commonly used size is 10 ml (two ampoules of 5 mg/5 ml). All patients undergoing intravenous sedation must have a flexible plastic cannula placed in a vein, so as to ensure reliable, continuous venous access throughout the procedure[13]. The most convenient cannula sizes are 20G and 22G.

Clinical procedure

It is important to ensure that the patient is fully prepared for the procedure and that the dental team is fully prepared for the patient. All the necessary equipment and drugs must be readily available. Nothing is more disconcerting to an anxious patient than having to wait whilst missing items are located or faulty equipment replaced. Having induced sedation, it is then important that the dentist is ready to proceed without delay.

The appearance of the clinical environment is also important in putting the patient at ease. Many dental surgeries are frankly alarming. It is important to avoid having cardiopulmonary resuscitation posters and anatomical diagrams displayed within the patient's line of vision and to keep threatening equipment covered. Someone must offer friendly support from the moment the patient enters the surgery. Having one person do this is better than relying on the whole team, as everyone may assume that it is someone else's responsibility.

Before any clinical procedure is started, it is important to check the patient's identity, medical history, and blood pressure. Written consent must have been obtained for both the procedure and the sedation. It is also imperative to confirm that the patient has a responsible adult escort, who is able and willing to look after the patient for the rest of the day. A patient, who is unable to provide a suitable escort, must not be sedated unless arrangements have been made for an overnight stay. If there are any doubts, it is better not to proceed with the use of sedation. A final check should be made to ensure that the patient has emptied their bladder.

The following description of the administration of intravenous midazolam (10 mg/10 ml) is appropriate for most fit and healthy adult patients between the ages of 16 and 65. However, even within this age group, variation in the response to sedation is common.

The dental chair should be adjusted to the supine position. Electromechanical monitoring must be established before the patient is sedated, in order to establish baseline readings. Pulse oximetry is mandatory[14]. Continuous blood pressure monitoring and an electrocardiogram (ECG) may be advisable for seriously unfit patients. If supplemental oxygen is indicated, this is the time to apply the nasal cannulae and turn on the oxygen (a flow of 2 litres per minute is sufficient).

A suitable vein must first be cannulated after appropriate skin preparation. The use of topical anaesthetic agents such as Ametop or Emla reduces the discomfort of venepuncture, but these creams must be applied some time before venepuncture in order to achieve good analgesia.

The prepared drug in a 10-ml syringe is attached to the port of the cannula and injected slowly, according to the regimen described below. The patient should be warned of a cold sensation at the needle site and perhaps also as the drug travels up the arm. Provided the sedationist is sure that the needle is correctly sited, the patient should be reassured that this sensation will pass within a short period of time. The injection must be stopped immediately if pain is felt radiating distally as this could indicate arterial injection.

A recommended titration regimen for intravenous midazolam sedation in healthy patients 16–65 years of age is to administer 2 mg (2 ml) injected over 30 seconds, pause for 90 seconds, and administer further increments of 1 mg (1 ml) every 30 seconds until sedation is judged to be adequate. Talk to the patient and watch for any adverse responses, in particular respiratory depression.

The correct dose has been given when there is a slurring of speech, and/or a slowed response to commands and the patient exhibits a relaxed demeanour. With midazolam, ptosis is an unreliable sign and so this should not be used to judge the adequacy of sedation. Some sedationists estimate the depth of sedation by asking the patient to close their eyes and then trying to touch the tip of their nose with an index finger. Inability to demonstrate the appropriate level of coordination is reputed to indicate that the patient is adequately sedated.

Patients over the age of 65 years often require much smaller doses of midazolam. A suggested administration regimen for these patients is 1mg injected over 30 seconds followed by a wait of at least 4 minutes, then additional 0.5-mg increments given every 2 minutes until sedation is adequate. Patients in this age group often need no more than 2 mg in order to provide more than an hour of sedation.

Local analgesia should be administered shortly after this state is attained. Approximately 30–40 minutes of sedation time is usually available and this should be more than adequate for most procedures. It is acceptable to top-up the sedation from time to time, if the procedure is prolonged, but this is rarely necessary during the first 20 minutes. Additional increments of midazolam should be small, 1 or 2 mg is usually adequate (less in the elderly).

At the end of the procedure, the patient should remain under the direct supervision of the sedationist or suitably trained recovery staff. No patient may be discharged until sufficiently recovered so as to be able to stand and walk without assistance. Although most patients will not be fit for discharge until at least 1 hour following the administration of the last increment of midazolam, there is no fixed time limit and recovery staff should be discouraged applying rigid criteria.

The patient should be discharged into the care of the escort, who must also be given written and verbal instructions. The patient should rest quietly at home for the remainder of the day and refrain from drinking alcohol, driving and operating machinery for a minimum of 8 hours. It is important to make the escort aware that the patient should be observed for the first few hours, not simply put to bed out of sight. It is unreasonable and unnecessary to demand that patients travel home by private rather than public transport.

Monitoring the sedated patient

In addition to any electromechanical devices (e.g. pulse oximeter), the sedationist and nurse must be constantly aware of the patient's respiratory rate and depth, the presence of airway obstruction, depth of sedation, and skin colour[10]. Periodic estimation of systemic arterial blood pressure and continuous ECG monitoring may be advisable for some unfit patients.

Respiratory rate is quite variable (12–20 breaths per minute in adults), but this is nearly always reduced during sedation and so must be monitored closely. The depth of breathing is also reduced. Apnoea may occur with an overdosage of (or idiosyncratic response to) midazolam. Such side effects are potentially life threatening if recognition and management is not swift. Some degree of respiratory depression is probably present in all sedated patients, but serious problems are most likely to occur immediately following induction.

Pulse oximetry measures the patient's arterial oxygen saturation and pulse rate from a probe, which is attached to the finger or ear lobe. The pulse oximeter detects changes in the patient's oxygen supply, oxygen uptake by the lungs, and the delivery of oxygen to the tissues via the circulation but does not monitor the adequacy of ventilation. Regardless, this it is a useful monitor of both respiratory and cardiovascular function. However, correct functioning can be affected by metallic nail varnish or excessive light falling on the probe. Oxygen saturations below 90% should be investigated and the cause corrected. Asking the patient to take several deep breaths resolves the majority of cases of midazolam-induced respiratory depression. If this fails, intermittent positive pressure ventilation (IPPV) should be instituted and the administration of flumazenil considered.

Bradycardia or tachycardia during sedation should be investigated. The former may be due to hypoxia or vagal stimulation, whilst the latter is often the result of painful stimuli. Most pulse monitors have audible alarms, which can be set to give audible and visible warning if the heart rate falls or rises beyond clinically acceptable levels. For ASA 1 and 2 patients, bradycardia and tachycardia alarm limits are normally 50 beats/min and 150 beats/min respectively.

Flumazenil (Anexate) antagonizes the action of midazolam, reversing the sedative, cardiovascular, and respiratory depressant effects (but not the amnesia). Although flumazenil is usually recommended for use only in emergency situations (e.g. benzodiazepine overdose), elective reversal may be necessary for some patients. In this case, it is imperative that the usual postoperative instructions for intravenous sedation are given and followed. Although flumazenil has a shorter half-life than midazolam, clinically significant re-sedation does not occur when midazolam is used for short clinical procedures.

Oral and intranasal sedation using midazolam[14-17]

Oral and intranasal sedation are useful where the patient is needle phobic and will not accept vene-puncture. The sedation produced may be adequate for the dental procedure to be carried out or it may then be necessary to administer intravenous sedation in the normal way.

The most commonly used drug is midazolam. In adults, the standard oral dose is 20 mg and the standard intranasal dose is 10 mg. Note that neither of these routes involves titration and so both are potentially less safe than intravenous sedation. Midazolam is has a bitter taste and so must be added to a strong-flavoured fruit juice for oral administration. Intranasal midazolam is much more rapidly absorbed than oral midazolam but may cause short-lasting nasal irritation, sneezing, and, occasionally, mild epistaxis. Intranasal midazolam is most effective when a high concentration formulation (40 mg/ml) is employed. This is not commercially available but is obtainable from some hospital pharmacies with a manufacturing

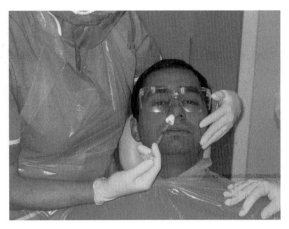

Figure 8.1 Mucosal atomization device (MAD) for the intranasal administration of midazolam for dental sedation.

facility. Figure 8.1 shows the intranasal administration of midazolam using a 1-ml syringe fitted with a mucosal atomization device (MAD).

The operative and postoperative management of patients, who have received oral or intranasal midazolam, is very similar to that for intravenous midazolam. The depth of sedation is similar but rather less predictable, monitoring with a pulse oximeter is mandatory, and the discharge and escort criteria are identical. It is recommended that patients who receive intranasal or oral sedation should have a cannula inserted as soon as adequate sedation has been achieved[4].

Although midazolam does not have a product licence for oral or intranasal administration, both routes are commonly used in dentistry and medicine. However, practitioners should not use these routes without appropriate training and clinical experience. Experience of cannulation and intravenous sedation are essential[4].

Alternative intravenous sedation techniques[4,18]

The following techniques must only be used by appropriately trained and experienced practitioners in an appropriate environment.

Opioid with midazolam

Patients, who are not adequately sedated using intravenous midazolam alone, may sometimes be successfully managed by administering a small bolus of an opioid drug prior to titrating the midazolam. Whilst it is usually preferable to use a single drug-sedation technique, using a combination technique may avoid the need for general anaesthesia.

The opioid selected should ideally have a shorter duration of action than midazolam so as to avoid prolonged recovery. For dentistry, fentanyl (Sublimaze) is now the most commonly used drug. It is administered as a slow 50-mcg fentanyl bolus. After 1 minute, appropriate titrated increments of midazolam are administered. It should be noted that the total dose of midazolam will be probably be considerably less that that required without the opioid.

All opioid drugs have the potential to cause dangerous respiratory depression necessitating prompt and effective management from the dental team. Nausea and vomiting are common and unpleasant side effects.

Propofol by operator-controlled infusion[19,20]

In subanaesthetic doses and when administered in an appropriate manner, propofol is a reliable and safe drug for intravenous sedation with a considerably shorter distribution half-life than midazolam. By comparison with midazolam, recovery is rapid and patients report feeling 'clear-headed' more quickly. Amnesia is often less profound. Propofol confers a greater degree of anxiolysis than sedation and patients appear less sleepy than with midazolam. When administered by continuous infusion, propofol is more controllable than titrated midazolam and the depth of sedation may be varied during the procedure. It is particularly useful both for very short cases and for long procedures. There are few contraindications to propofol but it should be avoided if there is known or suspected allergy to any of its components or for patients with epilepsy. There is still concern about the use of propofol for sedation in very young children.

Propofol infusion techniques are not suitable for use by an operator-sedationist. The technique may only be used by a second practitioner who has received specific training. For a fit adult of normal build, 30 mg of propofol (1%) is given by slow manual injection (this bolus is not weight-related) and an infusion started at an initial rate of 300 mg (30 ml) per hour. Sedation usually occurs within 1–2 minutes. The infusion rate may need to be adjusted during long procedures.

Particular care is needed with procedures lasting longer than 30 minutes in order to avoid too deep a level of sedation. Careful clinical monitoring and pulse oximetry is mandatory. Although respiratory depression may occur, it appears to be less marked than is the case with midazolam. As with all dental sedation techniques, the use of effective local analgesia is essential. The procedure for recovery is similar to that for midazolam. The criteria for discharge and instructions for after-care suggested for midazolam should be observed.

Patient-controlled infusion (PCI)[21,22]

Both midazolam and propofol have been used successfully in patient-controlled sedation (PCS) systems. An infusion pump with a demand system allows the patient to control the depth of sedation. Overdosage is prevented by a time-based lockout. In addition to making the patient feel more in control, PCS may optimize the level of sedation and thus reduce the incidence of both under- and oversedation.

Target-controlled infusion (TCI)[23]

TCI using propofol for dental sedation is currently under investigation and development and offers some promise. However, if these systems are to be effective the algorithms chosen to determine the infusion rate must be based on data from patients who suffer real dental anxiety/phobia.

Inhalational sedation using nitrous oxide/oxygen (relative analgesia)[24–27]

The use of nitrous oxide and oxygen in subanaesthetic concentrations was popularized as a method of sedation during the late 1940s. Machines which are designed to deliver a variable concentration of nitrous oxide in oxygen suitable are readily available.

Nitrous oxide has excellent anxiolytic, sedative, and analgesic properties, with little or no depression of myocardial function or ventilation. Induction and recovery are rapid and it has a wide margin of safety. Inhalational sedation may also be used to facilitate cannulation in some needle-phobic patients. The variation between individual patients is such that, whilst one person may be adequately sedated with 20% nitrous oxide, another individual may require in excess of 50%. A titration technique of administration is employed in order to avoid the risk of oversedation.

Because of the relatively poor solubility of nitrous oxide in blood and body tissues, there is rapid outflow of nitrous oxide across the alveolar membrane, when the incoming gas flow is stopped. This may dilute the percentage of alveolar oxygen available for uptake by up to 50%. This phenomenon is called diffusion hypoxia and is prevented by giving 100% oxygen for at least 2 minutes at the end of the procedure.

There are very few contraindications to inhalational dental sedation but they include nasal obstruction (e.g. cold, polyps, deviated septum), cyanosis at rest, poor cooperation, first trimester (12 weeks) of pregnancy, and fear of masks.

Equipment

Modern inhalational sedation (relative analgesia, RA) machines are similar to traditional Boyle's anaesthetic machines, but modified so as to make them safe for use by a dental seditionist (Figure 8.2).

Most portable inhalational sedation machines are designed to operate with two nitrous oxide and two oxygen cylinders for safety. A pin index system ensures that the nitrous oxide and oxygen gas cylinders cannot be accidentally interchanged. The popular MDM (Matrx Medical, Inc., Orchard Park, New York, USA) RA machine head has flow meters for nitrous oxide and oxygen, a control valve for regulating the total gas flow, and a mixture dial for adjusting the percentage of oxygen and nitrous oxide. All modern inhalational sedation machines are incapable of delivering a gas mixture containing less than 30% oxygen and also have a failsafe mechanism which shuts off the nitrous oxide if oxygen ceases to flow.

The mixed gases emerge at the common gas outlet to which the breathing system is connected. The

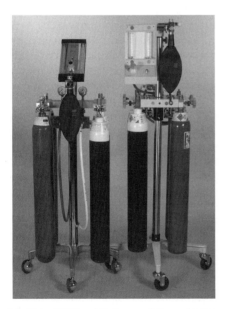

Figure 8.2 Matrx MDM and McKesson relative analgesia machines

reservoir bag is useful for adjusting the total gas flow to an individual patient's minute volume and also for monitoring respiration during treatment.

Although designs vary, all modern inhalational sedation breathing systems comprise an inspiratory limb, a nasal mask, and an expiratory limb. Nasal masks are available in a variety of styles and sizes. Older style breathing systems must be cold sterilized, but some of the newer materials are suitable for autoclaving. Modern nasal masks have both fresh gas and scavenging connectors.

Clinical procedure

Having checked that the inhalational sedation machine is working and that extra gas cylinders are available (or that piped gases are flowing), the patient is laid supine in the chair and the procedure explained.

The machine is then adjusted to administer 100% oxygen at a flow rate of 6 l/min and the correct size nasal mask selected. Patients often prefer to place the mask over their own nose. It is important to maintain a steady flow of conversation and encouragement. The oxygen flow rate (minute volume) may be checked by observing the movement of the reservoir bag. If there is under- or overinflating, the gas flow must be increased or decreased respectively. Ten per cent nitrous oxide is then added (90% oxygen) and the patient informed that he/she may feel light-headed, have changes in visual/auditory sensation, tingling of hands and feet, suffusing warmth, and a feeling of remoteness from the immediate environment. This concentration is maintained for one full minute, during which plentiful verbal reassurance is given. The concentration of nitrous oxide is increased by 10% for a further full minute (to a total of 20% nitrous oxide) and then in increments of 5% until the patient appears and feels sufficiently relaxed.

Nitrous oxide concentrations of between 20% and 50% commonly allow for a state of detached sedation and analgesia without any loss of consciousness or danger of obtunded laryngeal reflexes. At these levels, patients are aware of operative procedures and are cooperative without being fearful. If, after a period of relaxation, the patient becomes restless or apprehensive, it is probable that the concentration of nitrous oxide is too high.

Having carried out the dental procedure, the nitrous oxide is turned off and 100% oxygen administered for 2 minutes (to prevent diffusion hypoxia). Recovery is usually complete within 15–30 minutes.

Monitoring the sedated patient[14]

The sedationist and the dental nurse must be aware of the patient's respiration (rate and depth), the presence of airway obstruction, depth of sedation, and skin colour. Electromechanical devices (e.g. pulse oximeter, sphygmomanometer, ECG) are not indicated unless the patient has serious medical problems.

Nitrous oxide pollution and waste gas scavenging

Long-term exposure to nitrous oxide may result in an increased incidence of liver, renal, and neurological disease, and there is evidence of bone marrow toxicity and interference with vitamin B12 synthesis, which may lead to signs and symptoms similar to those of pernicious anaemia. For this reason, the UK Health and Safety Executive specify a maximum level of 100ppm of nitrous oxide time-weighted over 8 hours[28]. In order to achieve this level and so keep nitrous oxide pollution to a minimum, scavenging must be employed. Systems for use with active scavenging differ from those for use with passive removal of waste gases. Active scavenging is achieved by connecting the expiratory limb of the breathing system to a low power suction device, whilst passive scavenging often involves simply placing the open end of the expiratory tube as far away as possible, preferably outside the operating environment.

Sedation for younger patients

In the UK, inhalational sedation using a titrated dose of nitrous oxide in oxygen is the only completely tried and tested conscious sedation technique currently recommended for children under 12 years of age.

Intravenous sedation with midazolam has often been said to be reliably unpredictable in patients under 16 years of age and predictably unreliable below the age of 12. Some young patients sedate satisfactorily whilst others become disinhibited, more anxious, or even frankly aggressive. Despite a number of recent studies it has not been possible to identify any factors which may be used to predict the likelihood of success. Until more research has been carried out, therefore, intravenous midazolam should only be considered for children when other options have been considered. In any case, these techniques must only be used by experienced sedationists or anaesthetists working in an appropriate environment[4]. The use of flumazenil to manage a young patient with disinhibition following intravenous midazolam is not recommended as the data currently available suggests that the situation is often made worse rather than improved. Propofol is widely used for adult sedation but there are still reservations about its use for sedation in very young children.

Orally administered benzodiazepines such as temazepam and midazolam, appear to produce more reliable sedation for this age group. However, the time taken for the drug to act is much less predictable than with intravenous sedation owing to differences in the rate of gastric absorption, first-pass metabolism, and protein binding. Most patients become sedated somewhere between 10 and 30 minutes following oral administration. Midazolam appears to be the more predictable drug in this respect with a typical time of onset of about 12 minutes. Its widespread use in the UK in dental and medical disciplines has shown this to be a safe, appropriate, and effective technique. Orally administered antihistamines have been used for paediatric sedation in medicine for many years but their use in dentistry has been mostly limited to special care patients.

Benzodiazepines may also be administered intranasally and although this technique offers a number of advantages for certain groups, particularly very young patients, needle phobics, and those with disabilities, the route requires specific training and experience.

Whichever technique is used for paediatric sedation it is a requirement that the practitioner and the team are experienced in the use of the drug and its route of administration. It is important to remember that oral and intranasal sedation produces a similar level of sedation to that achieved by intravenous midazolam and so the pre- and postoperative instructions to the patient, monitoring, and arrangements for discharge must be identical to that for intravenous sedation. Oral sedation should not be regarded as a safer or easier option than intravenous sedation. In many ways it is potentially less safe owing to the poor predictability of onset, depth of sedation, and recovery.

Inhalational sedation using sevoflurane in oxygen, or a mixture of nitrous oxide and oxygen, is currently receiving research attention and it appears to be useful for younger patients[10]. At present, sevoflurane sedation must be administered only by practitioners trained in anaesthesia.

Complications of conscious sedation

Serious complications associated with carefully administered conscious sedation are rare. Minor problems are more common. Fortunately most minor problems are easily managed by a well-prepared dental team. Careful case selection, based on a detailed medical, dental, and social history, will often allow the dental team to anticipate potential difficulties and take appropriate action.

Respiratory depression

The most serious potential complication associated with intravenous sedation is respiratory depression. The effect is normally most pronounced during the first 10 or so minutes of sedation. It is also sometimes seen later if there is a lull in clinical activity. The difficulty in recognizing mild or even moderate respiratory depression underlines the necessity for continuous pulse oximetry in addition to careful clinical monitoring. However, patients who are receiving supplementary oxygen therapy can record apparently acceptable oxygen saturations despite significant hypoventilation secondary to sedation. Vigilance is paramount.

Management of midazolam-induced respiratory depression

Prompt action is necessary. Ask the patient to take several deep breaths. In the majority of cases, this will resolve the problem. If this fails summon help, open the airway (head tilt/chin lift or jaw thrust), and perform IPPV ventilation using a ventilating bag, preferably with an oxygen supply attached.

Administer flumazenil (500 mcg by slow intravenous injection) if there is no return to adequate spontaneous ventilation. Continue to ventilate and encourage breathing.

Airway obstruction

Obstruction of the airway may occur during any form of sedation. Excessive downward pressure from the dental practitioner without adequate support of the mandible during the extraction of molar teeth is a common cause. Accumulation of water and dental debris in the oropharynx can also be a problem. This is easily managed by the use of properly positioned high-volume suction.

Injection problems

Extravascular injection of midazolam is usually uncomfortable. If this occurs the cannula must be repositioned. Intra-arterial injection is rare and causes pain distal to the injection site. If this is suspected, the injection should be stopped and the cannula re-sited. Whilst painful, intra-arterial midazolam is unlikely to cause long-term sequelae. However, some sedative/analgesic agents can provoke severe spasm and may necessitate giving an antispasmodic such as papaverine.

Over-sedation and under-sedation

A small amount of oversedation with intravenous midazolam is not usually a serious problem. The most common effect is poor patient cooperation with the patient refusing to open his/her mouth and so treatment is delayed. Gross oversedation using midazolam may cause profound respiratory depression or even apnoea requiring prompt and effective management (discussed previously).

Mild oversedation with nitrous oxide is often more troublesome as the patient may feel panicky and reject further treatment. Oversedation of young children is particularly undesirable. Intentional undersedation, in the belief that it is safer, is pointless and may lead to increased dental phobia. Failing to provide an adequate depth of sedation is a common failure of the inexperienced sedationist.

Disinhibition

Many patients show signs of mild disinhibition when sedated with midazolam, for example, giggling, crying, talkativeness, or panic attacks which may seriously interfere with dental treatment. Firm management by the dental team may restore calm but further bouts may occur. Aggressive and abusive behaviour is probably another manifestation of disinhibition.

Paradoxical effects

Intravenous midazolam sometimes results in a paradoxical effect. The patient becomes more rather than less anxious and treatment may not be possible. This is particularly common in children and adolescents. The administration of more midazolam often makes matters worse and the effects of flumazenil are unpredictable. The best approach is to abandon treatment and allow the patient to rest quietly.

Prolonged recovery

Recovery from intravenous midazolam is variable due to variability in redistribution of the drug from the receptor sites (short-term recovery) followed by metabolism and excretion (long-term recovery). Some groups of patients, particularly those taking or using central nervous system depressant drugs have notoriously unpredictable recovery times. For the majority of these patients, management simply involves patience and careful monitoring. Flumazenil may be helpful but should not normally be used when the patient has psychiatric or medical conditions which involves treatment with potent central nervous system depressants or stimulants, in particular benzodiazepines.

Hypotension

All intravenous sedation drugs tend to cause a decrease in the systemic arterial blood pressure. Unlike respiratory depression, the fall in blood pressure is usually self-limiting and, as such, requires no active treatment. A patient with a naturally low arterial blood pressure should be moved slowly from the supine position to the sitting position to reduce the possibility of postural hypotension.

Hiccups

A small number of patients experience hiccups following intravenous sedation with midazolam. Most cases appear to be associated with either excessive midazolam or rapid injection (or both).

Sexual fantasies

Much has been written about the occurrence of sexual fantasies in patients receiving intravenous sedation using midazolam. The extent of the problem is unknown. The best advice which can be offered is to ensure that no sedated or recovering patient is ever left alone with only one member of the dental team.

Failure of sedation

Conscious sedation techniques are not always successful. Early recognition of impending failure is important in order to avoid starting a dental procedure which it may not be possible to complete. An open and honest discussion with the patient and their escort will reduce the disappointment of a failed sedation appointment. Alternative sedation techniques or general anaesthesia should be considered.

Conclusion

Conscious sedation, combined with regional anaesthesia, can offer a safer alternative to general anaesthesia for some oral and maxillofacial surgical procedures. Careful patient selection and evaluation is the key to a successful and satisfactory outcome. As the process is potentially dangerous in unskilled hands, sedation should only be conducted by those fully

trained and totally familiar with the techniques involved.

References

1. General Dental Council (UK). (2002) *The First Five Years. A Framework for Undergraduate Dental Education.* London: General Dental Council.
2. The Standing Dental Advisory Committee. (2003) *Conscious Sedation in the Provision of Dental Care. Report of an Expert Group on Sedation for Dentistry.* London: Department of Health.
3. *Commissioning Conscious Sedation Services in Primary Dental Care.* (2007) London: Department of Health.
4. *Standards for Conscious Sedation in Dentistry: Alternative techniques.* (2007) London: Faculty of Dental Surgery of the Royal College of Surgeons of England and the Royal College of Anaesthetists.
5. *Implementing ensuring safe sedation practice for healthcare procedures in adults.* (2001) London: Academy of Medical Royal Colleges.
6. General Dental Council (UK). (2005) *Standards for Dental Professionals.* London: General Dental Council.
7. *Conscious Sedation in Dentistry: Dental Clinical Guidance.* (2006) Dundee: National Dental Advisory Committee, Scottish Dental Clinical Effectiveness Programme.
8. *A Conscious Decision: Report of an expert group chaired by the Chief Medical and Dental Officer.* (2000) London: Department of Health.
9. *Conscious Sedation: A Referral Guide for Dental Practitioners.* (2001) London: Dental Sedation Teachers' Group in liaison with SAAD.
10. Averley PA, Girdler NM, Bond S, Steen N, Steele J. (2004) A randomised controlled trial of paediatric conscious sedation for dental treatment using intravenous midazolam combined with inhaled nitrous oxide or nitrous oxide/sevoflurane. *Anaesthesia,* **59,** 844–52.
11. Skelly AM. (1992) Sedation in dental practice. *Dental Update,* **19,** 61–7.
12. National Patient Safety Agency (2008) *Rapid Response Report (NPSA/2008/RRR011). Reducing risk of overdose with midazolam injection in adults.* London: National Patient Safety Agency.
13. The Royal College of Surgeons of England. (1993) *Guidelines for sedation by non-anaesthetists. Report of a Commission on the Provision of Surgical Services working party.* London: The Royal College of Surgeons of England.
14. Society for the Advancement of Anaesthesia in Dentistry. (1990) *Guidelines for physiological monitoring of patients during dental anaesthesia or Sedation.* London: Society for the Advancement of Anaesthesia in Dentistry.
15. Manley MCG, Skelly AM, Hamilton AG. (2000) Dental treatment for people with challenging behaviour: general anaesthesia or sedation? *Br Dent J,* **188,** 358–60.
16. Manley MCG, Ransford NJ, Lewis DA, Thompson SA, Forbes M. (2008) Retrospective audit of the efficacy and safety of the combined intranasal/intravenous midazolam

sedation technique for the dental treatment of adults with learning disability. *Br Dent J*, **205,** 523.

17. Boyle CA, Manley MCG, Fleming GJP. (2000) Oral midazolam for adults with learning disabilities. *Dent Update*, **27,** 190–2.

18. Wildsmith JAW, Craig DC. (2008) Conscious sedation for dentistry: an update. *Bull Roy Coll Anaesth*, **47,** 2405–7.

19. Rodrigo MRC, Jonsson E. (1989) Conscious sedation with propofol. *Brit Dent J*, **166,** 75–80.

20. Craig DC, Boyle CA, Fleming GJP, Palmer PA. (2000) Sedation technique for implant and periodontal surgery. *J Clin Periodontol*, **27,** 955–9.

21. Girdler NM, Rynn D, Lyne JP, Wilson KE. (2000) Patient controlled propofol sedation in phobic patients. *Anaesthesia*, **55,** 327–33

22. Leitch JA, Anderson K, Gambhir S, *et al.* (2004) A partially-blinded randomised controlled trial of patient-maintained propofol sedation and operator controlled midazolam sedation in third molar extractions. *Anaesthesia*, **59,** 853–60.

23. Leitch, JA, Sutcliffe N, Kenny GNC. (2003) Patient-maintained sedation for oral surgery using a target-controlled infusion of propofol - a pilot study. *Brit Dent J*, **194,** 43–5.

24. Roberts, GJ. (1990) Inhalation sedation (relative analgesia) with oxygen/nitrous oxide gas mixtures. 1. Principles. *Dental Update*, **17,** 139–46.

25. Roberts GJ. (1990) Inhalation sedation (relative analgesia) with oxygen/nitrous oxide gas mixtures. 2. Practical techniques. *Dental Update*, **17,** 190–6.

26. Crawford AN. (1990) The use of nitrous oxide-oxygen inhalation sedation with local anaesthesia as an alternative to general anaesthesia for dental extractions in children. *Brit Dent J*, **168,** 395–8.

27. Shaw AJ, Meechan JG, Kilpatrick NM, Welbury RR (1996) The use of inhalation sedation and local anaesthesia instead of general anaesthesia for extractions and minor oral surgery in children: a prospective study. *Int J Paed Dent*, **6,** 7–11.

28. Health and Safety Executive. (1998) *Occupational Exposure Limits*. London: Her Majesty's Stationery Office (HSMO).

9

Anaesthesia for dental surgery

Sean Williamson

Introduction

This chapter will concentrate on anaesthesia for procedures involving the gums and teeth including extraction (exodontia) and for the purpose of preservation or replacement of teeth. Removal of teeth for either caries or impaction is one of the commonest surgical procedures undertaken in the United Kingdom (UK). In the vast majority of cases the removal of teeth, and most other dental surgical procedures, can be carried out as day cases using local anaesthesia (Chapter 7) with or without sedation (Chapter 8). However, general anaesthesia is still a frequent request from both surgeon and patient.

Dentistry and general anaesthesia certainly have a long history of association (Chapter 1). Indeed, many of the early general anaesthetics were administered for dental extractions. The reliance on general anaesthesia in the UK, even for minor dental procedures, continued until the very late twentieth century with general anaesthesia being regarded as the normal method for providing painless dentistry. The sites for the administration of anaesthesia varied considerably, as did the practitioners themselves. It was not unusual to have the dental surgeon providing both anaesthesia and surgery simultaneously.

In the 1970s and 1980s, increasing concerns were raised over the level of safety associated with dental anaesthesia. Every year there were a number of deaths, often in healthy children undergoing simple procedures. At this time, hospital anaesthesia was progressively improving safety in a way that left dental surgeries wanting. The reasons were multi-factorial, including the fact that anaesthesia was often administered under conditions with substandard monitoring, assistance, and resuscitation equipment. Patients were often poorly prepared, and dental remuneration was such that it encouraged a high throughput of patients.

Increasing public and political concern resulted in a working party led by Professor David Poswillo[1] who subsequently made recommendations for the safe provision of general anaesthesia in dentistry outside of hospital in the UK. Poswillo recommended avoiding general anaesthesia for dental treatment wherever possible, that the same standards of personnel, monitoring, and equipment should apply whether anaesthesia is administered in a hospital or in a dental surgery, and that dental surgeries should be inspected and registered. Unfortunately many of the recommendations were not uniformly adopted. Despite an initial fall in the number of anaesthetics administered, this was followed by an increase both in anaesthetics and deaths[2].

In the late 1990s, following a number of high-profile deaths and a successful manslaughter prosecution, the UK General Dental Council (GDC) and the Royal College of Anaesthetists issued further guidance[3,4]. It was highlighted that general anaesthesia was often used inappropriately as a method of anxiety control in situations where local anaesthesia, with or without sedation, might be more appropriate.

Despite the clinical advice guiding decisions it is apparent that through the 1990s the need for general anaesthesia fluctuated with changing reports rather than being necessarily related to clinical need or patient choice[5]. Experience in Cardiff demonstrated a 19.6% rise in cases following Poswillo, followed by a 59.2% fall in cases following the GDC revised guidance.

The UK Royal College of Anaesthetists report[4] furthermore expressed again the expectation that the same standards (personnel, equipment, situation, etc.) should apply to dental anaesthesia as widely accepted for anaesthesia in other clinical settings. That these standards needed to be explicit may seem a surprise. Many anaesthetists working in dental anaesthesia at that time had considerable experience. However, a survey of practising anaesthetists in the UK in 1999 revealed only 16% used full monitoring and up to 30% did not have a specifically trained assistant or recovery staff. Furthermore, 71% did not obtain intravenous access as routine[6].

Subsequent recommendations, which remain current at time of print, addressed those personnel engaged in the administration of dental anaesthesia. It was proposed that only anaesthetists on the specialist register of the UK General Medical Council, trainees working under supervision in programmes accredited by the Royal College of Anaesthetists, and non-consultant career grade doctors working under the responsibility of a named consultant anaesthetist, could administer anaesthesia for dental surgery. In addition all anaesthetists in a training grade had to be able to demonstrate that they had devoted an appropriate part of their professional training to cases involving dental treatment.

Both the anaesthetists and dentists were expected to work with their own dedicated trained assistants. Patients were also to be recovered with appropriate monitoring and under the supervision of trained recovery staff. Wider training of both anaesthetists and dentists in alternative techniques of pain and anxiety control was suggested.

A marked reduction in the provision of general anaesthesia followed. In 2000, the UK Department of Health encouraged moves towards centralization of services to the hospital setting where clinical support and critical care facilities would be available. Finally, after 31 December 2001, the administration of general anaesthesia in dental surgeries in the UK was prohibited[7–9].

Indications for general anaesthesia for dental treatment

The reasons for choosing general anaesthesia are guided by the UK Department of Health and Royal College of Anaesthetists recommendations. Recommendations proposed that general anaesthesia should only be administered where no alternative existed. This in itself is interesting, as for many other procedures where local anaesthesia and general anaesthesia are both suitable, the patient may be given a choice provided they give appropriately informed consent.

Situations where general anaesthesia may be the only viable option include those in which it would be impossible to achieve adequate local anaesthesia and so

complete treatment without pain, such as the management of acute infection (e.g. acute dento-alveolar abscess). Similarly, patients who, because of problems related to age/maturity or physical/learning disability, are unlikely to allow safe completion of treatment and patients with long-term dental phobias are also thought to be unsuitable for treatment under local anaesthesia. The long-term aim in such phobic patients is the graduated introduction of treatment under local anaesthesia using, if necessary, an intermediate stage employing conscious sedation techniques. In practice, one of the main reasons for general anaesthesia is the inability to comply with the need for a still open mouth.

The initial referral for patients to have treatment with general anaesthesia comes from the general dental practitioner (GDP). Referrals for general anaesthesia tend to have a common pattern. In relevant studies of referral the commonest reasons are multiple extractions, severe anxiety, and age (i.e. children). Repeat referrals are common and there is often a history of low levels of cooperation. Estimates of complete lack of cooperation reach 23%[10]. Levels of dental anxiety are higher than in the general population. Carers of children requiring anaesthesia for dental treatment are likely to have poor oral health themselves as well as lower levels of education attainment[11]. The most important factor influencing choice is based on previous unpleasant dental experience[12]. Indices of dental health are higher. The decayed, missing, or filled teeth (DMFT) scores are higher and maternal educational achievement is lower[13]. Patients most often present with acute problems requiring surgical treatment[14] and therefore general anaesthesia is more likely to be indicated. However, the clinical rationale may differ between units and, as stated earlier, is often driven by external bodies.

The issue of repeat attendance creates longer-term problems. Up to 11% of children presenting at a young age are likely to return within 2 years for similar treatment[15]. Although this is a low frequency it is important to make the management of general anaesthesia be as smooth as possible in order to prevent problems at a later date with either dental anxiety or treatment avoidance with respect to parent or child. However, it is important at every stage of referral to consider moving towards sedation and away from general anaesthesia as those undergoing repeat general anaesthetics remain fearful of dentistry[16]. Patients with learning disability also present for dental anaesthesia. Although the majority of those with special needs can be cared for in general dental practice, those with profound disability and/or anxiety require a shared approach between dentist and anaesthetist.

Patient assessment

The initial screening of patients for general anaesthesia is performed by the referring dentist who should take a full medical history and discuss with the patient the risks of, and alternatives to, general anaesthesia[7]. Sedation should always be considered, although failed sedation is often an indication to proceed straight to a general anaesthetic. However, the final decision on whether a general anaesthetic has an acceptable risk/benefit ratio can only be made after direct consultation between the patient (or parent/legal guardian), the operating dental surgeon, and the anaesthetist. Therefore, anaesthetists should always be ready to discuss with dental colleagues policies for general anaesthesia, and their implications for an individual patient to allow efficient patient management. Preoperative assessment is the same as for any other operation (see Chapter 2). It is recognized that many adult patients with learning disability are more likely to experience mental health problems and are more prone to chronic illness, epilepsy, physical and sensory disabilities, and poor oral health.

Children

Children presenting for primary exodontia are often having their first visit to hospital. Repeated courses of antibiotics have often been given. There may be some oral conditions, such as lactose intolerance which make children more susceptible to caries due to drinking soya milk.

Preoperative assessment should include routine questioning of the parent/guardian. A detailed anaesthetic, surgical, and medical history should be taken, including drug history and allergies. The presence of coexisting acute medical problems, in particular respiratory tract infection, should be considered in the light of the pain and swelling being experienced by the patient. A risk/benefit analysis should be made. Airway examination should include a detailed assessment of loose deciduous teeth as these require particular care during airway manipulation prior to the operative dentistry. To find teeth misplaced during induction can be time consuming and these can cause obstruction to the airway (see Chapter 12). Particular

attention to fasting history is essential as patient cooperation is known to be variable[10].

Comorbidities in the paediatric population are often related to the root causes of the caries. Poor dental health is associated with poor diet and increased weight and obesity. Furthermore, there is an association with lower socioeconomic status independent of body mass index[17–21]. This association extends across children and adults presenting for dental treatment. The severity of dental disease is often worse in the obese patient than the non-obese. It is likely that other diseases associated with lower economic status, such as asthma, and household tobacco consumption also increase the frequency of childhood respiratory disease in the dental population as compared to other surgery. In addition, this paediatric population has a high incidence of respiratory tract infection, adenotonsillar, and nasal obstruction. Careful examination of the child may reveal new diagnoses as this may be an infrequent contact with the medical profession. One controlled study found a higher incidence of patent ductus arteriosus, aortic stenosis, ventricular septal defect, and obstructive sleep apnoea in the dental population compared to no new diagnoses in a non-dental control population. These were apparently fit asymptomatic children[22].

Patients with learning disaility

Learning disability may be associated with almost any other condition, both congenital and acquired. Patients with special needs as a result of learning disability have an increased prevalence of anaesthetic comorbidities. The major relevance of learning disability itself is the issue of consent (see Chapter 3). The most common medical conditions result from the same underlying cause of the disability. However, all diseases may be advanced as presentation with acute illness tends to be late and access to healthcare is poor. As such, standardized mortality rates are increased.

The incidence of epilepsy in this patient group is estimated at 30%, fifty times higher than in the general population[23]. Although the severity varies from patient to patient, labile poorly-controlled epileptic patients are a regular feature on a community dental operating list. Medications tend to have sedative side effects and recovery from anaesthesia, especially if premedication is necessary, may be prolonged. Poor oral health and poor diet often go hand-in-hand and obesity is common. Patients often need other planned surgical procedures throughout their lives and where possible, dental examinations and treatment by the community dental service should be coordinated with such coincidental procedures.

In addition to epilepsy and obesity, patients with learning disability often have a multiplicity of conditions of interest to the anaesthetist. These include deafness and visual loss causing communication problems, emotional and psychiatric problems making cooperation more difficult, gastrointestinal problems including reflux which may pose an additional aspiration risk, and respiratory disease due to recurrent clinical and subclinical aspiration. Orthopaedic problems, such as contractures, make venous access and patient positioning during surgery difficult. Airway difficulties are more common due to orthopaedic and neuromuscular problems[24] and airway examination may be difficult because of a lack of cooperation. For more information the reader should consult http://www.ncl.ac.uk/nnp/teaching/disorders/learning/ld_role.html

Cardiac disease

The presence of congenital heart disease should always be considered when dealing with patients with learning disability. Indeed, the most common non-cardiac procedure requiring general anaesthesia in patients with learning disability is dental practice[25]. Obvious associations with the more common developmental anomalies exist, for example atrioventricular septal defect and Down's syndrome. However, any cardiac anomaly may be present, both acyanotic and cyanotic. When a previously acyanotic shunt becomes reversed as in Eisenmenger syndrome, this causes particular concern for anaesthesia.

Congenital and acquired cardiac diseases of this type are also associated with an increased risk of infective endocarditis. Previously the use of antibiotics for prophylaxis was considered cheap, effective, and life saving[26]. However, although a bacteraemia is likely to be caused by dental extractions[27], this is also caused by the simple activity of cleaning and brushing the teeth[28]. The Working Party of the British Society for Antimicrobial Chemotherapy restricted the indications for antibiotic prophylaxis in 2006. They stated that there was a lack of association between the everyday bacteraemias and episodes of infective endocarditis and a lack of efficacy for antibiotic prophylaxis regimens. Antibiotics were limited to a single oral dose of either amoxicillin or clindamycin (if allergic to penicillin).

In 2008, the National Institute of Health and Clinical Excellence (NICE) issued UK guidelines for prophylaxis against infective endocarditis[29]. Healthcare professionals should regard people with acquired valvular heart disease with stenosis or regurgitation, valve replacement, structural congenital heart disease, including surgically corrected or palliated structural conditions but excluding isolated atrial septal defect, fully repaired ventricular septal defect or fully repaired patent ductus arteriosus, closure devices that are judged to be endothelialized previous infective endocarditis, and hypertrophic cardiomyopathy as being at risk of developing infective endocarditis. However, the advice from NICE is that antibiotic prophylaxis (including chlorhexidine mouthwash) is not required for the prevention of infective endocarditis as part of routine dental treatment. This advice specifically applies to adults and children with structural heart defects such as a valve replacement or hypertrophic cardiomyopathy, and those who have previously had infective endocarditis (whether or not they have an underlying cardiac problem) and related to any dental procedure. The NICE guidelines are a significant departure from previous established practice.

Consent

A consensus decision made it clear that a general anaesthetic should not be administered until a written consent has been obtained and all alternatives have been explored and the risks of the procedure explained to patient, parents, and carers[7].

Consent for the procedure should be taken by the surgeon and anaesthetist and all the procedures to be performed, while the patient is unconscious, should be explained in full prior to induction of anaesthesia. Parents, in particular, are understandably apprehensive that their child requires dental extractions under anaesthesia and many parents experience additional guilt that it is their fault that this intervention is required[30]. The surgical team will gain written informed consent for the procedure and may also raise the serious risks associated with anaesthesia. The language used in explaining the very small risk of death is important as the anxiety levels of both parents or carers and the patient tends to be high. Although the National Confidential Enquiry into Perioperative Death (NCEPOD 1990) quotes death rates solely attributable to anaesthesia as 1:187 000[31], a helpful booklet specifically advising parents on their child's dental anaesthetic published by the Royal College of Anaesthetists available via the internet[32] describes the risk of a life-threatening problem as about 1 in 400 000. 'This risk is considerably less than that of your child being seriously injured in a road accident'. Outpatient anaesthesia for dental surgery has been retrospectively quoted as 1:85 350 in dental clinics in the United States[33].

Anaesthesia consent should also specifically discuss the risks of nausea, vomiting, sore throat, dizziness, and dental trauma unrelated to the surgery. Clear advice on postoperative analgesic needs is useful at this stage. If rectal analgesia is the chosen method of administration for analgesia then specific informed consent must be sought[34].

The possible visual and hearing loss problems of those with special needs can make consent more difficult. More often it is due to intellectual impairment causing problems with understanding and processing information. Whilst this may, in its most severe form, present as completely absent communication, it is important to treat each patient as an individual and proceed in the first instance with formal introductions. Asking the patient their name and asking them to say who the carers are (that are often with them) is especially useful as this may reveal that the communication problem is entirely with articulating speech as opposed to understanding. It is not unusual to find that communication problems with health professionals are because health professionals are not listening.

The Mental Capacity Act 2005

It is not unusual for the following situations to exist simultaneously. A patient who is unable to give meaningful consent to medical procedures may also not be able to cooperate with carers when it comes to dental hygiene. Obesity and poor diet may coexist and it is therefore unsurprising that dental general anaesthesia is the most common indication for anaesthesia in the learning-disabled population. Acting in the patient's best interest is no longer a simple matter of two health professionals agreeing but does now need to take into account the Mental Capacity Act 2005 (see Chapter 3).

In principle, a person must be assumed to have capacity unless it is established that he/she lacks capacity and all steps have been taken to help him/her do so. Actions must be taken in the patient's best interests, but to determine these, the health professional must consider the beliefs and values that the patient may have if they had capacity or had previously had capacity. To determine this, those who should be consulted, include those involved in caring for the patient or any official legal representative.

Where there is no representative the National Health Service (NHS) body that wishes to carry out treatment must appoint an independent medical capacity advocate (see Chapter 3). They are appointed in order to help someone who lacks capacity have their views heard and their rights upheld. The majority of patients needing this service are likely to have learning difficulties, be older people with dementia, acquired brain injury, or mental health problems. It is important to understand that this is not necessarily best interests' advocacy and also that the advocate does not offer their own opinion or make the decisions. In order to make use of the provisions of this Act, further training is required[35,36].

The clinical setting

Following the reports of the 1990s it was apparent that the main problem experienced in community dental practice that led to the deaths of both adults and children under anaesthesia, was the lack of immediate high-quality critical care. Initial GDC guidance[3] defined that written protocols should be in place to define how high-quality care would be brought to the patient. The ultimate conclusion was that anaesthesia should take place in a hospital with critical care facilities on the same site including any clinics and outpatient departments maintained in association with any such hospital[7].

Equipment and drugs

Individual anaesthesia technique is undoubtedly the decision of the supervising consultant anaesthetist but should be well informed and consideration given to best practice[7]. The equipment used should be specifically designed for the purpose of anaesthesia in the dental setting and the monitoring used should adhere to nationally agreed standards. The equipment necessary for resuscitation should be instantly available and all equipment that is likely to be used should be checked before use. Single-use equipment should be used as per the manufacturer's instructions.

Premedication

Premedication prior to straightforward day-case anaesthesia is a matter of individual anaesthetist's preference. Children may benefit from anxiolysis during this very stressful time. However, premedication also carries a risk of inadvertent hyperactivity which can make the anaesthetic experience difficult for anaesthetist and carer[37]. Unfortunately those who have problems with anxiety and hyperactivity may be more affected by sedative premedication. The level of distress in both the child and adult population presenting for anaesthesia is higher than the norm. In one study, 42% of children were found to have high scores measured by the Children's Hospital of Eastern Ontario Pain Scale (CHEOPS) and 21% of adults displayed serious anxiety as measured by the dental anxiety scale[38]. Induction distress often carries into the postoperative period and makes subsequent dental general anaesthesia visits equally frightening.

Techniques

Clear instructions concerning fasting are essential. Topical anaesthesia for cannulation of both children and adults is sensible. Premedication for the most frightened patients, especially those who may be unable to cooperate in the anaesthetic room, is extremely useful. Benzodiazepines are the mainstay and the dosage should take into account other medications that the patient may already be taking.

The practice of dental anaesthesia regularly combines three complicating factors: children, bloody debris, and the airway. Unsurprisingly, the attractiveness of securing the airway with a gold-standard endotracheal tube is commonly chosen for the longer cases. However, it is often the case that experienced anaesthetists and dentists can manage the conflicting needs of keeping an airway open and clean, perform surgery, and not resort to endotracheal or nasotracheal intubation and all of its complications.

Patient positioning for dental surgery has been either sitting (chair) or supine. Each has advantages and disadvantages which individual proponents feel are vital. By and large the advantages of one are the disadvantages of the other. The supine position is the most popular as it is the most familiar position for all anaesthetists and as such, good practice is easily transferred from other practice. This fact similarly applies to the laryngeal mask airway for simple exodontias. The supine position favours venous return and results in greater cardiovascular stability and avoidance of hypotension, cerebral hypoperfusion, and hypoxia. This is especially problematic in the event of vagal bradycardia or fainting. Debris pooling in the pharynx is easier to clear and doesn't drain into the

larynx. The advantages of the sitting position are most apparently dental, especially the familiarity of the position for many dental procedures on awake patients. Gravity reduces venous return leading to less bleeding. Secretions, blood, and dental debris can drain anteriorly out of the mouth. Unknown gastric contents can remain in the stomach. Respiratory mechanics and physiology favour the sitting position.

Choice of airway

The choice of airway is dependent on a number of factors. The first decision, however, is whether there is an indication for endotracheal intubation. Broadly, these can be divided into patient, surgical, and anaesthetic factors.

Patient factors

Children under the age of 8 years usually have simple extractions of primary deciduous teeth and even a total clearance is likely to be of short duration. Endotracheal intubation may therefore carry an increased relative risk.

Adults and older children requiring general anaesthesia are more likely to have more preventative/restorative dentistry carried out in order to preserve teeth and reduce the need for a revisit for as long as possible. In principle, endotracheal intubation is preferred by many but is by no means an absolute requirement. Patients with learning disabilities and uncooperative patients are unlikely to have a clear surgical treatment plan as the dental surgeon may not have any chance to examine the mouth prior to anaesthesia. Again, the need for preventative/restorative dentistry is even more likely and therefore endotracheal intubation is preferred. Medical factors relevant to anaesthesia such as gastro-oesophageal reflux disease determine the choice of airway as in all surgical procedures.

Surgical factors

Dental treatment for primary exodontia is generally quick and the choice of airway is of less relevance to the dental surgeon. Permanent teeth may require more surgical leverage to extract dentally or require protracted surgical extraction. Surgeons are likely to prefer the maximum amount of room possible and nasal endotracheal intubation certainly provides this. Therefore any other airway presents an element of compromise on behalf of the surgeon. Conservations also require good surgical access. The time taken may be in excess of the time taken for dental extractions and the same compromise exists as discussed earlier.

Anaesthetic factors

Familiarity with airway technique is the main determinant. Nasal intubation with a north-facing preformed nasal tube (Figure 9.1) is normally safe as it provides good surgical access at the same time as protecting the airway from blood and debris from a surgical procedure inside the airway[39].

The laryngeal mask airway (see Chapter 4) is also suitable for most dental and oral surgical procedures but carries the constant risk of being accidentally dislodged and obstructed by the surgeon during surgery. Ease of insertion and removal as well as less airway morbidity must be balanced against the risk of airway loss during the procedure.

Nasal masks (Figure 9.2) are familiar to experienced dental anaesthetists and are suitable for many simple extractions. Again, the airway carries a constant risk of obstruction with as many as 30% causing problems with airway patency[40]. This technique requires two hands supporting the mandible and nasal mask. This coincidentally allows the anaesthetist's hands to function as a airway monitor and obstruction can be instantly recognized. The technique requires not only an experienced anaesthetist, but also a surgeon totally familiar with the difficulties associated with competing for the airway.

The laryngeal mask is now the most popular choice for the majority of simple dental cases. The choice of supraglottic airway has burgeoned in recent years. The original reusable mask was eminently suitable for

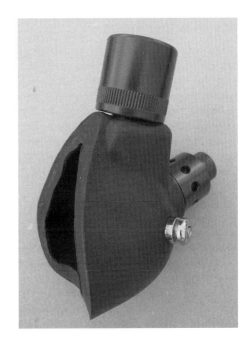

Figure 9.2 Nasal anaesthetic mask.

dental cases but, as with many newer versions, is rather bulky right in front of the mouth. The reinforced laryngeal mask is particularly useful (see Chapter 4) and although it is more difficult to place[41] than the ordinary mask, it is superior for this purpose. On comparing the reinforced laryngeal mask airway with the nasal mask, there were significantly fewer episodes of airway obstruction, better oxygen saturation, less tachycardia, and fewer arrhythmias in the reinforced laryngeal mask airway group. Single-use and reusable reinforced laryngeal masks have been demonstrated to have a similar performance when used for this indication[42].

The choice of tracheal tube needs to be considered before proceeding with dental and oral surgery. Preformed north-facing nasal RAE (Ring–Adair–Elwyn) tubes are particularly useful as they grant the surgeon the best access to the mouth. Although nasal intubation carries the additional complications of nasal trauma and haemorrhage (see Chapter 12) this is usually minor. For many anaesthetists regular nasal intubation using a fibreoptic laryngoscope in the elective setting is a vital way of retaining skills necessary to manage a subsequent difficult intubation. Oral south-facing preformed RAE tubes (Figure 9.1) are useful, especially in children and in adults with congenital or acquired haemostatic problems that could make epistaxis more likely.

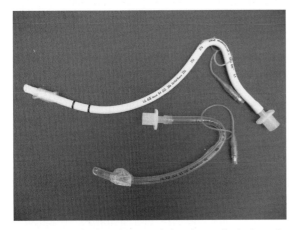

Figure 9.1 Tracheal intubation and dental anaesthesia. A north-facing Ring—Adair—Elwyn (RAE) nasotracheal tube (upper) and a south-facing oral RAE endotracheal tube (lower).

Choice of anaesthesia

General anaesthesia for dental and oral surgery in the hospital setting has the same choices as for all other day cases. Full monitoring is required[7] and the induction/anaesthetic room experience is usually well tolerated even by the most frightened of children and adults[43]. However, there may need to be a pragmatic acceptance that the patients in this population are known to be uncooperative with therapeutic interventions. Patients with learning difficulties are equally variable and require an individualized approach, although generally the techniques used will be the same[44,45].

The most important safety caveat is that airway examination in uncooperative patients may be less than ideal and this must be considered prior to induction and before administering a muscle relaxant.

An intravenous induction is certainly preferred. However, a gaseous induction with oxygen, nitrous oxide, and sevoflurane is a viable alternative especially when cooperation is less forthcoming. Involving parents and carers in deciding the best way forward is often valuable, especially in special needs dentistry. Their knowledge of how the patient may react in the anaesthetic room is easily transferable from other medical encounters[46]. Propofol is by far the most commonly used agent. For the shortest cases propofol alone may be used. The use of an opioid such as fentanyl is a matter for personal choice. It offers a reduction in induction agent's dose but increases opioid side effects such as respiratory depression and nausea. For longer cases fentanyl is certainly useful, especially prior to removal of impacted third molars.

Intramuscular induction with ketamine is more often needed on a dental surgery list than elsewhere in the hospital. The need for this is increased when oral sedation is refused but is usually a method of last resort. A dose of 5–10 mg/kg intramuscularly using the 50 or 100 mg/ml mixture usually has the desired effect.

Intubation usually requires a neuromuscular relaxant. The duration of the proposed surgery will influence the choice of drug. For the planned shorter procedure mivacurium offers some advantages for dental day-case surgery as it has a shorter duration and does not generally require antagonism with an anticholinesterase. The additional benefit may be reduced nausea. Historically suxamethonium was commonly used in this population for the benefits of short duration but mivacurium has a similar use without the myalgia[47]. There is little to choose between other medium-acting muscle relaxants. For longer procedures muscle relaxation is not necessarily required for surgical access and thus the predictable clearance of atracurium may offer some benefits[48].

Maintenance of anaesthesia is mostly with sevoflurane in either air or nitrous oxide. Dental anaesthesia and nitrous oxide have had the longest and most successful partnership in all of anaesthesia. Side effects such as nausea and vomiting during a short anaesthetic are balanced with the analgesic benefits and additive rapid anaesthesia effects which may be especially welcome when cooperation is limited. Sevoflurane offers the same advantages of halothane, previously the mainstay of dental anaesthesia, but without the same risk of arrhythmias.

Arrhythmias

Historically cardiac arrhythmias were a particular problem during dental extractions under general anaesthesia. Anxiety, sitting position, hypercarbia, endogenous and exogenous catecholamines combined with a light halothane anaesthetic proved particularly good at inducing cardiac arrhythmias. The incidence was as high as 50% and included life-threatening arrhythmias such as ventricular tachycardia[49,50]. Trigeminal stimulation brought about by the surgery is also implicated. The problem of arrhythmias during dental practice has historically been linked with the overtly high mortality. Subsequently the use of sevoflurane, even in the same circumstances, is much less arrhythmogenic and may be postulated as part of the reduction in deaths in the twenty-first century.

Throat pack

Throat packs are still commonly used in patients undergoing oral surgical procedures (Figure 9.3). They are useful in preventing blood and debris soiling the airway thus causing potential problems at emergence[51]. Virtually anything can be lost into the airway whilst operating, including fragments, whole teeth, surgical drill bits, and composite materials. The pack in theory thus reduces airway problems. The throat pack itself can be the cause of perioperative morbidity[52]. The safe placement of a pack under direct vision protecting the pharynx and nasopharynx must be accompanied by the safe removal of the pack once it is no longer required[53]. The complications and safe use of dental throat packs is discussed in Chapter 12.

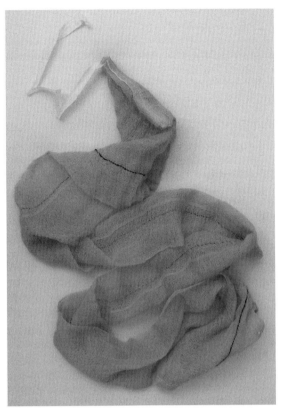

Figure 9.3 Ribbon throat pack. Deaths have been reported as a result of failing to remove the pack after oral surgery.

Postoperative complications

Pain

Much is written concerning the complications of dental surgery and anaesthesia, especially in children. The commonest complications are, unsurprisingly, pain, haemorrhage, sore throat, nausea, and sleepiness. Although minor complications are relatively frequent the severity of morbidity and postoperative admission rate is low[54]. The amount of pain and haemorrhage is related to the extent of the surgery[55,56]. The choice of anaesthetic technique may help alleviate these. In contradiction, the use of local anaesthesia intraoperatively has been shown both to provide postoperative analgesia[57] and also to make no difference to pain scores[58,59].

Local anaesthesia containing vasoconstrictors is a popular modality for pain relief with dental surgeons as it has the additional benefit of reducing haemorrhage. In practice, the vasoconstrictors used, along with local anaesthesia, may reduce the size of clot within the socket. Local anaesthesia carries the additional disadvantage that numbness is often distressing and can result in self-inflicted lip trauma (see Chapter 7)[60]. It has also been shown to cause dizziness postoperatively[61].

Historically, analgesia was not considered an important part of dental anaesthetic management. However up to 95% of paediatric patients[56] may experience moderate pain, with pain scores being highest in the immediate postoperative period. Pain relief should start in the intraoperative period and can be administered either orally or rectally provided previous consent has been given. Where no contraindications exist, diclofenac is superior to paracetamol[62], although a combination of a non-steroidal analgesic and paracetamol will provide the best results[63]. Advice on the dose and route of administration of paracetamol vary. However, regular 15 mg/kg orally is usually adequate. An alternative is 40 mg/kg rectally following induction. Although effectiveness is similar with either route, patient acceptability of the rectal route of administration varies[64]. The use of non-steroidal ant-inflammatory drugs are cautioned in the presence of asthma. Sevoflurane has been shown to cause postoperative agitation and tantrums which can be increased in frequency up to a week postoperatively[65].

Postoperative nausea and vomiting

Postoperative nausea and vomiting (PONV) is as much, if not more of a problem for this group of oral surgical patients as compared to other surgical patients. The combination of children anxiously gulping air during a stressful induction, swallowed blood, and early ambulation are potent causes of nausea. The incidence rises up to 30%[66] and is a cause of admission in approximately 1 in 25 patients. Follow-up of nausea and vomiting in this group shows that in a small number this persists for up to a week and may lead to a reluctance to eat and drink.

Treatment with ondansetron, cyclizine, and dexamethasone as a multimodal prophylaxis and treatment is likely to be helpful. Many other drugs, combination of drugs, and other modalities have been used over the years with variable results. The most important predictive factors associated with an increased risk of PONV are female gender, young patients (15–25 years old), non-smoking status, and the presence of predisposing factors such as prior history of motion sickness and/or PONV, vertigo, or migraine headaches. Other precipitating factors include the use of volatile anaesthetic agents, maxillary surgery, postoperative pain, and the use of post-operative analgesic opioid drugs.

Steroids

Dexamethasone is not just useful in the prophylaxis of PONV but is used in the prevention of trismus, oedema, and swelling, especially after surgery to remove third molars. It reduces analgesia requirements although not absolute pain scores. The dose should be 8 mg (or 100 mcg/kg) as a single bolus given at the start of surgery[67–69].

Conclusion

General anaesthesia for dentistry is not without risk and should not be undertaken as a first-line means of anxiety control. Consideration should always be given to the possibility of local anaesthetic techniques with or without conscious sedation. Patients requiring general anaesthesia for dental work are frequently children or individuals with learning disabilities. The standards of general anaesthesia for dentistry should be identical to those of general anaesthesia in any other setting[70].

References

1. Poswillo D. (1990) *General Anaesthesia, Sedation and Resuscitation in Dentistry. Report of an Expert Working Party for the Standing Dental Advisory Committee.* London: Department of Health.
2. Dental General Anaesthesia. (1995) *Report of a Clinical Standards Advisory Committee on General Anaesthesia for Dentistry.* London: Department of Health.
3. General Dental Council. (1998) *Maintaining Standards. Guidance to Dentists on Professional and Personal Conduct.* London: General Dental Council.
4. The Royal College of Anaesthetists. (1999) *Standards and Guidelines for General Anaesthesia for Dentistry.* London: The Royal College of Anaesthetists.
5. Hunter ML, Hunter B, Dhir AP, Shah B. (2002) General anaesthesia for exodontia in children: experience of a dental teaching hospital in relation to changes in national guidance. *Int J Paediatr Dent*, **12(4)**, 260–4.
6. Macmillan CSA, Wildsmith JAW. (2000) A survey of paediatric dental anaesthesia in Scotland. *Anaesthesia*, **55(6)**, 581–6.
7. *A Conscious Decision: Report of an expert group chaired by the Chief Medical and Dental Officer.* (2000) London: Department of Health.
8. Scottish Executive Health Department. (2001) *Guidance on General Anaesthesia and Sedation for Dental Treatment NHS (HDL (2001) 29).* Edinburgh: Scottish Executive Health Department.
9. Department of Health Welsh Executive. (2001) *General anaesthesia for dental treatment in a hospital setting with facilities for the provision of critical care. WHC (2001) 077.* Cardiff: Department of Health Welsh Executive.
10. Savanheimo N, Vehkalahti M. (2008) Preventive aspects in children's caries treatments preceding dental care under general anaesthesia. *Int J Paediatr Dent*, **18(2)**, 117–23.
11. MacCormac C, Kinirons M. (1998) Reasons for referral of children to a general anaesthetic service in Northern Ireland. *Int J Paediatr Dent*, **8(3)**, 191–6.
12. Savanheimo N, Vehkalahti M, Pihakari A, Numminen M. (2205) Reasons for and parental satisfaction with children's dental care under general anaesthesia. *Int J Paediatr Dent*, **15(6)**, 448–54.
13. Mac Cormac C, Kinirons M. (1999) Characteristics of children referred to a general anaesthetic service in Northern Ireland. *J Ir Dent Assoc*, **45(4)**, 119–23.
14. Albadri SS, Lee S, Lee GT, Llewelyn R, Blinkhorn AS, Mackie IC. (2006) The use of general anaesthesia for the extraction of children's teeth. Results from two UK dental hospitals. *Eur Arch Paediatr Dent*, **7(2)**, 110–15.
15. Albadri SS, Jarad FD, Lee GT, Mackie IC. (2006) The frequency of repeat general anaesthesia for teeth extractions in children. *Int J Paediatr Dent*, **16(1)**, 45–8.
16. Arch LM, Humphis GM, Lee GTR, (2001) Children choosing between general anaesthesia or inhalation sedation for dental extractions: the effect on dental anxiety. *Int J Paediatr Dent*, **11(1)**, 41–8.
17. Gerdin EW, Angbratt M, Aronsson K, Eriksson E, Johansson I. (2008) Dental caries and body mass index by socio-economic status in Swedish children. *Community Dent Oral Epidemiol*, **36(5)**, 459–65.
18. Alm A, Fåhraeus C, Wendt LK, Koch G, Andersson-Gäre B, Birkhed D. (2008) Body adiposity status in teenagers and snacking habits in early childhood in relation to approximal caries at 15 years of age. *Int J Paediatr Dent*, **18(3)**, 189–196.
19. Hong L, Ahmed A, McCunniff M, Overman P, Mathew M. (2008) Obesity and dental caries in children aged 2–6 years in the United States: National Health and Nutrition Examination Survey 1999–2002. *J Public Health Dent*, **68(4)**, 227–33.
20. Alm A. (2008) On dental caries and caries-related factors in children and teenagers. *Swed Dent J Suppl*, **195**, 7–63.
21. Ostberg AL, Nyholm M, Gullberg B, Rastam L, Lindblad U. (2009) Tooth loss and obesity in a defined Swedish population. *Scand J Public Health*, **37(4)**, 427–33
22. Rutherford J, Stevenson R. (2004) Careful physical examination is essential in the preoperative assessment of children for dental extractions under general anesthesia. *Pediatr Anesth*, **14(11)**, 920–3.
23. Bell GS, Sander JW. (2001) The epidemiology of epilepsy: the size of the problem. *Seizure*, **10(4)**, 306–14.
24. Mirón Rodríguez MF, García-Miguel FJ, Becerra Cayetano A, Cojo Del Peces E, Rueda García J, Gilsanz Rodríguez F. (2008) General anesthesia in

mentally disabled patients undergoing dental surgery. *Rev Esp Anestesiol Reanim*, **55(3)**, 137–43.

25. Lyons B, Motherway C, Casey W, Doherty P. (1995) The anaesthetic management of the child with Eisenmenger's syndrome. *Can J Anaesth*, **42(10)**, 904–9.

26. Gould IM, Buckingham JK. (1993) Cost effectiveness of prophylaxis in dental practice to prevent infective endocarditis. *Br Heart J*, **70**, 79–83.

27. Lockhart P, Brennan M, Sasser H, Fox Philip C, Paster B, Bahrani-Mougeot F. (2008) Bacteremia associated with toothbrushing and dental extraction. *Circulation*, **117(24)**, 3118–25.

28. Gould FK, Elliott TSJ, Foweraker J et al. (2006) Guidelines for the prevention of endocarditis: report of the Working Party of the British Society for Antimicrobial Chemotherapy. *J Antimicrob Chemother*, **57**, 1035–42.

29. NICE. (2008) *Antimicrobial prophylaxis against infective endocarditis. Clinical Guideline 64*. London: National Institute for Clinical Excellence.

30. Amin M, Harrison R, Weinstein P. (2006) A qualitative look at parents' experience of their child's dental general anaesthesia. *Int J Paediatr Dent*, **16(5)**, 309–19.

31. Buck N, Devlin H, Lunn J. (1987) *The Report of the Confidential Enquiry into Peri-operative Deaths*. London: Nuffield Provincial Hospitals Trust and the Kings Fund.

32. http://www.youranaesthetic.info (2009) London: The Royal College of Anaesthetists and The Association of Anaesthetists of Great Britain and Ireland.

33. D'Eramo EM, Bookless SJ, Howard JB. (2003) Adverse events with outpatient anesthesia in Massachusetts. *J Oral Maxillofac Surg*, **61(7)**, 793–800.

34. Mitchell J. (1995) A fundamental problem of consent. *BMJ*, **310**, 43–6.

35. http://www.dca.gov.uk/legal-policy/mental-capacity/mybooklets/booklet06.pdf.

36. *Mental Capacity Act 2005*. (2005) London: Her Majesty's Stationery Office.

37. Allen Finley G, Stewart S, Buffett-Jerrott S, Wright K, Millington D. (2006) High levels of impulsivity may contraindicate midazolam premedication in children. *Can J Anesth*, **53**, 73–8.

38. Hosey MT, Macpherson LM, Adair P, Tochel C, Burnside G, Pine C. (2006) Dental anxiety, distress at induction and postoperative morbidity in children undergoing tooth extraction using general anaesthesia. *Br Dent J*, **14(1)**, 39–43.

39. O'Connell J, Stevenson DS; Stokes MA. (1996) Pathological changes associated with short-term nasal intubation. *Anaesthesia*, **51(4)**, 347–50.

40. Bagshaw ONT, Southee R, Ruiz K. (1997) A comparison of the nasal mask and the nasopharygeal airway in paediatric chair dental anaesthesia. *Anaesthesia*, **52(8)**, 786–9.

41. George JM, Sanders GM. (1999) The reinforced laryngeal mask in paediatric outpatient dental surgery. *Anaesthesia*, **54(6)**, 546–51.

42. Flynn P, Ahmed FB, Mitchell V, Patel A, Clarke S. (2007) A randomised comparison of the single use LMA Flexible (TM) with the reusable LMA Flexible(TM) in paediatric dental day-case patients. *Anaesthesia*, **62(12)**, 1281–4.

43. Seed R, Boardman C, Davies M. (2006) Co-operation with pre-operative cardiovascular monitoring amongst children for chair dental general anaesthesia. *Ann R Coll Surg Engl*, **82(2)**, 207–9.

44. Hung WT, Liao SM, Ko WR, Chau MY. (2003) Anesthetic management of dental procedures in mentally handicapped patients. *Acta Anaesthesiol Sin*, **41(2)**, 65–70.

45. Mirón Rodríguez MF, García-Miguel FJ, Becerra Cayetano A, Cojo Del Peces E, Rueda García J, Gilsanz Rodríguez F. (2008) General anesthesia in mentally disabled patients undergoing dental surgery. *Rev Esp Anestesiol Reanim*, **55(3)**, 137–43.

46. Marshall J, Sheller B, Mancl L, Williams BJ. (2008) Parental attitudes regarding behavior guidance of dental patients with autism. *Pediatr Dent*, **30(5)**, 400–7.

47. Deehan S, Henderson D, Stewart K. (2000) Intubation conditions and postoperative myalgia in outpatient dental surgery: a comparison of succinylcholine with mivacurium. *Anaesth Inten Care*, **28(2)**, 146–50.

48. Rigg JD, Wilson AC, Pollard BJ. (1997) Mivacurium or vecuronium for muscular relaxation in day-case surgery. *Eur J Anaesthesiol*, **14(6)**, 630–4.

49. Thurlow AC. (1972) Cardiac dysrhythmias in outpatient dental anaesthesia in children. *Anaesthesia*, **27(4)**, 429–35.

50. Blayney MR., Malins AF, Cooper GM. (1999) Cardiac arrhythmias in children during outpatient general anaesthesia for dentistry: a prospective randomised trial. *Lancet*, **354(9193)**, 1864–6.

51. Whitley SP, Shaw IH. (1992) Dental throat packs and airway protection. *Anaesthesia*, **47(2)**, 173.

52. Tay JY, Tan WK, Chen FG, Koh KF, Ho V. (2002) Postoperative sore throat after routine oral surgery: influence of the presence of a pharyngeal pack. *Br J Oral Maxillofac Surg*, **40(1)**, 60–3.

53. http://www.rcoa.ac.uk/docs/Safety_Russell.ppt.

54. Enever GR, Nunn JH, Sheehan JK. (2000) A comparison of post-operative morbidity following outpatient dental care under general anaesthesia in paediatric patients with and without disabilities. *Int J Paediatr Dent*, **10(2)**, 120–5.

55. McWilliams PA, Rutherford JS. (2007) Assessment of early postoperative pain and haemorrhage in young children undergoing dental extractions under general anaesthesia. *Int J Paediatr Dent*, **17(5)**, 352–7.

56. Needleman HL, Harpavat S, Wu S, Allred EN, Berde C. (2008) Postoperative pain and other sequelae of dental rehabilitations performed on children under general anesthesia. *Pediatr Dent*, **30(2)**, 111–21.

57. Tan S, Ashley P, Gilthorpe M, Scheer B. Mason C Roberts G. (2004) Morbidity following dental treatment of children under intubation general anaesthesia in a day-stay unit. *Int J Paediatr Dent*, **14(1)**, 9–16.

58. Tordoff S, Brossy M, Rowbotham D, James J, James R, Raphael J. (1996) The effect of pre-incisional infiltration with lignocaine on postoperative pain after molar teeth extraction under general anaesthesia. *Anaesthesia*, **51(6)**, 585–7.

59. Macpherson A. (2007) Intra-operative local anaesthesia to reduce postoperative pain or distress in children after exodontia under general anaesthesia. *Evid Based Dent*, **8 (2)**, 45–6.

60. Chi D, Kanellis M, Himadi E, Asselin ME. (2008) Lip biting in a pediatric dental patient after dental local anesthesia: a case report. *J Pediatr Nurs*, **23(6)**, 490–3.

61. Atan S, Ashley P, Gilthorpe M, Scheer B, Roberts G. (2004) Morbidity following dental treatment of children under intubation general anaesthesia in a day-stay unit. *Int J Paediatr Dent*, **14(1)**, 9–16.

62. O'Donnell A, Henderson M, Fearne J, O'Donnell D. (2007) Management of postoperative pain in children following extractions of primary teeth under general anaesthesia: a comparison of paracetamol, Voltarol and no analgesia. *Int J Paediatr Dent*, **17(2)**, 110–15.

63. Gazal G, Mackie I. (2007) A comparison of paracetamol, ibuprofen or their combination for pain relief following extractions in children under general anaesthesia: a randomized controlled trial. *Int J Paediatr Dent*, **17(3)**, 169–77.

64. Rømsing J, Møiniche S, Dahl JB. (2002) Rectal and parenteral paracetamol, and paracetamol in combination with NSAIDs, for postoperative analgesia. *Br J Anaesth*, **88(2)**, 215–26.

65. Millar K, Asbury AJ, Bowman AW, Hosey MT, Musiello T, Welbury RR. (2006) The effects of brief sevoflurane-nitrous oxide anaesthesia upon children's postoperative cognition and behaviour. *Anaesthesia*, **61(6)**, 541–7.

66. Silva AC, O'Ryan F, Poor DB. (2006) Postoperative nausea and vomiting (PONV) after orthognathic surgery: a retrospective study and literature review. *J Oral Maxillofac Surg*, **64(9)**, 1385–97.

67. Markiewicz MR, Brady MF, Ding EL, Dodson TB. (2008) Corticosteroids reduce postoperative morbidity after third molar surgery: a systematic review and meta-analysis. *J Oral Maxillofac Surg*, **66(9)**, 1881–94.

68. Laureano Filho JR, Maurette PE, Allais M, Cotinho M, Fernandes C. (2008) Clinical comparative study of the effectiveness of two dosages of Dexamethasone to control postoperative swelling, trismus and pain after the surgical extraction of mandibular impacted third molars. *Med Oral Patol Oral Cir Bucal*, **13(2)**, 129–32.

69. Baxendale BR, Vater M, Lavery KM. (1993) Dexamethasone reduces pain and swelling following extraction of third molar teeth. *Anaesthesia*, **48(11)**, 961–4.

70. Cantlay K, Williamson S, Hawkings J. (2005) Anaesthesia for dentistry, *Cont Edu Anaesth Crit Care Pain*, **5(3)**, 71–5.

10

Anaesthesia for aesthetic surgery

Sandip Pal and Chandra Kumar

Introduction

There is evidence in the literature to suggest that plastic surgery originated in India more than 2500 years ago and it is believed that an ancient Indian surgeon, Sushruta, performed a rhinoplasty, the oldest plastic surgery operation, in 600 BC[1]. In ancient times, amputation of the nose was performed as a punishment for committing adultery, amongst other crimes. This explains the need for nasal reconstruction during that period. Sushruta, known as the 'father of Indian plastic surgery', wrote *Sushruta Samhita*, a compendium written in Sanskrit about most advanced surgical practices prevalent at that time. As well as introducing an ethical code, he highlighted all of the basic principles of plastic surgery, such as pedicle flap techniques, repair of ear lobe defects, and repair of both traumatic and congenital cleft lips. In addition he classified burns, described surgical instruments, the practice of mock operations, cadaveric dissection, and used wine to dull the pain of surgical incisions.

Aesthetic or cosmetic surgery on the face is performed to improve the appearance of the face and is one of the fastest growing medical practices in the United Kingdom. An increasing number of women as well as men are opting for cosmetic surgery to address dissatisfaction with their body image[2]. Physical appearance plays an important role in how we are perceived by others. Each individual has their own perceptions as to what constitutes beauty. This in turn is influenced by current standards and fashions in the society within which they live[3–5]. These issues have led patients to consider aesthetic surgery to enhance their self-esteem and attractiveness. As demands for aesthetic surgery increase, it becomes important to understand why patients are prepared to undergo invasive aesthetic surgery. Aesthetic surgery is performed both with and without surgical instruments, and sometimes both modalities are used.

Aesthetic procedures on the face

These procedures range from minor to major procedures and modality of anaesthesia (local anaesthesia [LA] with or without sedation or general anaesthesia [GA]) depends on the planned surgery. These procedures are both surgical as well as non-surgical. Surgical procedures may include reconstructive plastic surgery and removal of skin growths, scar revision, forehead lift, corrective eyelid surgery, facial reconstruction (facelift both laser and open, facial injuries), liposuction, jaw surgery (orthognathic surgery), corrective nose surgery (rhinoplasty), and ear surgery (otoplasty). Non-surgical procedures include the removal of pigmented lesions, tattoos, birth marks, treatment of vascular lesions, and botox injections. In adults, these procedures are usually carried out under LA but GA is invariably necessary for children. This chapter concentrates primarily on the anaesthetic management of aesthetic procedures requiring anaesthesia and the involvement of an anaesthetist.

Choice of anaesthesia and selection of patients

Anaesthesia for aesthetic surgery on the face poses many challenges for the anaesthetist due to the range of surgical procedures performed. Careful manipulation of physiology to achieve optimal surgical conditions, attention to anatomical details in securing the airway device, and close cooperation between anaesthetist and surgical team are vital. Anaesthetic techniques for aesthetic surgery may involve infiltration of LA agent, regional anaesthesia (RA) with or without intravenous sedation, or GA. A thorough preanaesthetic assessment is required to determine if the patient is suitable for GA, sedation, LA, or a combination of these. Any pre-existing medical condition should be optimized before embarking on anaesthesia and surgery. Patients who wish to have their surgery under LA, with or without sedation, should be prepared as for GA. This will facilitate intervention should the LA be inadequate. For example, the patient may be unable to lie still enough throughout the procedure or indeed become increasingly anxious, intolerant, or restless. The assessment and pre-optimization of the oral and maxillofacial surgery patient is discussed in detail in Chapter 2.

The profile of patients presenting for aesthetic surgery differs from that of other surgical patients because these patients are generally fit and healthy (American Society of Anesthesiologists [ASA] class 1 and 2). Anaesthetists should be aware of the psychological issues that surround these patients. The patient's expectations often go beyond what is possible surgically and consequently changes in their physical appearance alone may fail to fulfil their needs and even lead to deterioration in their psychological status. Patient's needs and expectations have to be explored and evaluated carefully before undertaking any surgical aesthetic procedures. The presence of an active psychotic disorder is commonly thought to contraindicate cosmetic surgery[3,4].

Local and regional anaesthesia

The basic requirements for all elective surgical procedures are that the patients be safe, comfortable, and stable. It is also desirable for them to be immobile and not too talkative, especially when the operative site is the face. LA by infiltration or nerve block has many advantages in aesthetic surgery and is often an ideal approach to painless surgery. It is important to understand the pharmacological properties of LA agents and other agents (see Chapters 7 and 21) used during LA. Readers are advised to read an authentic textbook of pharmacology for more details[7].

Local anaesthetic agents

LA agents reversibly inhibit signal transmission in the nerve by blocking sodium influx via protein-based sodium channels[6]. The agents used are manufactured as water-soluble hydrochloride salts. In an aqueous solution, each LA has a unique fixed dissociation constant (pKa) that determines the equilibrium between the charged cation and the uncharged base. It is the lipid-soluble uncharged base that freely diffuses through the lipid bilayer of neurons. After diffusing through the neuronal lipid bilayer, the LA molecule again dissociates into its basic and cationic forms. The charged cation then enters the protein-based sodium channel and renders the channel impermeable to sodium, thus preventing the propagation of action potentials and impulse conduction[8]. With time, depending on the pH, the lipid solubility, and protein binding, the LA diffuses out of the channel rendering the neurons once again susceptible to depolarization.

All LAs in clinical use consist of a benzene ring linked to a hydrocarbon chain by an ester or amide bond. Tetracaine, procaine, 2-chloroprocaine, and cocaine are ester-linked LAs. Amide-linked LAs include bupivacaine, mepivacaine, prilocaine, etidocaine, ropivacaine and lidocaine. Allergic reactions are more common with ester LAs. Allergic reactions to amides are rare. Esters such as benzocaine and procaine, break down to structures similar to p-aminobenzoic acid (PABA), a common component of cosmetics and sunscreens and should be avoided in patients with known sensitivity to such compounds.

The lipid solubility of LAs determines LA potency and is pH dependent. A high pH favours increased lipid solubility, anaesthetic potency, and speed of onset. Substitutions on the benzene ring or tertiary amine portion of the LA molecule alter its pKa value, lipid solubility, and protein binding, determining the speed of onset, potency, and duration of action, respectively.

Local anaesthetic additives
Sodium bicarbonate

Commonly used LAs in clinical use are poorly soluble in water; they are prepared as hydrochloride salts with commercial solutions having a pH in the range of 4 to 6. The addition of sodium bicarbonate can increase the rate of onset of some LAs by increasing the amount of lipid-soluble uncharged base, which readily penetrates neural tissue. It may also decrease the associated pain on injection as a result of neutralizing the pH. In practice, 1 ml of 8.4% sodium bicarbonate can be added to a 30 ml vial of 1% lidocaine or 0.2 ml can be added to a 30 ml vial of 0.25% bupivacaine. Adding further bicarbonate will result in precipitation of the LA.

Preservatives

Multidose vials of LA contain antimicrobial preservatives and can have potentially cytotoxic effects. The most frequently used antimicrobials are methyl-, ethyl-, and propyl-parabenzoates. Sodium ethylenediaminetetraacetic acid (EDTA), which has ion chelating properties, and anti-oxidants, are added to commercially available LAs to scavenge divalent cations and prevent oxidation thus retarding LA degradation. Preservative-free preparations are available and recommended for patients suspected of having allergy with any of these preservatives.

Epinephrine

Low concentrations of the vasoconstrictor epinephrine can be added to LAs. This has the effect of prolonging the duration of anaesthesia and decreasing systemic absorption, thus minimizing the risk of attaining toxic blood levels. The addition of 5 mcg epinephrine to 1ml of LA produces the commonly used 1:200 000 concentration. It must be used with caution in patients known to suffer from coronary vascular disease.

Hyaluronidase

By catalysing the hydrolysis of hyaluronic acid, a major constituent of the interstitial barrier, hyaluronidase lowers the viscosity of hyaluronic acid, thereby increasing tissue permeability. It is commonly used in diluted form during liposuction but the exact recommended dose is not clear[9]. However, in clinical practice it is not unusual to see 1500 IU mixed with 1000 ml of 0.9% sodium chloride.

Regional anaesthesia

RA implies blockade of peripheral nerves or nerve. The sensory nerve supply of the face is complex (see Chapter 6) and multiple nerves may need to be blocked to achieve good anaesthesia. There are relatively few absolute indications for RA in aesthetic surgery, as opposed to merely being an option. In general terms, RA techniques can be advantageous by reducing the overall stress of surgery and anaesthesia, providing better postoperative pain control, decreasing the incidence of postoperative nausea, vomiting, and dysphoria, and possibly improving wound healing. There can also be compelling reasons for avoiding GA in unfit or high-risk patients. Alternatively supplementing GA with some form of RA can give ideal conditions for surgery. Although safer than GA, RA is not without its complications. Complications of RA (see Chapters 7 and 21) include neurotoxicity, allergy, and systemic toxicity, the details of which can be found in any standard pharmacology or anaesthetic textbook.

Conscious sedation

Modern anaesthetic medications are extremely short acting and have minimal side effects. Fast emergence and early discharge have become normal practice. Conscious sedation describes a state that allows patients to tolerate unpleasant procedures while maintaining adequate cardiorespiratory function and the ability to respond purposefully to verbal commands and tactile stimulation, and is described in detail in Chapter 8. Conscious sedation allows patients to tolerate, and sometimes forget, unpleasant procedures by relieving anxiety, discomfort, or pain. Too much sedation can rapidly convert conscious sedation into a state of GA and expose the patient to the risks associated with an unsecured airway and a lack of protective reflexes. This is the reason why conscious sedation should only be employed in the presence of a competent trained clinician, invariably an anaesthetist, in an environment where the patient's vital signs can be continuously monitored and where resuscitation equipment is immediately available.

General anaesthesia

Preoperative anaesthetic considerations

The assessment and preoptimization of the oral and maxillofacial surgery patient is discussed in detail in Chapter 2. GA has been popular for major aesthetic surgery but RA and conscious sedation are increasingly popular. The proposed surgery can dictate the anaesthetic modality. For example, rhinoplasty is almost always done under GA although LA has been advocated, whereas most adult patients will accept LA and conscious sedation for a pinnaplasty. Not all aesthetic surgical procedures can be performed under LA or RA. Lengthy operations and having to maintain uncomfortable positions for a prolonged period of time can deter even the most motivated of patients. Concomitant sedation may help alleviate this discomfort but should be used judiciously. Oversedation must be avoided, especially in the elderly. Disinhibition, agitation, dysphoria, and unconsciousness can result from excessive sedation[10]. In terms of cardiovascular stability and recovery from anaesthesia, there are distinct advantages of using a target-controlled infusion of propofol or remifentanyl to sedate patients. If the surgery is to be carried out under LA, the anaesthetist must ensure that the patient understands the procedure and its risks. In addition they must be capable of cooperating, have no known allergies to the proposed LA agents, and be able to maintain the required operative position without undue discomfort and hazard for the duration of surgery.

Anaesthetic considerations for a specific aesthetic surgery

Brow lift and blepharoplasty

Brow lift is the resuspension of the brows and elimination of upper facial rhytids to help give a youthful appearance of the upper face. It usually has better cosmetic results when combined with upper blepharoplasty. Blepharoplasty is the surgical rejuvenation of the periorbital region to eliminate the tired and aged appearance of the eyes. Blepharoplasty involves resection of skin, orbicularis muscle, and fat.

Blepharoplasty as an isolated procedure is often performed under LA with or without sedation. Patient cooperation may be needed in opening and closing the eye during the procedure to ensure good results. This procedure can also be done by carbon dioxide laser but must be done under safety parameters of eye protection and fire and burn prevention (see below).

Infiltration of LA is performed carefully avoiding haematoma and injection into the muscle. The injection is usually performed by the surgeon. Occasionally GA is required on indication or at the patient's request.

Combined brow lift and blepharoplasty is routinely performed under GA. A simple laryngeal mask airway (LMA) anaesthesia following intravenous induction and spontaneous ventilation with inhalational agent is commonly employed.

Rhinoplasty

Rhinoplasty is the surgical manipulation of the nasal form for aesthetic and or functional improvement. When surgery is combined with nasal septal surgery it is called septorhinoplasty. Patients usually request reduction of nasal hump, reduction, augmentation, or improved tip definition. The exact surgical procedures from surgical perspective are different and it is either performed as open or closed technique depending on the patient's requirements and the surgeon's preference. An open approach utilizes a transcolumellar incision to allow elevation of a nasal skin flap, degloving the lower alar cartilages for direct and wide exposure of the nasal frame. The closed approach utilizes intercartilaginous, intracartilaginous,

infracartileginous, rim, hemitransfixion, and transfixion incisions.

Although septoplasty can be performed under LA, rhinoplasty or septorhinoplasty is routinely preformed under GA. The essential surgical requirements include patient immobility, clear surgical field (minimum bleeding), and smooth recovery. GA with an oral endotracheal tube or flexible LMA with either spontaneous or controlled ventilation can be used. LA and packing of nostrils are also used with GA.

It is important to know the anatomy and sensory nerve supply of the face (see Chapter 6) before embarking on LA. The nose is supplied by the ophthalmic division and maxillary division of the trigeminal nerve. The skin of the nose is supplied by the supratrochlear branch of the frontal nerve of the ophthalmic; the anterior ethmoidal branch of the nasociliary (ophthalmic); and the infraorbital branch of the maxillary. The fifth nerve provides the sensory supply to the anterior one-third of the septum, and the lateral walls are innervated by the anterior ethmoidal branch of the nasociliary nerve. The long sphenopalatine nerves from the sphenopalatine ganglion, innervates the posterior two-thirds of the septum and lateral walls.

The nasal cavities are packed with gauze soaked in 4–5% cocaine. Paste is also applied to the area of sphenopalatine ganglion behind the middle turbinate. The mucosa will become avascular as a result of the vasoconstrictor properties of cocaine. Cocaine is a powerful vasoconstrictor so adrenaline is not necessary. Alternatively, Moffett's solution, a mixture of 2 ml of 8% cocaine hydrochloride, 2 ml of 1% sodium bicarbonate, and 1 ml of 1 in 200 000 adrenaline solution is used.

Blockade of the sphenopalatine ganglion gives a good surgical field. If the septum is to be operated on, 2 ml of 1% lidocaine with adrenaline should be injected into the columella and base of the septum as this area is covered by squamous epithelium which will not absorb the topically applied agents. In fact, use of the combination may precipitate cardiac arrhythmias and should be avoided.

GA for rhinoplasty can include total intravenous anaesthesia (TIVA) with remifentanil which allows greater flexibility in quickly modulating the blood pressure by altering the rate of the remifentanil infusion. Alternatively, conventional intravenous induction with propofol followed by inhalational agents will suffice. Maintaining a head-up posture during surgery and recovery reduces venous congestion and bleeding. Recent trends have been to use a classic or flexible

LMA for rhinoplasty. It must be remembered that the laryngeal mask does not protect the airway in an anaesthetized patient and consequently many anaesthetists still prefer to use a cuffed endotracheal tube (Ring–Adair–Elwyn [RAE] tube). The endotracheal tube or LMA must be taped to the patient's chin to keep it out of the surgeon's field of vision. The usual perioperative precaution for surgery in the head and neck region applies. A significant blood pooling can occur in the nasopharyngeal area when nasal osteotomies are used to narrow or straighten the nasal dorsum. A throat pack is used to protect the airway from blood and to reduce the amount of blood which can enter the oesophagus and then into the stomach. Any ingested blood in the stomach is a well-known factor for postoperative nausea and vomiting. Attention must be paid to removing the throat pack at the end of procedure. Even though the throat pack is soaked with saline, it is still very abrasive to the oesophageal mucosa and the patient usually complains of a sore throat postoperatively. The application of a surgical splint or dressing of the nose is an art and varies with surgeon's preference. Most surgeons also pack both nostrils. The patient should be only allowed to wake up when the splint has stiffened and contoured. Postoperative recovery should be smooth and excessive coughing will increase bleeding. Equally, the patient must be fully awake before the extubation as application of a face mask will be very difficult, especially when nostrils are packed. Postoperative pain is not a major problem but mouth dryness due to mouth breathing may be distressing.

Surgical facelift (rhytidectomy)

Surgical facelift is performed to reduce facial folds and wrinkles to create a more youthful appearance. Surgical facelift involves removing excess fatty tissue of the face, tightening of underlying facial muscles, and smoothing facial skin. Facelift surgery is categorized as full, lower, or mid or mini facelift. Incisions are commonly made above the hairline following the natural facial creases (e.g. the line where the ear meets the side of the face), so that any scarring forming after the face lift will remain unseen. Facial skin is separated from the underlying tissue. Excess fat and skin are removed, and the surrounding muscles are tightened to improve the contours and appearance of the patient's face. Redundant skin is excised. The skin is then repositioned with stitches or staples, and the treated area is wrapped in bandages. Facelift surgery may be combined with forehead lift, upper and/or lower blepharoplasty, removal of submental or submandibular fat, and liposuction. The procedure is also combined occasionally with septorhinoplasty.

Most patients are usually aged 45–65 years and they are generally fit and well. Often simple facelift surgery can be performed using LA with or without sedation but GA is always an option. Patients must be assessed before GA. The procedure may be unpredictable, especially if the facelift is combined with other surgical procedures. The patient's head is usually nearer the anaesthetic machine and easy access to an intravenous access must be ensured. TIVA or propofol induction, followed by inhalational agent is suitable. Securing the airway is an important factor. The airway can be maintained with a reinforced LMA or an endotracheal tube (RAE). The usual perioperative precautions for surgery in the head and neck region apply. The use of LA infiltration helps. To avoid hypothermia, warming blanket should be used. The continued use of muscle relaxant is avoided if intraoperative testing of VII nerve function is intended.

Liposuction of face

Liposuction or lipoplasty is a body contouring procedure which is done in almost any area of the body, including the face. The subcutaneous fat is aspirated via a small skin incision with a specialized blunt-ended cannula. The most common method of liposuction is the use of a power suction canister or spring-loaded syringes especially for the face. The area of liposuction is usually instilled with saline mixed with LA, epinephrine, and other adjuvants. Fibrous area is difficult to suction and is less conducive to the spread of the tumescent fluid. An ultrasonic suction device can help liquefy the fat and makes subsequent suction of fat easier. However, an ultrasonic device can increase seroma formation and produce heat injury to the skin. The suction cannulae and syringes vary in sizes and lengths. An appropriate sized cannula is inserted in the least visible area through the skin incision and is moved backwards and forwards in repetitive fashion to break the fat tissue and then suction is applied.

Patients are usually fit and well but adequate anaesthesia is essential. Liposuction involving a small area can be performed under LA with or without sedation. However, if area involved is larger, GA may be necessary. The use of LMA after intravenous induction, spontaneous ventilation, and maintenance with a modern inhalalational anaesthetic agent usually suffice. Alternatively TIVA may be used. Postoperative pain is not a major problem and simple analgesics are required.

Dermabrasion

Dermabrasion is used to minimize the appearance of fine wrinkles, acne, scars, and sun damage by carefully scraping away the top layers of the skin. The purpose of dermabrasive surgery is to reorganize or restructure the collagen of the papillary dermis without injuring the reticular dermis. Dermabrasion was first introduced by Kromayer in 1905, who observed that if superficial mechanical injury did not penetrate the reticular dermis, scarring would not occur. The technique originally involved the use of cylindrical knives for treating scars and other cosmetic defects[11]. Later methods involved the use of rasps, burrs, and punches. Kromayer also described the use of carbon dioxide snow and ether to produce anaesthesia and rigidity prior to dermabrading. Dermabrasion can be performed with sandpaper, wire brush, scalpel, or laser. The thickness of skin layers varies greatly from one area to another, and although all areas may be dermabraded without scarring, it is the face that is ideally suited to dermabrasion. Scars which are raised above the skin are particularly susceptible to dermabrasion. Concerns regarding the incidence of postoperative infection have made it less popular in recent years. Although this procedure has been performed for a long time, and is almost always done using a small, sterilized electric sander, now laser techniques have become popular as they can be applied with much greater precision. The development of carbon dioxide laser dermabrasion has allowed greater control of the procedure and has the advantages of facilitating a bloodless field and being much less painful than surgical dermabrasion.

The anaesthetic technique for dermabrasion is similar to that for a facelift. The procedure is usually short and endotracheal intubation is not required. The use of LMA and intravenous induction and spontaneous ventilation with modern inhalational agents is routine. The procedure can be uncomfortable in the immediate postoperative period and the skin may remain indurated for several weeks.

Otoplasty (pinnaplasty or correction of prominent ears)

Prominent ears are usually an isolated finding. Prominence is examined in thirds to determine where the prominence lies. The surgery is tailored to correct the specific excesses. The antihelical fold is flattened and may require reshaping. The surgery usually involves an elliptical skin incision behind the ear, dissection, cartilage scoring or resection, and mattress suturing. A porous polyethylene implant may be used if cartilage is deficient.

The majority of patients are children and the anaesthetic considerations are as for any other paediatric anaesthetic (see Chapter 19). Surgery can be performed under simple laryngeal mask anaesthesia. Adult patients will accept LA for pinnaplasty. LA can be achieved by infiltrating each ear with 10 ml of 1% lidocaine with 1:200 000 epinephrine. GA technique in adult is similar to that required of a facelift or blepharoplasty (see earlier sections). As the dermatomes supplying the back of the ears correspond to the vomiting centre in the brain, the incidence of postoperative nausea and vomiting (PONV) is much higher in these patients and prophylactic antiemetic should be considered. This must be explained to the patient in the preoperative consultation. Postoperative pain usually requires non-steroidal and simple analgesics. Dressing should be firm without being excessively tight. Scalp discomfort and itching can cause discomfort.

Aesthetic procedures by lasers

Laser physics

Laser is increasingly used for aesthetic and non-aesthetic procedures in both paediatric and adult practice. There are numerous textbooks devoted to lasers and their development and readers should consult an authentic textbook for further details. A recent land mark article by Takac et al.[11] contains a very good description of lasers and their applications in clinical medicine.

Laser is electromagnetic radiation falling between infrared and ultraviolet on the spectrum mainly in the visible light spectrum. Properties of laser light are monochromacity (the same colour), coherence (all of the light waves are in phase both spatially and temporally), and collimation (all rays are parallel to each other and do not diverge significantly even over long distances). Lasers were first conceived by Einstein in 1917 when he wrote 'Zur Quantum Theorie der Strahlung' (the quantum theory of radiation) which led to the concepts of stimulated and spontaneous emission and absorption[12]. Later in 1958, Arthur Schawlow and Charles Townes extended lasers into the optical frequency range[13]. In simple terms, a laser is a device that emits light or electromagnetic radiation through a process called stimulated emission and its acronym is Light Amplification by Stimulated

Emision of Radiation. To understand the above concept, it is necessary to understand the basic physics of the atom. If an excited atom is struck by another photon of energy before it returns to the ground state, two photons of equal frequency and energy, travelling in the same direction and in perfect spatial and temporal harmony, are produced. This phenomenon is termed stimulated emission of radiation. An external power source (or 'pumping system' which may be optical, mechanical or chemical) hyperexcites the atoms in the laser medium so that the number of atoms possessing upper energy levels exceeds the number of atoms in a power energy level, a condition termed a population inversion. These atoms then spontaneously emit photons of light. The laser chamber or optical cavity contains an active lasing medium which usually determines the name of each laser. There are four types of lasing material commonly employed: 1) solid state lasers use a solid matrix material such as a ruby crystal; 2) gas lasers use a gas or mixture of gases such as helium, argon, and carbon dioxide; 3) dye lasers employ a complex organic dye in liquid solution or suspension such as rhodamine; 4) semiconductor lasers use two layers of semiconductor substances such as gallium arsenide. The energy from the electromagnetic spectrum can be described in terms of wavelength, frequency, and energy.

Wavelength

Wavelength is the distance from peak to peak, or trough to trough, of a wave and is measured in the unit of microns (millionths of a metre) or nanometers (nm, thousandths of a micron). The wavelength determines the colour of the beam, the amount of energy the photons will carry, and hence determines how a beam will interact with the tissues of the body. The wavelengths of commonly used clinical lasers range from far infrared, near infrared, visible beams, through to ultraviolet beams (Table 10.1).

Frequency

Frequency is inversely related to wavelength in the following way:

Frequency (f) = speed of light (3 × 108 ms)/wavelength

The frequency of visible light is very high and is expressed in tera Hz (tera = 10^{12}).

This also explains the concept of 'frequency doubling', for example, neodymium:yttrium aluminium garnet (Nd:YAG) laser normally emits at 1064 nm or

Table 10.1 Lasers in used in aesthetic surgical practice

Laser	Spectrum	Wavelength (nm)
Carbon dioxide (CO_2)	Far infrared	10 600
Neodymium:yttrium aluminium garnet (Nd:YAG lasers)	Near infrared	1064
Alexandrite	Deep ultraviolet	755
Ruby	Visible	694
Potassium titanyl phosphate (KTP)	Green	126
Excimer laser	Ultraviolet	126–337[1]*

* Dependent on the molecule used.

can be frequency doubled to emit at 532 nm using a crystal such as potassium titanyl phosphate (or 'KTP') crystal. For this reason it is also referred to as 'KTP laser'.

Pulse repetition frequency (PRF)

Pulse repetition is the number of pulses emitted in one second quoted in hertz (Hz). All matter in the universe is made up of atoms which consist of negatively charged 'electrons' orbiting around a positively charged nucleus. Exciting atoms to emit photons can produce light. To produce laser light, atoms of some material such as a gas, a liquid dye, or a crystal rod must be excited. If an electron absorbs energy it can go on to a higher level and be in an 'excited state'. Energy can be delivered into an atom by an electrical power supply or flash of light. By doing so the atom becomes unstable, hence the electron returns to a lower level spontaneously by emitting a photon. The photon released in this way can stimulate another electron to release its photon and so on. These photons have identical energy and frequency and travel in 'phase' or coherence.

Laser construction

A laser consists of a gain medium inside a highly reflective optical cavity, an energy supply to the gain medium to stimulate continuous emission releases the light as a laser beam. Principal components of a laser include gain medium, laser pumping energy, high reflector, output coupler, and laser beam

Gain medium

The gain medium is a material of controlled purity, size, concentration, and shape with properties that allow it to amplify light of a specific wavelength by stimulated emission. It can be in any state, either a gas, liquid, or solid. Argon, helium, carbon dioxide, and krypton are in gaseous form, Ng:YAG, ruby and alexandrite are solids, and rhodamine a liquid.

Laser pumping energy

The process by which supplied energy amplifies the light is called 'pumping'. The energy source is typically an electrical current or light at a different wavelength provided by a flash lamp.

High reflector

In its simplest form, the laser optical cavity consists of two mirrors arranged such that light bounces back and forth, each time passing through the gain medium.

Output coupler

One of the two mirrors in the cavity, called the 'output coupler' is partially transparent and allows some of the light to pass through and escape as a beam of light.

Laser beam

The laser beam generated is a beam of coherent electromagnetic radiation which is of uniform wavelength, parallel, non-divergent, and undirectional in the same phase. Different gain medium produce different types of laser beam. The output of a laser varies with respect to time. Beams can be emitted as continuous constant-amplitude output, known as continuous wave (CW), or as a single pulse or series of pulses.

The length of time the laser beam is activated is known as the pulse duration and is measured in seconds. It determines how tissues will react to light of specific wavelength. Many systems deliver pulses with a fixed or variable pulse delay between the pulses to maximize effectiveness, at the same time minimizing damage to adjacent tissues.

Many medical laser systems can be Q-switched whereby the population inversion is allowed to build up by making the optical cavity conditions (the 'Q') unfavourable for generating a laser beam. Then, at the desired level of pump energy stored in the laser medium, the 'Q' is adjusted, electro- or acousto-optically to more favourable conditions, releasing the pulse. This results in high peak powers as the average power of the laser is packed into a few nanoseconds. For achieving an even greater density of power, modelocking can be deployed. In modelocking extremely short pulses of laser are emitted in the order of tens of picoseconds down to less than 10 femtoseconds such

as in a titanium sapphire laser. This achieves extremely high power density suitable for ablation applications.

The types of lasers used in clinical practice use a variety of laser media and energy pumps. Some clinical lasers use a gaseous medium such as carbon dioxide, argon, krypton, or helium-neon and are pumped by electric discharge through the gas. Gas layers may produce a continuous or an intermittently pulsed output. Other lasers use solid rods of laser-passive material containing small quantities of ionic impurities, known as dopants, which are the actual laser materials. Dopants commonly used for their laser potential include chromium (ruby laser), neodymium (Nd), and holmium (Ho). A synthetic crystal YAG is commonly used as a passive host matrix. Lasers are also made from dyes in liquid media and semiconductors. A list of different lasers used for surgical procedures is included in Table 10.2.

Laser safety

In the United Kingdom, the Medicines and Healthcare products Regulatory Agency (MHRA) is the executive body responsible for protecting and promoting public health and patient safety. The MHRA have published guidance on the safe use of lasers in the medical environment[14]. Most lasers used in medical practice are in Class 4, so a formal educational and safety programme must be completed before using such devices

Table 10.2 Laser applications in aesthetic surgery

Lesion	Laser
Port-wine stain	Pulsed dye
Tattoo removal	Pulsed ruby
Facial telangiectasis	Pulsed dye
Small-vessel disorders	Pulsed dye
Haemangiomas	Pulsed dye
Large haemangiomas	CW Nd:YAG

Epidermal pigmented lesions:
  Lentgines
  Café au lait macules
  Melanocytic naevi
	QS ruby
	QS Nd:YAG
	QS Alexandrite

Facial resurfacing	Carbon dioxide lasers.
Hair removal	QS Nd:YAG (plus topical carbon) Ruby Alexandrite

CW, continuous wave; QS, Q-switched

in the clinical setting. Illuminated signs indicating lasers are in use must be obvious outside the entrance to the clinical area. All staff must be trained in the use of lasers and be totally familiar with the dangers to both patient and personnel. Staff should wear masks to protect from inhalation of vaporized laser smoke and appropriate goggles to protect their eyes (see next section). Means of actively scavenging laser smoke should be deployed.

Effects of exposure to laser

Lasers are potentially dangerous technologic devices; hence their clinical use is subject to regulation. Light can interact with body tissues as it gets transmitted, scattered, or absorbed by the tissues. The effect of a particular laser on body tissues depends on the nature of the tissue being irradiated, the power density of the beam, and the wavelength. Selective photothermolysis refers to the concept of targeting a chromophore in a specific manner utilizing the light energy to cause a temperature medicated localized injury in a manner that avoids damage to adjacent non-targeted tissues[15,16].

Eyes

The eye is particularly susceptible to damage from laser beams either directly or through reflection. The optical gain of the eye can result in an extremely concentrated area of radiant energy falling on the cornea or retina. This can result in permanent damage in a matter of seconds. Carbon dioxide can cause serious corneal injury whereas argon, KTP, and Nd:YAG lasers may burn the retina.

The eyes of both patient and theatre personnel should always be protected by approved laser safety glasses appropriate to the laser modality in use (laser specific or wavelength specific). Regular eyeglasses may be sufficient but contact lenses are not. Protective eyewear must be undamaged and have permanent labels with wavelength and optical density tolerance, side shields, damage threshold of greater than 10 seconds, no surface reflection, good fit, and approval from the laser safety officer of the hospital. If protective eye glass interferes with the operative field then moistened sterile eye pads and towels should protect the patient's eyes. Scleral shields are also available in case where surgery is performed near or on the eyelids. All operating room windows must be covered with an opaque material that will absorb the appropriate wavelength of the lasers in use and specially designed warning signs should be posted.

Tissue damage

Misdirected laser energy may damage an organ or large blood vessel. Vessels larger than 5 mm are not coagulable by laser. With an Nd:YAG system it is impossible to assess immediately or accurately because organ damage or bleeding may not occur until oedema and necrosis have become maximal several days later.

Fire hazard

Many items used in the operating theatre, such as drapes, gowns, sponges, plastic cannula, endotracheal tube, LMA, infusion giving set, are made of materials that can be a fire hazard if not kept from interaction with high intensity laser beam heat. Protection from fire can be prevented by using fire retardant (or moist drape), availability of water basin, availability of a fire extinguisher, use of non-alcohol containing prep solutions, avoiding plastic and rubber instruments, fire-resistant endotracheal tube or LMA, and keeping the inspired oxygen concentration to a minimum. If the endotracheal tube or LMA is not fire retardant, it should be covered with aluminium foil or saline wet swabs. The endotracheal tube provides the least leakage of oxygen to the area and is the best option of securing an airway. It is important to avoid the use of metal and reflective materials.

Atmospheric contamination or smoke inhalation

The destruction of cells by laser releases smoke, carbon particles, and fine particulates smaller than 0.31 microns which can be transported and deposited in the alveoli. Many staffs do not like smells. Carbon dioxide lasers seem to produce more smoke because of vaporization of tissues. An ordinary surgical face mask is not sufficient in preventing particulate inhalation and the use of a powerful smoke evacuator at the surgical site is recommended.

Skin cooling devices

When a laser is used clinically the skin absorbs some light from the laser spectrum which is then converted to heat, producing side effects or damage to adjacent tissue. To prevent this, the heat must be dissipated rapidly from the tissues. This can be achieved by pre-treatment cooling using ice packs or with damp gauze. The alternative, a Dynamic Cooling Device (Candela), can be used which allows a burst of cryogenic spray to be fired for a fraction of a second before the laser is delivered. Simultaneous cooling with water-cooled tips or moving air systems have also been used with success. Post-treatment cooling can be achieved with damp gauze, ice packs, moving air gel, and creams. This has the added benefit of reducing redness and is soothing for the patients.

Laser resurfacing of face

Carbon dioxide laser is commonly used for resurfacing surgery and this is preferred to surgical facelift to avoid scarring and for quicker recovery. Laser resurfacing reduces fine lines, wrinkles, and skin discolouration. It is also used for facial scarring due to acne or injury. The skin healing is quicker and the connective tissue becomes stronger, hence tightening the facial skin. The duration of surgery may take hours as the skin layers are lasered several times.

Preoperative clinical considerations

A general medical history should be obtained prior to treatment, including information on wound healing, any bleeding diathesis, history of infectious diseases, particularly hepatitis and human immunodeficiency virus (HIV) infection. The presence of HIV proviral DNA has been demonstrated in the laser plume generated by carbon dioxide laser irradiation of HIV-infected tissue culture[17].

Anaesthesia

Most patients experience only a transient stinging sensation during laser or intense pulsed light source treatment that is well tolerated, thus limiting the need for anaesthesia. However, cumulative pulses may produce increasing and intolerable discomfort. Anaesthesia is often required in young children or individuals with large lesions. In many instances, use of topical anaesthetics such as eutectic mixtures of LA (EMLA) or Ametop cream alone is sufficient. Application of a thick layer of LA cream under an occlusive dressing for 60 minutes followed by removal 10–30 minutes before treatment is necessary for maximal effectiveness. If needed, local infiltration or regional nerve block may be performed with lidocaine. Epinephrine should generally be avoided during local infiltration of haemangiomatous lesions because it may constrict the targeted vessels. Premedication with hypnotics, sedatives, or analgesics may be required in anxious patients.

Where GA is unavoidable for aesthetic laser procedures, then minimally explosive mixtures of inspired gases, such as air with less than 30% supplementary oxygen, should be used. Only dedicated laser protective airway devices should be used and protected from accidental direct contact with the laser beam by means of saline soaked dressings. Endotracheal cuffs should be filled with saline rather than air. Intravenous induction and controlled ventilation with an endotracheal tube and inhalational agent or TIVA is a standard anaesthetic technique in routine use.

Postoperative care

Postoperative pain or discomfort is essentially like a severe burn. Intraoperative analgesia and its continuation in the postoperative period is important for keeping the patient pain-free. Occlusive ointment and analgesic provide pain relief. PONV may occur and should be prevented and treated as soon as possible. Patients may shiver and this is usually associated with long duration of surgery.

Laser for other procedures

Laser treatment is popular and is used for a wide variety of other maxillofacial aesthetic procedures. The choice of laser modality is in part influenced by the lesions to be treated (see Table 10.2).

Removal of pigmented lesions

Every person has a few obvious brown spots on their skin. Freckles, 'age spots', 'liver spots', and various birthmarks are just a few of the commonly known marks, generally referred to as pigmented lesions. Melanin is what gives our skin its colour. We all have varying amounts of melanin. Pigmented lesions are dark in colour simply because melanin is abnormally concentrated in one area of the skin. High concentrations of melanin can be due to various factors. Pigmented lesions can be successfully lightened or removed with modern laser technology. A laser is designed to produce one or more specific light wavelengths which are preferentially absorbed by the pigment. Pigmented lesions are either lightened or removed when the laser light passes through the skin but is absorbed by abnormal concentrations of melanin. The rapid absorption of light energy causes the destruction of the melanin. This reduction in local concentration leaves the treated skin looking uniform in colour and texture.

Removal of tattoos

Tattoo ink is removed by using a specific wavelength which passes through the skin but is absorbed by the ink. The rapid absorption of light energy causes the tattoo ink to destruct and it is then removed by the body's natural filtering systems.

Removal of birthmarks and other lesions

Port-wine stain birthmarks respond remarkably well to laser treatment. The abnormal blood vessels that cause these marks are reduced in size by the laser. This results in a lightening of the treated area. Skin growths, facial 'spider veins', and warts respond to laser surgery. Most situations take more than one laser treatment, but some respond to a single treatment.

Treatment of vascular lesions

The pulsed dye laser delivers an intense but gentle burst of yellow light to the skin. The light is specifically absorbed by the blood vessels in the dermis. These blood vessels are coagulated and then reabsorbed by the body during the natural healing process.

Botox injection

Botox injections are usually performed for frown lines, smile lines, forehead lines, brow lift, laugh lines, jaw muscles, neck horizontal lines, excessive sweating and body odour, facial contouring. This procedure is usually performed in an office setting or the high street. Botox is derived from a purified protein and can be used in adults below 65 years of age for medical and aesthetic indications. Botox temporarily blocks the release of acetylcholine, preventing the muscles from contracting and enabling them to relax[18]. During treatment, very small doses of botox are administered via a few tiny injections into the muscles responsible for frown lines between the brows. The procedure takes approximately 10 minutes and there is minimal downtime afterward. Discomfort is minimal and brief. Botox injections are performed with or without injection of LA agents and the help of an anaesthetist is not required.

Wrinkles

Pulse Repetition Frequency (PRF) is designed to rejuvenate the skin by removing pigment and stimulating collagen and elastin production. PRF is helpful for fine facial wrinkles, large pores, and post-acne scarring, pigmentation, prominent blood vessels, and unwanted hair.

Conclusion

Aesthetic surgery provides many challenges for the anaesthetist. The procedures can range from a minor to major surgery requiring prolonged anaesthesia. Success or failure of aesthetic surgery not only depends on surgical skill but also on careful selection of the anaesthesia technique.

References

1. Rana RE, Arora BS. (2002) History of plastic surgery in India. *J Postgrad Med*, **48**, 76–8.
2. Sarwer DB, Pertschuk MJ, Wadden TA, Whitaker LA. (1998) Psychological investigations of cosmetic surgery patients: a look back and a look ahead. *Plast Recon Surg*, **101**, 1136–42.
3. Sarwer DB. (1997) The obsessive cosmetic surgery patient: a consideration of body image dissatisfaction and body dysmorphic disorder. *Plast Surg Nurs*, **17**, 193–209.
4. Sarwar DB, Wadden TA, Pertschuk MJ, Whitaker LA. (1998) Body image dissatisfaction and body dysmorphic disorder in 100 cosmetic surgery patients. *Plast Reconstr Surg*, **101**, 1644–9.
5. Ben Simon GJ, McCann JD. (2008) Cosmetic eyelid and facial surgery. *Surv Ophthalmol*, **53**, 426–42.
6. Butterworth JF, Strichartz GR. (1990) Molecular mechanisms of local anaesthesia: a review. *Anesthesiology*, **72**, 711–34.
7. Calvey TN, Williams NE. (2008) *Principles and Practice of Pharmacology for Anaesthetists*, 5th edn. Chichester: Wiley.
8. Caterall WA. (1995) Structure and function of voltage-gated ion channels. *Ann Rev Biochem*, **64**, 493–531.
9. British Medical Association and Royal Pharmaceutical Society of Great Britain. (2009) *British National Formulary*, 57th edn. London: Pharmaceutical Press.
10. Fiset L, Milgrom P, Beirne OR, Roy-Byrne P. (1992) Disinhibition of behaviour with midazolam: report of a case. *J Oral Maxillofac Surg*, **50**, 645–9.
11. Takac S, Stojanović S. (1999) Characteristics of laser lights. *Med Pregl*, **52**, 29–34.
12. Einstein A. (1917) Zur quantum theorie der strahlung. *Physikalische Zeitschrift*, **18**, 121–8.
13. Schawlow AL, Townes CH. (1958) Infrared and optical masers. *Phys Rev*, **112**, 1940–9.
14. MHRA. (2008) *Device Bulletin. Guidance on the safe use of lasers, intense light source systems and LEDs in medical, surgical, dental and aesthetic practices. DB 2008(03)*. London: Medicines and Healthcare products Regulatory Agency.
15. Anderson RR and Parish JA. (1983) Selective photothermolysis: precise microsurgery by selective absorption of pulsed radiation. *Science*, **220**, 524–7.
16. Anderson RR. (1994) Laser-tissue interactions. In: Goldman MP, Fitzpatrick RE.(eds). *Cutaneous Laser Surgery: The Art and Science of Selective Photothermolysis*. St Louis, MO: Mosby-Year Book Inc, pp. 1–18.
17. Baggish MS, Poiesz BJ, Joret D, *et al.* (1991) Presence of human immunodeficiency virus DNA in laser smoke. *Laser Surg Med*, **11**, 197–203.
18. Flynn TC. (2009) Use of intraoperative botulinum toxin in facial reconstruction. *Dermatol Surg*, **3**, 182–8.

11

Infection and oral and maxillofacial surgery: implications for anaesthesia

Ian D. Clement

Introduction

This chapter looks at the anaesthetic management of patients presenting with orofacial infection. It will examine the pathophysiology of oral and dental infection and the associated local and systemic effects. This includes a discussion on the recognition and management of sepsis syndrome and the postoperative care of these patients in a critical care environment. In addition, the anaesthetic implications of patients with transmissible bloodborne infections presenting for maxillofacial surgery will be considered.

Infection of the oral cavity, including dental caries, dental abscess, and gingivitis, is one of the commonest diseases in the world. Management of these conditions rarely involves the anaesthetist. Standard management includes improved oral hygiene, antibiotics, and drainage under local anaesthesia. However, when this fails, or when serious local or systemic infection develops, then the anaesthetist will become involved. Infection in the head and neck requiring surgical intervention represents a major part of the emergency workload in maxillofacial surgery units.

Pathophysiology of dental and oral infections

Dental caries are caused by the action of acid-producing bacteria on the dental enamel, causing it to dissolve. Once through the enamel the infection passes through the dentine and into the pulp, causing pulpitis. Infection can then track through the pulp to the root apex and into the alveolar bone of the mandible or maxilla, leading to the formation of a periapical abscess. In a recent study of odontogenic infection[1], the clinical focus of infection was found to be the maxillary dentition in 30% of cases and the mandibular dentition in 70% of cases. Having reached the medullary bone, the infection may then erode through the cortical plate and into the surrounding tissues. From this point the infection may either resolve, become localized, forming an abscess, or may spread. Spreading infection will follow the line of least resistance through the fascial planes and into adjoining structures. The direction of spread is to some extent predictable based upon knowledge of the anatomy. Pus arising from the root apices of the lower teeth, perforating the lingual surface of the mandible, may drain intraorally if the apices of the teeth lie above the bony attachment of the mylohyoid muscle (incisors, canines, and premolars), or extraorally if they lie below it (second and third molars), draining through the skin or spreading through the superficial submandibular tissues. Infection arising in the mandibular molars may spread posteriorly into the lateral pharyngeal space. From here infection may spread to regions where the consequences of local infection can be very serious. Infection spreading upwards to the base of the skull may spread intracranially, potentially resulting in cavernous sinus thrombosis. Infection spreading downwards may cause glottic inflammation and airway obstruction, or may spread into the thorax resulting in mediastinitis. Infection arising in the root apices of the maxillary teeth may spread into the maxillary sinuses, the infraorbital soft tissues, or via the venous circulation into the cranium, again risking cavernous sinus thrombosis.

Necrotizing ulcerative gingivitis, also known as Vincent's angina or trench mouth, is a polymicrobial infection of the gums leading to inflammation and necrosis of gum tissue. It is caused by an overgrowth of normal oral bacteria as a consequence of poor oral hygiene combined with other factors such as poor diet and smoking. Management involves improved oral hygiene and antibiotics. Left untreated, the infection can spread, leading to complications such as osteomyelitis.

Microbiology

Dental caries are thought to be caused most commonly by serotypes of *Streptococcus mutans* (*cricetus, rattus, ferus, sobrinus*), although *Lactobacilli* also contribute to enamel decay by production of acid. Spreading odontogenic infection is usually polymicrobial and is caused by those organisms present as part of the normal oral flora (Table 11.1). Any combination of these organisms may be isolated in more severe odontogenic infection, although approximately 75% of isolates tend to be anaerobes (*Bacteroides, Fusobacterium, Actinomyces*).

Patients with an uncomplicated dental abscess who are otherwise well do not usually require antibiotics. However, the spectrum of patients presenting to the anaesthetist will have more severe local or spreading infection, which justifies early and effective antimicrobial therapy. Since a significant proportion of the isolates may be resistant to penicillin, then an intravenous cephalosporin such as cefuroxime, combined with metronidazole, would be a reasonable choice. The use of cephalosporins in patients with a history of penicillin allergy is controversial[2] and, if it is felt necessary to use an alternative, then clindamycin would be an appropriate choice.

Epidemiology

Dental caries is the most common chronic disease in the world. Improved public understanding of the need for good dental hygiene, combined with the widespread addition of fluoride to drinking water, led to a 39% reduction in dental caries in the UK between 1970 and 1980. With appropriate dental treatment carious teeth should not progress to the formation of dental abscess. Nevertheless, the lifetime prevalence of dental abscess has been estimated at anywhere between 5% and 46%. There is some evidence that the incidence of severe odontogenic infection requiring hospital admission may have increased in the UK in recent years[3]. Analysis of hospital episode statistics showed that the number of admissions in the UK for drainage of dental abscess almost doubled between 1998 and 2006. The average age of these patients was 32 years. It has been suggested that this increase may be a consequence of a reduction in access to routine dental care in the UK during this time period. A major risk factor for carious dental disease and odontogenic infection is lower socioeconomic status. Many of the patients presenting for surgery with odontogenic infection, although relatively young, will have a higher than average prevalence of other significant comorbidities, including obesity, smoking, drug and alcohol misuse, and poor nutritional status.

Complications of odontogenic infection

Dental cysts and osteomyelitis

Undrained dental abscesses may eventually resolve, leaving a fluid-filled cyst within the bone. These can lead to recurrent infection, and patients may present for surgical excision of the cyst. Alternatively, dental abscesses may progress to cause an osteomyelitis in the surrounding bone. This can be very painful and can cause significant bony destruction and deformity, requiring surgical excision and reconstruction. Where the mandible is involved, mouth opening can be significantly compromised. These patients are at risk of haematogenous spread of infection to distant sites and may develop systemic sepsis.

Maxillary sinusitis

Infection arising in the root apices of the maxillary teeth may spread into the maxillary sinuses or the infraorbital soft tissues. Maxillary sinusitis can cause fever, pain, and tenderness, and may require treatment with antibiotics.

Table 11.1 Microorganisms implicated in odontogenic infections

Streptococcus species
Staphylococcus aureus
Bacteroides species
Fusobacterium species
Actinomyces species
Haemophilus influenzae

Ludwig's angina

Ludwig's angina is a potentially life-threatening condition characterized by a rapidly spreading cellulitis of the tissues of the floor of the mouth. The term angina is derived from the Greek word meaning 'strangling', and the eponym relates to the German physician who first described the condition in 1836. The infection is odontogenic in 90% of cases and most commonly arises from the lower third molars. Other causes include trauma to the floor of the mouth, recent tooth extraction, pericoronitis (infection of the gums surrounding partially erupted lower third molars), peritonsillar abscess, and postprocedural infection after piercing of the frenulum. Impaired immunity is a major risk factor, but the condition can arise in otherwise healthy individuals. The commonest organisms involved are the *Actinomyces* species, although other oral pathogens are frequently involved. The patients may be severely septic, with pain and tenderness around the submandibular region. The infection can lead to boardlike swelling of the submandibular tissues and elevation of the tongue, leading to drooling, dysphonia, and ultimately to airway obstruction. The airway will not reliably improve with induction of anaesthesia, and awake fibreoptic intubation is frequently required, either for surgery or airway protection.

Cavernous sinus thrombosis

Periapical abscesses affecting the maxillary incisor and canine teeth can lead to spread of infection via the facial veins into the cranium. This can lead to septic thrombosis in the veins of the cavernous sinus behind the eye and at the base of the brain. It is estimated that 10% of cases of cavernous sinus thrombosis begin as a dental infection, the remainder being the result of sinusitis or superficial infection in the midface. Patients may present with headache, fever, periorbital oedema, exophthalmos, and chemosis. *Staphylococcus aureus* is the commonest organism, although when dental infection is the cause then other organisms are likely to be implicated. Treatment is with high dose, broad spectrum intravenous antibiotics and systemic anticoagulation. Surgical treatment of the underlying source of infection, such as dental abscess, is also required. Mortality is high at around 20% even with optimal treatment.

Mediastinitis

The fascial planes of the neck are contiguous with those of the mediastinum. In consequence, downward spread of infection arising from the head and neck into the mediastinum can occur very readily. The initial infection is frequently odontogenic and is therefore likely to be polymicrobial with a preponderance of anaerobes. The descending infection is often associated with multiple abscesses and gas formation within the tissues of the neck and mediastinum. These patients can become very unwell and may develop severe sepsis and multiorgan failure (see below).

Symptoms of retrosternal or pleuritic chest pain in the presence of neck infection may suggest mediastinal spread. Chest radiograph may show pleural collections or basal consolidation but CT scan of the neck and chest should be performed early if there is clinical suspicion. This will demonstrate soft tissue swelling within the neck, particularly in the retropharyngeal and supraglottic regions, and the presence of any gas within the tissues. Fluid collections and abscesses within the mediastinum or pleural space will be identified. Corsten *et al.*[4], in a case series and literature review of mediastinitis caused by descending neck infection, described a mortality rate of 31% in a group of patients with an average age of 38 years. Patients who underwent early thoracic surgery for drainage of the mediastinal collections, in addition to drainage of neck collections and intravenous antibiotics, had a significantly better outcome than those in whom mediastinal drainage was delayed or did not happen. This underlines the importance of early CT imaging of the chest in these patients.

Airway compromise

Spreading odontogenic infection can lead to compromise of the airway by a variety of mechanisms. Patients with abscesses of the lower second or third molars may develop airway problems as a consequence of infection spreading posteriorly and inferiorly into the retropharyngeal and supraglottic tissues. Infection may also spread into the masseter muscles leading to trismus. Osteomyelitis of the mandible may lead to bone destruction and limitation of mouth opening which, whilst not compromising the airway, may make management of the airway more difficult. In Ludwig's angina, the hardening and swelling of the tissues of the floor of the mouth and the elevation of the tongue, combined with impaired swallowing, can predispose the patient at risk of either airway obstruction or aspiration. In these patients conventional intubation is likely to be impossible, and airway management is challenging (see below). Patients with septic shock may have obtunded reflexes to the extent that they require airway protection.

Systemic sepsis

The systemic inflammatory response syndrome (SIRS) is a clinical state which arises as a result of the pathophysiological response to an insult such as infection, trauma, burns, or pancreatitis. The SIRS criteria have been agreed by international consensus[5], and SIRS is said to be present when at least two of the four SIRS criteria have been met (Table 11.2). Sepsis is defined as SIRS in the presence of suspected or documented infection. Septic shock is present when hypotension refractory to fluid resuscitation leads to evidence of inadequate organ perfusion, such as altered mental state, oliguria, and lactic acidosis. The exact process involved in this chain of events is complex and is still not fully understood. The loss of homeostasis within the vascular endothelium plays a critical role in the development of a pathologically vasodilated state, with increased capillary permeability and loss of fluid from the circulation. The role of the endothelium in the regulation of the clotting cascade is also disturbed, leading to coagulopathy and microvascular thrombosis. These processes frequently result in a patient who is shocked as a consequence of both vasodilatation and hypovolaemia. The basic principles of management in this situation are as follows:

- Oxygen
- Restoration of the circulation through a combination of fluid resuscitation and vasopressor therapy to restore an adequate blood pressure and oxygen delivery to the major organs[6]
- Broad spectrum antibiotics. Delay in the time to administration of effective antimicrobials after the onset of septic shock has been shown to increase mortality significantly, so this should be seen as a priority[7]
- Surgery to excise or drain the septic focus.

Table 11.2 Criteria for diagnosis of systemic inflammatory response syndrome (SIRS)

Criterion	Values
Temperature	<36˚C or >38˚C
Pulse rate	>90 /min
Respiratory rate	>20 /min
White cell count	<4 or >12 × 10^9/L

Odontogenic infection can frequently lead to the development of sepsis. Handley et al.[1] found that amongst patients presenting to a regional maxillofacial unit with odontogenic infection, 61% met the criteria for sepsis. Patients with septic shock from odontogenic infection can present a major challenge to the anaesthetist, requiring emergency surgery in the context of unstable physiology and a difficult airway. The perioperative management of these patients is discussed below.

Perioperative management of patients undergoing surgery for odontogenic infection

Many patients with dental abscess can be managed in the community with surgical drainage under local anaesthesia. However, patients with more severe odontogenic infection are likely to require management in hospital, which may well include urgent or emergency surgery under general anaesthesia.

Preoperative management

The spectrum of patients presenting for surgery will vary widely, from those with a simple localized infection with no systemic sequelae to patients with extensive local tissue damage, airway compromise, and septic shock. The patient population is typically younger adults, but comorbidities related to drug and alcohol misuse are more common in this population and should be sought. In patients with evidence of a systemic inflammatory response, a careful assessment of fluid status needs to be made. Patients may have been unwell and unable to drink adequately due to pain and swallowing problems for some time before presenting to hospital. Increased capillary permeability and fluid loss related to sepsis can compound this problem. Intravenous fluid administration prior to surgery may well be required. Patients with septic shock may have acute renal failure and clotting abnormalities, and need a full range of blood tests prior to theatre. Careful assessment of the airway is required in patients with signs of spreading infection. Mouth opening limited by swelling or trismus related to infection cannot be reliably expected to improve following induction of anaesthesia and there needs to be a low threshold for the use of fibreoptic intubation in these patients. Patients with Ludwig's angina develop firm, woody swelling of the tissues, including the tongue, which is likely to make conventional laryngoscopy impossible. If there is a suspicion of spread of infection to the mediastinum, then there is an indication for CT of the neck and chest to seek drainable collections. However, these patients are likely to be significantly compromised and it may be necessary to resuscitate the patient and secure the airway before going for CT.

Perioperative management

The management of the patient is clearly heavily dependent upon the clinical state at the time of surgery. Patients with an uncomplicated dental abscess could be adequately managed using conventional intravenous induction, nasal endotracheal tube, and throat pack to collect pus and debris. Intravenous antibiotics, including anaerobic cover (e.g. cefuroxime and metronidazole), should be given. Patients with spreading infection and signs of sepsis will need much more careful management. If the preoperative assessment has suggested that conventional laryngoscopy may be difficult, then awake fibreoptic intubation is probably the method of choice. If this is not possible and the airway is in peril, then awake tracheostomy under local anaesthesia is another option, although if the tissues on the anterior surface of the neck are infected this may be difficult. Patients with septic shock may need vasopressors to support the blood pressure following induction of anaesthesia. Invasive monitoring with arterial and central venous lines and urinary catheter for urine output measurements may well be required.

Postoperative management

Patients with uncomplicated dental abscess will be extubated at the end of surgery and observed on the ward postoperatively. Those with more severe infection may need to remain intubated and ventilated either because the airway itself remains compromised by the infection or because the overall clinical state precludes extubation. These patients will clearly need to go to a critical care unit postoperatively. Patients with clear signs of systemic sepsis should ideally be observed in a critical care environment postoperatively even if they are extubated at the end of the case. The critical care management of septic shock is outside the scope of this book, but some of the principles will be outlined. The Surviving Sepsis Guidelines[8] provide a useful appraisal of the evidence in this area. The initial management, as already outlined, includes measures aimed at optimizing tissue oxygen delivery (oxygen therapy, fluid resuscitation, and vasopressor therapy). At the same time, measures to identify and treat the infection are initiated, including blood cultures, broad spectrum antibiotics, and surgery for drainage and debridement of infected issues. Despite these measures, patients with septic shock frequently go on to develop multiorgan failure, requiring numerous modalities of organ support.

Circulatory support

Fluid therapy to ensure an adequate circulating volume is crucial. Unfortunately, the endpoints for this therapy are not always clearly defined and will depend on the circumstances. For example, urine output is often a useful marker but ceases to be so in the context of acute renal failure related to sepsis. The response of the central venous pressure (CVP) to a fluid challenge, or the variation in the pulse pressure or volume with respiration, are reasonable endpoints but are subjective in their interpretations. Patients in the early phases of septic shock can have significant ongoing fluid requirements as a result of increased capillary permeability. There is little evidence to support the use of one particular type of fluid over another. Crystalloids are safe and cheap. Synthetic colloids are also frequently used. The pathologically vasodilated state often seen in these patients can be managed with noradrenaline (norepinephrine). However, hypotension is sometimes refractory to high doses of noradrenaline (>0.4 micrograms/kg/min), and in this situation the addition of low dose vasopressin is sometimes helpful[9]. The use of corticosteroids (hydrocortisone 200 mg daily) in severe sepsis became popular following a study by Annane et al.[10], but a more recent study[11] suggests this treatment has no effect on mortality.

Respiratory support

This patient population frequently goes on to develop acute respiratory distress syndrome (ARDS). This condition is characterized by patchy bilateral infiltrates on chest X-ray, hypoxaemia, and reduced lung compliance. These patients often require prolonged respiratory support. The use of a lower tidal volume ventilator strategy (6 ml/kg ideal body weight) has been shown to reduce mortality compared with higher tidal volumes[12].

Renal support

Acute renal failure develops in a significant proportion of patients with septic shock. Renal function usually recovers over a timescale of 1–3 weeks, but patients require renal replacement therapy during this time. The modality most commonly used in UK critical care units is continuous venovenous haemo-filtration (CVVH).

Nutrition and glucose control

Early nutrition, preferably via the enteral route, is accepted as the standard for all critically ill patients. Hyperglycaemia is common in these patients and there is much interest in the benefit of maintaining tight glycaemic control with the use of insulin infusion. The major benefit seen in some of the earlier studies has not been replicated in subsequent clinical trials[13,14].

Other measures

There is some evidence to support the use of recombinant activated protein C in patients with severe sepsis[15]. However, this agent carries an increased risk of bleeding and would need to be used with caution in patients following maxillofacial surgery. Oversedation should be avoided in these patients. Nursing the patients with 30° head-up tilt helps to reduce secondary ventilator-associated pneumonia[16]. Frequent positioning of patient which avoid pressure sores, stress ulcer prophylaxis, and deep vein thrombosis prophylaxis are all important. Evidence of ongoing sepsis requires prompt action, including further imaging, removal or change of intravascular catheters and further surgery if necessary.

Septic shock remains a condition which is frequently associated with a poor outcome. International studies frequently demonstrate 28-day mortality rates in the range of 30–40% in these patients. Those patients that do survive may be left with physical or psychological needs requiring long-term support.

Maxillofacial surgery in high risk patients

The subgroup of patients presenting for surgery for odontogenic infection has a much higher risk for the presence of transmissible infections, including human immunodeficiency virus (HIV), hepatitis B and C, and tuberculosis. It is a fundamental responsibility of every practising anaesthetist to minimize the risk of these infections being transmitted either between patient and anaesthetist, patient and other members of the theatre team, or between patients. Every hospital has a statutory requirement to enforce effective infection control procedures. The Association of Anaesthetists of Great Britain and Ireland has published guidelines on infection control in anaesthesia[17].

Patients with a history of intravenous drug use present a particular set of challenges. They are at high risk of infection with transmissible bloodborne viruses. Many will have been tested, but previous negative serology does not rule out recently acquired infection and these patients should always be treated as high risk irrespective of their serological status. Venous access may be very difficult to obtain. The patients themselves can sometimes advise of the best sites, but it is sometimes necessary to use a central vein to secure good access. Patients who have been heavy users of opiates will exhibit tolerance to therapeutic opiates and may need significantly higher doses to achieve adequate analgesia. These patients should not be denied adequate opiate medication during the perioperative period. Patients on regular methadone should generally have this continued if possible whilst in hospital.

Antibiotic prophylaxis in maxillofacial surgery

It is generally accepted (previous concept) that certain groups of patients with cardiac conditions are at increased risk of developing infective endocarditis. This includes patients with the following conditions:

- Cardiac valve replacement
- Structural congenital heart disease, including surgically corrected conditions, but excluding isolated atrial septal defect, fully repaired ventricular septal defect or fully repaired patent ductus arteriosus
- Previous infective endocarditis.

Since the mid 1950s it has been standard practice to offer antibiotic prophylaxis to patients with these conditions undergoing dental procedures. This practice has been based on a number of assumptions. These include an assumption that the dental procedure may cause a bacteraemia, that the bacteraemia may lead to infective endocarditis, and that antibiotic prophylaxis will prevent endocarditis from developing. The evidence underlying these assumptions was studied in detail by the UK National Institute for Health and Clinical Excellence, leading to the publication of a guideline in 2008[18]. Although studies suggest that dental treatment may well lead to a transient bacteraemia, there is some evidence that normal toothbrushing and many other daily activities can cause similar bacteraemias. The evidence for a causal link between dental treatment and the subsequent development of endocarditis is weak, and there is even less evidence that antibiotic prophylaxis is of any benefit. The authors felt that, given the available evidence, the routine use of antibiotic prophylaxis had the potential to do greater harm through anaphylaxis and increasing microbial resistance. The guideline recommends that antibiotic prophylaxis should not be used in routine dental treatment. The risk of infective endocarditis from an odontogenic source can best be minimized by maintaining good oral hygiene, regular check ups and prompt dental treatment when required. Patients with severe or spreading odontogenic infection are likely to be on antibiotics anyway. In patients at risk of infective endocarditis, it is important to choose antibiotics which will effectively cover the likely pathogens in infective endocarditis, including *Streptococci, Staphylococcus aureus,* and *Enterococci.*

Conclusion

Patients requiring surgery for maxillofacial infection can present a number of challenges to the anaesthetist. The problems of managing a potentially difficult airway can be compounded by the requirement for emergency anaesthesia in patients with significant systemic disturbance and a high prevalence of major comorbidities.

References

1. Handley T, Devlin M, Koppel D, McCaul J. (2009) The sepsis syndrome in odontogenic infection. *JICS,* **10(1),** 21–5.
2. Pegler S, Healy B. (2007) In patients allergic to penicillin, consider second and third generation cephalosporins for life threatening infections. *BMJ,* **335,** 991.
3. Thomas SJ, Hughes C, Atkinson C, Ness AR, Revington P. (2008) Is there an epidemic of admissions for surgical treatment of dental abscesses in the UK? *BMJ,* **336,** 1219–20.
4. Corsten MJ, Shamji FM, Odell PF *et al.* (1997) Optimal treatment of descending necrotising mediastinitis. *Thorax,* **52,** 702–8.
5. Muckart DJ, Bhagwanjee S. (1997) American College of Chest Physicians/Society of Critical Care Medicine Consensus Conference definitions of the systemic inflammatory response syndrome and allied disorders in relation to critically injured patients. *Crit Care Med,* **25(11),** 1789–95.
6. Rivers E, Nguyen B, Havstad S *et al.* (2001) Early goal-directed therapy in the treatment of severe sepsis and septic shock. *N Engl J Med,* **345,** 1368–77.
7. Kumar A, Roberts D, Wood K *et al.* (2006) Duration of hypotension before initiation of effective antimicrobial therapy is the critical determinant of survival in human septic shock. *Crit Care Med,* **34,** 1589–96.
8. Dellinger RP, Levy MM, Carlet JM *et al.* (2008) Surviving Sepsis Campaign: International guidelines for management of severe sepsis and septic shock. *Crit Care Med,* **36,** 296–327.
9. Russell J, Walley K, Singer J *et al.* (2008) Vasopressin versus norepinephrine infusion in patients with septic shock. *N Engl J Med,* **358,** 877–87.
10. Annane D, Sebille V, Charpentier C *et al.* (2002) Effect of treatment with low doses of hydrocortisone and fludrocortisone on mortality in patients with septic shock. *JAMA,* **288,** 862–71.
11. Sprung C, Annane D, Keh D *et al.* (2008) Hydrocortisone therapy for patients with septic shock. *N Engl J Med,* **358,** 111–24.
12. ARDS Network. (2000) Ventilation with lower tidal volumes as compared with traditional tidal volumes for acute lung injury and the acute respiratory distress syndrome. *N Engl J Med,* **342,** 1301–8.
13. Van den Berghe G, Wouters P, Weekers F. (2001) Intensive insulin therapy in the critically ill patients. *N Engl J Med,* **345,** 1359–67.
14. The NICE-SUGAR Study Investigators. (2009) Intensive versus conventional glucose control in critically ill patients. *N Engl J Med,* **360,** 1283–97.
15. Bernard G, Vincent J-L, Laterre P-F *et al.* (2001) Efficacy and safety of recombinant human activated protein C for severe sepsis. *N Engl J Med,* **344,** 699–709.
16. Drakulovic M, Torres A, Bauer T *et al.* (1999) Supine body position as a risk factor for nosocomial pneumonia in mechanically ventilated patients: a randomised trial. *Lancet,* **354,** 1851–8.
17. Association of Anaesthetists of Great Britain and Ireland. (2008) Infection control in anaesthesia. *Anaesthesia,* **63,** 1027–36.
18. National Institute for Health and Clinical Excellence. (2008) Prophylaxis against infective endocarditis. *NICE Clinical Guideline* **64.**

12

Oral and maxillofacial related injuries and hazards during anaesthesia

Hilary Turner and Ian Shaw

Introduction

Major catastrophic sequelae such as death or permanent injury following general anaesthesia are thankfully rare. However, inadvertent damage to teeth, intraoral soft tissues, and morbidity associated with throat packs and nasal intubation represent some of the most commonly reported oral and maxillofacial related injuries. This chapter will be limited to discussion of these injuries. For a wider discussion of the hazards and complications of anaesthesia, the reader should consult the literature[1,2].

Dental damage

Less serious complications of anaesthesia, such as damage to teeth, can be of major significance to the individual patient. Inadvertent dental damage represents the single most commonly reported anaesthetic related injury, accounting for over a third of all compensatory claims against anaesthetists. Although often individually fiscally moderate, the cumulative cost is substantial.

The reported incidence of dental damage during anaesthesia has been retrospectively reported as 0.05–12%[3,4]. This, however, may be a substantial underestimate[5]. Obvious damage to teeth during anaesthesia will be noted by the anaesthetist at the time of injury. Alternatively, the patient may report damage to their teeth postoperatively. In a prospective study of 745 patients who underwent general anaesthesia, preoperative and postoperative examination by a dentist reported an incidence of oral trauma as high as 18%, of which two-thirds was damage to natural or prosthetic teeth[4]. The implication is that, without expert examination, minor injuries such as enamel microfractures may pass unnoticed[6,7].

Dental anatomy

An appreciation of normal developmental dental anatomy is necessary for an understanding of the mechanism of dental injury during anaesthesia. Humans have 20 deciduous teeth, also known as 'milk' or 'baby' teeth, which are replaced by 32 permanent teeth by the second decade of life. The deciduous teeth in each quadrant are identified by the letters A to E, working outwards from the midline. Permanent teeth are identified by the numbers 1 to 8 in a similar manner. To reduce the likelihood of misidentification of teeth during treatment, the World Dental Federation has proposed an alternative international nomenclature system in which the tooth number is prefixed by a 1, 2, 3, or 4, corresponding to upper right, upper left, lower left and lower right quadrants, respectively (Chapter 13, Figure 13.8).

Anatomically, each tooth is divided into two distinct parts, an exposed crown and a hidden embedded root (Figure 12.1). The boundary between the two parts is known as the cementoenamel junction. Depending on their functional role and the intended axis of applied force, teeth can have single or multiple roots. Within each tooth is a central pulp cavity covered in dentine, a hard elastic avascular mineralized tissue composed of collagen and water. The pulp cavity contains blood vessels and nerves. The dentine of the crown is protected by an outer layer of enamel of varying thickness which extends from the tip of the tooth to the cementoenamel junction. Enamel, which is thickest at the biting edge of the tooth and thinnest near the gingival margin, is the hardest substance in the body and is composed of tightly packed rods or prisms containing crystalline calcium phosphate known as hydroxyapatite. Although of considerable integral strength, enamel is brittle and is susceptible to shatter under abnormally applied shearing forces.

Below the cementoenamel junction the dentine of the anatomical root is covered with cementum, a specialized bony substance composed of collagen and hydroxyapatite. Adherent to the cementum is the collagenous periodontal ligament which suspends each tooth independently within a socket of alveolar bone. The ligament facilitates a slight degree of movement during mastication, so allowing adjacent touch and pressure receptors to relate sensory information critical to the masticatory process via central mechanisms.

Overlying the alveolar bone is the keratinized epithelium of the jaws, or gingiva, in contrast to the non-keratinized oral mucous membrane. Inflammation and infection of this soft tissue caused by bacterial plaque is an important coexisting factor in anaesthetic related dental damage, particularly when associated with underlying bone loss as seen in periodontitis (see below).

In a patient with normal dentition, when the teeth are brought together the lower mandibular teeth will lie symmetrically and slightly lingually to the upper

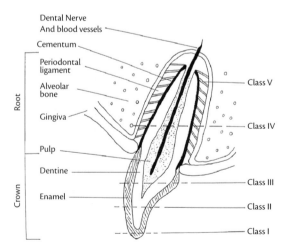

Figure 12.1 Structure of normal tooth and site of injury. Each tooth has an exposed crown and embedded hidden root. Injuries to teeth are categorised into Classes I to V depending on the site of injury (see Table 12.3).

maxillary teeth. A slight incisor overbite is normal, with about one-third of the upper incisors covering the lower incisors. The upper and lower teeth are designed to meet during mastication. Molars, which have up to three roots, are in the position of maximal mechanical advantage adjacent to the powerful muscles of mastication. Teeth tolerate substantial applied axial forces in the intended physiological vector better than lesser abnormally applied lateral forces. For further detail the reader should consult the literature[8].

Aetiology of dental injury during anaesthesia

Whilst the majority of dental injuries during anaesthesia are reported following laryngoscopy, endotracheal or nasotracheal intubation[3,4,9], about 25% occur on emergence when injury is most commonly associated with extubation or the use of oropharyngeal airways[3,10,11], laryngeal masks, bite blocks, or suction catheters. Emergence dental injuries are more likely to involve the lower teeth[12,13] and often pass unnoticed by the anaesthetist[4]. Diagnostic laryngoscopy or the instrumental assisted passage of a nasogastic tube in an anaesthetized patient can also result in sustained abnormally applied forces leading to dental or soft tissue trauma.

The upper left central incisors are the most vulnerable teeth to damage during anaesthesia[12,15] (Figure 12.2). The preponderance of left-sided injuries is thought to reflect the fact that most anaesthetists are right-handed. Typically, although not exclusively, dental damage is usually limited to a single tooth[9,16]. Teeth have different dental axes depending on their function. Incisors are mono-rooted teeth with a forward dental axis and small cross-sectional area designed to withstand considerable biting forces along their axis. Upper premolar and molar teeth have two or three roots, respectively, and are designed to withstand substantial aligned forces along a vertical dental axis. Lower premolar and molar teeth have one or two roots, respectively. Any alteration in the vector of the force applied, such as strong vertical forces applied to incisors, makes them more vulnerable to damage[10,17].

Forces involved in laryngoscopy

Dental injuries during general anaesthesia are typically caused by direct contact of the upper anterior teeth with the rigid blade of the laryngoscope. In addition to predisposing patient factors (see below), dental injury

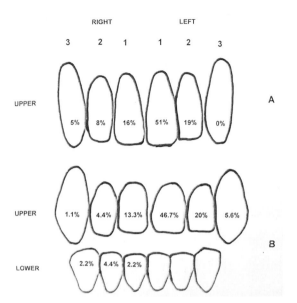

UPPER

5%   8%   16%   51%   19%   0%

A

UPPER

1.1%   4.4%   13.3%   46.7%   20%   5.6%

B

LOWER

2.2%   4.4%   2.2%

Figure 12.2 Distribution of dental damage following general anaesthesia as reported by [A] Lockhart et al [3] and Jaw-Jen Chen et al [B] [4]. The upper incisors are the most vulnerable teeth accounting for two-thirds of the reported injuries. Adapted from Owen and Smith [25] with permission.

is associated with the characteristics of the laryngoscope blade[18] in use and the skill of the anaesthetist. The proximity of the upper anterior incisors to the laryngoscope blade during optimal view of the vocal cords has been studied. The forces exerted on the upper teeth vary with the design of the laryngoscope[19]. In consequence, modifications to laryngoscope blades with the intention of minimizing contact with the upper teeth have been proposed[20–22]. Alternative protective strategies have included the application of compressible adhesive tape[23] and foam cushions[24] to the upper surface of the laryngoscope blade[25]. The use of plastic-bladed scopes may confer some protective advantage[26]. Electronic warning devices for the prevention of dental injury during laryngoscopy have been developed[27] but have not been widely accepted.

The inadvertent use of the upper incisors as a fulcrum during difficult intubation is a well recognized pre-sequel to dental injury, although when intubation is difficult this is regarded as inevitable by some[28]. Forces of 30–65 Newtons (N) or greater exerted on the maxillary incisors during laryngoscopy have been recorded[18,28,29] but the sensitivity of the measuring devices was questioned following subsequent reports of mean axial forces of 20 N[21,30]. Regardless, the

applied forces are substantial. Putting this into perspective, a gallon of water exerts a force of 37 N. The patient's body mass index, height, weight[21,30,31], and Mallampati Score appear to correlate with the overall force applied when using a MacIntosh blade, but less so with the McCoy modified blade[21,30]. Patients of increasing age required less applied force for intubation.

Oropharyngeal airways

Oropharyngeal airways have been implicated in 20% of anaesthetic related dental injuries[32]. Masseter spam and teeth clenching are not uncommon following anaesthesia with volatile agents[13,33]. During emergence, the masseter muscles can exert considerable forces (of up to 80 N)[9] which are normally absorbed by the multi-rooted molar and premolar teeth. In the presence of a midline placed oropharyngeal airway, the molar teeth are unable to meet, resulting in the transfer of the vertical jaw clenching forces forward through the anterior mono-rooted incisors[13]. The common practice of using an oropharyngeal airway as a bite guard to protect an endotracheal tube or laryngeal mask airway may therefore put incisor teeth at an increased risk of fracture or impaction[10,13,17]. A similar mechanism of injury could also result from biting hard on a midline placed suction catheter. Placing a bite block between the premolar or molar teeth, rather than adjacent to the incisor teeth, would in theory be less likely to result in dental damage.

Predisposing factors and anaesthetic related dental injury

Localized infection and inflammation

Healthy teeth are robust and capable of withstanding considerable force and pressure. Although factors predisposing to dental injury during anaesthesia are multifactorial, a prime contributory factor is pre-existing dental or intraoral disease, which increases the risk of injury fivefold[3,4,11]. Dental caries resulting in enamel loss, dentine softening, cavity formation, and previous injury can all weaken teeth, making them susceptible to fracture or dislodgement even with minimal applied force.

After dental caries, periodontal and gingival disease are the most prevalent worldwide diseases in adults. Bacterial plaque which has accumulated in the crevices between the teeth and gums can give rise to

Table 12.1 Factors predisposing to dental injury during anaesthesia

Anaesthetic related factors

    Oropharyngeal airways

    Emergency anaesthesia

    Difficulty in maintaining airway

    Increasing Mallampati score

    Laryngoscopy

    Endotracheal intubation

    Suction catheters

    Emergence teeth clenching

Patient related factors

    Patient characteristics

    Age

    Obesity (BMI)

Oral and maxillofacial anatomy

    Isolated teeth

    Missing teeth

    Abnormally positioned teeth

    Limited mandibular mobility

    Maxillary protrusion and incisor overbite

    Limited neck movement

Dental pathology

    Previous dental damage

    Dental caries

    Periodontal disease

    Gingival disease

Previous restorative and prosthetic dental treatment

    Bridges

    Crowns

    Implants

    Orthodontic braces

    Anterior dental restorations

Systemic disease (see Table 12.2)
Drug therapy (see text)

inflammation of the gums and loss of the supporting underlying alveolar bone. Patients with abnormal dentition are especially prone to plaque accumulation. If left unattended plaque can thicken, become mineralized, and provide a localized anaerobic environment in which bacteria can proliferate. Periodontitis, which is invariably painless, is caused by an aggressive immune and inflammatory response to the bacteria resident on the tooth's surface. Released collagenases destroy the adjacent bony support, predisposing to dental avulsion. Avascular root-filled teeth become brittle and devitalized, making root fracture or dislodgement, even with minimal force, more likely. Associated risk factors include poorly controlled diabetes, osteoporosis, arteriosclerosis, smoking, and an individual genetic predisposition. Patients whose anterior segments have significant decay, advanced periodontitis, or are shedding deciduous teeth (see below) are the most prone to anaesthetic related damage[4] (Table 12.1).

Systemic diseases with intraoral manifestations

Many systemic diseases have intraoral manifestations which can exacerbate periodontal disease, so weakening the teeth and gums, and making them susceptible to damage during anaesthesia[34–36] (Table 12.2). The mechanisms by which systemic disease can influence the pathogenesis of periodontal disease are unclear but may involve a modification of the host's normal immune response. Adequate saliva production is a prerequisite for optimal dental health. Conditions in which saliva production is diminished or absent are often associated with dental disease and a vulnerability to injury during anaesthesia.

Medication and dental disease

Chronic medication can result in dental discoloration, structural damage or intraoral manifestations that predispose to dental injury during anaesthesia. The drugs most implicated are those formulated in sugar-containing vehicles and drugs which lower the intraoral pH such as aspirin and powdered antiasthmatic medication. Anticholinergics, antidepressants, and antipsychotics all result in decreased saliva secretion, predisposing to periodontitis. Over one-third of patients on the immunosuppressant cyclosporin, nifedipine, and anticonvulsants such as phenytoin will experience gingival overgrowth which may undergo

Table 12.2 Systemic conditions with oral manifestations which may be associated with an increased risk of dental damage during anaesthesia.

Some systemic diseases predispose to dental disease resulting in weakened teeth and friable surrounding soft tissues.

Systemic condition	Intra-oral manifestations
Gastro-oesophageal reflux	Lowers intra-oral pH
Smoking	Increased susceptibility to periodontal disease
Osteoporosis	Periodontal disease, demineralization and reduced bone density
Poorly controlled diabetes mellitus	Gingivitis and periodontal disease due to angiopathy
HIV infection	Necrotizing gingivitis, destruction of alveolar bone due to peridontitis and accelerated dental caries
Pregnancy	Hormonal modification of the host's response to dental plaque can make pregnant females more prone to gingivitis in the second trimester
Hypophosphataemia	Impaired enamel formation
Blood dyscrasias	Periodontitis, gingivitis and loose teeth bone loss associated with neutropenia
Xerostomia	Reduced salivary flow accelerates dental caries and increases risk of periodonitis
HIV and AIDS	
Sjogrens syndrome	
Radiotherapy	
Vitamin C deficiency (scurvy)	
Trisomy 21	Deficient tooth fixation due to an abnormal periodontal ligament
Osteogenesis imperfecta	Suboptimal dentine formation and brittle enamel

subsequent local inflammatory changes. Localized irradiation can also result in a loss of bony support.

Patients who chronically misuse illegal drugs have a high incidence of periodontal disease. Cocaine and methamphetamine mixed with saliva creates a highly acidic environment, resulting in erosion of enamel and dental caries, often in a very short period of time. Heroin causes a craving for sweet and sugary foods, and ecstasy induces xerostoma, a prerequisite to periodontal disease. Patients on supervised withdrawal programmes are often prescribed methadone. In order to make methadone palatable, it is formulated in concentrated sugary syrup which partly explains why such patients often have very poor dental health and frequently require a dental clearance. For a comprehensive discussion of this topic, the reader should consult Tredwin et al.[36].

Age

Between the age of 6 and 12 years, a child's deciduous teeth are progressively replaced by permanent adult teeth and children of this age will have mixed dentition

present. Deciduous teeth have shorter roots than adult teeth. As the erupting permanent tooth develops, the root of the overlying deciduous tooth undergoes resorption, leading to a loss of structural bony support. Adult teeth take up to 3 years before they are fully embedded and reach optimal strength[5]. As a result, children between the ages of 5 and 10 are at the greatest risk of inadvertent dental damage during anaesthesia[4,5]. It is a commonly held misconception that because deciduous teeth will be replaced in time, damage to them is of less concern. Injury to a deciduous tooth can easily damage the developing underlying permanent tooth, and loss of the tooth may delay or result in premature eruption of the permanent tooth[5]. This may give rise to crowding and dental misalignment which can require orthodontic treatment in later years. Anaesthetists should therefore treat deciduous teeth with the same respect they would show permanent teeth[5,17].

Although the elderly are at greater risk of dental injury[12], this is not always reflected in the literature as many patients in the past would have been wholly or partially edentulous. Although the forces applied during laryngoscopy appear to be less with increasing age, the overall incidence of dental injury is high, reflecting the increased incidence of dental and periodontal disease in the elderly. Bony support of teeth declines with age. With greater health education and the availability of dental services, a significant number of elderly patients have retained some or all of their teeth, making them at greater risk than previously.

Abnormal oral and maxillofacial anatomy

The anatomical relationship between the upper and lower incisors can have a significant effect on their tolerance to applied forces. Misaligned teeth resulting in malocclusion are more likely to be exposed to abnormal forces[37]. Traditionally there are three classes of dental malocclusion as described by Angle's classification, the details of which can be found in any standard dental textbook[38]. Class II relationships, or retrognathia, are of greatest concern to the anaesthetist[5]. Malocclusion, retarded mandibles, prominent anterior teeth, anterior crowding, and high dental arches can all increase the risk of dental damage during anaesthesia. Where the upper incisors are severely proclined or irregular, visualization of the vocal cords during laryngoscopy can be very difficult, encouraging the inadvertent use of the incisors as a lever fulcrum. Patients with malocclusion are also more susceptible to dental and periodontal disease on account of the difficulties in providing effective dental hygiene.

Isolated teeth, which lack the support of adjacent teeth and may also have the same pathological condition as the missing teeth[37,39], are vulnerable to damage or dislodgement during laryngoscopy by the passage of the endotracheal tube and positioning of a laryngeal mask.

Prosthetic dental restorations

The anaesthetist may encounter several forms of dental restoration, such as single or multiple crowned teeth, fixed bridges, surface veneers, removable partial or complete dentures, and dental implants[5]. Pathologically weakened teeth, either from disease or previous restoration, are unable to withstand the forces tolerated by healthy teeth[9]. Although modern dental resins and porcelain are very robust, excessive pressure from a laryngoscope blade or via an oropharyngeal airway can result in fragmentation. Gold, as a restorative material, seems to be more robust, with fewer patients reporting dental damage following anaesthesia. In one

retrospective study, previously filled teeth accounted for 50% of those damaged during anaesthesia[9].

Whilst the cosmetic result of dental restorations may be pleasing to the patient, the prosthetic tooth is unable to withstand the forces accommodated by a normal healthy tooth. The commonest site for crowned restorations is the upper incisors, further compounding the risk[13], particularly during recovery from an anaesthetic. Prosthetic dental restorations, such as crowned teeth, involve cavity preparation which removes some of the tooth's original structure and replacement with resins and metal supporting posts (see Chapter 13). The remaining tooth structure, whilst restored, may not be optimally healthy. Prosthetic restorations are designed primarily to withstand axial loading forces along the line of the tooth such as those experienced in chewing. Applied lateral or shearing forces are tolerated poorly (Figure 12.3).

The type of restoration can also influence the consequences of the injury. Where a crowned tooth has a long metal supporting post within the tooth cavity, excessive applied force can result in vertical splitting of the tooth. Crowns with short metal retaining posts are more prone to dislodgement if excessive non-axial force is applied, whilst both restorations are vulnerable to root fractures.

On account of the minimal preparation involved, the cosmetic application of thin veneers to visible teeth has become very popular. Veneers are 0.5–1 mm thick laminates of porcelain, ceramic or a composite of both, the former being the most popular on account of its enhanced strength. The veneer is bonded to either the tooth enamel or underlying dentine, the former creating a much more stable bond[5]. As veneers are bonded only to healthy teeth, abnormally applied

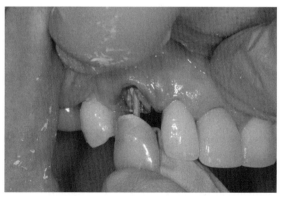

Figure 12.3 A crown and post dislodged during laryngoscopy

Table 12.3 Classification of dental injury during anaesthesia

Dental injuries are classified into six classes according to the level of the damage. Classes I, II and VI constitute the majority of iatrogenic anaesthetic related injuries which are invariably associated with underlying dental and periodontal disease.

Class	Site of injury	Features	Dental treatment
Class I	Fracture through dental enamel	Commonest injury. Damage to tooth surface. Painless and may go unnoticed by the anaesthetist. Patient may complain of feeling a new irregular tooth edge with their tongue.	May require filing to smooth tooth edge or prosthetic capping. Non-urgent dental referral
Class II	Fracture into dentin	Invariably painful, especially to extremes of temperature. Fracture site will show a yellow discolouration as the sub-enamel layer is exposed. Exposed dentin is porous and renders the pulp susceptible infection, especially in children who only have a thin layer of dentine.	Dental emergency. Requires prompt dental referral.
Class III	Fracture into tooth pulp	Exquisitely painful as fracture penetrates the densely innervated tooth pulp. Typically anterior teeth involved. Exposed pulp at risk of infection.	Requires urgent dental referral and treatment. Treatment can be complex necessitating root canal evacuation followed by metal post insertion and overlying crown placement or restoration.
Class IV	Fracture of tooth root	Typically associated with an unstable tooth as a result of periodontal disease.	Surgical extraction of damaged tooth
Class V	Subluxation (displacement) of a tooth	Tooth becomes loose and dislodged although retained within the alveolar bone. Subluxation can interrupt the blood supply to the tooth	Provided the tooth still has periodontal support it can be stabilized by splinting into original position. If support is lost then surgical extraction may be necessary.
Class VI	Avulsion of entire tooth	Complete dislodgement of the tooth representing a serious aspiration risk. Essential to recover tooth. Invariably associated with periodontal disease.	Dental emergency. Prompt re-implantation may be possible provided there is no significant coexisting periodontal disease.

forces, especially of a levering nature, will risk chipping the veneer or shearing the comparatively weaker bond between the tooth and the overlying veneer. Bridges, which involve prosthetic teeth being interconnected with supporting bands of metal, are particularly at risk of displacement if excessive shearing force is applied[5,9].

Classification of dental injury

Dental trauma is divided into six categories[40] depending on the anatomical site of the injury (Figure 12.1 and Table 12.3). Although all injuries can occur during anaesthesia—Class I, II, and VI are the most common. An understanding of the implications of the nature and site of the injury is important if effective corrective dental treatment is to be provided.

Prevention of anaesthetic related dental injury

Ideally, prevention of anaesthetic related dental injuries should start with an attempt to attain optimal dental and gingival health. Routine preanaesthetic dental examination of all patients has been proposed[6,41,42] but dismissed as unworkable. Whenever possible, any remedial and restorative dental treatment should be undertaken prior to elective anaesthesia and surgery. In reality, this is often unattainable and unrealistic. Patients who present with poor dental health will invariably have a long history of dental neglect and poor intraoral hygiene which is unlikely to be changed during the immediate preoperative period. Concerns have also been raised as to the lack of availability of dental care possibly leading to a greater incidence of anaesthetic related dental damage[11]. Patients attending anaesthetic preassessment clinics should have their oral cavity and teeth carefully inspected for risk factors such as dental caries, loose teeth, and periodontal disease[10,42]. When risk factors are identified, an explanation of your concerns should be given to the patient and, time permitting, they should be encouraged to attend their dentist for treatment.

Protective mouthguards

The use of a protective mouthguard to minimize dental injury to upper incisors during laryngoscopy and intubation has long been established[3]. One study claimed that 90% of reported dental injuries were preventable had the patient's dental state been correctly assessed preoperatively and a mouthguard used intraoperatively[3]. Despite this, the use of protective mouthguards by anaesthetists is still not routine practice[3,9,41,43] in recognition of the fact that their use can make laryngoscopy and intubation difficult, particularly for less experienced anaesthetists[44]. When the anaesthetist has identified especially vulnerable dentition, the reported usage of mouthguards increases sharply[3].

The most commonly used anaesthetic mouthguards are bulky and commercially manufactured to a standard design. A less common but superior alternative is a preformed custom-made mouthguard which fits the patient's dentition precisely. The thinner preformed mouthguards are less like to impede intubation and have been shown successfully to dissipate the forces applied to teeth during laryngoscopy[42]. Unfortunately, the measured protective effect correlated with the increasing bulk of the mouthguard negates any advantage. The use of a mouthguard therefore does not obliterate the risk of dental damage during anaesthesia[42]. Indeed, their efficacy and routine use has been questioned[39,45]. Whilst their use may offer protection against superficial chipping of dental enamel, it will not prevent the avulsion of loose teeth.

Immediate management of a damaged tooth during anaesthesia

When a tooth is damaged during the course of anaesthesia, a full explanation must be given to the patient, the details of which are then recorded in the patient's notes.

The immediate management of teeth damaged during anaesthesia will depend upon the extent of the injury (Table 12.3). For superficial damage, such as chipped enamel (Class I), a routine dental appointment will suffice. As Classes II–VI injuries are at risk of secondary infection, they should receive expert attention within 24 hours. Class II and III injuries can be extremely painful, prompting the patient to present for treatment immediately.

Subluxed deciduous teeth should not be replaced in their sockets as they are prone to fuse with alveolar bone in an abnormal manner. Subluxed or avulsed permanent teeth, however, require urgent treatment if the tooth is to remain viable. Once a subluxed tooth has been repositioned, the tooth socket should be compressed firmly between the thumb and forefinger for 1 minute and the tooth temporarily splinted back into position to avoid further movement[46]. Movement can endanger the blood supply, resulting in an avascular tooth. The patient should be started on oral penicillin and urgently referred to a dental surgeon for definitive stabilization.

No action is necessary if a deciduous tooth has been avulsed other than to inform the parents. In contrast, an avulsed permanent tooth constitutes a dental emergency. Typically, there is coexisting dental caries and/or periodontal disease. Regardless, an attempt should be made to salvage the tooth and preserve the periodontal ligament. A tooth deprived of its blood supply becomes increasingly unviable after 30 minutes, so speed is of the essence.

Reimplantation is only possible if the tooth remains viable. The avulsed tooth and socket should be immediately lavaged in sterile isomolar normal saline (never water) and inspected. Provided the tooth is intact and there are no root fractures, the tooth should be immediately returned to the socket by holding the crown and taking great care to avoid touching the root. When immediate reimplantation is not feasible, the tooth should be stored in sterile isomolar saline or milk and the patient referred urgently to a dental surgeon. Reimplantation of a tooth in a patient partially recovered from a general anaesthetic always carries the risk displacement and aspiration.

An unaccounted for dislodged tooth, or fragment of tooth, can be life-threatening if inhaled on extubation[49]. It is essential to recover the tooth and any fragments. If a tooth, or part of a tooth, is unaccounted for, then X-rays of the head, neck, and chest in two planes should be taken[45] (Figure 12.4).

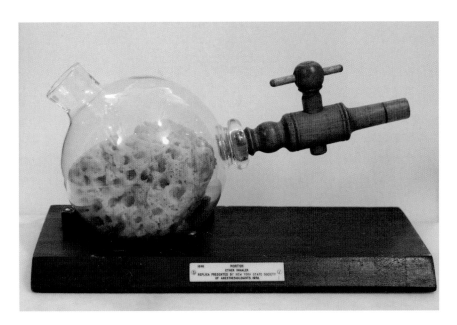

Plate 1

Morton's ether inhaler, as used in one of the first successful demonstrations of general anaesthesia in October 1846. (Photograph reproduced with the kind permission of the Association of Anaesthetists of Great Britain and Ireland.) See also Figure 1.1.

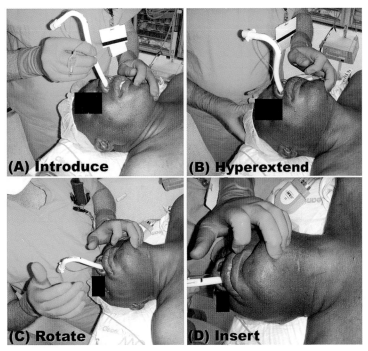

Plate 2

Blind nasal intubation. See also Figure 4.5.

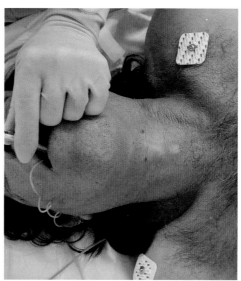

Plate 3

Transillumination. See also Figure 4.6.

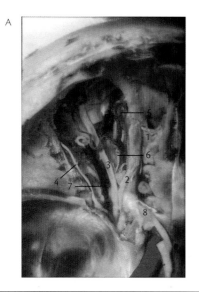

A

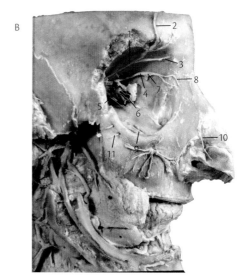

B

1	Superior oblique muscle	4	Lacrimal nerve
2	Trochlear nerve	5	Ophthalmic artery
3	Frontal nerve dividing into	6	Nasociliary nerve
	supraorbital and	7	Superior ophthalmic vein
	supratrochlear nerves	8	Optic nerve

1	Frontal nerve	7	Anterior ethmoidal nerve
2	Supra-orbital nerve	8	Infratrochlear nerve
3	Supratrochlear nerve	9	Infra-orbital nerve
4	Nasociliary nerve	10	External nasal nerve
5	Ciliary ganglion	11	Zygomaticofacial nerve
6	Short ciliary nerves		

Plate 4

A Orbit viewed from above showing distribution of nerves **B** View of medial wall of orbit showing distribution of nerves. See also Figure 6.4.

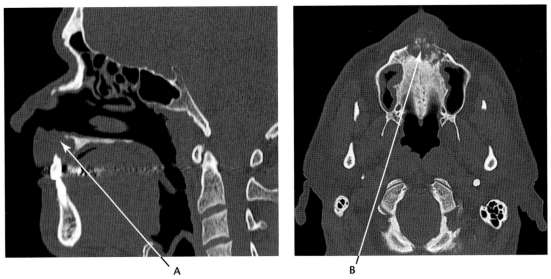

Plates 5 and 6

Sagittal (left) and axial (right) conventional non-contrast-enhanced CT sections of an osteosarcoma (arrows) at the level of the hard palate imaged in 2D. Appreciation of its dimensions and erosive extent can be more easily seen in the CT cross-sections. See also Figure 13.3.

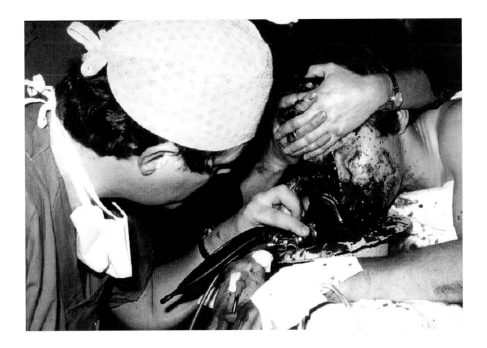

Plate 7

Gunshot wound to face. The patient was best able to maintain a clear airway lying supine and was induced in this position. See also Figure 14.2.

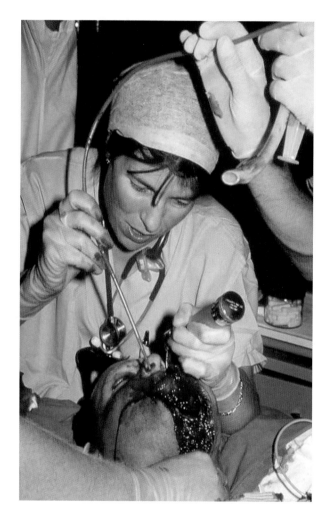

Plate 8

Intubation using a bougie with cricoid pressure applied. See also Figure 14.3.

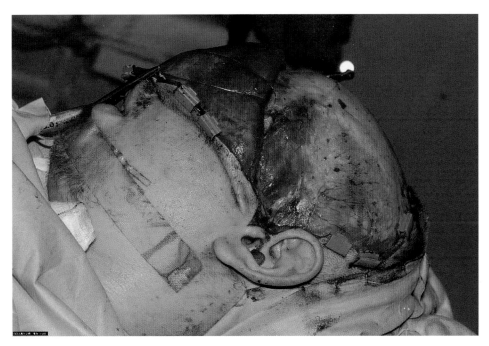

Plate 9

Reflected coronal flap to gain surgical access to the orbital bone. Oral endotracheal tube visible. See also Figure 14.7.

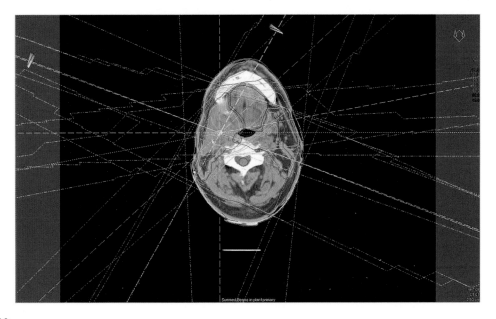

Plate 10

This shows a typical conformal head and neck treatment plan using multiple linear accelerator beams summated giving maximum dose to a right oropharyngeal tumour and minimal spinal cord dose (courtesy of Mr Nick Willis). See also Figure 17.2a.

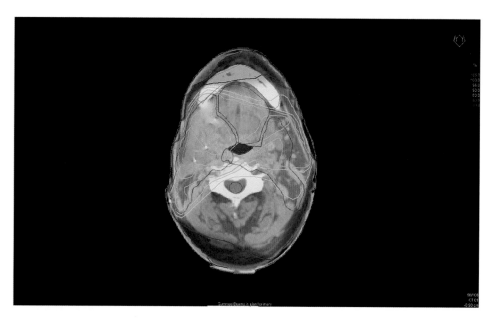

Plate 11

Shows the high-dose area in colour wash (courtesy of Mr Nick Willis). See also Figure 17.2b.

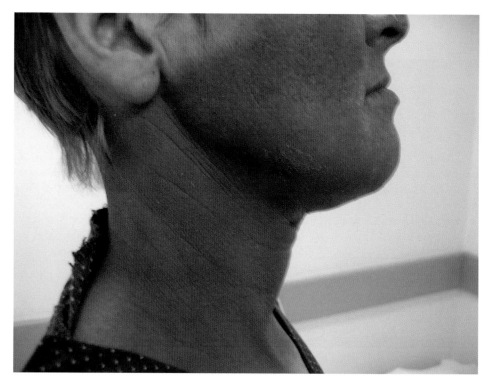

Plate 12

A pigmented radiotherapy skin reaction. See also Figure 17.6.

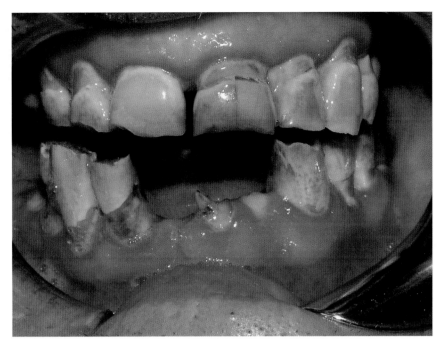

Plate 13

Radiation caries (courtesy of Dr Stewart Barclay). This shows extensive radiotherapy caries with the lower incisors having snapped off. See also Figure 17.7.

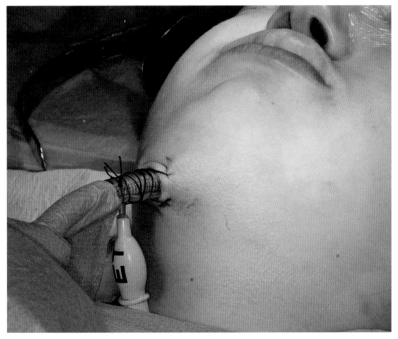

Plate 14

Submental tracheal tube. See also Figure 18.2.

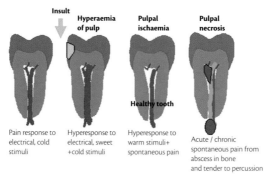

Insult
Hyperaemia of pulp
Pulpal ischaemia
Pulpal necrosis

Healthy tooth

Pain response to electrical, cold stimuli

Hyperesponse to electrical, sweet +cold stimuli

Hyperesponse to warm stimuli+ spontaneous pain

Acute / chronic spontaneous pain from abscess in bone and tender to percussion

Plate 15

The stages and characteristics of dental pulpal pain. See also Figure 22.1.

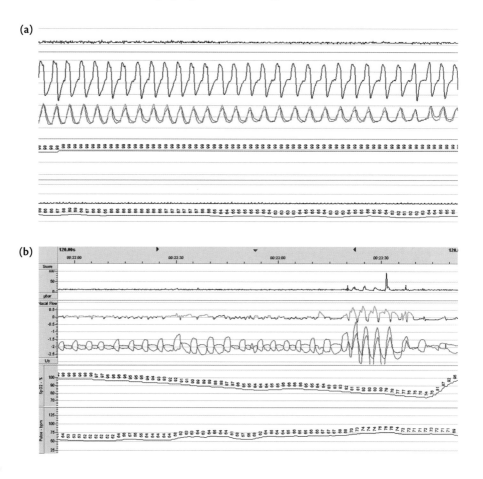

Plate 16

a A sample from a normal respiratory study. The blue waveform is airflow, the red is rib cage movement, and the green is abdominal movement. Both red and green traces are in phase, indicating normal respiratory effort. Oxygen saturation is below with the values inserted, and the heart rate trace is the lowest on the printout. **b** This sample is using the same montage as normal (Plate 16a), but paradoxical movements of rib cage and abdominal wall and absent airflow show complete obstruction. There is a gasping resolution with large tidal airflow and normalization of ventilation. The characteristic delay between the obstructive event and the fall in oxygen saturation is clearly seen. See also Figure 23.3.

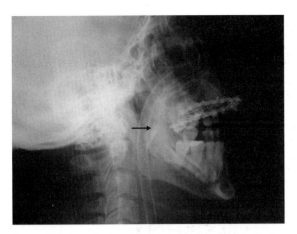

Figure 12.4 An avulsed tooth lodged in the vallecula anterior to a nasotracheal tube (arrow). The tooth, present prior to induction, was noted to be missing at the onset of surgery and could not be located necessitating a lateral skull X-ray. In this position, airway aspiration of the tooth following extubation would have been very likely. It is essential to account for any missing dental fragments resulting from anaesthetic related injuries (photo by courtesy of Mr J Adams)

Damage or dislodgement to prosthetic teeth and fittings should be attended to within a few days of injury. It is important to ensure that all detached fragments have been recovered. Of concern is the fact that some prosthetic materials are not radiolucent, making the location of fragments difficult.

Oral soft tissue injuries

Damage to intraoral soft tissue as a consequence of general anaesthesia is common and, while rarely life-threatening, there are significant problems that can develop. Trauma is not only associated with the use of a laryngoscope and endotracheal intubation but is also seen with laryngeal mask airways (LMA), Guedel airways, bite blocks, suction catheters, and throat packs. The incidence of oral injuries associated with anaesthesia and endotracheal intubation is as high as 18%[4], with minor dental injury accounting for the majority. However, over 6% of the 745 cases in this study had soft tissue injuries such as contusions of the lip, gingiva, and edentulous ridge. This figure could be much higher if postoperative sore throat was considered as a form of pharyngeal soft tissue injury; the incidence of this was approximately 40% after intubation, greater than 65% if blood was found on the laryngoscope[49], and 20–42% after LMA placement[50].

Lip injuries are most commonly caused by laryngoscopy and include haematomas, lacerations, and generalized oedema which, although usually self-limiting, cause inconvenience and discomfort. A malpositioned or overinflated LMA can compress the lingual artery, resulting in cyanosis of the tongue and loss of taste. Similarly, loss of tongue sensation secondary to compression of the lingual nerve during overzealous laryngoscopy is well recognized. Multiple case reports of gross tongue swelling or macroglossia exist, and some have resulted in life-threatening airway obstruction requiring prolonged intubation[51]. Several contributory factors are thought to be involved, including positioning of the patient, prolonged procedures, and anything that causes compression on the base of the tongue resulting in arterial and venous compromise and massive oedema. Thus prolonged intraoral surgery and the use of pharyngeal packs and bite blocks are risk factors[52,53].

The uvula is also vulnerable to injury which can follow compression by an oral or nasal endotracheal tube, LMA or as a result of a suction injury resulting in oedema and subsequent necrosis. There are several case reports of injury to the uvula secondary to suctioning the tip of the uvula into the Yankauer sucker, which is usually associated with higher suction power[54,55]. These patients complain of a severe sore throat and gagging or choking caused by the uvula touching the back of the tongue. Conservative treatment results in resolution after a few days with the necrosed area sloughing off. Suctioning with a narrower-tipped Yankauer with smaller side holes than the traditional wide-tipped, larger side holed catheter has also been reported to have caused soft tissue injury to the tonsillar pillars, and pharyngeal soft tissue with bleeding and aspiration of small amounts of tissue[56]. Ideally, suctioning would always be under direct vision but this is not practical immediately prior to extubation when airway reflexes and muscle tone have returned. Care should always be taken to use the lowest power of suction that achieves optimal results.

Although rare, several cases of pharyngeal perforation, which can result in death following mediastinitis, have been reported[57]. Laryngoscopy and difficult passage of endotracheal tubes account for most cases, but both nasogastric tube placement and suctioning have been implicated, particularly in the paediatric setting[58].

Hoarseness postoperatively can be due to damage to the laryngeal muscles and suspensory ligaments or minor lacerations and abrasions to the cords. More severe lesions can result and are usually related to difficult and traumatic intubation with the use of adjuncts such as stylets and bougies. Symptoms usually settle without intervention, but hoarseness can be permanent following unilateral cord paralysis which is thought to be due to compression on the recurrent laryngeal nerve from the cuff of a poorly positioned endotracheal tube in the subglottic larynx[59]. It can be seen that soft tissue injuries can occur during induction, maintenance, and emergence of anaesthesia and a wide variety of pathologies can result.

Injuries associated with throat packs

Throat packs are in common use in dental, maxillofacial, and ENT surgery to pack the oropharynx and nasopharynx. The pack itself usually consists of variable amounts of coarse green gauze which is moistened and supplied in rolls 180 cm long and 10 cm wide (Figure 9.3). The aim of throat packs is to absorb any blood which is not adequately aspirated, thus preventing drainage of this blood into the stomach and leaking of blood around the cuff of an endotracheal tube (ETT) with subsequent contamination of the trachea. It has been shown that a cuffed ETT cannot provide 100% protection from aspiration and so prolonged pooling of blood in the pharynx is undesirable[60]. Methods of inserting pharyngeal packs vary, with some users preferring Magill forceps and others digital insertion. To avoid tearing the frenulum, particularly during blind insertion, the tongue should always be displaced. The placement of throat packs is implicated in grazes to the soft and hard palate, and tears to the frenulum and posterior pharyngeal wall. These injuries are often missed as direct laryngoscopy is not routinely performed. These can occur even after apparently atraumatic insertion and, on occasions, cause bleeding[61]. It is thought that this is why some studies have shown a high incidence of sore throat associated with pharyngeal packs. Fine et al.[62] reported an 80% incidence of sore throat in patients with pharyngeal packs and a zero incidence with no packing. This study was small, with only 25 patients, and a similar study in 62 patients by Tay et al.[63] found conflicting results with no difference in the incidence or severity of sore throat when throat packs were used. Basha et al.[64] prospectively studied 100 patients having nasal surgery and found a higher incidence of sore throat in those with a throat pack, although this did not delay discharge. They also found that the incidence of postoperative nausea and vomiting (PONV) was unaffected by the presence of a throat pack.

Pharyngeal packs can also damage the pharyngeal plexus and have resulted in macroglossia due to compression ischaemia and subsequent oedema as previously discussed[53]. Potentially the most catastrophic hazard of a pharyngeal pack is in neglecting to remove it on completion of the anaesthetic, which could result in airway obstruction and asphyxiation following extubation. There are sporadic reports in the literature relating to airway obstruction, including a paediatric fatality[65] and another child presenting with acute respiratory distress in recovery in which the causative throat pack was promptly discovered and removed without consequence[66]. There were three cases of retained throat packs in 2007 reported in the United Medical News Australia, all of which involved a change in anaesthetic personnel and a lack of documentary evidence of pack insertion. In one case the pharynx had been suctioned under direct vision, but the heavily bloodstained pack was unseen. Fortunately, all packs were expelled several hours postoperatively with no morbidity. Retained throat packs may become lodged in the nasopharynx or swallowed and present problems postoperatively. A pack lodged in the nasopharynx for many weeks caused nasal obstruction and bilateral foul discharge, and was discovered on nasendoscopy. Similarly, a swallowed throat pack risks causing bowel obstruction and, potentially, perforation.

Careful thought must always be given to minimize the risk of complications arising from the use of throat packs. It is wrong to assume that all oral, maxillofacial, dental, and ENT cases require a throat pack. The intended benefits of throat pack insertion should always be considered for each individual patient and balanced against the perceived risks. Concern over the lack of uniform practice as regards ensuring removal of packs has recently been discussed at a Royal College of Anaesthetists Safety Conference. Several methods have been advised, including visual checking systems such as labelling or marking the patient's forehead with the mark to be removed when the pack is removed, labelling the airway device, tying the pack to the airway device, or leaving part of the pack protruding. There is no method to suit all situations; for example, intraoral surgery may not allow either tying the pack to the airway or leaving part outside the mouth. Documentary based solutions were also discussed, including a two-person checking system on insertion and removal. One potential solution would be to include the throat pack in the surgical count and introduce a uniformity in practice throughout the country.

Injuries associated with nasal intubation

Nasotracheal intubation is a common anaesthetic technique which facilitates access during oral, dental, and maxillofacial surgery. There are well described complications of both oral and nasotracheal intubation, some of which have been previously discussed in relation to soft tissue injuries. However, there are some issues particularly pertinent to nasotracheal intubation which need to be considered. In addition, modern dedicated nasotracheal tubes are intentionally made of a softer and more pliable material, making them more prone to extraneous compression and kinking during oral and maxillofacial surgery.

Indications for a nasal ETT include maxillofacial surgery, oropharyngeal, and dental surgery, as well as being useful in rigid laryngoscopy and microlaryngeal surgery. Awake fibreoptic intubation almost invariably involves the nasal route and can be useful in a wide variety of situations when direct laryngoscopy is difficult (Chapter 4).

Assessment of the nasal airway is important if local injury is to be avoided, and attempts should be made to identify any optimal nare. Nasal septal deviations and hypertrophied turbinates are common, but identification of patency problems through patient history, and specifically enquiring about airflow obstructive symptoms, will not reliably predict the best nostril to intubate[67].

Nasendoscopy can identify asymptomatic nasal abnormalities, but few anaesthetists are sufficiently familiar with this technique to incorporate it into routine practice. Consequently, it may be difficult to predict the best nostril[68].

Epistaxis

Epistaxis is the most common complication encountered during nasal intubation, usually resulting from mucosal tears in the anterior part of the nasal septum—Little's area[69]. Avulsion of polyps, especially in asthmatics, trauma to tonsils, adenoids, or the posterior pharyngeal wall can result in bleeding which, at its worst, can be torrential and life-threatening. The reported incidence of epistaxis varies widely from 18 to 66%[70,71], although the majority of these cases were minor bleeding, with some classifying blood-tinged saliva as a significant event.

There is a higher risk of epistaxis if too large a nasotracheal tube is used, repeated attempts are required, and if excessive force is applied when difficulty is experienced during navigating the tube through the nasal passages[72]. Various methods to reduce epistaxis have been proposed, including thermosoftening of the tube, alternative tube materials, and the use of vasoconstrictors. It is commonplace to lubricate the tube and apply vasoconstrictors to the nostril such as phenylephrine, ephedrine, cocaine or oxymetazoline which are usually combined with lidocaine. The literature fails to support any significant difference in efficacy between these agents in reducing the incidence of epistaxis following intubation[73].

Introducing sequential nasopharyngeal airways of increasing size to dilate a nasal passage prior to intubation is thought by some to reduce trauma and bleeding[74], but others believe there is greater potential to damage the delicate mucosa and cause more bleeding than with direct intubation[75].

Despite attempts to minimize the risks, significant nasal bleeding can still occur. Blood within the airway not only obscures vision but can obstruct the airway, especially if large clots have formed, which can cause bronchospasm, laryngospasm, and impede adequate ventilation. This becomes a particular hazard if direct laryngoscopy is suboptimal. This latter scenario is highlighted in a case report where epistaxis occurred on advancing the nasal ETT through a vasoconstricted nostril[76]. On direct laryngoscopy, there was an unpredicted Cormack and Leherne grade 4 view. The presence of copious blood in the airway made ventilation difficult and negated the use of a fibreoptic scope to facilitate endotracheal intubation. Emergency cricothyroidotomy was necessary to facilitate oxygenation. Visualization of the larynx and fibreoptic intubation was only then achievable after the haemorrhage was brought under control by nasal tamponade. Prior laryngoscopy to assess the adequacy of the laryngeal view before introducing a nasotracheal tube has been proposed as a means of reducing the risk of the aforementioned situation. Having evaluated the airway, fibreoptic devices can then be used if required without the risk of blood obscuring the view. These also allow the anaesthetist to make a judgement that, if nasal haemorrhage does occur, laryngeal intubation will be readily acheivable.

Epistaxis resulting from nasotracheal intubation is usually self-limiting and can invariably be controlled by either the pressure of the nasal tube or through insertion of an absorbent nasal tampon and sitting the patient upright. More persistent haemorrhage may necessitate inserting a Foley catheter and applying a tamponade by means of inflating the cuff.

Structural injuries associated with naso-tracheal intubation

Avulsion of nasal polyps, inferior and middle turbinates, and tumour have all been reported as resulting in airway and nasotracheal tube obstruction. Less common injuries include submucosal placement and creating false submucosal passages, usually when there have been repeated attempts to pass the tube through the nose. This can lead to retropharyngeal abscess formation, and consideration should be given to the use of antibiotics if a pharyngeal tear is identified[77]. Similarly, use of prophylactic antibiotics in susceptible patients with valve replacements should be considered as nasotracheal intubation can be associated with a bacteraemia[78].

Prolonged nasal intubation can lead to pressure necrosis of the nostrils and septum, retropharyngeal abscess formation, and paranasal sinusitis.

Eye injuries during oral and maxillofacial surgery

Although a detailed discussion of eye injuries associated with general anaesthesia is beyond the scope of this chapter, patients undergoing oral and maxillofacial surgery are at an increased risk from such injuries[79]. The eyes, which are often hidden from view by operative drapes, are in close proximity to the surgical field, making them vulnerable to both physical insult and inadvertent instillation of antimicrobial skin preparations. The eyes are at particular risk during laser surgery (Chapter 10). Eye injury has been reported as accounting for 3% of all compensatory claims against anaesthetists, of which 35% are corneal abrasions[80]. Fortunately most, but not all, recover without permanent visual impairment.

In one study, 59% of patients had incomplete eye closure following the induction of anaesthesia[81], so protective measures should always be adopted. Common techniques for protecting the eyes during oral and maxillofacial surgery include taping the eyes shut, with or without protective ointment, protective ointment alone, methycellulose drops, and goggles. There is no evidence that one technique is superior to another.

Conclusion

Injuries to the oral and maxillofacial structures are some of the commonest iatrogenic anaesthetic related injuries reported. Even apparent minor injuries can be a source of considerable discomfort, inconvenience, and expense to the patient. In this respect, damage to teeth and intraoral soft tissues during laryngoscopy are foremost. It is important that anaesthetists are familiar with the risk factors that can predispose to injuries of the oral cavity and maxillofacial region during anaesthesia.

Acknowledgements

The authors would like to thank Mr James Adams, Consultant in Oral and Maxillofacial Surgery, and Dr Claire Storey for their help and advice in the preparation of this chapter.

References

1. Aitkenhead AR. (2005) Injuries associated with anaesthesia. A global perspective. *Br J Anaesth*, **95**, 95–109.
2. Hove LD, Nielsen HB, Christoffersen JK. (2006) Patient injuries in response to anaesthetic procedures: cases evaluated by the Danish Patient Insurance Association. *Acta Anaesthesiol Scand*, **50**, 530–5.
3. Lockhart PB, Feldbau EV, Gabel RA, Connolly SF, Silversin JB. (1986) Dental complications during and after tracheal intubation. *J Am Dent Assoc*, **112**, 480–3.
4. Chen J-J, Susetio L, Chao CC. (1990) Oral complications associated with endotracheal general anaesthesia. *Anaesthesia Sinica*, **28**, 163–9.
5. Abraham R, Kaufman J. (1999) Dental damage during anaesthesia. In: Kaufman L, Ginsburg R. (eds) *Anaesthesia Reviews 15*, Chapter 12. Edinburgh: Churchill Livingstone, 158–200.
6. Chadwick RG, Lindsay SM. (1996) Dental injuries during general anaesthesia. *Br Dent J*, **180**, 255–8.
7. Simon JH, Lies J. (1999) Silent trauma. *Endod Dent Traumatol*, **15**, 145–8.
8. Standring S. (1999) Oral cavity. In: *Gray's Anatomy*, 39th edn. Edinburgh: Elsevier Churchill Livingstone, pp. 581–608.
9. Burton JF, Baker AB. (1987) Dental damage during anaesthesia and surgery. *Anaesth Intensive Care*, **15**, 262–3.
10. Kok PHK, Kwan KM, Koay CK. (2001) A case report of a fractured healthy tooth during use of Guedel oropharyngeal airway. *Singapore Med J*, **42**, 322–4.
11. Watts J. (2008) NHS dentist shortage may have adverse effects for anaesthetists. *Anaesthesia*, **63**, 1377.
12. Givol N, Gershtansky Y, Halamish-Shani, T *et al.* (2004) Perianesthetic dental injuries: analysis of incident reports. *J Clin Anesth*, **16**, 173–6.
13. Tolan TF, Westerfield S, Irvine D, Clark T. (2000) Dental injuries in anaesthesia: Incidence and preventive strategies. *ASA Meeting Abstracts*; A1133.
14. Bory EN, Goudard V, Magnin C. (1991) Tooth injuries during general anesthesia, oral endoscopy and vibro-massage. *Actual Odontostaomatol*, **45**, 107–20.
15. Newland MC, Ellis SJ, Peters KR *et al.* (2007) Dental injury associated with anaesthesia: a report of 161,687 anesthetics given over 14 years. *J Clin Anaesth*, **19(5)**, 339–45.

16. Bergan RP. (1972) Law and medicine. Lost or broken teeth. *J Am Med Assoc*, **221,** 119–20.

17. Dornette WH, Hughes BH. (1959) Care of teeth during anesthesia. *Anesth Analg Curr Res*, **38(3),** 206–15.

18. Hastings RH, Hon ED, Nghiem C, Wahrenbrock EA. (1996) Force and torque vary between laryngoscopists and laryngoscope blades. *Anesth Analg*, **82(3),** 462–8.

19. Bito H, Nishiyama T, Higarhizawa T, Sakai T, Konishi A. (1998) Determination of the distance between the upper incisors and the laryngoscope blade during laryngoscopy: comparisons of the McCoy, the Macintosh, the Miller and the Belscope blades. *Masui*, 47(10), 1257–61.

20. Watanabe S, Suga A, Asakura N et al. (1994) Determination of the distance between the laryngoscope blade and the upper incisors during direct laryngoscopy: comparison of a curved, an angulated straight, and two straight blades. *Anesth Analg*, **79,** 638–41.

21. McCoy EP, Mirakhur RK, Rafferty C, Bunting H, Austin BA. (1996) A comparison of the forces exerted during laryngoscopy. The MacIntosh versus the McCoy blade. *Anaesthesia*, 51(10), 912–15.

22. Lee J, Choi JH, Lee YK et al. (2004) The Callander laryngoscope blade modification is associated with a decreased risk of dental contact. *Can J Anaesth*, 51(2), 181–4.

23. Ghabash MB, Matta MS, Mehanna CB. (1997) Prevention of dental trauma during endotracheal intubation. *Anesth Analg*, **84,** 230–1.

24. Lisman SR, Shepherd NJ, Rosenberg M. (1981) A modified laryngoscope blade for dental protection. *Anesthesiology*, **55,** 190.

25. Owen H, Waddell-Smith, I. (2000) Dental trauma associated with anaesthesia. *Anaesth Intensive Care*, **28,** 133–45.

26. Itoman EM, Kajioka EH, Yamamoto LG. (2005) Dental fracture risk of metal vs plastic laryngoscope blades in dental models. *Am J Emerg Med*, **23(2),** 186–9.

27. Ho AMH, Hewitt G. (2000) Warning devices for prevention of dental injury during laryngoscopy. *J Clin Monit Comput*, 16(4), 269–72.

28. Bucx MJL, Snijders CJ, van Geel, RT et al. (1994) Forces acting on the maxillary incisor teeth during laryngoscopy using the MacIntosh laryngoscope. *Anaesthesia*, **49(12),** 1064–70.

29. Bucx MJL, van Geel, RTM, Wegener JT, Robers C, Stijnen T. (1995) Does experience influence the forces exerted on maxillary incisors during laryngoscopy? A manikin study using the MacIntosh laryngoscope. *Can J Anaesth*, **42,** 144–9.

30. McCoy EP, Austin BA, Mirakhur RK, Wong KC. (1995) A new device for measuring and recording the forces applied during laryngoscopy. *Anaesthesia*, **50(2),** 139–43.

31. Bishop MJ, Harrington RM, Tencer AF. (1992) Force applied during tracheal intubation. *Anesth Analg*, **74,** 411–14.

32. Vogel C. (1979) Dental injuries during anaesthesia and their forensic consequences. *Anaesthetist*, **28(7),** 347–9.

33. Quinn JB, Schulthesis LW, Schumacher GE. (2005) A tooth broken after laryngoscopy: Unlikely to be caused by the force applied by the anaesthesiologist. *Anesth Analg*, **100,** 594–6.

34. Kinane DF, Marshall GJ. (2001) Periodontal manifestations of systemic disease. *Aust Dent J*, **46(1),** 2–12.

35. Swinson B, Witherow H, Norris P, Lloyd T. (2004) Oral manifestations of systemic diseases. *Hosp Med*, **65(2),** 92–9.

36. Tredwin CJ, Scully C, Bagan-Sebastian, J-V. (2005) Drug induced disorders of teeth. *J Dent Res*, **84(7),** 596–602.

37. Owen H. (2002) Anaesthesia and dental trauma. *Anaesth Intensive Care Med*, **3,** 253–5.

38. Houston WJB, Stephens CD, Tulley WJ. (1992) The classification of occlusion and malocclusion. In: *A Textbook of Orthodontics*, 2nd edn. Oxford: Wright Butterworth Heinemann, pp. 42–53.

39. Skeie A, Schwartz O. (1999) Traumatic injuries to teeth in connection with general anaesthesia and the effect of use of mouthguards. *Endo Dent Traumatol*, **15,** 33–6.

40. Clokie C, Metcalf I, Holland A. (1989) Dental trauma in anaesthesia. *Can J Anaesth*, **36,** 675–80.

41. Chydillo SA, Zukaitis JA. (1990) Dental examinations prior to elective surgery under anesthesia. *New York State Dent J*, **56(9),** 69–70.

42. Monaca E, Fock N, Doehn M, Wappler F. (2007) The effectiveness of preformed tooth protectors during endotracheal intubation: An upper jaw model. *Anesth Analg*, **105,** 1326–32.

43. Hoffmann J, Westendorff C, Reinert S. (2005) Evaluation of dental injury following endotracheal intubation using the Periotest technique. *Dent Traumatol*, **21,** 263–8.

44. Aromaa U, Pesonen P, Linko K, Tammisto T. (1988) Difficulties with tooth protectors in endotracheal intubation. *Acta Anaesthesiol Scand*, **32,** 304–7.

45. Whitley S, Shaw IH. (1992) Dental throat packs and anaesthesia. *Anaesthesia*, **47,** 173.

46. Welbury R. (1994). Dental pain, infection, haemorrhage and trauma. In: Hawkesford J, Banks JG (eds). *Maxillofacial and Dental Emergencies*, Chapter 2. Oxford: Oxford University Press, pp. 7–34.

47. Nicholson MJ. (1965) Endobronchial aspiration of a tooth. A case report. *Anesth Analg*, **44,** 355–7.

48. Nakahashi K, Yamamoto K, Tsuzuki M et al. (2003) Effect of teeth protector on dental injuries during general anaesthesia. *Masui*, **52(1),** 26–31.

49. Monroe MC, Gravenstein N, Saga-Rumley, S. (1990) Postoperative sore throat: Effect of oropharyngeal airway in orotracheally intubated patients. *Anesth Analg*, **70,** 12–16.

50. Brimacombe J, Holyoake L, Keller C. (2000) Pharyngolaryngeal, neck and jaw discomfort after anaesthesia with the face mask and laryngeal mask airway at high and low cuff volumes in males and females. *Anesthesiology*, **93,** 26–31.

51. Kuhnert SM, Faust RJ, Berge KH, Piepgras DG. (1999) Postoperative macroglossia: Report of a case with rapid resolution after extubation of the trachea. *Anesth Analg*, **88,** 220–3.

52. McAllister RG. (1974) Macroglossia—a positional complication. *Anesthesiology*, **40**, 199–200.

53. Kawaguchi M, Sakamoto T, Ohnishi H, Karasawa J. (1995) Pharyngeal packs can cause massive swelling of the tongue after neurosurgical procedures. *Anesthesiology*, **83**, 434–5.

54. Das PK, Thomas W. (1980) Complication of pharyngeal suction. *Anaesth Intens Care*, **8**, 375.

55. Bogetez M, Tupper B, Vigil C. (1991) Too much of a good thing. Uvular trauma caused by overzealous suctioning. *Anesth Analg*, **172**, 125–6.

56. Podeschi DM, Sprague DH. (1991) Additional factor related to suction trauma. *Anesth Analg*, **73**, 238.

57. Domino KB, Posner KL, Caplan RA, Cheney FW. (1999) Airway injury during anaesthesia. A closed claims analysis. *Anaesthesiology*, **91**, 1703.

58. Patnaik S, Raju U, Arora M. (2007) Neonatal pharyngeal perforation. *Med J Armed Forces India*, **63**, 275–6.

59. Hagberg C, Georgi R, Krier C. (2005) Complications of managing the airway. *Best Pract Res Clin Anaesthesiol*, **19**, 641–59.

60. Seraj MA, Ankutse MN, Khan FM, Siddiqui N, Ziko AO. (1991) Tracheal soiling with blood during intranasal surgery. *Mid East J Anaesthiol*, **11**, 79–89.

61. Parry MG, Glaisyer H, Enderby DH. (1997) Prevention of trauma associated with throat pack insertion. *Anaesthesia*, **54**, 444–53.

62. Fine J, Kaltman S, Bianco M. (1998) Prevention of sore throat after nasotracheal intubation. *J Oral Maxillofac Surg*, **46**, 946–7.

63. Tay JY, Tan WK, Chen FG, Koh KF, Ho V. (2002) Postoperative sore throat after routine oral surgery; influence of the presence of a pharyngeal pack. *Br J Maxillofac Surg*, **40**, 60–3.

64. Basha SI, McCoy E, Ullah R, Kinsella JB. (2006) The efficacy of pharyngeal packing during routine nasal surgery—a prospective randomized controlled study. *Anaesthesia*, **61**, 1161–5.

65. Crawford BS. (1977) Prevention of retained throat pack. *Br Med J*, **49**, 1029.

66. Najjar MF, Kimpson J. (1995) A method for preventing throat pack retention. *Anaesth Analg*, **80**, 208.

67. Smith JE, Reid AP. (2001) Identifying the more patent nostril before nasotracheal intubation. *Anaesthesia*, **56**, 258–62.

68. Williamson R. (2002) Nasal intubation and epistaxis. *Anaesthesia*, **57**, 1033–4.

69. Dauphinee K. (1988) Nasotracheal intubation. *Emerg Med Clin North Am*, **6**, 715–23.

70. Watanabe S, Yaguchi Y, Suga A, Asakura N. (1994) A bubble tip tracheal tube system—its effects on incidence of epistaxis and ease of tube advancement in the subglottic region during nasotracheal intubation. *Anesth Analg*, **78**, 1140–3.

71. Kim YC, Lee SH, Noh GJ et al. (2000) Thermosoftening treatment of the nasotracheal tube before intubation can reduce epistaxis and nasal damage. *Anesth Analg*, **91**, 78–701.

72. O', JE, Stevenson DS, Stokes MA. (1996) Pathological changes associated with short term nasal intubation. *Anaesthesia*, **31**, 347–50.

73. Katz RI, Hovagim AR, Finkelstein HS et al. (1990) A comparison of cocaine lidocaine with epinephrine and oxymetazoline for prevention of epistaxis on nasotracheal intubation. *J Clin Anaesth*, **2**, 16–20.

74. Kay J, Bryan R, Hart HB, Minkel DT, Munshi C. (1985) Sequential dilatation; a useful adjunct in reducing blood loss from nasotracheal intubation. *Anesthesiology*, **63**, A259.

75. Adamson DN, Theisen FC, Barrett KC. (1988) Effect of mechanical dilatation on nasotracheal intubation. *J Oral Maxillofac Surg*, **46**, 372–5.

76. Piepho T, Thierbach A, Werner C. (2005) Nasotracheal intubation: look before you leap. *Br J Anaesth*, **6**, 859–60.

77. Divatia JV, Bhowmick K. (2005) Complications of endotracheal intubation and other airway management procedures. *Ind J Anaesth*, **4**, 308–18.

78. Valdes C, Tomas I, Alvarez M et al. (2008) The incidence of bacteraemia associated with tracheal intubation. *Anaesthesia*, **63**, 588–92.

79. Anderson DA, Braun TW, Herlich A. (1995) Eye injury during general anaesthesia for oral and maxillofacial surgery: Etiology and prevention. *J Oral Maxillofac Surg*, **53**, 321–4.

80. Gild WM, Posner KL, Caplan RA, Cheney FW. (1992) Eye injuries associated with anaesthesia; A closed claims analysis. *Anesthesiology*, **81**, 273–4.

81. Battra YK, Bali IM. (1977) Corneal abrasions during general anaesthesia. *Anesth Analg*, **56**, 363.

13

Oral and maxillofacial imaging for the anaesthetist

Neil Heath and Iain Macleod

Introduction

The oral and facial structures are a problematical area for both the anaesthetist and maxillofacial surgeon as the oral cavity and nasal passages provide a common portal for both airway access and surgical intervention. Obviously an understanding of the anatomy of these structures and their variations is essential. In addition, the jaws provide radiographic challenges by virtue of their unique anatomy.

Dental imaging is a specialist area, which utilizes radiographic techniques that are unusual in their acquisition. For example, the use of non-screen film for intraoral views that give high resolution images is the main way in which teeth and their supporting structures are demonstrated. Such techniques include bitewings, periapical, and occlusal views.

The dental panoramic tomogram (DPT), sometimes called the orthopantomogram (OPG) is the 'work horse' of jaw imaging. However, this view has unusual anomalies which are created by virtue of the way it is formed. These units produce an image of the dental arches using a variation on the technique of tomography that involves rotating the X-ray tube and film, producing blurring of the structures on either side of the centres of rotation.

In dental panoramic tomography, a horseshoe-shaped in-focus plane (focal trough) is created by moving the centre of rotation during the exposure. Care must be taken in patient positioning to ensure that the teeth lie within the trough otherwise, the resultant image will be distorted.

Advances in dental imaging include cross-sectional modalities such as modified dental panoramic views, conventional computed tomography (CT) and cone beam CT scans[1]. Cone beam CT is a new process that, when compared with conventional CT, uses a lower radiation dose and a cross-sectional imaging technique which acquires a volume of data that can be presented in a number of formats, e.g. panoramic or as axial, coronal, or sagittal slices similar to those seen using conventional CT.

The use of magnetic resonance imaging (MRI) is becoming invaluable in helping to characterize neoplasia presenting in the head and neck. Cysts, inflammatory lesions, and bone pathology can also be assessed using this modality. MRI is now the gold standard for investigation of temporomandibular joint (TMJ) pathologies owing to its ability to resolve and demonstrate the complexities of the internal features of this atypical joint.

Cross-sectional imaging has simplified much of the clinical problem-solving carried out in the oral and maxillofacial region. The remainder of this chapter will address some of the key aspects of oral and maxillofacial imaging now available.

Radiological anatomy

As in all areas of radiology, in order to recognize the abnormal/pathological, the normal must first be appreciated. The DPT is a commonly used view and consequently the anatomy it demonstrates is shown in Figures 13.1 and 13.2.

Pathology that was once only assessable from conventional images is now more frequently assessed from cross-sectional images such as CT (Figures 13.3a and b; see also Plates 3 and 4). Yet more recently, imaging modalities allowing three-dimensional reformatting of the initial 'raw data' can be viewed from any angle.

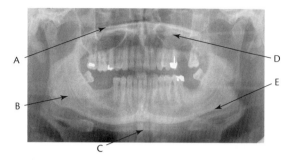

Figure 13.1 Dental panoramic tomogram or orthopantomogram. Ghost shadows of the: **A** left hard palate; **B** left lower border of mandible; **C** cervical spine. True projection of: **D** is the true left hard palate; **E** the true left lower border of mandible.

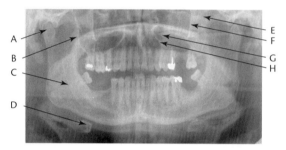

Figure 13.2 Dental panoramic tomogram of a partially dentate patient. **A** Right condylar; process; **B** right coronoid process; **C** right inferior dental canal; **D** hyoid bone; **E** posterior wall of the left maxillary sinus; **F** zygomatic buttress; **G** displaced root in maxillary antrum; **H** inferior border of left maxillary antrum.

This data can be linked to a computer-aided design/computer-aided manufacturing (CAD/CAM) process to allow the build up of accurate resin models of the structures imaged (Figure 13.4). These types of models can allow preplanning for surgery such as preforming of titanium fixation plates and for dentofacial implant planning.

A detailed discussion of the physics of such scanning equipment is beyond the scope of this chapter; however, examples of current imaging modalities will be shown.

Many excellent texts are available covering the more intricate details of oral and maxillofacial radiology[2,3]. The emphasis in this chapter will therefore be on applied radiological imaging anatomy with some relevant pathological examples.

Craniofacial anatomy revisited

The face has special importance, as personality, emotion, and the basic necessities of respiration and digestion are all facilitated at least initially in and around the craniofacial area. Direct exposure to the external environment of neural tissue (the eyes) happens in the face. The eyes and their supporting structures are all too often victims of such contact!

Regarding the mouth, the anaesthetist must give special consideration to the potential hazards of the teeth when securing an airway, as dental disease and the presence of overt or occult inflammatory disease can easily be overlooked. Invariably,

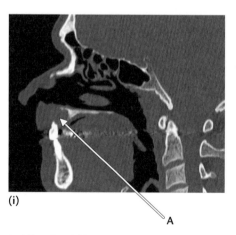

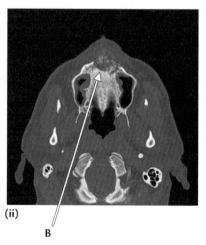

Figure 13.3 Sagittal (i) and axial (ii) conventional non-contrast-enhanced CT sections of an osteosarcoma (arrows) at the level of the hard palate imaged in 2D. Appreciation of its dimensions and erosive extent can be more easily seen in the CT cross-sections. See also Plates 5 and 6.

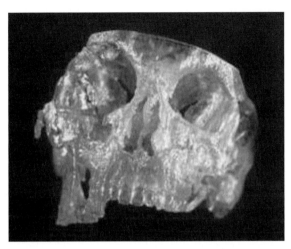

Figure 13.4 Resin model constructed from the 3D CT scan data. This can assist in presurgical planning.

cross-sectional scans of the head and neck will contain images of the cervical spine and the convolutions of the upper respiratory tract, which can be helpful when carrying out preoperative anaesthetic risk assessments.

The facial skeleton is a delicate, lightweight, scaffolding with more rigid bony buttresses, which allow for a 'protective crumple zone' in the event of trauma. Dissipation of forces that may potentially injure the brain in its protective calvarial 'box' is thus facilitated. These thin, bony buttresses are aligned vertically and support horizontal bony platforms that run across the face. Two examples of these horizontal planes run from the right supraorbital and infraorbital ridges across the midline to the left. Within this scaffolding, the paranasal sinuses provide mucosal lined, air-filled spaces. The paranasal sinuses allow for an overall reduction in the weight of the skull, give resonance for the voice and, some would argue, are a means of humidifying and warming air on its way to the lungs. Radiologically, these are low density features.

Changes in the appearances of the paranasal sinuses and mastoid air cells on imaging may give vital clues to the clinician who may suspect infection, tumour, or trauma.

The three main vertical facial buttresses to be appreciated are:

◆ Naso-maxillary buttress

◆ Zygomatico-maxillary buttress

◆ Pterygo-maxillary buttress.

These dense struts of bone provide the thickened bony pillars around which the rest of the face is supported (Figure 13.5). Normal suture lines in the oral–maxillofacial and base of skull should be appreciated so that they are not confused with pathology (Figures 13.6 and 13.7).

The teeth and their supporting structures

There is a degree of clinical myth and mystery around the subject of the dentition.

Apart from an obvious source of intense pain, the teeth provide a special hazard to the anaesthetist. The accidental fracturing of an anterior tooth or dislodging of a crown or post-retained restoration can be cause for litigation. Patients may wear small partial, dental prostheses that, if not noted at the time of admission, may become dislodged at operation with obvious potential for medical complications and legal ramifications. Dentures are usually made from acrylic, which is radiolucent and may be difficult to locate if no metal clasps (fastener) are present to give away its location on a radiograph. Crowns form a special hazard, especially if the underlying tooth is diseased as this may lead to fracture or dislodgement during intubation (Chapter 12). The anaesthetist therefore requires a broad appreciation of the teeth and dental

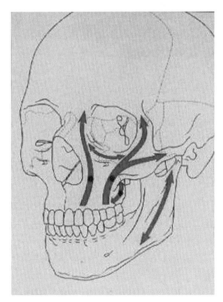

Figure 13.5 Three main bony buttresses of the maxillofacial area: the nasomaxillary, zygomatico-maxillary, and the pterygo-maxillary.

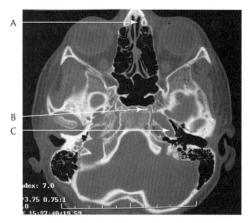
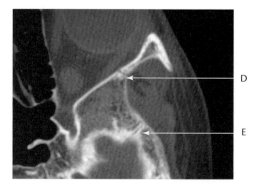

Figure 13.6 Axial CT sections showing normal anatomy and fracture mimics (left) and left posterior orbit (right). **A** Nasomaxillary suture; **B** petroclival fissure; **C** left carotid canal; **D** left sphenozygomatic suture; **E** left sphenotemporal suture.

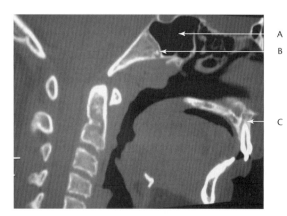

Figure 13.7 Fracture mimics. The normal sagittal skull base as seen on CT in a young adult. The spheno-occipital synchondrosis fuses at age 25 years and should not be mistaken for a fracture. **A** Sphenoid sinus; **B** spheno-occipital synchondrosis; **C** nasopalatine canal.

structures so that risk can be assessed and effective communication between clinicians can be made.

Dental nomenclature

Primary (deciduous), mixed, and secondary (adult) dentitions may be encountered depending on the maturity of the patient. The Federation Dentate International (FDI) system of dental nomenclature is now accepted to denote the position and type (class) of

tooth. This method is computer-friendly in that each tooth is given a two-digit number (Figure 13.8).

In an adult arch there are usually two incisors, a canine, two premolars, and three molars in each quadrant. The first digit in the system denotes the quadrant 1–4, each quadrant being numbered in a clockwise fashion. The adult quadrants are denoted by 1, 2, 3, and 4. Where present, each of the eight teeth in each quadrant are then ascribed a number 1–8 running posteriorly, thus giving a second digit. For example, an upper first incisor on the patient's right side is given the quadrant digit 1 and the arch location 1, denoting tooth 11. Similarly, a lower left third molar will be denoted 38.

In the primary dentition any teeth present are given the quadrant prefix, again in a clockwise fashion, 5 (upper right), 6 (upper left) 7 (lower left) and 8 (lower right). This time the dentition is made up of two incisors, a canine, and a first and second molar tooth. These are denoted in the arch as 1 through 5, again running posteriorly.

Alveolar bone is specialist bone that supports the teeth. In it are located Sharpey's fibres, specialized collagen bundles that make up the periodontal ligament. This is represented as a radiolucent line around the tooth root on imaging. If intact and unaffected by physiological or pathological processes, it should be 1 mm thick (Figure 13.9). If this is widened by infection/cyst or trauma, then the integrity of the tooth support may be compromised. In the traumatized dentition, a partially extruded upper anterior tooth may give rise to a risk of foreign body inhalation.

Permanent teeth															
upper right								upper left							
18	17	16	15	14	13	12	11	21	22	23	24	25	26	27	28
48	47	46	45	44	43	42	41	31	32	33	34	35	36	37	38
lower right								lower left							

Deciduous teeth (baby teeth)															
upper right								upper left							
		55	54	53	52	51	61	62	63	64	65				
		85	84	83	82	81	71	72	73	74	75				
lower right								lower left							

Figure 13.8 The Federation Dentate International (FDI) system of dental nomenclature.

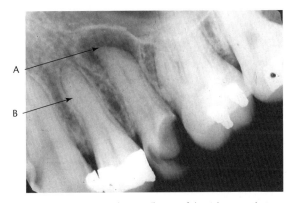

Figure 13.9 A periapical (intraoral) view of the right premolar area where **A** shows an infected root (periapical periodontitis) in the first premolar; and **B** shows a healthy root with a thin radiolucent ligament space bounded closely by an intact lamina dura (radio-opaque) thin line.

Imaging the facial skeleton

In the past, investigation of the facial skeleton was limited to using the following conventional radiographic views.

Caldwell's view

Posteroanterior (PA) or occipitofrontal (OF) skull view with 20° caudad angulation of the X-ray tube (OF 20 view). This mainly shows the upper third of the face and frontal sinuses with the skull vault.

Waters view

Occipitomental (OM) view to show the mid third of the face. This is achieved by angling the patient's head so that the dense petrous ridge is projected inferior to the lower borders of the maxillary sinuses.

Occipitomental (OM) 30 view

This used the same head position as the OM with a 30° caudad angle on the X-ray tube to give a further demonstration of the mid third of face, free of the dense petrous bone.

Lateral facial view

In the lateral facial view, both sides of the face are superimposed. This allows a crude assessment of the anteroposterior extent of any pathology.

Submentovertex view (SMV)

The SMV view is a full axial conventional radiographic technique, designed to outline the zygomatic arches in profile from below. It is sometimes called a 'jug handle' view. This can be a very difficult technical feat for both patient and radiographer!

Although some centres still use these radiographic projections, the advent of low dose conventional CT and the arrival of cone beam CT has revolutionized the investigation of the maxillofacial skeleton.

Magnetic resonance imaging (MRI)

MRI is a non-ionizing modality and a well established tool in the diagnostic armoury. MRI is particularly good at discriminating soft tissue structures and tissue/facial planes depending on the sequence requested. With this technique, tumour characterization and the extent of a lesion/mass can be appreciated fully.

In acute trauma, MRI does have limitations. Accessibility by the injured patient, comparatively lengthy scan times, and the necessity to respect the strength of the magnet can make the CT scanner a more practical option. Specialized equipment and training of the anaesthetic team are required before gaining entry to the MRI suite.

Specialist interpretative skills are now utilized by the viewing clinician to maximize the diagnostic yield from these cross-sectional modalities.

Trauma imaging

Imaging oral and maxillofacial trauma includes the spectrum of predominantly dentoalveolar trauma through to full scale craniofacial trauma.

Dento alveolar trauma

A tooth may undergo a fracture of any of its component structures, including the root, dentine or enamel only. Prostheses (dentures) may be *in situ* at the time of injury which will result in forces being exerted in a non-classical distribution, so altering any expected fracture pattern. Fractured or dislodged dentures may have metallic components and so be easily appreciated on a radiograph/scan, or be made of acrylic plastic with a relatively low radio-opacity which is more difficult to see. Acrylic may be difficult to appreciate on the standard chest film if dislodged. Recognition of the fate of any lost dental fragment is important—'count and account'. A fragment can potentially be inhaled, ingested or embedded into surrounding orofacial soft tissues (Figure 13.10).

Increasingly, patients are undergoing restorative treatments with titanium implants, which are radio-dense and which, if dislodged, as with luxated teeth, can provide a potential for an inhaled foreign body. Significant cost implications can occur if these types of restorations undergo iatrogenic damage! Intraoral films with a low kVp technique may be useful in localization of these fragments if impaction in the immediate soft tissues of the face is suspected; alternatively, ultrasound may help in their location.

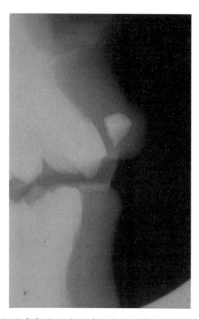

Figure 13.10 Soft tissue lateral projection showing a fragment of tooth embedded in the upper lip as a result of trauma. Counting and accounting for fragments of teeth in trauma is essential.

Classical description and distribution of facial fractures

The mechanism of facial injury is important. It cannot be assumed that the oral and maxillofacial region is the only focus of trauma. Brain, cervical spine, and life-threatening trauma to the thorax or abdomen may take precedence with regard to imaging and patient management. For the purposes of classification, tissue trauma to the oral and maxillofacial structures will be dealt with in four sections—the upper third, mid third, lower third of face, and dentoalveolar fractures.

Trauma to the upper third of the face

The upper third of the face is that skeleton above the supraorbital margin. The frontal sinuses are intimately related at their deep surface to the dura and frontal lobes of the brain. Soft tissue swelling will often accompany trauma to this area. The tendency for the young child to injure this area is greater than that of an adult owing to the comparative prominence of this region as the developing facial skeleton grows downwards and outwards.

In the developed frontal sinus, radiography can demonstrate the difference in density represented by an air–fluid level in a supine patient (using a horizontal beam lateral projection of the skull/facial bones). Blood from the trauma settles in the frontal sinus with air above it, and the horizontal rays of the X-ray beam run tangentially along this interface. Coincidentally, reviewing the cervical spine depicted in lateral projection is recommended in such an injury. A formal cervical imaging assessment may be required.

Before the advent of isocentric skull units, fronto-occipital views (also called AP views) were carried out if the patient was on a casualty trolley. More ideally, occipitofrontal projections (so-called PA) provide the view at 90° in assessing the frontal sinus. Increasingly, however, injury to the brain has been recognized as being of primary concern and so cross-sectional imaging using CT is employed as a first line modality. Any breach of the inner frontal sinus wall, with involvement of the dura or brain parenchyma, needs to be recognized.

Trauma to the mid third of the face

The area of the mid third of the face brings a set of unique challenges in planning and executing adequate imaging. An understanding of the classical fracture distribution and the potential for anatomical superimposition when using conventional radiography are crucial to answering the clinical questions posed by facial trauma.

Rene Le Fort (1869–1951), a French surgeon, first described the patterns of facial bone injuries in 1901 and his name has become inextricably associated with their classification. All the Le Fort fractures involve the pterygoid processes of the sphenoid, and their classical descriptions are given below. It should be remembered that it is the adult patient, where facial maturation has resulted in forward growth of the face, that is more likely to sustain a mid third facial injury. In addition, the most common fractures of the facial skeleton are to the nasal bones and zygomatic complex.

In reality, facial fractures often do not obey the classical rules, and combinations of fracture patterns can present depending on the mechanism and direction of injury, especially if significant force has been experienced (Figure 13.11).

Le Fort I (Guerin fracture)

This is a transverse (horizontal) maxillary fracture caused by a blow to the premaxilla. The fracture line involves the alveolar ridge, lateral aperture of the nose, and inferior wall of the maxillary sinus. The Le Fort I fracture results in detachment of the dentoalveolar process of the maxilla with any teeth contained within this arch.

This can result clinically in an 'anterior open bite' (mouth gagged open) appearance owing to the unopposed action of the pterygoid muscles. Incidentally, often it will be accompanied by a midline palatal fracture. Clinically, haematoma will be appreciated in the upper buccal sulci (lateral to the upper teeth), with a loss of resonance on tooth percussion (sounds like a 'cracked china cup') and mobility of the lower maxilla.

This injury may compromise the airway by posterior bony displacement, giving rise to compression or through the massive haemorrhage that will result if the palatine arteries are transected.

The surgeon, when advancing or setting back the upper jaw in orthognathic surgery, will induce this fracture deliberately.

Le Fort II

This is the so-called 'pyramidal fracture'. The midface is in essence acting as a crumple zone to absorb the traumatic forces and so protects the calvarium (skull-cap). This class of fracture may be unilateral, the fracture line passing through the posterior alveolar ridge, medial orbital rim and across the nasal bones (either just superior or just inferior to the nasal bones). The result is a separation of the mid portion of the face with the fracture line involving the floor of the orbit, hard palate, and the nasal cavity (Figure 13.12).

Le Fort III

The fracture path follows an essentially horizontal course through the nasofrontal suture, maxillofrontal suture, the orbital wall, zygomatic arch, and separates the entire face from the base of the skull leading to craniofacial dysjunction. There is a very real risk of intracranial infection from this injury.

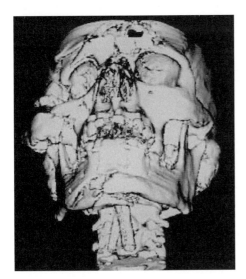

Figure 13.11 CT stereolithogram showing the maxillofacial area in 3D and a complicated right-sided facial and skull fracture.

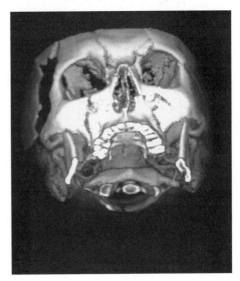

Figure 13.12 A complicated Le Fort II type injury as seen on a 3D reconstruction from conventional CT data.

Le Fort II and III fractures will result in extensive periorbital bruising, the so-called 'panda eye appearance', with significant soft tissue response to this injury.

Imaging the above in 2D using OM, OM 30 and lateral facial views gives very limited information. CT at an early stage will give definitively more detailed information of soft and hard tissues.

Other fractures which involve the midface

Zygoma fractures

The zygomatic bones are prominent and, as such, may be exposed to trauma readily.

Trauma to this area has been termed zygomatic complex, malar or trimalar fracture (Figures 13.13 and 13.14). Various classifications of injury to this bone have been offered.

Displacement or rotation of the zygoma is of prime concern to the surgeon.

The trimalar fracture is a bit of a misnomer in that the zygoma has four points of articulation. This bone has sutural union with the maxilla, temporal, frontal, and, often forgotten, the sphenoid bone. Any of the four sutural joints, the zygomatico-temporal, the zygomatico-frontal, the zygomatico-maxillary, and the spheno-zygomatic may be involved in its fracture.

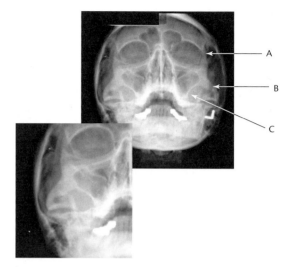

Figure 13.14 OM view designed to show the mid third of the face. The 'elephant's trunk appearance' of the zygoma is a helpful diagnostic sign. **A** Zygomatico-frontal suture; **B** zygomatic arch; **C** lateral wall of the maxillary sinus.

Fractures of the zygomatic arch tend to occur at the weakest point along this rim of bone that bounds the infratemporal fossa laterally, specifically a point 1.5 cm posterior to the zygomatico-temporal suture. The arch can be bowed inwards or fully displaced with three distinct breaks into a W-type shape when viewed from below.

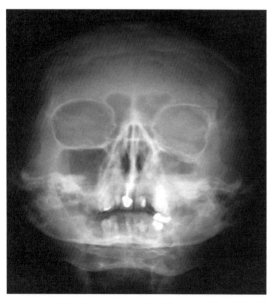

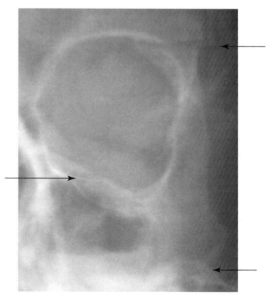

Figure 13.13 Trimalar fracture or tripod fracture of the zygoma (arrows give the location of the fractures). Any fracture of the articulation with the sphenoid bone will not be appreciated on this view.

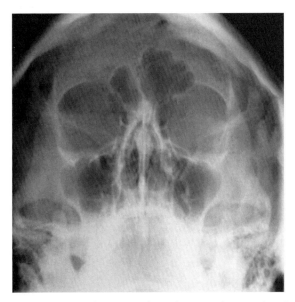
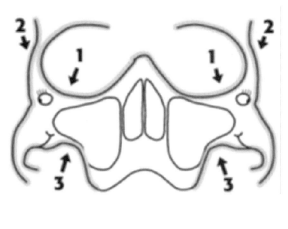

Figure 13.15 Numbers 1, 2, and 3 outline areas that may show bony discontinuities. The elephant's head is shown. Note the smooth outline of the 'trunk' in the non-fractured situation.

Significant fractures with displacement or rotation of the zygoma will present with predictable signs and symptoms. Prior to swelling, a depression in the cheek may be appreciated clinically. Soft tissue swelling may obscure this feature. Typical signs and symptoms may include the loss of sensation in the infraorbital nerve distribution. Zygomaticotemporal and zygomaticofacial nerves (branches of the maxillary division of trigeminal) that exit the lateral border of this bone may also be affected, giving cheek paraesthesia.

The fracture lines can follow a path seen on imaging to travel through the lateral wall of the maxillary sinus, orbital rim close to the infraorbital foramen. The fracture line will involve the floor of the orbit, and, if significant force is used, most if not all of the above-mentioned sutural joints would be disrupted. Orbital involvement via the attachment of the suspensory ligament of Lockwood will lead to double vision and ophthalmoplegia. The traumatic impression of the zygomatic arch against the normally free-moving coronoid process will disrupt jaw opening. This will have obvious anaesthetic access implications.

OM, OM 30, SMV (submentovertex), and reverse Townes views have been the mainstay of conventional imaging of the zygoma. The 'elephant trunk sign', where an imaginary outline of an elephant head and trunk, which, if not continuous in its smooth outline, may denote a fracture of the zygoma to even the most junior casualty officer, is one of the more useful radiological aids to diagnosis in the OM view (Figure 13.15). Access to CT allows full appreciation of this type of injury and the potential impact on the base of the skull.

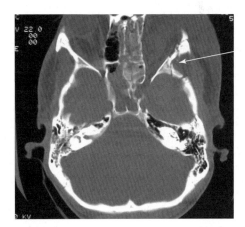

Figure 13.16 Axial CT of the left orbital complex. Significant force was involved, causing a complex fracture involving the lateral orbital wall with a 'tristar fracture' of the left greater wing of sphenoid (arrow). This will have significant implications for the muscles of mastication which attach here. Blood in the ethmoid and sphenoid sinuses can be noted, together with massive soft tissue swelling.

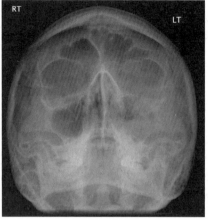

OM view

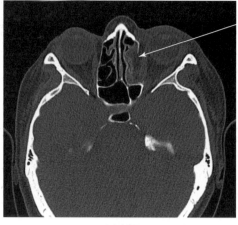

Axial CT

Figure 13.17 Occipitomental (OM) (left) and axial (right) CT of trauma to left orbitomeatal complex. A clear understanding of the injury is gained from the cross-sectional image. The thin medial wall has fractured, with herniation of the medial rectus muscle and periorbital fat into this space (arrow).

The involvement of the sphenoid bone in the so-called sphenotemporal buttress indicates that significant force has been experienced (Figure 13.16).

Nasal fractures

Nasal fractures are the third most common of all fractures to occur and the commonest facial fracture. Despite this, they are frequently underassessed with resultant functional and cosmetic sequelae. The latter include the typical flattened 'boxer's nose' to the malaligned nose. The former results in poor nasal airway patency, deviation of the nasal septum, and septal haematoma. Significant problems can arise if the adjacent ethmoidal complex is involved—nasoethmoidal injury (Figure 13.17). These can result in significant haemorrhage to the anterior ethmoidal arteries, CSF leakage, communication with intracranial tissues, and traumatic telecanthus if the medial canthal ligament becomes dislodged from its native position. As with all trauma, the first assessment is essentially clinical, but these injuries may also be apparent on the facial radiographs already discussed. It is unusual nowadays to take specific radiographs to asses a 'simple' fractured nose.

The isolated orbital floor fracture (blow out fracture)

During trauma to the eye, the globe is protected at the time of impact as a result of the orbital floor or inner medial orbital surface giving way in preference. Classically, a squash ball or a ball with a similar dimension with sufficient velocity could cause this injury to the unprotected eye. This mechanism of injury is an example of a 'fail safe' which gives classical signs on imaging. Signs and symptoms include diplopia on upward gaze, as the eyeball struggles to rotate against its tethered inferior rectus and inferior oblique muscles.The infraorbital nerve is often involved because of its close proximity.

Historically, an undertilted OM view was used which allowed the central X-ray to pass tangentially just inferior to the lower orbital rim. This highlighted a

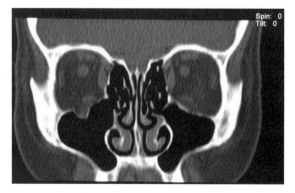

Figure 13.18 This is a CT coronal section showing a blow out fracture of the right orbital floor with herniation of orbital floor contents into the maxillary antrum.

'tear-shaped drop' of radio-opacity (infraorbital fat) against the air-filled (radiolucent) background of the maxillary sinus. This represented the inferior orbital contents herniating into the maxillary sinus. It was a difficult projection to perfect and demanded a degree of image interpretation skill, especially if accompanying haemorrhage degraded the classical teardrop sign (Figure 13.18).

Often the maxillary sinus involved would completely opacify with blood.

The ethmoid sinuses are frequently involved given their close proximity to the thin medial orbital wall (lamina papyracea). Post-traumatic changes can bring about enophthalmos. Today CT, in coronal section, makes this injury more easily diagnosable.

Mandible and temporomandibular joint (TMJ) trauma

The mandible is an unusual bone in that it spans the midline and articulates with the skull base via the TMJs. These are sliding hinge joints, with two joint compartments separated by a fibrocartilage disc. The TMJs are atypical joints both in their anatomy and the

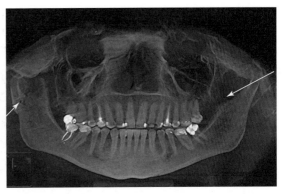

Figure 13.19 A panoramic style image constructed from the raw data of a cone beam CT acquisition (Sirona, Galileos). Arrows show an example of a contra coup injury/fractured right neck of condyle and bilateral coronoid fractures. This image is devoid of ghost images that appear on the conventional panoramic view.

dynamics of their function. One joint's movement elicits movement on the contralateral joint.

The mandibular condylar neck is a particularly weak point, which will fracture in order to dissipate forces directed towards the cranial base. Other areas of potential weakness in the mandible include those

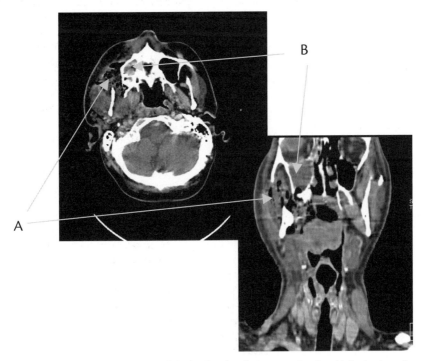

Figure 13.20 Axial and coronal conventional CT scan of the head and neck. An aggressive dental infection in an immunocompromised patient giving rise to a right-sided necrotizing fasciitis. Note the loss of normal fatty planes, **A** the presence of gas in the tissues, and **B** opacification of the right maxillary sinus with pus and infected secretions.

spanned by teeth such as the lower canine or third molar regions. Unerupted teeth are common and can facilitate a fracture through the bone in these regions. The angle of the mandible is an especially common site of fracture as a result of both a change in direction of the bone and the frequent presence of unerupted third molars. Fractures are classified as displaced or undisplaced.

When inspecting the dental panoramic for mandibular trauma, remembering the fact that the mandible can fracture in two sites is essential. The 'contra coup injury' is often noted with a body/ramus and condyle fracture combination (Figure 13.19).

The danger to the airway is particularly acute if the fracture segments experience posterior or medial displacement by muscle action, or if swelling due to oedema and haemorrhage effaces the upper respiratory tract.

Infection and tumours affecting the oral and maxillofacial region

Infections of the oral and maxillofacial regions are common (Chapter 11).

The changes in the jaws noted on imaging can be non-specific. Dental infections can cause marrow changes and erosions of cortical bone often associated with more sinister pathology. Severe infections do occur on occasion and, in the immunocompromised, may spread into the surrounding tissues (Figure 13.20).

There are numerous types of neoplasia that can affect the dentofacial region[4].

Those affecting the jaws are usually classified as odontogenic (those arising from toothbearing tissues)

and non-odontogenic. Both groups of neoplasia are again subdivided into benign and malignant. Odontogenic tumours are rare, with the most likely encountered being the ameloblastoma.

Malignant neoplasms affecting the orofacial region are most commonly of primary origin; for example, the squamous cell carcinoma (Chapter 16), lymphomas or, more rarely, osteosarcomas. In addition, the mandible can be the site for metastatic deposits, particularly from malignancies of the breast, thyroid, lung, brochi, renal, bowel, ovary and prostate.

Other common tumours affecting the oromaxillofacial region include salivary tumours, about which the reader would be advised to consult one of the more specialist texts[2,3].

Conclusion

Dental and maxillofacial radiology is a specialist complex area of radiology which can often be problematical for the non-radiologist. An appreciation of some of the complexities in obtaining and interpreting the radiological images is useful for those anaesthetists treating oral and maxillofacial surgical patients.

References

1. Zöller JE, Neugebauer J. (2008) *Cone-beam Volumetric Imaging in Dental, Oral and Maxillofacial Medicine.* Germany: Quintessence Publishing.
2. Larheim TA, Westesson P-L. (2006) *Maxillo-facial Imaging.* Berlin: Springer.
3. Ahuja A, Evans R, King A, van Hasselt CA. (2003) *Imaging in Head and Neck Cancer, a practical approach.* London: GMM.
4. Soames JV, Southham JC. (2005) *Oral Pathology*, 4th edn. Oxford: Oxford University Press.

14

Anaesthesia for maxillofacial trauma

Joy Curran

Introduction

Maxillofacial trauma is a vitally important area of trauma management. Four of five of our vital senses are contained within the face—sight, hearing, smell, and taste. Also, scarring and disfigurement to the face deeply affects our sense of self and our front to the world.

The aetiology of facial trauma has shifted in the more developed world towards assault being the most common cause (at around 36–41%), closely followed by road traffic accidents (RTAs)(25–32%). Other causes listed in order of frequency are falls (mainly in the extremes of age), sport, occupational injuries, and gunshot wounds[1,2].

As a group, 55–70% of patients with significant facial trauma will have other serious injuries[2,3]. Looking at it the other way around, 30% of severely injured trauma patients also had maxillofacial trauma[4]. The most common isolated fracture reported is the nose which serves as the 'crumple zone' for the face when hit from the front (Figure 14.1). Those patients with injuries resulting from gunshots and RTAs had higher injury severity scores (ISS)[2,3].

One study from an American level 1 trauma centre looked at those patients with maxillofacial injuries and an ISS of over 12[2]. They found that 43.7% of patients also had cerebral haematoma, with subdural being the most common. The second most commonly associated injury was pulmonary trauma, in particular contusions. Forty-two per cent of patients required intubation and 14% required a tracheostomy at some point. With regard to cervical spine injuries, 5% also had a cervical fracture and a quarter of these had neurological deficit. Looking at significant trauma injuries in Canada between 1992 and 1997[3], 17% of patients with

an ISS score of over 12 had maxillofacial injuries. The entire group had some kind of head injury with altered conscious level and 11% had a cervical spine injury.

Ophthalmic injury has been strongly linked to not wearing a seatbelt, increasing the risk from 2% up to 20% in one review[5]. Blindness is associated with 0.5–3% of midfacial fractures[5]. Upper and midfacial fractures are associated particularly with smell or taste disturbances. In one Italian series, about one-third of those who had treatment for upper third and mid third fractures suffered long-term disturbances of smell or taste[6].

Assessment and triage

Major injuries of the head and neck should be seen initially by a full trauma team. Patients are assessed using the ABCs of trauma management with the airway as priority one, maintenance of cervical spine immobilization and oxygenation following on logically from this. Haemorrhage control of facial injuries has an immediate impact on the airway and oxygenation, and must therefore be dealt with as a matter of urgency.

The most senior help possible is needed with the airway management, as repeated attempts at intubation will worsen the situation. If maxillofacial or ear, nose, and throat (ENT) assistance is not a routine part of the trauma team, they should be summoned. Early ophthalmic review is also required, as rapid facial and periorbital swelling may mean that the eyes cannot be inspected for some time. Also, as previously alluded to, the risk of head injury is high, necessitating early neurosurgical input.

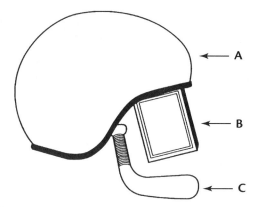

Figure 14.1 The brain is protected by the relative strength of the skull bones from a blow to zone A, whilst the flimsy structure of the nasal bones acts as a crumple zone absorbing the energy from a blow to zone B. The effect of a blow to zone C is to crack at the symphysis or angle of the mandible and also to transmit pressure upwards to the coronoid process and TMJ joint.

If unrestrained in a RTA or on a motor cycle, the patient is at risk from uncommon laryngeal/tracheal injuries. A high index of suspicion must be maintained. In a large US study between 1992 and 2004, only 37 of 16 465 patients with head, neck, or facial injuries were diagnosed with laryngeal fracture. However, 20 of these needed definitive airway control. Fourteen required tracheostomy, five endotracheal intubation, and one underwent cricothyroidotomy[7]. Laryngeal fracture is rare on account of the elastic nature of the larynx; however, it does become more calcified with age and may then fracture more readily.

Airway injuries can range from the life-threatening, such as a disrupted larynx which needs immediate intubation, to the patient with slight swelling and dysphagia who may only require observation. Observation is critical since maximal swelling will not occur for around 24–48 hours after injury. Only air bubbling through a wound and subcutaneous emphysema are pathognomonic signs for airway injury. Soft signs to watch for are stridor, respiratory distress, dysphagia, and hoarseness. The latter two can be signs of oesophageal or tracheal trauma.

The pathognomonic signs of vascular injury may be less reliable. These include haematoma, especially if there is expanding, active haemorrhage from the wound (arterial), bruit/thrill (arteriovenous fistula), pulse deficit, and distal ischaemia or neurological deficit. Current guidelines and the literature suggest four-vessel angiography with computerized tomography (CT) only if the patient has clinical signs and is haemodynamically stable. If unstable, then surgical exploration is indicated[8].

Since a proportion of maxillofacial trauma patients have cervical spine injury (6.7%) and the spine may not have clearance prior to intubation, there is a need to protect the spine from unnecessary movement[9,10].

Emergency airway management

In an emergency situation, oral endotracheal intubation is the route of choice. A comparative study on cadavers[11] looking at the effects of manual inline stabilization and traction on oral intubation using different laryngoscope blades, the intubating laryngeal mask airway (ILMA), and the fibrescope (both oral and nasal) found that all airway interventions cause spinal movement, including facemask ventilation[10,11]. Traction in the presence of cervical instability causes significant distraction that is damaging to the spinal cord and should be avoided. Manual inline stabilization and oral intubation gave conflicting results but there was less cervical movement with manual inline stabilization than with a rigid cervical collar in place. The presence of a cervical collar, tape, and sandbags also impeded optimal visualization of the laryngeal inlet, with 64% reporting Cormack and Lehane Class 3 and 4 laryngeal views. This compared to 22% reported Class 3 and 4 views when only manual inline stabilization was adopted[12]. The ILMA and fibreoptic approaches, although causing significantly less movement, were more time-consuming[13]. Currently data is unavailable to differentiate between tracheostomy or cricothyroidotomy.

Clinicians should use the techniques with which they are most familiar and that are appropriate to the situation whilst keeping cervical movement to a minimum. Recent data indicate that direct laryngoscopy and intubation are unlikely to cause significant movement, but that manual inline stabilization may not fully immobilize injured segments[14].

In one study, 22% of patients with significant facial trauma and higher Le Fort fractures required a tracheostomy for airway control, as did 10 out of 23 patients with Le Fort III injuries[15]. There has been some work looking at elective tracheostomy in patients with documented cervical spine injuries. An Israeli group followed up 38 such patients for an average of 18 months and found no deterioration following percutaneous tracheostomy. They stressed the importance of an experienced surgeon, avoiding neck extension but using a 'gentle rostral traction of the larynx' (towards the nose)[16].

The use of the LMA in an emergency is debatable since it may worsen pharyngeal and laryngeal trauma, and does not protect the airway sufficiently from stomach contents and lower airway haemorrhage. As an emergency holding measure it probably has a place, particularly when facial disruption makes face mask ventilation difficult.

Transtracheal jet ventilation is another option for short-term oxygenation, but care must be taken to avoid hypercapnia and barotrauma, particularly if there is a concurrent intracranial injury.

A great deal of work is currently being carried out using new hand-held fibreoptic devices and we wait to see which will emerge as the most reliable and useful in these difficult scenarios (Chapter 4). However, work which conforms to the guidelines laid out in the excellent meta-analysis and review by R. Mihai of different airway aids is rare[17]. In a comparative unblinded study of the glidescope, the Pentax AWS, the Trueview EVO2, and the Macintosh laryngoscope, a small group of experienced anaesthetists used a mannequin to compare normal, rigid cervical spine, and tongue oedema scenarios. They found that the Pentax AWS performed best, probably owing to the side channel through which the endotracheal tube is placed before starting[18].

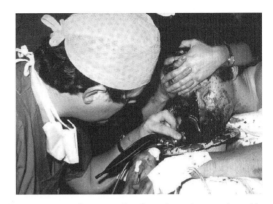

Figure 14.2 Gunshot wound to face. The patient was best able to maintain a clear airway lying supine and was induced in this position. See also Plate 7.

A strategy for airway control should be formulated promptly and all immediate clinical personnel involved in the patient's care made aware of the intended procedure. A fibreoptic laryngoscope may be of little benefit in the presence of active haemorrhage. Summon senior anaesthetic and surgical help. Sufficient skilled anaesthetic assistance is mandatory for the induction of anaesthesia and maintaining cervical immobilization when necessary. It always helps to plan for the worst case scenario.

Practical points for emergency room intubation

Acute airway management in maxillofacial injuries can be challenging (Figure 14.2; see also Plate 5) and requires a coordinated team effort. Head injury and reduced consciousness will also dictate the need for direct airway control. The Glasgow Coma Score (GCS) should be regularly monitored since progressive airway obstruction is a risk. A GCS score of less than 8 indicates the need for intubation.

A patient with facial trauma may have other problems affecting the airway (Figure 14.3; see also Plate 6), e.g. blood, haematoma, foreign bodies, lost or broken teeth (see Figure 13.10), dentures, bony fragments, displaced bone, vomit, tongue injuries, and tissue oedema. Around a quarter of patients with Le Fort fractures present with either airway obstruction or decreased respiration requiring immediate airway control.

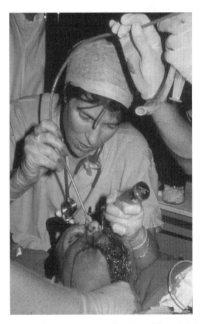

Figure 14.3 Intubation using a bougie with cricoid pressure applied. See also Plate 8.

- Administer high-flow O$_2$ at 100%. Use a Guedel airway if needed

- Establish large bore venous access

- Patient should rest the voice as much as possible

- Where necessary, maintain manual inline mobilization as far as possible

- In the absence of cervical injury, allow the patient to adopt the best position for draining any haemorrhage (Figure 14.2)

- Ensure effective suction

- Establish standard monitoring

- Have available a variety of laryngoscope blades and endotracheal tubes

- Preload a bougie onto an endotracheal tube

- Have available an LMA, ILMA, criocothyroidotomy or tracheostomy kit

- Perform a rapid sequence anaesthetic induction (release cricoid pressure if laryngeal view inadequte for intubation)

- Maintain adequate blood pressure, normocapnia after intubation.

Antibiotics, antacids, and steroids are given, the last to reduce inflammation and fibrosis.

Blunt facial trauma

Most facial fractures will cause minor bleeding from the nose or mouth. In general terms, it is rare to have circulatory shock from maxillofacial injuries alone, and if significant resuscitation is ongoing then other sources of blood loss should be sought. Generally, this is a slow venous bleed and is controlled with a nasal pack or direct pressure to the wound. A steady flow of blood from the nose and mouth with profound cheek swelling is probably the result of a closed injury to the middle third. Occasionally, a major bleed will occur which needs careful packing of the posterior and anterior nasal spaces after airway control (Figures 14.4 and 14.5). Commonly this bleeding is from the end branches of the maxillary artery at the level of the pterygopalatine fossa and from the common carotid at the level of the skull base. Bleeding can often be seen as haematoma of the buccal mucosa. If packing is ineffective and the haemorrhage persists, then facial fractures should be repaired if possible. In the cardiovascularly unstable patient an alternative approach is to ligate the relevant

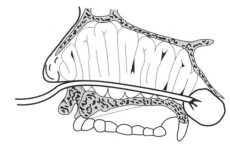

Figure 14.4 Nasopharyngeal pack. The pack sits in the nasopharyngeal space to prevent blood from flowing down to the trachea and oesophagus.

arteries, although this can be inadequate as the face has a strong collateral circulation. Recently, blunt facial trauma and haemorrhage guidelines (Figure 14.6) recommend angiographic embolization when alternative methods have failed[19].

Bleeding from the ear can be caused by a fracture at the base of the skull or a fracture of the condylar head which has been forced backwards and torn the external auditory meatus.

Penetrating trauma

There are two main categories of penetrating facial trauma to consider: gunshot wounds and stab wounds. The higher the velocity of the gunshot, the greater the tissue damage and loss. There is also proportionately more swelling with high energy injury. The velocity depends on the type of weapon, torque of the bullet, and also the distance that the bullet has travelled. Transcervical gunshots cause very significant damage as might be expected. South African data suggests around half of gunshot victims have vascular injuries, of which most will need proactive airway management. A quarter will have spinal cord injuries, but only 9% had facial fractures. Laryngeal and pharyngeal injuries are very rare, constituting only 2%[20].

In contrast, stab wounds cause cleaner wounds with less tissue damage. A review of the management of penetrating neck injury looked at the issues surrounding those cases which did not have obvious signs of injury. In the absence of any neurological deficit, this group of patients may be better managed without a cervical collar which could obscure from view any expanding haematoma[21]. The generally accepted classification of injuries to the neck was described by Roon

(a)

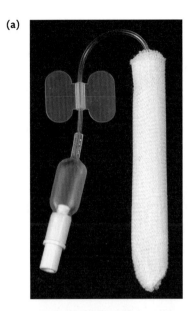

(b)

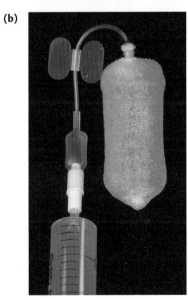

Figure 14.5 Alternative method of nasal packing in epistaxis using a pneumatic nasal tamponade (Rapid Rhino™). **a** Deflated; **b** inflated.

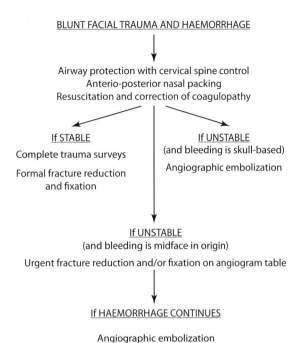

BLUNT FACIAL TRAUMA AND HAEMORRHAGE

↓

Airway protection with cervical spine control
Anterio-posterior nasal packing
Resuscitation and correction of coagulopathy

If STABLE

Complete trauma surveys

Formal fracture reduction
and fixation

If UNSTABLE
(and bleeding is skull-based)

Angiographic embolization

If UNSTABLE
(and bleeding is midface in origin)
Urgent fracture reduction and/or fixation on angiogram table

↓

If HAEMORRHAGE CONTINUES

Angiographic embolization

Figure 14.6 Management of blunt facial trauma[19].

Pharyngeal and oesophageal injury

Digestive tract injury is a rare occurrence but if undiagnosed beyond 24 hours has a much higher morbidity from mediastinitis[24]. Symptoms and signs are vague but dysphagia, odynophagia (painful swallowing), haematemesis, central chest pain radiating to the back, and drooling should make the clinican alert to such a potentially serious injury[25]. It should always be considered, even following minor penetrating trauma of the neck, and excluded with a swallowing/water-soluble dye test[26].

Neurological deficits should be monitored with the AVPU scale (A, alert; V, responds to vocal stimuli; P, responds only to painful stimuli; U, unresponsive to all stimuli), together with the pupillary reactions. The GCS should also be measured at frequent intervals.

Ophthalmic assessment

Damage to the eye and the neuronal pathways can occur directly or from external compression. Periorbital oedema may limit eye examination, but every effort should be made to examine the visual acuity, visual fields, pupillary size, and reflexes. The eyes should be inspected for conjunctival or fundal

and Christiansen (Table 14.1)[22]. With no obvious signs of vascular injury and stable vital signs, even patients with penetrating trauma to Zone 2 can be investigated with CT angiography rather than surgical exploration as has been advocated in the past. The same recommendations apply to children with penetrating neck injuries[23].

Table 14.1 Roon and Christensen's[22] classification of penetrating injuries to the neck

---

ZONE 1: From the clavicles to the cricoid cartilage

Zonal structures:

Common and internal carotid artery

Jugular veins

Subclavian and vertebral arteries

Subclavian and innominate veins

Oesophagus

Trachea

Lung

Spinal cord

ZONE 2: From the cricoid cartilage to the inferior border of the mandible

Zonal structures:

External and internal carotid arteries

Internal jugular veins

Subclavian arteries

Vertebral arteries

Trachea

Larynx

Pharynx

Oesophagus

Spinal cord

ZONE 3: From the inferior border of the mandible to the base of the skull

Zonal structures:

External and internal carotid arteries

Internal jugular veins

Vertebral arteries

Basilar arteries

Salivary and parotid glands

Trachea

Oesophagus

Spinal cord

Cervical vertebrae

Cranial nerves IX–XII

---

haemorrhage, penetrating injury, lens dislocation, and ocular entrapment. The latter will be evident by inability to move the eyes through a full range of normal movements.

If there are any concerns regarding ocular damage, the ophthalmologist should be contacted promptly since early diagnosis correlates favourably with the preservation of visual accuity. Serial examination of function is vitally important. A progressive loss of vision indicates urgent surgical exploration and decompression of the optic nerve. In addition to surgical intervention, the anti-inflammatory effects of high dose steroids may be necessary to preserve the function of the optic nerve, the most common cause of visual loss[27].

Dural tears and cerebrospinal fluid leaks

A dural tear is possible with all midface and above fractures. It is reported to occur in 4.6% of patients with maxillofacial trauma[28] at the cribriform plate and can present with cerebrospinal fluid (CSF) rhinorrhoea. Fracture of the temporal bone in the middle cranial fossa may result in otorrhoea that can track along the Eustachian tube to give 'paradoxical' rhinorrhoea. Soft tissue oedema may prevent the leakage of CSF which can then become apparent after a few days when the swelling subsides.

Definitive diagnosis can be difficult. CSF classically causes tram lines on the face or a halo effect on bedding. This is due to blood coagulating and CSF continuing to flow. However, a mix of blood and tears or saliva can give the same effect. Measurement of beta-2 transferrin is the most sensitive test as it is only found in the CSF, perilymph, and vitreous humor. Fine cut CT scans may show CSF fistulae, but MRI scanning is more accurate and is the preferred modality[28].

Most cases of CSF leakage stop spontaneously and the majority after the fractures have been fixed. Persistent CSF leaks should be referred to the neurosurgical team and are usually treated by lumbar drainage followed by surgery if necessary.

Antibiotic prophylaxis is usually given, but good CSF penetration is unreliable and there is growing concern regarding bacterial resistance. Since the main risk is meningitis, many clinicians are reluctant to withhold antibiotic treatment. One retrospective analysis of 160 patients with traumatic CSF fistulae showed a 30.6% incidence of meningitis if untreated, 4% of which were fatal. Formal dural repair reduced the incidence of meningitis to 2%[29].

The implications for the anaesthetist are unclear. Certainly passage of an endotracheal tube into the cranium has occurred (although there is only one case following facial trauma reported in the literature) and been associated with a fatal outcome[30]. As regards facial injuries, there is no real need to consider the nasal route for intubation in the acute situation. However, for definitive surgery to have good results, nasal intubation is necessary for optimal intraoperative occlusion. Although the studies have limitations, there is no evidence that nasal intubation following facial trauma increases the risk of CSF contamination over and above that which has already occurred[31,32]. Alternative strategies for endotracheal intubation in facial trauma are discussed further below.

Pain control

With the exception of mobile fracture of the mandible, even extensive facial trauma does not cause a large amount of pain. Simple analgesics such as non-steroidal anti-inflammatory drugs (NSAIDs) with paracetamol and/or codeine are usually sufficient. Acute pain often subsides with the fixation of the fractures.

Elective or semi-urgent anaesthesia

Facial fractures can be unilateral or bilateral and follow specific lines of structural weakness and are described in Chapter 13. The timing of definitive repair of facial injuries will depend on prioritization in the presence of other significant injuries. Ideally, eye injuries should be treated first followed by soft tissue toilet and suture (within 12 hours). Most fractures will be fixed via other incisions, so the repair to the soft tissues should be considered as definitive. Mandibular fractures are very painful and inhibit swallowing, and should be fixed within 24–48 hours. Other fractures, in particular midfacial and orbital, may need CT scanning to assess them adequately and should ideally be fixed by 7–10 days after injury. Delays beyond this time increase the likelihood of suboptimal fixation and misalignment.

Definitive repair of maxillofacial fractures usually occurs through intraoral, subconjunctival, or scalp incisions. In complex cases, 3D imaging is used to allow intraoperative navigation-guided fixation. Mandibular fractures are generally more painful and often prevent swallowing and do not usually necessitate CT images.

Anaesthesia for facial trauma

Of particular interest to the anaesthetist is the mechanism of the trauma and the possibility of a head, cervical spine, or other injury. A history of drug or alcohol abuse should be sought as these conditions are often related to the circumstances leading up to the injury.

Airway assessment

Assessment of the airway should include the normal inspection for deformity, swelling, dental damage or loss, nasal patency, mouth opening, Mallampati score, and neck movements. For fractures within 10–14 days, limited mouth opening is usually due to trismus caused by pain and will disappear after induction. There are, however, a few situations when inability to open the mouth may not be due to pain and trismus alone. Late presentation of an infected fracture with submasseteric pus and also rarely central dislocation of a temporomandibular joint (TMJ) into the temporal fossa, a fractured zygoma which obstructs the coronoid process of the mandible, can give rise to serious limitation of mouth opening which persists even after the induction of anaesthesia and therapeutic neuromuscular paralysis. These latter patients need very careful preoperative evaluation (Chapter 4).

Intubation

Before commencing anaesthetic induction, it is essential to discuss the operative plan with the maxillofacial surgeon. If in doubt, ask the surgeon if there is any mechanical reason why the mouth might not open fully following anaesthesia. In most cases of midfacial fractures, temporary dental intraoperative occlusion is required and an oral tube will prevent this unless there is a sufficient gap in the patient's dentition. Some complex injuries, however, may require the application of intraoperative intermaxillary fixation (IMF) which will prevent access to the oral cavity postoperatively, with major implications for the anaesthetist and patient. For zygomatic and orbital surgery, a south-facing Ring-Adair-Elwyn (RAE) tube is suitable. The latter often involves surgical access to the superior orbital fractures via a coronal flap which allows the scalp to be reflected down over the face (Figure 14.7; see also Plate 7). Panfacial fractures involve both the structural bones and smaller bones of the nasal complex, which means that access to the nose as well as occlusion is needed. If the proposed surgery cannot be carried out with an oral endotracheal tube, the alternative options are formal tracheostomy (Chapter 5), a nasal fibreoptic intubation under direct vision (Chapter 4), or a submental intubation (Table 14.2).

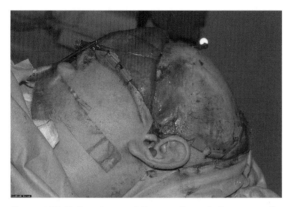

Figure 14.7 Reflected coronal flap to gain surgical access to the orbital bone. Oral endotracheal tube visible. See also Plate 9.

Submental intubation

Submental intubation involves passing the endotracheal tube through a surgical incision in the floor of the mouth (Figure 14.8). Since it was first described in 1986 by Hernandez Altemir[33], it has been successfully used in the anaesthetic management of both trauma and elective orthognathic patients with a low complication rate[34–36]. The literature reports two abscesses in the floor of the mouth following submental intubation but both resolved with local conservative treatment[35]. In another report two patients subsequently required a tracheostomy for respiratory failure. Interestingly, 14 patients of this series of 25 were ventilated postoperatively for over 24 hours with no problems[36].

There are a number of practical points to consider with regard to submental intubation. Owing to the acute angle from the submental insertion of the tube to the trachea, an armoured tube is recommended to prevent kinking. The endotracheal tube associated with the ILMA is the easiest to use for submental intubation as the tube is reinforced and has a detachable connector. Once exteriorized, the tube is secured at the neck by a surgical suture. Movements of the neck will have an exaggerated effect on the distal end of the tube in the trachea, and both accidental extubation and bronchial intubation have been reported. Positioning of the tube at a midway point between the carina and vocal cords is therefore important. In complex cases the position of the endotracheal tube may need to be changed intraoperatively.

Maintenance of anaesthesia

For maintenance of anaesthesia a total intravenous technique using propofol and remifentanil has a number of advantages. It allows rapid awakening with early return of glottic reflexes, immediate assessment of conscious level, and cooperation with eyesight testing after zygomatic and orbital floor work. It is also less emetogenic than the volatile agents. Deliberate hypotension is of limited benefit in the majority of cases and is contraindicated if there has been a concomitant head injury. The general principles for control of intracranial pressure (ICP) suffice (head-up tilt, normocapnia, and rehydration).

Surgical manipulation of the mid third of the face can be associated with a severe reflex bradycardia.

Table 14.2 Comparative advantages and disadvantages of tracheostomy, nasal intubation, and submental intubation for securing the airway following facial trauma

Advantages		
Tracheostomy	**Nasal intubation using the fibrescope**	**Submental intubation**
Avoids controversial nasal route. Allows preoperative IMF. Better for long-term ventilation	Allows intraoperative IMF. Avoids an extra surgical procedure. Avoids a surgical scar	Technically easy. Allows intraoperative IMF. Low complication rate. Said to be a cosmetically acceptable scar
Disadvantages		
Tracheostomy	**Nasal intubation**	**Submental intubation**
Most invasive of the techniques. Extra procedure. Risks of haemorrhage, tracheal damage—stenosis, tracheomalacia, and infection	Requires the use of a fibreoptic scope. Poor for prolonged postoperative ventilation and weaning. The nose must be unblocked. Risks of nasal haemorrhage, sinusitis, and unproven possibility of an increase in the infective complication of meningitis	Many surgeons are unfamiliar with technique. Not good in prolonged ventilation and weaning. If an armoured tube is used, then reintubation may be necessary as the connector does not detach from the tube

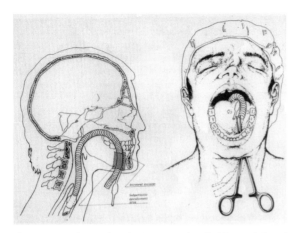

Figure 14.8 Submental intubation. Reproduced with permission of Elsevier. © 1986.

Levering, in an attempt to reduce a depressed zygomatic arch fracture, is of particular note in this respect.

Once fixed many facial fractures are often associated with only moderate pain so large doses of opiates are unnecessary. Intravenous NSAID administration and intravenous tramadol is a good alternative or addition since it causes less sedation and respiratory depression than morphine. Mandibular fractures and orbital repairs which go behind the eye are, however, exceptions and often require opiate analgesia. The use of local anaesthesia by the surgeon is helpful in this respect. A throat pack is used to prevent accumulation of blood in the oropharynx. Although endotracheal tubes are cuffed seepage of blood into the lungs can occur and cause bronchial blockage. It is important that mechanisms are in place to prevent accidental pack retention. To this end it is recommended that the pack is part of the surgical pack count and its insertion and removal recorded separately.

Extubation strategies

Extubation should be considered as carefully as intubation. There are a number of patients who will need to stay ventilated for neurosurgical considerations or other injuries received. If the patient is to be extubated, the degree of oedema and airway compromise must be carefully evaluated; further swelling can occur up to 48 hours after the initial injury. Patients with hyoid fractures have a very high risk of airway obstruction owing to secondary oedema and should be left intubated for at least 24 hours before evaluating the degree of swelling.

The position of any residual nasal packs must be checked since they can migrate down into the pharynx and cause considerable airway irritation and, occasionally, complete airway obstruction (Chapter 12). Oropharyngeal suction to remove any residual blood clots, secretions and throat pack is mandatory prior to extubation.

Peroperative remifentanil has found widespread acceptance for oral and maxillofacial anaesthesia and has undoubtedly made difficult extubation easier[37]. Once the remifentanil has been discontinued, the patient will reliably wake up, obey commands, and tolerate extubation smoothly under its residual narcotization. All Le Fort II or III fractures are at risk postoperatively from further swelling or haemorrhage which may compromise the airway and will require specialist nursing care, preferably on a high dependency unit or similar facility for 12–24 hours postoperatively.

Dog bites

In children, 78% of dog bites received are on the face, in contrast to adults which are mainly on the limbs. In one year there were 902 children under the age of 9 years admitted to hospital in England because of dog bites and there continue to be occasional deaths[38]. Because of dog's high masticatory forces in the order of 50–100 kg/cm^2, there is often severe tissue contusion with large areas of devitalized tissue. In contrast, domestic cat bites tend to have a deeper puncture wound with a very high risk for deep-sited infection. The main preoccupation for animal bites is the prevention of infection. Consequently, rapid cleansing is needed with high intensity flushing. This should be carried out as a matter or urgency with minimal delay. Routine simple anaesthetic technique is used and intravenous antibiotics are indicated if infection occurs[38].

Gunshots

Gunshot wounds to the face require thorough cleansing. The absorbed energy of high velocity bullets causes massive tissue necrosis; however, owing to the excellent blood supply to facial tissues a surprising amount can survive. CT scanning, plus or minus angiography, is the most useful investigation for evaluation of this type of injury. Residual metal fragments can, however, cause some distortion of the image. Gunshot wounds must be cleansed as for dog bites above, debrided as little as possible, and then simultaneous soft tissue revision and closure is advised[39,40].

Conclusion

The patient with maxillofacial trauma can be a considerable challenge to the anaesthetist. With minimal notice, they can be called upon to secure an airway acutely following oral and maxillofacial trauma. The situation often requires specialized skills and equipment. A systematic and ordered approach to what can be a frightening situation is essential.

References

1. Erdmann D, Follmar KE, Debruijn M et al. (2008) A retrospective analysis of facial fracture etiologies. Ann Plast Surg, 60(4), 398–403.
2. Alvi A, Doherty T, Lewen G. (2003) Facial fractures and concomitant injuries in trauma patients. Laryngoscope, 113 (1), 102–6.
3. Hogg NJ, Stewart TC, Armstrong JE, Girotti MJ. (2000) Epidemiology of maxillofacial injuries at trauma hospitals in Ontario, Canada, between 1992 and 1997. J Trauma Injury Infect Crit Care, 49(3), 425–32.
4. Hayter JP, Ward AJ, Smith EJ. (1991) Maxillofacial trauma in the severely injured patients. Br J Oral Maxillofac Surg, 29(6), 370–3.
5. Ashar A, Kovacs A, Khan S, Hakim J. (1998) Blindness associated with midfacial fractures. J Oral Maxillofac Surg, 56, 1146–50.
6. Renzi G, Carboni A, Gasparini G, Perugini M, Becelli R. (2002) Taste and olfactory disturbances after upper and middle third facial fractures: a preliminary study. Ann Plast Surg, 48(4), 355–8.
7. Verschueren DS, Bell RB, Bagheri SC et al. (2006) Management of laryngo-tracheal injuries associated with craniomaillofacial trauma. J Oral Maxillofac Surg, 64(2), 203–14.
8. Brywczynski JJ, Barrett TW, Lyon JA, Cotton BA. (2008) Management of penetrating neck injury in the emergency department: a structured literature review. Emerg Med J, 25, 711–15.
9. Hackl W, Hausberger K, Sailer R et al. (2001) Prevalence of cervical spine injuries in patients with facial trauma. Oral Surg Oral Pathol Oral Radiol Endod, 92(4), 370–6.
10. Crosby ET. (2006) Airway management in adults after cervical spine trauma. Anesthesiology, 104, 1293–318.
11. Brimacombe J, Keller C, Kunzel KH et al. (2000) Cervical spine motion during airway management: A cinefluoroscopic study of the posteriorly destabilized third cervical vertebrae in human cadavers. Anesth Analg, 91, 1274–8.
12. Heath KJ. (1994) The effect of laryngoscopy of different cervical spine immobilization techniques. Anaesthesia, 49, 843–5.
13. Gercek E, Wahlen BM, Rommens PM. (2008) In vivo ultrasound real-time motion of the cervical spine during intubation under manual in-line stabilization: a comparison of intubation methods. Eur J Anaesthesiol, 25(1), 29–36.
14. Ollerton JE, Parr MJA, Harrison K, Hanrahan B, Sugrue M. (2006) Potential cervical spine injury and difficult airway management for emergency intubation of trauma adults in the emergency department—a systematic review. Emerg Med J, 23, 3–11.
15. Bagheri SC, Holmgren E, Kademani D et al. (2005) Comparison of the severity of bilateral Le Fort injuries in isolated midface trauma. J Oral Maxillofac Surg, 63(8), 1123–9.
16. Nun AB, Orlovsky M, Best LA (2006) Percutaneous tracheostomy in patients with cervical spine fractures—feasible and safe. Interact Cardio Vasc Thorac Surg, 5, 427–9.
17. Mihai R, Blair E, Kay H et al. (2008) A quantitative review and meta-analysis of performance of non-standard laryngoscopes and rigid fibreoptic intubation aids. Anaesthesia, 63, 745–60.
18. Malik MA, Donoghe CO, Corney J et al. (2009) Comparison of the glidescope, the Pentax AWS and the Trueview EVO 2 with the macintosh laryngoscope in experienced anaesthetists. A mannequin study. Br J Anaesth, 102(1), 128–34.
19. Ho K, Hutter JJ, Eskridge J et al. (2006) The management of life-threatening haemorrhage following blunt facial trauma. J Plastic Reconst Aesth Surg, 59, 1257–62.
20. Milner A. (2008) The airway in face, head and neck injury. SAJAA, 14(1), 52–7.
21. Brywczynski JJ, Barrett TW, Lyon JA, Cotton BA. (2008) Management of penetrating neck injury in the emergency department: a structured literature review. Emerg Med J, 25, 711–15.
22. Roon AJ, Christensen N. (1979) Evaluation and treatment of penetrating cervical injuries. J Trauma, 19, 391–4.
23. Vick LR, Islam S. (2008) Adding insult to injury: neck exploration for penetrating pediatric neck trauma. Am Surg, 74(11), 1104–6.
24. Luqman Z, Khan MA, Nazir Z. (2005) Penetrating pharyngeal injuries in children: trivial trauma leading to devastating complications. Pediatr Surg Int, 21(6), 432–5.
25. Rathlev NK, Medzon R, Bracken ME. (2007) Evaluation and management of neck trauma. Emerg Med Clin N Am, 25, 679–94.
26. Nel L, Jones LW, Hardcastle TC. (2009) Imaging the oesophagus after penetrating cervical trauma using water-soluble contrast alone: simple, cost-effective and accurate. Emerg Med J, 26(2), 106–8.
27. Palmer O, Whittaker V, Pinnock C. (2006) Early perioperative care of the acutely injured maxillofacial patient. Oral Maxillofac Surg Clin N Am, 8, 261–73.
28. Bell RB, Dierks EJ, Homer L et al. (2004) Management of cerebrospinal fluid leak associated with craniomaxillofacial trauma. J Oral Maxillofac Surg, 62(6), 676–84.
29. Eljamel MS, Foy PM. (1990) Acute traumatic CSF fistulae: the risk of intracranial infection. Br J Neurosurg, 4(5), 381–5.
30. Marlow TR, Goltra DD, Schabel SI. (1997) Intracranial placement of a nasotracheal tube after facial fracture: a rare complication. J Emerg Med, 15, 87–91.

31. Rosen CL, Wolfe RE, Chew SE. (1997) Blind nasotracheal intubation in the presence of facial trauma. *J Emerg Med*, **15,** 141–5.

32. Weitzel N, Kendall J, Pons P. (2004) Blind nasotracheal intubation for patients with penetrating neck trauma. *J Trauma Injury Infect Crit Care*, **56(5),** 1097–101.

33. Altemir H. (1986) The submental route for endotracheal intubation. A new technique. *J Maxillofac Surg*, **14(1),** 64–5.

34. Schütz P, Hamed HH. (2008) Submental intubation versus tracheostomy in maxillofacial trauma patients. *J Oral Maxillofac Surg*, **66(7),** 1404–9.

35. Meyer C, Valfrey J, Kjartansdottir T, Wilk A, Barriére P. (2003) Indication for and technical refinements of submental intubation in oral and maxillofacial surgery. *J Cranio-Maxillofac Surg*, **31(6),** 383–8.

36. Caron G, Paquin R, Lessard M, Trèpanier CA, Landry P-E. (2000) Submental endotracheal intubation: An alternative to tracheotomy in patients with midfacial and panfacial fractures. *J Trauma*, **48(2),** 235–40.

37. Hohlrieder M, Tiefenthaler W, Klaus H *et al.* (2007) Effect of total intravenous anaesthesia and balanced anaesthesia on the frequency of coughing during emergence from the anaesthesia. *Br J Anaesth*, **99(4),** 587–91.

38. Morgan M, Palmer J. (2007) Dog bites. *BMJ*, **334,** 413–15.

39. Kaufman Y, Cole P, Hollier L. (2008) Contemporary issues in facial gunshot wound management. *J Craniofac Surg*, **19 (2),** 421–7.

40. Vayvada H, Mederes A, Yilmaz M *et al.* (2005) Management of close-range, high-energy shotgun and rifle wounds to the face. *J Craniofac Surg*, **6(5),** 794–804.

15

Facial, oral, and airway thermal injuries and anaesthesia

Tim Vorster

Introduction

The remit in this chapter, and rationale for inclusion in this book, is to discuss facial and oral burns management for anaesthetists. The pure surgical aims of treating facial and oral burns are identical to the treatment of burns elsewhere on the body, that is to excise non-viable burned tissue, allow viable tissue that has the capacity to heal quickly, to heal in a time-frame that will make scaring minimal, and to cover debrided areas with skin grafts or skin substitutes in order to maximize cosmetic and functional result.

However, facial and oral burns are seldom an isolated injury, and are often a harbinger of more immediate life-threatening insults to the patient as a whole. Acute thermal airway burns are seldom encountered without an associated facial burn, and require the immediate attention of a skilled anaesthetist. Other aspects of the 'smoke inhalation complex' will also be commonly involved and require assessment and appropriate treatment prior to any evacuation to a Burn Unit. Though not all patients with facial burns will have an associated inhalation burn, the vast majority of inhalation injury patients do have a facial burn. The presence itself, of a full thickness facial burn, has been shown to be an independent indicator of a significant increase in the probability of death, when compared with similar size burns elsewhere (logistical regression coefficient 0.70)[1]. It is proposed that this is due to the close association between this type of burn and the presence of an inhalation injury. Those who suffer facial and oral burns are very fortunate, if it can be said under such circumstances, to escape with these as their only cutaneous thermal injury. Facial burns are often just a small part of the overall burn seen in patients with massive thermal injuries. Also, it must be noted, a significant number of burn victims will have other injuries and coexisting pathologies that will need evaluating, and appropriate management.

This chapter is designed to give a brief outline of burns treatment, with a specific emphasis on inhalation injury and the airway management in these cases. Within the limits of the chapter, a somewhat holistic approach to the subject of burns injuries in general, rather than just injuries in an isolated anatomical area is warranted.

It will briefly touch on burns resuscitation, but the reader is advised to consult other textbooks specifically dealing with all aspects of burns treatment for a more thorough overview [2]. An alternative is to enrol in the Emergency Management of Severe Burns (EMBS) course run in the United Kingdom (UK) via The British Burn Association[3].

Epidemiology

Though minor cutaneous burns are extremely common, in the UK deaths from burns are rare and becoming more so[4]. In the United States (US), with a population of 300 million, the American Burn Association (ABA) estimates that 500 000 burns are seen a year in US emergency departments, of which 40 000 were admitted as inpatients, 25 000 of these to specialized burn centres. Approximately 2500 of these had burns over 30% total body surface area (TBSA). 4000 patients died, with 75% of these dying before reaching hospital[5].

Inhalation injury occurs in approximately 10–20% of patients admitted to burn centres, increasing in frequency with increasing burn size. Inhalation injury, age, and burns size are the three most commonly cited predictive factors for prolonged ventilation, hospital stay, and death in burn patients[6–9].

Isolated inhalation injury, or inhalation injury with a minor cutaneous burn has a mortality rate of 0.3–5%[10,11]. However, the large ABA National Burn Repository 2007 database shows that the presence of an inhalation injury increases the risk of death in patients under 60, with burns under 20%, by 15 times[12]. With increasing age, and increasing burn size, the mortality increases dramatically, so that a patient older than 60, with a burn greater than 40% total body surface area (TBSA) and an inhalation injury has a predicted mortality of 90% in one study[10]. This compares with a predicted mortality of 30% without the inhalation element.

The relative rarity of inhalation injuries, and especially those related to major burns, make it unlikely for non-specialist to see many of these patients during their training, or subsequently. It is this fact that can make dealing with these cases even more difficult than it might be.

Although major burns and inhalation injury are rare they may be associated with a concurrent major cutaneous burn and high mortality.

An acute major burn admission to an emergency department

Acute major burn patients are an assault on the senses and emotions of all hospital staff. Visually they may be dramatic, they may overwhelm the olfactory senses, and one may have a patient screaming in agony. Emotionally, we all tend to sympathize with our patients, and few things can be as dramatic as dealing and empathizing with your first major burn victim.

Even hardened Accident and Emergency staff, anaesthetists, and surgeons can easily be distracted by the burn and forget to deal with these patients in the systematic way they would deal with other trauma victims. Most, if not all, burn units will have stories about missed injuries and pathologies turning up in patients referred to their units. Injuries seldom overlooked in other trauma situations such as cervical spine instabilities, thoracic emergencies, abdominal crises, long-bone fractures, myocardial infarcts, or potentially fatal concurrent drug overdoses, have all been anecdotally reported to have been missed by referring hospitals.

Cutaneous burns, per se, are in effect best left to the secondary survey of any major burn. It is best to initially 'ignore' the burn, and make sure your team concentrate on the whole patient! While gathering a quick history from the patient, relatives or ambulance staff, a full Advanced Trauma Life Support (ATLS) trauma survey is essential. The normal trauma team approach of the ABC(DEF) primary survey is mandatory until knowledge of the injury rules out such aspects as cervical spine protection. Common sense will tell us that an alert and orientated burn victim giving a history of a scald and without further trauma does not need a cervical collar. However, this is something that must be ruled out, rather than overlooked.

Burn victims may have jumped out of an upstairs window to escape a fire, may have been thrown across a room in a blast, or have been assaulted prior to immolation. If one does not know what happened, the presence of immediate life-threatening complications of polytrauma must be sought and discounted before treating a patient as an isolated burn. Seven per cent of burn admissions have been reported to have an associated polytrauma[13].

Though uncommon, it is not rare for suicidal patients to attempt their goal through self-immolation. On top of any ATLS management, thought should be given to any concurrent suicide attempt. All such patients should have blood sent for paracetamol and salycilate levels. Though jaundice at day 3 or 4 of a major burn may be more difficult to see through an eschar, an overlooked paracetamol overdose in a burn patient will still have the same outcome as one in a non-burn patient. Both could equally well be treated if detected early enough.

Burns occurring in the extremes of age are also often more likely a 'symptom' of other pathologies. Toddlers with colds are more likely to be seen with scalds than well children. More importantly, burns in the elderly may be caused by the effects of arrhythmias, myocardial infarcts, or cerebral vascular accidents. The burn in these patients, especially if minor, may be the least important pathology as far as longevity is concerned.

Dramatic as major burns are, they should not distract the team from treating the patient as a whole. Associated trauma or medical conditions must be dealt with systematically.

Primary survey: ABCDEF

Airway (cervical spine control)

Apnoeic patients and those with decreased consciousness and unable to maintain their own airway patency should be intubated forthwith. The possibility of impending airway compromise due to inhalation injury must be considered and continuously re-evaluated. This will be discussed later in this section. All burns patients should receive continuous high-dose humidified oxygen. Cervical spine control is mandatory until the history, examination, or radiological evidence rule out a neck injury.

Breathing

The chest and neck must be fully exposed, examined, and auscultated. A history of a blast or other trauma will make haemo/pneumothorax or other intrathoracic injury more likely. Inhalation injury, as discussed later, often shows little clinical signs initially, but may exacerbate existing pulmonary pathology, such as asthma. A high respiratory rate is a key finding. Pulse oximetry should be undertaken, but a blood gas analysis will be needed to check its validity.

Beware full thickness burns to the neck, abdomen, and chest. When a burn injury affects the whole of the dermis, the skin loses its elasticity and the ability to expand. In full thickness burns to the neck, oedema formation around the injury may lead to compression of the structures within the neck and airway obstruction. This is of greatest importance in children who have smaller diameter airways in the first place. When the trunk is extensively burned, the resulting decrease in compliance may reduce ventilation. In adults this is seen with circumferential burns of the chest. In children, who are abdominal breathers, this can occur with isolated anterior burns of the chest and upper abdomen. An escharotomy, a surgical incision down to subcutaneous fat, may be needed as a matter of urgency to avoid airway obstruction, to alleviate ventilatory embarrassment, or to prevent iatrogenic barotrauma secondary to mechanical ventilation.

Circulation

Tachycardia, delayed capillary refill (greater than 2 seconds) or tachypnoea may be early signs of cardiovascular inadequacy, though pain or the need for limb escharotomy may account for the first two signs. Hypotension is as always a late sign. Circulatory inadequacy may be secondary to the burn, but other causes such as associated trauma must be sought, especially in those who do not respond to the burn fluid resuscitation.

Disability

Alcohol and drug intoxication are common causes of accidents leading to burns. Though these may be a cause of a decreased level of consciousness, carbon monoxide poisoning, shock due to other causes, and head injuries must be excluded in all patients who present with an obtunded mental state.

Exposure

While all patients should be examined from head to toe, burns victims lose heat quickly through radiation and evaporation, and all possible means should be used to minimize heat loss and subsequent hypothermia.

Fluid resuscitation

Formal fluid resuscitation is recommended in adult burns over 15% TBSA, and in children with burns over 10%. Until the age of 10 years children have different body proportions, with larger head to limb ratios. An age specific burn body chart should be used for children under this age. A rough guide is that the patient's palmar area is one percent TBSA. Burn size is calculated from the 'Rule of Nines' or from a burn body chart. In the acute burn, fluids should be started at the time of primary survey, and formally calculated when appropriate. The subsequent fluid requirements can appear extravagant, especially in children, and it is useful to have them reviewed and agreed on by the local Burn Unit. This is often best done by faxing the unit a completed burn body chart, so they may agree the percentage of the burn involved and the fluid resuscitation volumes.

Ideally, two large-bore cannulae should be sited through unburned skin. In very large burns this may be difficult and central access via the groin, which is often spared even in massive burns, is a useful alternative. In current practice the standard fluid regimen in the UK is the Parkland formula. Fluid resuscitation is calculated as 3–4 ml Hartmann's solution/kg/% burn. Of this, the first half is given in the first 8 hours *from the time of injury*. The second half is given over the next 16 hours. In adults additional maintenance fluids are not required.

Children under 25 kg, with a greater surface to mass ratio, should receive additional maintenance fluid (4 ml/kg for first 10 kg, plus 2 ml/kg for next 10kg, plus 1 ml/kg for subsequent weight). In our unit we give such children Parkland plus maintenance fluid for the first 8 hours, then 50% of Parkland plus normal maintenance for the following 16 hours. Any further fluid requirements should be with judicious use of colloids.

Adequacy of fluid resuscitation should be monitored clinically, primarily by urinary output. This makes catheterization mandatory in these large burns. We aim for a urine output of 0.5 ml/kg/hour in adults and 1ml/kg/hour in children. The exception to this is in patients with haemoglobinuria or myoglobinuria where we aim for 1–2 ml/kg/hour, using sodium bicarbonate and mannitol.

Inhalation injury, in addition to a cutaneous burn, is associated with an increased fluid resuscitation requirement. However, further fluid should be given cautiously as there is an increasing suggestion that over-resuscitation results in increasing lung and tissue oedema with a deleterious outcome.

Pain

Burns hurt! Pain should be treated with incremental doses of intravenous opiates, given cautiously as necessary. The intramuscular route should never be used, as peripheral circulatory changes associated with burn shock will render absorption unpredictable.

Radiology

If appropriate, a full trauma screen of cervical spine, chest, and pelvis should be undertaken.

Secondary survey

History

An 'AMPLE' (Allergies, Medical, Past illnesses, Last meal, Events/Environment related to injury) history should be obtained. A burn history should be sought, in particular duration of exposure, type of clothing worn, temperature, and nature of fluid if scald, and adequacy of first aid measures. An inhalation history (see later) should also be taken, as well as any other relevant history of blast, ejection, assault, or other trauma.

Examination

A full examination from head to toe is required, including the eyes, which are commonly overlooked, and the back, where further burn is again commonly overlooked. The limbs should be carefully examined for the need for escharotomies, looking for circumferential burns, and the signs of decreasing limb perfusion (pain, paraesthesia, pulselessness, and paralysis).

Monitoring

Pulse oximetry, electrocardiogram, and blood pressure monitoring are minimum standards. Arterial lines are generally essential for large burns, where non-invasive blood pressure monitoring may be difficult, and facilitate regular blood gas analysis. Central venous access will generally be used in those requiring intensive care treatment. Cardiac output monitoring is usual in a Burn Unit Intensive Care, but may be useful to guide therapy if there is a delay in transfer to such a unit. Temperature monitoring, usually via a temperature urinary catheter (incorporating a temperature probe), is useful and may guide warming in a hypothermic patient.

Burn wounds

By the nature of the injury, burns are initially sterile. They do, of course, ultimately provide an ideal medium for bacterial colonization and bacterial growth. Initially they should be wrapped in a plastic cling film wrap until advice is sought from the local Burn Unit. Tetanus prophylaxis should be given in those who are currently not fully immunized.

Referral to a Burn Unit

The National Burn Care Group and British Burn Association have identified the specific injuries and criteria which should automatically trigger referral to a Burn Unit (Table 15.1.)[14].

Even the transfer of physiologically stable patients can be dangerous, and should be done carefully with adequately trained personnel, monitoring appropriate to the patient (this may require arterial line and central venous pressure monitoring), a full range of emergency drugs and equipment, and after discussion with the Burn Unit. The main worry is the airway, which should be secured if there is any doubt of deterioration during transfer, or cardiovascular collapse. Large-bore cannulae should be in place and securely fixed, and inotropes available if necessary.

Inhalation injury
Diagnosis of inhalation injury

Diagnosis or suspicion of inhalation injury is initially from the history:

What was the nature of the burn?

A flame, blast, or steam injury may lead to an inhalation injury. A scald is very unlikely to have an

Table 15.1 Criteria for referral to a specialist Burn Unit

Burn greater than 10% TBSA in adults
Burn greater than 5% TBSA in children
Burns of special areas: face, hands, feet, genitalia, perineum, and major joints
Full thickness burns greater than 5% TBSA
Electrical burns
Chemical burns
Burns with associated inhalation injury
Circumferential burns of the limbs or chest
Burns at the extremes of ages
Burn injury in patients with pre-existing medical disorders which could complicate management, prolong recovery, or effect mortality
Any burn patient with associated trauma

inhalation element unless associated with a significant steam injury. An exception to this is a full thickness scald to the neck, especially in a child, which may cause airway obstruction due to the loss of the elasticity of the skin and subsequent oedema within the neck.

Was the fire in an enclosed space?

A history of fire or smoke in an enclosed space should raise suspicion of an inhalation injury. The longer the entrapment in such an environment, the stronger the suspicion of injury. Burns sustained in the open air will be less likely to have a high chance of such an injury, though petrol immolation and prolonged burning of clothing may add to the risk.

Was the patient unconscious at scene?

Any history of unconsciousness should raise suspicions of the patient suffering a significant inhalation injury. An unconscious patient loses the protective ability to breath-hold and to extricate themselves quickly. The cause of the unconsciousness may also be directly due to an inhalation injury (see next section).

Signs of inhalation injury (Table 15.2)

Burns around the *face* and *mouth* and *singed nasal hairs*, while not pathognomic of an inhalation injury, indicate proximity to the heat source, and are strongly associated with a thermal airway inhalation injury. They also have the potential to increase the difficulty of any subsequent intubation attempt. The swelling and oedema of facial burns can be extremely impressive in

the first few hours and days of an injury and if intubation is warranted to secure an airway, it should be done ideally before this is problematic.

The standard exceptions are facial scalds (without a significant steam injury, or oral ingestion of burning liquids) and 'flash flame' burns. If the patient can give a history of a single flash of heat/flame, no oral involvement, and the telltale sparing of the 'smile' lines around the eyes ('crow's feet') and nasolabial folds, they are unlikely to have significant airway injury.

Soot in the mouth and nose are suggestive of smoke inhalation, but not as important as *blistering, oedema,* or *burn within the oral cavity*. The latter should be taken extremely seriously. A *'brassy' cough, respiratory difficulty, wheeze,* or an *altered or hoarse voice* are all indicative of an inhalation injury. A conscious patient complaining of an altered voice, especially where they are subjectively describing worsening of voice quality should also be taken seriously. A report of difficulty in swallowing is also strongly indicative.

Carbonaceous secretions seem to be less exact than other signs and should be regarded as an indicator to exposure but not more.

Examination

Dyspnoea, wheeze, cyanosis, inspiratory stridor, and *increased respiratory rate* are rare presenting signs but must be dealt with quickly. Confusion and restlessness, though these may be due to other causes, may indicate hypoxia and the requirement for urgent treatment.

Initial investigations

Blood gas analysis and carboxyhaemoglobin levels are mandatory as a baseline, and to evaluate any degree of carbon monoxide poisoning. Carboxyhaemoglobin levels may be extrapolated to the time of injury using a nomogram. A chest X-ray should also always be taken routinely.

Table 15.2 Suspicion of inhalational injury

Flame, blast, or steam injury
Injury in an enclosed space
Unconsciousness at scene
Burns to the face, neck, nose, or mouth
Soot in the mouth or nose
A cough, respiratory difficulty, or wheeze
A hoarse voice or difficulty in swallowing

Mechanism of inhalation injury

Inhalation injury is caused by either direct thermal damage to the airway, or by the effects of the products of combustion, or both. The products of combustion can be broken down into those due to toxic non-particulate gases, and those due to particulate smoke. This gives the traditional description of a triad of toxic gases, injury above the cords, and injury below the cords, which make up the 'smoke inhalation complex'. It is thus divided into three modalities on pathophysiological and anatomic differences. While some may only suffer one aspect of the complex, many patients will have a range of symptoms and pathology involving at least two of the modalities.

Systemic gaseous toxins

Deaths at the scene of a fire are often attributed to the victim being 'overcome by the effects of smoke'. It is actually unlikely that these unlucky people are killed by smoke, but instead die of hypoxia. The hypoxia is due to a decreased availability of oxygen found during a fire, with oxygen concentrations decreasing to 10–15% in a burning building[15,16]. In addition, gaseous systemic toxins lead to a decreased tissue availability of oxygen. Burning the materials found in modern life produces many toxic products of combustion. The two we are primarily concerned with in this role are carbon monoxide and hydrogen cyanide.

Carbon monoxide toxicity

Carbon monoxide is a leading cause of smoke-related fatalities, causing up to 80% of deaths[17,18]. Carbon monoxide is rapidly transported across the alveolar membrane and preferentially binds to haemoglobin. It has an affinity with haemoglobin 210 times that of oxygen, reducing oxygen carriage and therefore the delivery of oxygen to the tissues[19]. It shifts the oxygen dissociation curve to the left, so bound oxygen is released poorly to tissues. The affinity of carbon monoxide for myoglobin causes myocardial depression, hypotension, and arrhythmias[20]. It also binds to hepatic and other cytochromes and causes peroxidation of cerebral lipids[19].

Neurological signs include confusion, disorientation, visual changes, syncope, seizures. and coma. Arrhythmias and myocardial infarction may be provoked in those with coronary heart disease. The extent of injury is dependant on the concentration of carbon monoxide, the duration of exposure, and an individual's underlying health status. Long term, the delayed development of neuropsychiatric impairment is often a serious complication for survivors[19].

Normal carboxyhaemoglobin levels in an average person are less than 5%, but may be up to 9% in a heavy smoker. Serious toxicity is often associated with carboxyhaemoglobin levels above 25%, and the risk of fatality is high with levels over 70%. However, no consistent dose response effect has been found between levels and clinical effects[21]. Therefore, carboxyhaemoglobin levels provide a guide to exposure levels (and predictors of the chance of other inhalation injuries), and do not reliably predict clinical course or outcome[22].

Pulse oximeters cannot generally distinguish between oxyhaemoglobin and carboxyhaemoglobin, and should not be relied on until carboxyhaemoglobin levels are in the normal range.

Treatment

Oxygen

The half-life of carboxyhaemoglobin is 320 minutes breathing room air at sea level. This is reduced to 80 minutes with the administration of 100% oxygen[23]. Therefore, all suspected or confirmed cases of carbon monoxide poisoning should have high-flow (humidified) oxygen via a tight fitting non-rebreathing mask. Intubation is called for in those who are comatose and unable to maintain their own airway, or in those with thermal damage to their upper airway (see later).

Hyperbaric oxygen

Hyperbaric oxygen therapy has been used to treat carbon monoxide poisoning and results in even faster displacement of carbon monoxide from the blood. At three atmospheres of oxygen the half-life of carboxyhaemoglobin is 23 minutes. This treatment has been shown to be most likely ineffective if started more than 6 hours after exposure[24].

Does displacing the carbon monoxide from haemoglobin improve cell survival or neurological status in the long term? There are six randomized controlled trials involving hyperbaric oxygen therapy for carbon monoxide poisoning. A Cochrane database showed four of these did not give improved long-term benefit, and two did. It concluded that there was no evidence that the use of hyperbaric oxygen reduced the incidence of neurological sequalae[25].

Hyperbaric oxygen may have a place in the management of severe carbon monoxide poisoning, but the logistics of transfer and treatment in the severely burned are formidable. It should be considered for patients with a carboxyhaemoglobin level greater than about 40% or 20% in pregnant women. In practice it is rarely performed.

Prognosis

Acutely, carbon monoxide poisoning tends to either kill at scene or allow recovery as it is washed out of the system. This may require supportive treatment to deal with seizures, cardiac abnormalities, pulmonary oedema, or acidosis, but for each moment post exposure the situation improves. However, long-term neuropsychiatric problems may occur in up to 30% of these patients[26].

Cyanide toxicity

Oral cyanide poisoning leads to a rapidly developing coma, apnoea, cardiac dysfunction, severe lactic acidosis, and associated high mixed venous oxygen and low arteriovenous oxygen content difference[27]. There is controversy about whether cyanide toxicity has any role in mortality or morbidity in the victims of fire[28].

Those who do not believe in the cyanide poisoning theory of smoke inhalation point to the fact that levels in fire recreations are low[29], it is a normal metabolite[30,31], it is released by many organs after death[31], and that data on fatal levels is highly variable[32,33].

Proponents of cyanide poisoning in smoke inhalation note that cyanide is found in smoke, in the blood of fire victims[34-38], and the knowledge that oral cyanide poisoning mirrors the metabolic acidosis seen in some fire victims.

Whatever the outcome of the debate, cyanide poisoning would be synergistic with concurrent carbon monoxide poisoning and the hypoxic air found during a fire, and this may explain why sublethal levels of carbon monoxide and cyanide are found in some deaths from fire. Symptoms are similar to carbon monoxide poisoning, with severe acidosis and an obtunded patient.

Diagnosis

Blood samples can be taken, but there is presently no quick test, and for other than post mortem or research purposes serve no direct patient benefit. A severe metabolic acidosis, high venous oxygen saturation, and a narrow arteriovenous oxygen gradient may be signs of potential poisoning. However, in any case of a metabolic acidosis in a burn patient, it must be first assumed to be due to under-resuscitation, carbon monoxide poisoning, or unrecognized concomitant trauma. Only once these have been ruled out should the possibility of cyanide poisoning be ruled in.

Treatment

Supportive therapy is the mainstay of treating suspected cyanide toxicity. 'Antidotes' such as dicolalt edetate, hydroxycobalamin, thiosulphate, sodium nitrite, amyl nitrate, dimethylaminophenol are available, but are not without their own, occasionally fatal, side effects. Use of these agents in an inhalation injury should only be on the advice of the local Burn Unit.

Thermal damage to the airway

It is the thermal injury component of the smoke inhalation triad that has the potential to become the anaesthetist's worst nightmare. The 'can't ventilate, can't intubate' scenario is caused by direct heat injury by the hot air, gases, or vapours to the oropharynx and upper airway. Because the heat exchange capabilities of the upper airway are so efficient, even super-heated air is rapidly cooled before reaching the lower respiratory tract. This is therefore often referred to as injury above the cords. The thermal damage to the airway depends on the heat capacity characteristics of the gas or vapour and the duration of exposure. Dry gases have less injurious effects than saturated vapours at the same temperature. Burns below the glottis are extremely rare and only occur if super-heated soot particles or steam are inhaled.

The thermal injury (Table 15.3) produces immediate injury to the mucosa, causing oedema, erythaema, and ulceration. Oedema forms rapidly due to a combination of altered hydrostatic pressures, increased vascular permeability, and cytokine and free radical release[39-46]. Though oedema will form spontaneously, it is accelerated by fluid resuscitation, especially over-aggressive fluid resuscitation. Anecdotal evidence from unintubated patients received at the Royal Darwin Hospital more than 24 hours following the Bali bombings of 2002, showed that suboptimal fluid resuscitation may have been fortuitous in maintaining the airway patency in several patients with an airway burn. Once more aggressive fluid resuscitation was implemented there was an increase in airway oedema, and the necessity for expert airway skills to urgently secure these airways[47]. However, fluid should not be withheld as delayed fluid resuscitation (greater than 2 hours) has been shown to increase the rates of sepsis,

Table 15.3 Thermal injury

A thermal burn to the oropharynx can lead to rapid complete airway obstruction

Diagnosis is on history, signs, and careful examination

Early, though not hasty, intubation is the treatment of choice

Late intubation is dangerous and may be very challenging

The airway oedema will usually resolve in 3–5 days, and providing no further indication for ventilation, the patient can safely be extubated after careful examination of the airway

renal failure, cardiac arrest, multiorgan failure, and death[48].

The effects of an airway burn are caused by increasing oedema leading to direct airway obstruction and ultimately occlusion. Airway oedema may not be maximal until up to 24 hours, but will usually manifest itself within 2–6 hours.

Consequence of an airway burn

Airway burn may lead to airway obstruction due to intraoral and laryngeal oedema and swelling. This is often complicated by anatomical distortion of the face and neck due to burn and subsequent oedema of theses areas. Oral oedema will also lead to a decreased ability to clear secretions and with impaired protection from airway aspiration injury.

Clinical signs

Signs of potential impending airway obstruction include erythema and oedema of the mucosa in the mouth; significant facial burns; carbonaceous sputum; singed nasal hairs; and an altered or hoarse voice. Pulse oximetry and blood gas analysis are of little predictive power, as these will only be significantly altered in a pre-terminal state.

Symptoms

Altered voice, perceived difficulty in swallowing, and oropharyngeal pain may be present prior to extremis. Other symptoms, stridor, dyspnoea, increased work of breathing, tracheal tug, intercostal recession, paradoxical breathing pattern or cyanosis, do not appear until it is nearly too late.

Treatment

The possibility of pending airway obstruction must be considered continuously while administering high-dose humidified oxygen. This must be done in an environment where urgent intubation can be safely performed. Change in voice quality may be a sign of progressive oedema, and should be monitored in those who are initially felt not to warrant early intubation. In addition, these patients should have a gentle examination of the oropharynx using a spatula or laryngoscope, to rule out erythema, oedema, or blistering. Nasendoscopy, after adequate preparation of the nose with local anaesthetic, will also allow direct visualization of the posterior oropharynx. These procedures may need repeating if there are any changes in symptomology.

If, however, there are major suspicions or signs of a direct thermal burn, the treatment of choice is early, semi-urgent intubation. A wait and see approach is only justifiable in those where a true airway burn is believed to be unlikely. All Burn Units would prefer to receive a live intubated patient and extubate them, than a dead one. Even more important is the management of any transfers. If there were doubt about a patient's airway, it would be better to either electively intubate them prior to transfer, or delay the transfer until such time as the airway is known to be safe. The last place to tackle a rapidly obstructing airway is in the back of a moving ambulance.

Intubation

If a thermal injury to the oropharynx is confirmed or strongly suspected, the patient should be intubated early. A large-bore endotracheal tube should be placed to secure the airway, allow airway toilet, and ensure optimal management of secretions. Though a semi-urgent procedure, a patient with no symptoms of imminent airway loss should be allowed a few moments with loved ones where possible. It is one of the few times where one can have a completely lucid patient, and know that it is not inconceivable that you may be the last person who ever speaks to them while they are conscious. This is especially true in large burns with inhalation injury, where those who die will seldom come off a ventilator prior to their demise.

Late intubation in extremis should be avoided at all costs. It necessitates the presence of the most skilled anaesthetist experienced in difficult airway available at short notice, the full array of difficult airway adjutants, and a surgeon or anaesthetist capable of inserting a subglottic airway (cricothyroid or tracheostomy) very quickly.

Prognosis

Airway oedema, though maximal at 24 hours, will usually take 3–5 days to resolve. During this time the tube should be left in place (it could be disastrous to change it), and the oedema left to settle. Once there is a good leak around the tube, the airway has been examined to show resolution of the oedema, and providing the patient's vital signs and ventilation allow it, they may be extubated.

'Smoke' injury to the lungs

Inhalation of particulate smoke past the vocal cords makes up the third component of the inhalation injury complex, also referred to as injury below the cords. The carbonaceous material present in the smoke particles is not thought to be directly responsible for subsequent damage, but serves as a carrier for other agents[49]. The exact nature of the associated toxic products of combustion depends on the materials incinerated. Common materials such as cotton and polyvinyl chloride produce multiple toxic compounds including aldehydes, the oxides of sulphur and nitrogen, hydrochloric acid, and carbon monoxide[50,51]. Toxic compounds in the smoke cause redox reactions, a chemical tracheobronchiolitis, and local or systemic cytokine release. This causes an oedematous tracheobronchial mucosa[52], de-epithelization, shedding of the epithelial lining, and formation of pseudomembranous casts[53]. These casts are composed of mucous, cellular debris, fibrinous exudates, polymorphonuclear leucocytes, and clumps of bacteria. Pulmonary compliance is markedly decreased[54], and surfactant is inactivated causing microatelectasis and a ventilation perfusion mismatch.

Though pathological changes occur almost immediately following inhalation of smoke, hypoxia, rales, rhonchi, and wheezes are seldom present on admission. Chest X-rays are almost always unremarkable on day 1, though two-thirds of patients develop changes of diffuse or focal infiltrates, or pulmonary oedema by day 5–10[55].

Diagnosis

Diagnosis is by clinical suspicion in the first instance, confirmed in most centres by bronchoscopic findings of soot, mucosal necrosis, airway oedema, and inflammation[56,57]. Some centres use xenon scanning[58], which can evaluate true parenchymal damage not identified on bronchoscopy alone.

Management

Apart from supportive treatment, the mainstay of therapy is via various nebulizer regimens. Patients should be given humidified oxygen, guided by serial blood gas analysis, have early chest physiotherapy, and be started immediately on the local nebulizer protocol.

Nebulizers

Though the mainstay of active treatment for smoke inhalation, there is very limited data on the efficacy of these various treatments. In a survey of UK Burn Units carried out by our unit[59], the majority of units used nebulized agents, though few had written protocols in place. Of those using nebulized agents most used salbutamol, and either heparin, N-acetylcystine, or sodium bicarbonate. Other agents used included dornase-alpha, ipratropium, and prostacycline.

Salbutamol

Salbutamol is useful in helping with the bronchospasm resulting from the chemical bronchitis, especially in those with pre-existing reactive airway disease. It can also be used prior to N-acetylcystine to prevent it inducing bronchospasm.

Heparin

Heparin is used to break down fibrin deposits, which form a major part of cast-like plugs that can obstruct the bronchioles. Evidence for the use of heparin in burns is probably the most robust, though largely carried out in animal models of smoke inhalation. A retrospective study in children has shown it to be effective in paediatric patients when combined with N-acetylcystine.

N-acetylcystine

N-acetylcystine is a powerful mucolytic agent, but also is an irritant to the respiratory tract and can cause bronchospasm. It is also a free radical scavenger.

Bicarbonate

Bicarbonate is a mucolytic, and is also used in the hope that it may buffer some of the toxic compounds within the smoke and hence decrease the inflammatory cascade produced by the redox reactions.

As stated, evidence in human burns is largely weak or non-existent for these nebulizer regimens, and thus there is little consensus for which to follow.

Our unit uses an ongoing hourly nebulizer regimen consisting of 5 ml 2.1% bicarbonate, followed by salbutamol, then N-acetylcystine. This is continued until there is no soot seen on bronchoscopy or the patient stops coughing up carbonaceous sputum. This is usually around day 5.

Though purely anecdotal, 'plugging', which was a constant cause of desaturation in these patients, is now very rarely seen in our unit, and unpublished mortality figures compare favourably to published ones.

Primary referral centres are advised to contact their local Burn Unit for advice and to discuss their local protocols. Important factors to be considered in inhalational injuries are summarized in Table 15.4.

Intubation

Particulate smoke inhalation victims without any associated upper airway thermal burn, and with a normal conscious level, do not need or benefit from immediate or prophylactic intubation (Table 15.5). Having said this, a high level of suspicion for upper airway burn must be maintained in any patient with signs of smoke inhalation. Instead, these patients should be carefully monitored with serial blood gas analysis and continuous pulse oximetry. As stated, hypoxia is rarely an initial feature of particulate smoke inhalation, and is usually delayed until day 3 or 4. Deterioration in blood gases and increasing requirements for supplemental oxygen indicate the need for rapid elective intubation. However, if continuous positive airway pressure or other forms of non-invasive ventilation are available in an otherwise stable patient, these should be explored initially.

Though often ultimately necessary, intubation and ventilation for prolonged periods is a bad prognostic sign. The ABA National Burn Repository 2008[5] shows a vast increase in pneumonia, adult respiratory distress syndrome, septicaemia, and organ failure for those ventilated more than 4 days. Galeiras et al.[60] also propose that early intubation with or without inhalation injury in burn patients, is predictive for mortality, and that inhalation injury per se is not an independent risk factor. Though these do not distinguish between cause and effect, it is well known that mechanical ventilation, and especially ventilator-acquired pneumonia, are associated with a higher mortality in all patients[61]. Thus, if intubation can be avoided, it is best avoided. In reality the majority with a significant cutaneous burn complicating an inhalation burn will need a prolonged period of ventilation.

Mechanical ventilation should be implemented with lung protective strategies, low pressure, low tidal volumes, and appropriate levels of positive end-expiratory pressure. Nebulizers should continue once ventilated, and bronchoscopy performed daily for microbiological samples and bronchial toilet. A ventilator care bundle approach with head up 30 degrees and sedation holds should be commenced and early tracheostomy considered.

Early extubation is always the main goal in treating these patients. But it must be noted that many of these patients also suffer from significant cutaneous burns. The treatment of the latter vastly complicates the treatment of the inhalation element of these burns patients. They will often require multiple major debridement and grafting operations and regular dressing changes over a period of days or months. While this in itself provides many opportunities for a 'second hit' phenomena, it also makes timing of extubations difficult. This inevitably elongates time on a ventilator, and combined with multiple blood transfusions, bacteraemias and the like, contribute to the increasing mortality seen in these patients with increasing size of burn.

Prognosis

Deaths are invariably due to multiorgan failure, preceded by sepsis and pneumonia[62]. Deaths tend to fall into a small early group, within a week or so, or a larger late group at 3 weeks or longer. The early group

Table 15.4 Important considerations in inhalational injury

The symptoms from inhalation of smoke particles are often delayed for several days
Ongoing cytokine release, oedema, and pseudomembranous cast formation cause an increasing perfusion mismatch and deterioration in lung function
Intubation is a bad prognostic sign and all reasonable attempts to avoid this (if uncomplicated by a thermal airway burn) should be investigated first
Intubation is in reality often needed, but the aim should be extubation as soon as safe
Nebulizer regimen are widely used, under-validated, but largely thought to be beneficial
Death is a common outcome, but survivors can be left with little residual pulmonary morbidity

Table 15.5 Top tips for intubating burn patients

If in doubt intubate! Early extubation in a Burn Unit is better than an emergency difficult intubation
If a semi-urgent intubation is required in a pink, fully conscious, and respiratorily undistressed patient, allow the patient a brief time to speak with relatives first if possible
A patient with stridor or respiratory distress will be a difficult airway until proved otherwise. Intubation should be performed quickly, but after mustering the most appropriate anaesthetist available and a full range of airway adjutants including a cricothyroid needle/airway
A rapid sequence induction is usually warranted in these patients
Suxamethonium is allowed and safe to use in the first 24 hours
Never cut the endotracheal tube. This is especially important in facial burns. These can swell dramatically and leave a cut tube apparently disappearing down the throat of the victim. Changing tubes in a thermal inhalation injury is fraught with danger
Document the grade of intubation, any evidence of soot or oedema, or airway abnormality. This will help the receiving hospital in planning treatment
Tubes are precious and should be firmly secured. At the same time, the tube tie should not cause damage or obstruct venous blood return and increase facial oedema. Therefore if a tube tie is used it must be secure, but loosely tied, somewhat of an oxymoron. An ideal alternative is to tie it to a dental wire placed securely to a stable tooth

often die of rapid overwhelming sepsis or a systemic inflammatory response syndrome picture, and sudden multiorgan failure. The late group tend to show a steadier decline in overall organ function, associated with several septic episodes interspersed with times of improvement. Ultimately they seem to 'run out of reserves'.

Survivors either tend to make a quick recovery over a week or so (mainly those with small cutaneous burns), or a slow recovery interspersed with septic episodes, over a few weeks or months. Survivors however, can be left with few chronic problems secondary to the inhalation injury. Chronic airway disease is relatively rare in adults[63,64]. Children however, may show decreased pulmonary function for up to 10 years post injury[65]. Subglottic tracheal stenosis is not uncommon in those intubated for long periods but can be reduced by minimizing cuff pressures in endotracheal or tracheostomy tubes.

Intensive care therapy

Intensive care treatment is similar to that of 'normal' intensive care patients. Burn management requires special emphasis on early nutritional support, stress ulcer prophylaxis until full enteral feeding is established, micronutrient support, thromboprophylaxis, mandatory patient isolation, 'heightened' paranoia for infection control, thermoregulation, acute and chronic pain issues, and early psychological input to patients and relatives.

Though there is conflicting data as to benefit[66–68] we strive for 'early' placement of tracheostomy in all patients who will require prolonged ventilation. This is only done through unburned or grafted skin, and for this reason the priority at any initial operation is to debride and graft the front of the neck. Once the graft has healed it is usually inserted percutaneously. It allows a decreased level of sedation, easier pulmonary toilet, and ideally early mobilization even in ventilated patients.

Patients may spend weeks or months in intensive care, with multiple septic episodes, multiple staged operations, and even more dressing changes. Relatives should be informed that it will be an emotional rollercoaster of highs and lows, and be always warned that death is a real possibility.

Immediate major burn debridement

Early debridement is now the standard aim in most Burn Units. The operative aim is to debride and graft the burn wound as quickly and efficiently as possible while maintaining stable patient haemodynamics. By excising the full thickness areas of the wound it is hoped that there will be a decreased cytokine production, less wound infections, and hence a decrease in mortality and morbidity. As yet this has not been shown definitively, but has the advantage of reduced blood loss when compared with late debridement[69]. Despite this, large excisions can have extensive and rapid blood loss, and planning is needed to take this into account. The wound is then covered with skin from non-burned areas of the patient (autograft), or dressed with donated cadaver skin (allograft), or with a synthetic skin substitute or other dressing. Once healed, the patient's skin can be reharvested from previous donor sites and applied to areas that had been previously temporarily dressed.

Fine judgement is often required as to the timing of operations in the critically ill burn patient. Often a sick patient may be better off after surgery and so it goes ahead, while some patients will need a delay to optimize their physiology prior to any further insult.

General considerations for anaesthesia for burns excision and grafting

Although large burns could be considered the 'glamorous' aspect of burn surgery, the majority of burn patients have smaller burns that are uncomplicated with inhalation injury. The burns case mix is often far from representative of the general population. Patients at the extremes of age suffer proportionally more burns than the general population, as do those with pre-existing morbidities such as epilepsy, alcohol or drug dependency, or psychiatric illness. Adults, but more commonly children, with burns are not infrequently the victims of non-accidental injury. Below are some general aspects that need careful consideration:

Venous access

This can be difficult in those with significant burns, burns to the limbs, and in small infants. The usual sites for venous access, including central access, are frequently burned, or may have been put out of action during any resuscitation phase. Femoral access is often possible when other sites are not available. If a major debridement is planned, at least two large-bore cannulae should be sited as blood and fluid loss can be rapid and considerable (see later).

Airway problems

As with any other patient requiring a general anaesthetic, the airway should be evaluated for predicted difficult intubation or mask ventilation (see Chapter 4). Acute burns to the face will make mask ventilation problematic and intubation may also be made more difficult. A chronic burn to the face and neck may result in limited mouth opening and a reduced neck extension making intubation predictably difficult. It is especially important to re-evaluate the airway in

long-stay patients who present for surgery regularly. 'Familiarity breeds contempt' is an apt saying for these patients, who may be a grade one intubation on a Monday, but due to rapid neck contractures may be closer to a grade four by Friday. Though rare, some of these patients will be best suited to securing their airway with an awake intubation prior to induction of anaesthesia.

Blood loss

Blood loss can be a significant problem in major burn excisions. A very rough guide is 100 ml of blood loss for every 1% surface area excised. With improved surgical techniques, and an ever-decreasing transfusion trigger, the massive blood transfusion requirements of old are now seldom seen. Realization that the avoidance of hypothermia has an important role in normalizing blood clotting, has also improved the situation. However, blood should be cross-matched for all but the smallest excisions, and certainly available for debridements approaching 10%.

Temperature

Burn patients lose heat quickly due to a combination of radiation and evaporation from the burn wound. During surgery this is compounded by the skin prep prior to surgery, the large exposed areas often required, the lengthy operations, the loss of core–periphery homeostasis caused by anaesthetic agents, and the administration of large volumes of intravenous fluids often required. This is even worse at the extremes of ages.

Any resulting hypothermia is likely to increase the already high metabolic rate of major burns, increase surgical bleeding, wound infection, pulmonary infection, cardiac function, and results in increased morbidity and mortality.

Core temperature should be monitored carefully in all but the shortest operations and all measures taken to maintain it at levels 'normal' for that patient. Hypermetabolic, hyperthermic patients are probably best kept close to their starting core temperature.

Despite making it uncomfortable for staff, theatre temperature should be above 27°C and areas of the body not being operated on covered. Forced air warming devices should be used, though they may be of little value if insufficient areas of the patient are available for coverage. Alternative devices such as under-body forced air devices, warming mattresses, and radiant heaters should be used as appropriate. All fluids must be administrated via a fluid warmer. Pre-warming of patients should also be strongly considered. If hypothermia still occurs, it may be better to delay or suspend surgery while more extreme measures such as warm bladder irrigation are used to achieve normothermia.

Drugs

Pathophysiological changes after a burn injury alter patients' normal pharmacokinetics. Absorption, bioavailability, protein binding, volumes of distribution, and clearance are all affected[72]. These alterations are dependant on the size of the burn, and the time since the burn[73].

Initially the hypovolaemia leads to a hypoperfusion state, and absorption of drugs given by any route other than the intravenous route is delayed and unpredictable[74]. Albumin levels decrease, and plasma protein binding of albumin-bound drugs is decreased, resulting in an increased free fraction of drug with a larger volume of distribution[75]. Most anaesthetic agents are not protein bound and with the effects of the major haemodynamic changes seen in burns, clinically the pharmacology of anaesthetic drugs is minimally altered. In addition, fluid loss to the burn wound and general oedema can decrease plasma concentrations of many drugs below those expected.

After this initial phase there is increased blood flow to the kidneys and liver and increased drug clearance[76]. These alterations in drug pharmacokinetics show a wide patient-to-patient variability and may require alterations in the dosing of various drugs to suit the individual patient[73,77]. This is often clinically relevant in the dosing of various antibiotics.

Anaesthetic drugs
Suxamethonium

Suxamethonium is safe to use in the first 24 hours after a major burn. After this time it is contraindicated because it is associated with a profound acute hyperkalaemia, which may result in cardiac arrest. It is caused by a proliferation of extrajunctional acetylcholine receptors leading to a resistance to non-depolarizing muscle relaxants and the hypersensitivity to suxamethonium[70]. The effect is proportional to the total burns surface area. The drug data sheet states that the 'greatest risk of hyperkalaemia is from about day 5 to 70 days after injury and may be further prolonged if there is delayed healing due to persistent infection'. It is unclear how long it should be avoided, but figures of 9 months to 2 years are quoted in several texts.

Non-depolarizing muscle relaxants

All the non-depolarizing agents have been used successfully. There is a greatly increased ED_{50}, proportional to the size of the burn. If complete paralysis is required (e.g. complex eye surgery) neuromuscular blockade should be monitored carefully. A 'rapid sequence induction' can be achieved either with high-dose opiates (alfentanil/remifentanil) or with a dose of 1.5 mg/kg of rocuronium[71].

Volatile agents

Sevoflurane has replaced halothane as the inhalational agent of choice for gaseous induction. The incidence of halothane hepatitis was very small in burns patients, despite multiple uses at short intervals, probably relating to the immunocompromised state. The choice of anaesthetic agents does not seem to appear to influence the outcome from anaesthesia for burn surgery. The dose requirements for all anaesthetic agents are generally increased in the burns population due to their hypermetabolic state and hyperdynamic circulation. Minimum alveolar concentration (MAC) values are raised and the duration of action is decreased.

Opiates

Opiates given in conjunction with paracetamol and NSAID, where appropriate, are the mainstay of analgesia for burn wounds and postoperatively. Tolerance can develop quickly and with the hyperdynamic metabolism shown with large burns, doses required can be impressive. In a recent case, a large-burn patient required a dose of remifentanil of 4.5 mcg/kg/min to reduce spontaneous ventilation rate <20 breaths/minute.

Opiates cause side effects. As well as nausea, the major side effect, often overlooked in all surgical specialties, is constipation. Traditionally this is overlooked until this causes a problem before instituting appropriate therapy. All intensive care patients and all burns patients on regular opiates need appropriate prophylactic aperients charted regularly.

Tramadol

Tramadol can be a dramatically effective analgesic in some patients seemingly resistant to other analgesics.

Patient monitoring during anaesthesia

Monitoring burn patients, especially those with large burns, can be difficult. This is not helped by surgeons who may be working on all available sites, or by procedures such as a 'shower' dressing change, where electrical safety issues may severely limit what can be monitored. Compromise is the norm.

Electrocardiogram

Electrodes may float off in a sea of blood, ooze, or oily dressing. Staples through the electrode, or direct attachment to a staple or wire suture are often used.

Pulse oximeter

Pulse oximeter probes are often difficult to place, and ear probes to the cheek or even tongue can be useful.

Blood pressure

Blood pressure cuffs can be difficult to place, and occasionally arterial lines are needed for even small surgical procedures.

Capnography

End-tidal carbon dioxide measurement assumes added importance in the face of the difficulties previously listed.

Temperature

Temperature monitoring is important in all but the smallest case, and is most easily done in large cases with the aid of a temperature catheter.

Urinary catheters

Urinary catheters are used in all major cases, and urine output monitored throughout surgery.

Invasive monitoring

Central venous and arterial pressure monitoring are routine for all major excisions. As stated earlier, the groin is often the only non-burned access for these, making it important that they are inserted with scrupulous asepsis and by an experienced operator—the paucity of sites to reliably place these lines makes them less than ideal for novices to practise on.

Cardiac output monitors

Cardiac output monitors are especially useful in patients undergoing major debridements, where blood loss is difficult to calculate.

Postoperative anaesthetic care

It is difficult to anticipate the degree of fluid loss that will occur postoperatively. The haematocrit, haemoglobin concentration, urinary output, core–peripheral temperature gradient, and blood gas analysis are all indicative, but need staff who are aware of their meaning, and who will treat the patient

appropriately. All major debridements should be treated in a High Dependency Unit, or Intensive Care setting where the staffing and skills required to monitor and treat these patients are appropriate.

Good postoperative analgesia is a must, and feeding should be resumed early if it has been stopped in theatre.

Psychological care of the burn patient

Burn patients have many reasons to have major psychological problems following their injury. The mechanism of injury is always traumatic and may result in 'flash backs' and a degree of post-traumatic stress disorder. All patients will be disfigured to some degree and even in those in whom this is minor or relatively temporary this can be devastating. Patients are often faced with the knowledge that they are embarking on a series of operations, which in some instances can go on for decades. Disfigurement as a result of facial burns in particular can cause considerable psychosocial distress and adversely affect the patient's quality of life. Fears over long-term function, mobility, appearance, and employment issues are also common. Skilled psychological help is often required, but it is also very much a team effort for all the disciplines involved in their care. An anaesthetist who takes the time to sort out analgesic issues and who makes any operative visits pleasant will be rewarded with a more cooperative and easier to manage patient. An early 'bad' experience in the anaesthetic room may haunt all who go after.

Long-term management and problems of subsequent anaesthesia

Patients who have suffered major burns often endure years of corrective surgery following their discharge from the acute event. They are also just as likely as anyone else to have an acute abdomen or other event that requires urgent or elective surgery.

As in any patient a careful history and full examination should be performed prior to anaesthesia.

Special consideration needs to be taken of any potential difficult airway. Facial and neck burns can lead to reduced mouth opening and neck contractures. Evaluating neck extension is vital, as a reduced ability to extend the neck is associated with a reduction in the Mallampati score to four if severe. It can occasionally be severe enough to make any 'plan B' of a surgical airway impossible. It is vital to assess each patient on their own merits and if concerned, enrol the foremost airway specialist available, and the full range of difficult airway adjutants.

While most postburn patients will be straightforward, those with a neck contracture are probably best dealt with by an initial awake fibreoptic intubation. Even this may be tricky in the extreme case, and there are patients in whom a local anaesthetic surgical release of their neck contracture is needed even prior to this.

Vascular access may be a significant problem in some postburn patients and may necessitate obtaining central access prior to anaesthesia.

Suxamethonium is best avoided in patients who have suffered major burns within a year or two of surgery.

Conclusion

Burn patients, especially those with large burns or an inhalation burn, will need the dedicated and professional services found at a regional Burn Unit. Here they will hopefully be treated successfully and return to a functionally normal and happy life.

However, to get this opportunity, they first must rely on the professionalism and skills of the staff at the receiving hospital. A trauma team who can see past the burn and treat the patient is essential. An anaesthetist who can do this, and consider and appropriately treat any inhalation injury is vital. This is especially important in those who may be at risk of impending upper airway obstruction from a thermal airway burn. Though there are often major hurdles for these patients to overcome, it would all be academic if they were not treated appropriately in the first instance.

References

1. Wachtel TL, Frank DH, Frank HA. (1981) Management of burns of the head and neck. *Head & Neck Surg*, **3**, 458–74.
2. Herndon DN. (2007) *Total Burn Care*, 3rd edn. London: Elsevier Saunders.
3. The British Burn Association. Available online at http://www.britishburnsassociation.co.uk
4. Goldacre M, Duncan M, Cook-Mozaffari P, Davidson M, McGuiness H, Meddings D. (2006) *Burns in England 1996 to 2004. Mortality Trends. Unit of Health-Care Epidemiology.* Oxford University and South-East England Public Health Observatory.
5. American Burn Association Burn Incident Fact Sheet and National Burn Repository 2008. Available online at http://www.ameriburn.org/resources_factsheet.php
6. Smith DL, Cairns BA, Ramadan F, *et al.* (1994) Effect of inhalation injury, burn size, and age on mortality: a study of 1447 consecutive burn patients. *J Trauma*, **37**, 655–9.
7. Shirani KZ, Pruitt BA Jr, Mason AD Jr. (1987) The influence of inhalation injury and pneumonia on burn mortality. *Ann Surg*, **205**, 82–7.
8. Sellersk BJ, Davis BL, Larkin PW, Morris SE, Saffle JR (1997) Early prediction of prolonged ventilator dependence in thermally injured patients. *J Trauma*, **43**, 899–903.
9. Tredget EE, Shankowshy HA, Taerum TV, Moysa GL, Alton JD. (1990) The role of inhalation injury in burn trauma. A Canadian experience. *Ann Surg*, **212**, 720–7.
10. Ryan CM, Schoenfeld DA, Thorpe WP, *et al.* (1998) Objective estimates of the probability of death from burn injuries. *N Engl J Med*, **338(6)**, 362–6.
11. Edelman DA, White MT, Tyburski JD, Wilson RF. (2006) Factors affecting prognosis of inhalation injury. Journal of Burn Care & Research, **27(6)**, 848–53.
12. American Burn Association, National Burn Repository 2007 Report. Available online at hppt://www.ameriburn.org/2007NBRAnnualreport.pdf
13. Dougherty W, Waxman K. (1996) The complexities of managing severe burns with associated trauma. *Surg Clin N Am*, **76(4)**, 923–58.
14. National Burn Care Group. Available online at http://www.nbcg.nhs.uk/EasySiteWeb/GatewayLink.aspx?alld=39993
15. Cohen MA, Guzzardi LJ. (1983) Inhalation products of combustion. *Ann Emerg Med*, **12**, 628–32.
16. Demling RH. (1991) Physiological changes in burn patients. In: Wilmore DW, Brennan MF, Harken AH, Holcroft JW, Meakins JL. (eds) *American College of Surgeons Care of the Surgical Patient*. New York: Scientific American, Inc.
17. Ernst A, Zibrak JD. (1998) Carbon Monoxide poisoning. *N Engl J Med*, **339**, 1603–8.
18. Raub JA, Mathieu-Nolf M, Hampson NB, Thom SR. (2000) Carbon monoxide poisoning – a public health perspective. *Toxicology*, **145(1)**, 1–14.
19. Weaver LK. (1999) Carbon monoxide poisoning. *Crit Care Clin*, **15**, 297–317.
20. Ganong WF. (1995) *Review of Medical Physiology*. East Norwalk, CT: Appleton and Lange.
21. Hardy KR, Thom SR. (1994) Pathophysiology and treatment of carbon monoxide poisoning. *J Toxicol Clin Toxicol*, **32(6)**, 613–29.
22. Scheinkestel CD, Bailey M, Myles PS, *et al.* (1999) Hyperbaric or normobaric oxygen for acute carbon monoxide poisoning: a randomised controlled clinical trial. *Med J Aust*, **170(5)**, 203–10.
23. Peterson JE, Stewart RD. (1970) Absorption and elimination of carbon monoxide in inactive young men. *Arch Environ Health*, **21**, 165–71.

24. Goulon M, Barios A, Rapin M. (1969) Carbon monoxide poisoning and acute anoxia due to breathing of hydrocarbons. *Ann Med Interne*, **120**, 335–49.

25. Juurling DN, Buckley NA, Stanbrook MB, et al. (2005) Hyperbaric oxygen for carbon monoxide poisoning. *Cochrane Database Syst Rev*, **1**, CD002041.

26. Weaver LK, Hopkins RO, Howe S, Larson-Lohr V, Churchill S. (1996) *Undersea Hyperb Med*, **23**, 215–19.

27. Klaassen CD. (1996) *Casarett and Doull's Toxicology: The Basic Science of Poisons*, 5th ed. New York: McGraw-Hill.

28. Barillo DJ. (2009) Diagnosis and treatment of cyanide toxicity. *J Burn Care Res*, **30(1)**, 148–51.

29. Davies JWL. (1986) Toxic chemicals versus lung tissue – an aspect of inhalation injury revisited. *J Burn Care Rehabil*, **7**, 213–22.

30. Anderson RA, Harland WA. (1982) Fire deaths in the Glasgow area. III. The role of hydrogen cyanide. *Med Sci Law*, **22**, 35–40.

31. Symington IS, Anderson RA, Thomson I, Oliver JS, Harland WA, Kerr JW. (1978) Cyanide exposure in fires. *Lancet*, **2**, 91–2.

32. Curry AS, Price DE, Rutter ER. (1967) The production of cyanide in post mortem material. *Acta Pharmacol Toxicol*, **25**, 339–44.

33. Caravati EM, Litovitz TL. (1988) Pediatric cyanide intoxication and death from an acetonitrile-containing cosmetic. *JAMA*, **260**, 3470–2.

34. Silverman SH, Purdue GF, Hunt JL, Bost RO. (1988) Cyanide toxicity in burned patients. *J Trauma*, **28**, 171–6.

35. Clark CJ, Campbell D, Reid WH. (1981) Blood carboxyhaemoglobin and cyanide levels in fire survivors. *Lancet*, **1**, 1332–5.

36. Whetherell HR. (1966) The occurrence of cyanide in the blood of fire victims. *J Forensic Sci*, **11**, 167–73.

37. Barillo DJ, Goode R, Rush BF, Lin RL, Freda A, Anderson EJ. (1986) Lack of correlation between carboxyhemoglobin and cyanide in smoke inhalation injury. *Curr Surg*, **43**, 421–3.

38. Barillo DJ, Rush BF, Goode R, Lin RL, Freda A, Anderson EJ. (1986) Is ethanol the unknown toxin in smoke inhalation injury? *Am Surg*, **52**, 641–5.

39. Lund T, Wiig H, Reed RK. (1988) Acute post burn edema: role of strongly negative interstitial fluid pressure. *Am J Physiol*, **255**, H1069–74.

40. Arturson G. (1979) Microvascular permeability to macromolecules after thermal injury. *Acta Physiol Scand Suppl*, **2**, 111–22.

41. Lund T, Onarkeim H, Reed R. (1992) Pathogenisis of edema formation in burn injuries. *World J Surg*, **16**, 2–9.

42. Lund T, Reed RK. (1986) Microvascular fluid exchange following thermal skin injury in the rat: changes in extravascular colloid osmotic pressure, albumin mass water content. *Circ Shock*, **20**, 91–104.

43. Matsuda T, Tanaka H, Reyes HM, et al. (1995) Antioxidant therapy using high dose vitamin C: reduction of post resuscitation fluid volume requirements. *World J Surg*, **19**, 287–91.

44. Yoshioka T, Monafo W, Ayvazian VH, Deeitz F, Flynn D. (1978) Cimetidine inhibits burn edema formation. *Am J Surg*, **136**, C81–5.

45. Nwariaku FE, Sikes PJ, Lightfoot E, Mileski WJ, Baxter C. (1996) Effect of a bradykinin antagonist on the local inflammatory response following thermal injury. *Burns*, **22**, 324–7.

46. Barrow R, Ranwiez R, Zhang X. (2000) Ibuprofen modulates tissue perfusion in partial thickness burns. *Burns*, **26**, 341–6.

47. Palmer DJ, Stephens D, Fisher DA, Spain B, Read DJ, Notaras L. (2003) The Bali bombing: the Royal Darwin Hospital response. *Med J Aust*, **179**, 358–61.

48. Barrow RE, Herndon DN. (2000) Early fluid resuscitation improves outcomes in severely burned children. *Resuscitation*, **45(2)**, 91–6.

49. Zikria BA, Budd DC, Floch F, Ferrer JM. (1975) What is clinical smoke poisoning? *Ann Surg*, **181(2)**, 151–6.

50. Dowell AR, Kilburn KH, Pratt PC. (1971) Short-term exposure to nitrogen dioxide. Effects on pulmonary ultrastructure, compliance, and the surfactant system. *Arch Intern Med*, **128(1)**, 74–80.

51. Einhorn IN. (1975) Physiological and toxicological aspects of smoke produced during the combustion of polymeric materials. *Environ Health Perspect*, **11**, 163–89.

52. Head JM. (1980) Inhalation injury in burns. *Am J Surg*, **139(4)**, 508–12.

53. Walker HL, McLeod CG, McManus WF. (1981) Experimental inhalation injury in the goat. *J Trauma*, **21(11)**, 962–4.

54. Nieman GF, Clark WR, Wax SD, Webb SR. (1980) The effect of smoke inhalation on pulmonary surfactant. *Ann Surg*, **191(2)**, 171–81.

55. Putman CE, Lkoe J, Matthay RA, Ravi CE. (1977) Radiographic manifestations of acute smoke inhalation. *Am J Roentgenol*, **129(5)**, 865–70.

56. Wanner A, Cutchavaree A. (1973) Early recognition of upper airway obstruction following smoke inhalation. *Am Rev Respir Dis*, **108(6)**, 1421–3

57. Moylan JA, Adib K, Birnbaum M. (1975) Fibreoptic bronchoscopy following thermal injury. *Surg Gynecol Obstet*, **140(4)**, 541–3.

58. Moylan JA, Wilmore DW, Moulton DE, Pruitt BA. (1972) Early diagnosis of inhalation injury using 133 xenon lung scan. *Ann Surg*, **176(4)**, 477–84.

59. Prior K, Nordmann G, Sim K, Mahoney P, Yhomas R. (2009) Management of inhalational injuries in UK burns centers – a questionnaire survey. *J Intens Care Soc*, **10(2)**, 141–4.

60. Galeiras R, Lorente JA, Pertega S, et al. (2009) A model for predicting mortality among critically ill burn victims. *Burn*, **35**, 201–9.

61. Van der Kooi TI, de Boer AS, Mannien J, et al. (2006) Incidence and risk factors of device-associated infections and associated mortality at the intensive care in the Dutch surveillance system. *Intens Care Med*, **33(2)**, 271–8.

62. Saffle, JR, Sullivan JJ, Tuohig GM, Larson CM. (1993) Multiple organ failure in patients with thermal injury. *Crit Care Med*, **21(11)**, 1673–83.

63. Demling RH. (1987) Smoke inhalation injury. *Postgrad Med*, **82(1)**, 63–8.

64. Cahalane M, Demling RH. (1984) Early respiratory abnormalities from smoke inhalation. *JAMA*, **251(6)**, 771–3.

65. Mlcak R, Desai MH, Robinson E, *et al.* (2000) Inhalation injury and lung function – a decade later. *J Burn Care Rehabil*, **21(1)**.

66. Saffle JR, Morris SE, Edelman LRN. (2002) Early tracheostomy does not improve outcome in burn patients. *J Burn Care Res*, **23(6)**, 431–8.

67. Palmieri TL, Jackson WRRT, Greenhalgh DG. (2002) Benefits of early tracheostomy in severely burned children. *Crit Care Med*, **30(4)**, 922–4.

68. Griffiths J, Barber VS, Morgan L, Young JD. (2005) Systematic review and meta-analysis of studies of the timing of tracheostomy in adult patients undergoing artificial ventilation. *BMJ*, **330**, 1243.

69. Desai MH, Herndon DN, Broemeling L, Barrow RE, Nichols RJ, Rutan R. (1990) Early burn wound excision significantly reduces blood loss. *Ann Surg*, **211(6)**, 753–62.

70. Marathe PH, Dwersteg JF, Pavlin EG, Haschke RH, Heimbach DM, Slattery JT. (1989) Effect of thermal injury on the pharmacokinetics and pharmacodynamics of atracurium in humans. *Anesthesiology*, **70**, 752–5.

71. Han TH, Martyn JAJ. (2009) Onset and effectiveness of rocuronium for rapid onset of paralysis in patients with major burns: priming or large bolus. *BJA*, **102(1)**, 55–60.

72. Martyn JA. (1986) Clinical pharmacology and drug therapy in the burned patient. *Anesthesiology*, **65**, 67–75.

73. Jaehde U, Sorgel F. (1995) Clinical pharmacokinetics in patients with burns. *Clin Pharmacokinet*, **29**, 15–28.

74. Ziemniak JA, Watson WA, Saffle JR, Russo J Jr, Warden GD, Schentag JJ. (1984) Cimetidine kinetics during resuscitation from burn shock. *Clin Pharmacol Ther*, **36**, 228–33.

75. Martyn JA, Abernethy DR, Greenblatt DJ. (1984) Plasma protein binding of drugs after severe burn injury. *Clin Pharmacol Ther*, **35**, 535–9.

76. Bonate PL. (1990) Pathophysiology and pharmacokinetics following burn injury. *Clin Pharmacol*, **35**, 535–9.

77. Boucher BA, Hickerson WL, Kuhl DA, Bombassaro AM, Jaresko GS. (1990) Imipenem pharmacokinetics in patients with burns. *Clin Pharmaco Ther*, **48**, 130–7.

16

Anaesthesia for oral and maxillofacial malignancy

Anjum Ahmed-Nusrath, Seema Pathare, and Stephen Bonner

Pathology

Oral cancer is the sixth most common cancer worldwide and accounts for approximately 2% of all cancer-related deaths. Approximately 5000 new cases are diagnosed annually in the United Kingdom. In recent years, trends show a significant increase in the incidence of oral cancer in young males (aged under 40 years)[1].

The distribution of head and neck cancer is shown in Figure 16.1. Squamous cell carcinoma accounts for 90% of all malignant head and neck tumours, but a wide variety of other tumours and premalignant states may also present in this region (Table 16.1). Patients with oral cancer have a 10% risk of having a synchronous primary elsewhere in the aerodigestive tract. Almost 60% of patients present with advanced disease. Lesions in the head and neck region spread primarily by the lymphatic system and distal metastasis occur relatively late in the course of the disease. In all, 30–40% of patients with head and neck cancer have persistent or recurrent locoregional disease after completion of definitive treatment. Despite advances in cancer treatment, the overall 5-year survival rates for cancer of the oral cavity and pharynx have remained unchanged at around 55%[2].

The main predisposing factors are smoking and alcohol, which seem to have a synergistic effect. Chewing betel nut, tobacco, and poor oral hygiene are significant risk factors for oral cancer. In addition, more recent evidence is emerging of a link between viral infection with human papilloma virus 16 and oral cancer. Immunosuppression in solid-organ transplant recipients is also an important risk factor in a small subgroup. Head and neck cancer occurring in transplant patients tends to affect a younger group of patients and is more aggressive with a poorer outcome as compared to the general population. Cancer progression has been associated with loss of tumour suppressor oncogenes p16 and p53 and an increase in epidermal growth factor receptor, which is being investigated as a biomarker for the disease[3].

Management options

Head and neck cancer is staged on the basis of the tumour, node, and metastases (TNM) system (Table 16.2), which is useful in planning treatment and predicting outcome. Ideally, all cancer patients are seen at multidisciplinary team meeting comprising oncologists, surgeons, and radiologists who objectively assess and agree on the optimum management strategy.

The treatment depends on the patient's age, general medical condition, and tolerance, acceptance and compliance of the proposed treatment plan. The principal treatment options remain elective surgery and radical radiotherapy.

Traditionally, the primary modality of treatment has been surgery for squamous cell carcinoma of the oral cavity supplemented by adjuvant radiation therapy when indicated (in the majority of Stage III and IV cases). Although surgery with postoperative radiation remains the cornerstone in treatment, with recent advances in chemoradiation protocols and greater understanding of importance of organ preservation, the role of radiotherapy in the management of head and neck cancer is increasing[4] (see Chapter 17).

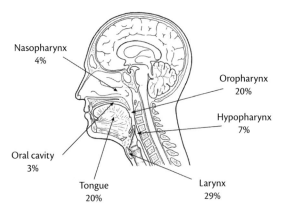

Figure 16.1 Anatomical distribution of cancer in the head and neck region. Salivary gland tumours form 8% of tumours seen in the head and neck region and the rest are secondaries to the neck.

Current evidence suggests that results of surgical excision are superior for lesions involving anterior tongue, mandible, and buccal mucosa as compared to those achieved with radical radiotherapy. For cancer of the base of tongue, oropharynx, and hypopharynx the survival figures are broadly similar with both modalities of treatment[5].

However, the overall medical condition and ability of the patient to tolerate an optimal therapeutic programme are important factors which govern the choice of treatment. The perioperative morbidity and mortality remain uniformly high with advancing age and associated cardiopulmonary conditions with extensive surgical treatment. This is where the anaesthetist should play a vital part in the multidisciplinary team in deciding the treatment plan. The potential benefits of surgical intervention in cancer patients must be weighed against the risks of surgery and alternative non-surgical therapeutic options must be explored.

Surgical management

Surgical management depends again upon the size, location, and type of tumour.

T1 lesions are excised and repaired with local flap reconstruction. Lesions of T2 and higher level require extensive resection. Elective neck dissection is advocated where nodal disease is present on either clinical or radiological examination or where the risk of spread to the nodes exceeds 20%. The majority of head and neck tumours metastasize in a predictable fashion to levels I–IV in the neck and rarely to other levels (Figure 16.2). Traditionally, radical neck dissection used to be performed, where the superficial and deep cervical fascia

Table 16.1 Histopathological subtypes of oral and maxillofacial cancer

Premalignant lesions
Erythroplakia
Leucoplakia
Lichen planus
Submucous fibrosis
Oral cavity, pharynx, and tongue
Squamous cell cancer
Verrucous cancer
Spindle cell carcinoma
Lymphoepithelial carcinoma
Salivary gland
Acinic cell cancer
Mucoepidermoid carcinoma
Adenocystic carcinoma
Vascular tissue
Hemangiopericytoma
Hemangiosarcoma
Tooth
Ondontogenic carcinoma
Ondontogenic sarcoma
Odontogenic myxoma
Bone
Osteosarcoma
Chondrosarcoma
Other tumours
Lymphoma
Burkitt's tumor
Kaposi's sarcoma
Neurofibroma

along with the lymph nodes within it were removed along with the sternocleidomastoid muscle, internal and external jugular vein, submandibular gland, and spinal accessory nerve. However, more recently radical neck dissection has lost favour because of a higher incidence of complications[6]. These include massive facial oedema, cerebral oedema resulting from the removal of internal jugular vein, and severe restriction of shoulder function caused by the excision of accessory nerve. In the 1990s, several studies showed that the integrity of neck dissection and subsequent

Table 16.2 Staging of head and neck cancer based on the tumour, node, and metastases (TNM) classification

T	Tumour size
T0: no primary tumour is present	
Tis: carcinoma *in situ*	
T1: the tumour is 2 cm or less	
T2: the tumour is 4 cm or less	
T3: the tumour is larger than 4 cm	
T4: the tumour is larger than 4 cm, and it has deeply invaded surrounding structures	
N	**Lymph node involvement**
N0: no lymphatic nodes involved	
N1: ipsilateral lymph node, less than 3 cm size	
N2: one or more ipsilateral lymph node, size less than 6 cm	
N3: few ipsilateral or contralateral nodes, size more than 6 cm	
M	**Distant metastases**
M0: no metastases are present	
M1: the cancer has spread to distal organs	
Stage grouping	
Stage I:	T1N0M0
Stage II:	T2N0M0
Stage III:	T3N0M0
	T1 or T2 or T3N1M0
Stage IV:	T4N0 or N1M0
	Any T, N2, or N3M0
	Any T, any N, M1

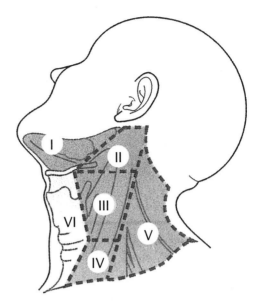

Figure 16.2 Distribution of neck nodes in head and neck cancer.

1) Primary closure with or without local flap
2) Pedicled flap
3) Free flap transfer
4) Use of alloplastic materials and osteointegrated implants.

Primary closure

Primary closure and skin grafting is only possible in small defects. After extensive resection, pedicled or free flap repair is needed which aims to improve not only the cosmetic appearance but more importantly to restore the complex functions of upper aerodigestive tract, particularly swallowing and speech.

Pedicled flaps

The commonly used pedicled flaps in the head and neck region are pectoralis major, deltopectoral, and temporalis flaps. Skin and muscle is raised from the donor area and rotated with the vascular pedicle as a pivot point to cover the defect. Unlike free flaps, the blood supply comes from its own vascular pedicle. As there is no microvascular anastomosis, the length of the operation is reduced significantly.

The disadvantages of a pedicled flap is that in the majority of cases, the type of tissue that is needed to reconstruct is not available, and contouring of the flap is difficult, which leads to a bulky flap with poor functional results. Furthermore, blood supply at peripheral areas is less robust leading to a high rate of partial dehiscence and flap necrosis. Pedicled flap

clinical outcome is not compromised by selective neck dissection; consequently, this approach is preferred for N0 and N1 tumours[7].

In selective neck dissection, only the nodal tissue from level I to IV is dissected, however, the critical non-lymphatic structures such as the spinal accessory nerve, the internal jugular vein, and sternocleidomastoid muscle are preserved. In extensive nodal disease these structures may have to be sacrificed to remove tumour metastases.

Reconstruction

The different methods available for reconstruction following tumour resection are:

Table 16.3 Commonly used free flaps in oral and maxillofacial cancer surgery

Free flap	Advantages	Potential problems
Radial forearm flap	Thin pliable tissue Ideal for repair of intraoral soft tissue Technically easy to harvest	Risk of radial bone fracture in osteocutaneous flap
Fibular free flap	Method of choice to reconstruct mandible Limited morbidity at donor site—limited sensory loss and dorsiflexion of great toe Simultaneous dual-team approach	Limited muscle and cutaneous tissue bulk Cannot be used in peripheral vascular disease
Iliac crest flap (deep circumflex iliac flap)	Large tissue bulk available for repair of through and through defects	Significant postoperative pain at donor site Advanced skill requirement Long-term gait problems, femoral nerve damage
Free jejunum transfer	Reconstruction of circumferential defects of hypopharynx and cervical oesophagus Mucus secretion alleviates xerostomia and improves swallowing	Additional minilaparotomy needed Difficult to monitor postoperatively Jejunum does not tolerate ischaemia well
Scapular flap	Wide range of tissue types available Both intraoral and cutaneous cover for complex resections	Simultaneous two-team approach not possible, increasing operating time Intraoperative repositioning needed Shoulder weakness

transfer is technically less demanding and suitable for high-risk patients with significant comorbidity.

Free flaps

A free flap is a composite block of tissue which is removed from the donor site and transferred to a distant recipient site where its circulation is restored by microvascular anastomosis. This is in contrast to a 'pedicled' flap in which tissue remains attached to the donor site keeping the 'pedicle' intact as a conduit for blood supply. For all free flaps, the artery and vein are reconnected to recipient vessels in the neck.

Free flaps may be soft tissue flaps which have muscle and skin, free visceral flaps, e.g. free jejunum transfer for reconstruction of oropharynx, and composite flap where vascularized bone is grafted, e.g. radius, fibula, iliac, or scapular graft for reconstruction of mandible.

Free flaps are the preferred option in reconstruction because of greater ability to match the resected tissue (like for like), suitable contour to match the defect, and a robust blood supply. The main disadvantage is that the surgery is technically demanding with prolonged operating time. Intensive postoperative monitoring is needed to ensure flap perfusion and additional morbidity of the donor site is also seen.

Commonly used free flaps used in head and neck reconstruction are listed in Table 16.3.

Stages of free flap transfer

The stages during flap transfer include initial dissection, flap elevation and clamping of vessels, period of primary ischaemia when there is no blood flow in the flap and intracellular metabolism is entirely anaerobic, and reperfusion after anastomosis of artery and vein.

Free flaps rely on small vascular anastomosis for perfusion and this makes them extremely vulnerable to hypoperfusion and ischaemia. All flaps undergo a period of primary ischaemia during harvest. This in part triggers a reperfusion injury which results in microcirculatory sludging, release of inflammatory mediators and vasospasm with reduction in blood flow in the initial 8–12 hours[8]. Flap failure is most commonly due to formation of thrombus at the anastomosis site, which in turn is related to the quality of vessels and the technical skill of the surgical team. Duration of primary ischaemia is a critical determinant of ischaemic complications[9].

Arterial vasospasm and extrinsic compression of the pedicle have also been identified as crucial factors in flap failure. Vessels that are used for anastomosis are generally 1–4 mm in diameter and any vasoconstriction can lead to critical ischaemia. Interstitial oedema from tissue handling and excessive fluids could also contribute to poor perfusion.

Free flaps are different from normal tissues in several respects. There is no lymphatic drainage in the flap tissue. Hence, reabsorption of interstitial fluid is minimal and this makes the flap tissue highly vulnerable to interstitial oedema. Transplanted vessels in a free flap have no sympathetic innervation but are still able to respond to physical stimuli such as cold, handling, and local and humoral factors including circulating catecholamines. The impaired autoregulation in flap tissue also predisposes to vasospasm[10].

Contraindications to free flap transfer

Poorly controlled diabetes leads to increased microvascular atherosclerosis, impaired wound healing, and delayed neovascularization of the flap. Patients with significant cardiac disease may not tolerate prolonged surgery with large fluid shifts and these patients may be better served with less ambitious reconstruction.

Collagen vascular disease is a relative contraindication with a high incidence of anastomotic thrombosis especially during active vasculitis. Free flap transfer may not be acceptable to some Jehovah's Witness patients. The only absolute contraindication for free flap transfer is sickle cell disease and polycythaemia because of high failure rate from a combination of microcirculatory sludging and hypercoagulability.

Physiology of microcirculation

A basic understanding of the physiology of microcirculation and the unique features of free flap is essential for anaesthetic management[11]. Hagen–Poiseuille's law quantitatively relates the laminar flow of a liquid through a rigid tube to the driving pressure. The equation describing this relationship is:

$$\text{Blood flow} = \frac{\Delta P \, \pi r^4}{8 \eta l}$$

where ΔP is the pressure difference across the tube, i.e. the perfusion pressure, r is the radius of the tube, l the length of the tube and η the viscosity of the liquid.

Although the microcirculation is too complex for a strict application of the formula, we can see that any change in perfusion pressure, cross sectional area, and viscosity will have an influence on flap flow. Pressure gradient depends on mean arterial blood pressure and pressure in the interstitial space. As the flow depends on the fourth power of the radius, halving the diameter will lead to a 16-fold reduction in flow rate.

In addition, Laplace's law states that diameter of the vessel also depends on the transmural pressure. Transmural pressure is decreased by a decrease in intraluminal pressure (hypotension, hypovolaemia) or an increase in extravascular pressure (oedema, haematoma).

The relationship between viscosity and haematocrit is non-linear. Viscosity rises steeply when the haematocrit levels rise above 40%. Viscosity also depends on plasma proteins, temperature, and aggregation of cells. A reduction in viscosity is accompanied by an increase in velocity of erythrocytes. This increases the shear stress on the capillary endothelial cells, which is believed to be a crucial local factor in regulating capillary circulation[12].

An additional factor which can affect microcirculation is the pulse pressure. A good pulse pressure in the microcirculation ensures a greater period of capillary patency for the same mean arterial pressure (MAP) because of relaxation of precapillary sphincter. Peripheral vasoconstriction produces a damping of the pressure wave and in addition to reduction in total flow makes the flow less effective.

These physiological principles are the rationale of haemodynamic interventions taken to improve blood flow in both pedicle and free flap transfer. Basic principles of patient management in free flap transfer are to maintain the patient warm and vasodilated, with a well filled circulation, adequate pulse pressure, free from pain and shivering which may lead to sympathetic stimulation and vasoconstriction, and with a haematocrit around 0.30 to optimize microcirculation through optimal rheology.

Anaesthetic management

The patient may present for initial examination under anaesthetic and panendoscopy as part of diagnostic workup or for definitive surgery for excision of tumour with immediate or delayed reconstruction.

Preanaesthetic assessment

The aims of preassessment are to detect potential difficulty in intubation because of the tumour or its treatment, coexisting medical problems, and decide on suitable options for surgery.

Airway

Preoperative evaluation should aim to assess the site and extent of the tumour and to detect any symptoms

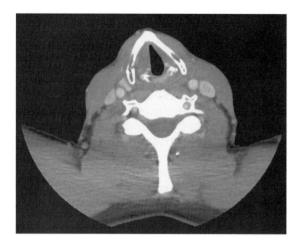

Figure 16.3 Hypopharyngeal tumour with ipsilateral vocal cord palsy.

of obstruction, which may be indicative of significant distortion of airway (Figure 16.3) or direct laryngeal involvement with tumour with implications for safe induction of anaesthesia (Figure 16.4). Patients should be asked about recent change in voice, hoarseness, dysphagia, and dyspnoea on lying flat. Old anaesthetic charts and notes of previous operations should be reviewed. Stridor, recent onset of snoring, or obstructive sleep apnoea are ominous signs and may indicate airway obstruction.

The tongue may be fixed and immobile in cancer arising from the base of tongue and floor of mouth potentially leading to airway obstruction and difficult intubation (Figure 16.5). Large pedunculated and mobile supraglottic lesions can obstruct the laryngeal

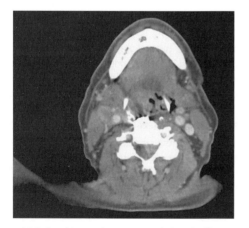

Figure 16.4 Oropharyngeal tumour producing significant airway obstruction at level of larynx with erosion of cervical vertebra.

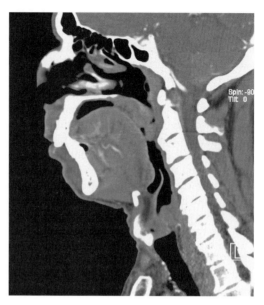

Figure 16.5 Upper airway obstruction caused by tumour of soft palate.

inlet with loss of muscle tone after induction of general anaesthesia[13]. Infiltration of hyoepiglottic ligament and stylohyoid ligament by hypopharyngeal tumour can cause fixation of epiglottis. Among the effects of radiotherapy in the head and neck region (Table 16.4) is fibrosis, which produces thick woody non-compliant tissue which is very difficult to elevate during direct laryngoscopy as well as severe limitation in mouth opening (Figure 16.6) (see Chapter 17).

Radiological investigations such as CT scan and MRI should be reviewed for information about the location of tumour and severity of airway obstruction. Awake nasal endoscopy is a simple bedside (or anaesthetic room) test which gives vital information about the size, mobility and site of lesions and degree of airway obstruction. The real time view of the supraglottis and the laryngeal inlet obtained is useful in planning the approach to airway management. However, it must be remembered that air passages visible in an awake patient in the sitting position via the bronchoscope, may narrow or disappear altogether as muscle tone is lost with general anaesthesia

Comorbidity

Patients are often malnourished from dysphagia caused by the tumour per se, dietary habits (e.g. alcoholism), systemic effects of chemotherapy, and radiation mucositis. Preoperative malnutrition has been shown to

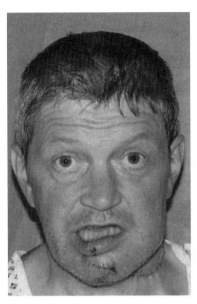

Figure 16.6 Severely limited mouth opening following radiotherapy and radical neck dissection and free flap surgery for oral squamous cell carcinoma. Securing the airway in such circumstances usually involves an awake fibreoptic intubation.

correlate with impaired wound healing and infection. Nutritional status should be corrected in the time preceding surgery and the enteral route is preferred if feasible. A specialist dietician should be involved wherever possible. With history of alcohol abuse, a detoxification regimen should be commenced if possible, in order to avoid postoperative withdrawal[14].

Patients with head and neck cancer are usually elderly with a history of smoking and alcohol abuse. There is a high prevalence of smoking-related respiratory disease, coronary artery disease, and peripheral

Table 16.4 Effects of radiotherapy

Acute effects	Late effects
Oropharyngeal mucositis	Decreased neck extension
Laryngeal oedema	Trismus
Xerostomia	Temporomandibular joint ankylosis
	Laryngeal chondronecrosis
	Swallowing dysfunction
	Osteoradinecrosis of mandible
	Hypothyroidism
	Systemic immunosuppression

vascular disease. Old age per se is not a contra-indication for free flap surgery; however, coexisting cardiac and respiratory disease increases the incidence of complications and flap failure[15].

With a history of heavy smoking, cardiorespiratory assessment is necessary. Although functional capacity may be assessed clinically, formal cardiopulmonary exercise testing is more accurate for stratification of risk. Patients with an anaerobic threshold lower than 11 ml/min/kg are at high risk of postoperative cardiac complications after major surgery and alternative treatment options may have to be explored.

Routine preoperative tests include full blood count and chemistry profile including liver function tests, clotting studies, chest radiography, and an electrocardiogram. If the patient is elderly or has a history of smoking it is advisable to obtain pulmonary function tests, perform cardiopulmonary exercise testing, and a nutritional assessment including determination of total serum protein, albumin, and transferrin levels.

Airway management

A north preformed nasal endotracheal tube (Figure 9.1) is commonly used to facilitate surgical access to the oral cavity for the majority of oral and maxillofacial cancer operations. The tube should be carefully secured to avoid dislodgement during surgery.

These patients present significant airway challenges and intubation and even mask ventilation may be difficult. Decisions regarding airway management in these patients is often between asleep induction, intravenous if no loss of airway is anticipated, inhalational spontaneously breathing if there is a potential to lose controlled ventilation, or awake fibreoptic intubation. If there are any markers to suggest that conventional direct laryngoscopy or mask ventilation is likely to be difficult then an awake technique should be considered, which is the standard method for management of an anticipated difficult airway (see Chapter 4). However, it is worth remembering that awake fibreoptic intubation is a relative contraindication in the presence of significant airway stenosis and severe stridor, particularly if the larynx is not visible on diagnostic nasal endoscopy.

In patients with severe upper airway distortion or impending obstruction, awake surgical tracheostomy under local anaesthesia may be the safer option. Note that extubation and re-intubation can also present significant problems in this patient population and will be discussed later.

Role of tracheostomy

Elective tracheostomy at the start of surgery under general anaesthesia is critical if postoperative airway compromise is anticipated[16]. The indications for elective tracheostomy include possibility of postoperative airway oedema and prevention of aspiration.

Significant oedema with potential to cause airway obstruction is likely after resection of the posterior two-thirds of the tongue, mandible, and oropharynx. This is from a combination of tissue handling and impaired venous and lymphatic drainage. The airway can also be compromised by large bulky flaps. Aspiration of blood and secretions is likely with mechanical difficulty in swallowing, after excision of base of tongue, total glossectomy, and oropharyngeal resection. Damage to lower cranial nerves during neck dissection or from compression by the tumour also causes impairment in swallowing[17]. Therefore, elective tracheostomy is indicated for airway protection.

In major head and neck cases, tracheostomy has several advantages: the airway is secure; oral hygiene is improved with more effective bronchial toilet. The reduction in dead space and airway resistance assists in weaning from mechanical ventilation in the typical head and neck cancer patient with a history of heavy smoking and associated chronic obstructive airway disease. Additional benefits are decreased requirement of sedation, improved patient comfort with better mobility, and communication. Tracheostomy enables safe transfer to theatre and the airway is secure in the event of flap failure or haemorrhage in the immediate postoperative period[18].

However, tracheostomy carries its own risks and should not be a blanket policy for all major head and neck resections[19,20]. Recent studies show that it is not needed after uncomplicated maxillectomy unless a bulky flap is used for reconstruction[21]. Postoperative oedema after bilateral modified neck dissection is not significant and tracheostomy is generally not required[17]. Kruse-Lösler and colleagues have proposed a scoring system to predict need of tracheostomy in the postoperative period based on tumour size, location, coexisting respiratory disease, and alcohol consumption, but this has not been validated[22].

Postoperative ventilation for a short period through an oral or nasal endotracheal tube is an option if tracheostomy is to be avoided[23]. Submental intubation (Figure 14.8) is an absolute contraindication in cancer cases because of high incidence of orocutaneous fistula[24].

Intraoperative considerations
Venous access and monitoring

Head and neck cancer resection carries risk of major blood loss so large-bore venous access is needed.

In addition to standard monitoring, invasive arterial and central venous pressure, urine output, and temperature monitoring is also indicated. Arterial pressure monitoring is recommended to allow safe manipulation of blood pressure and facilitate sampling for serial blood gas analysis and haematocrit measurement. Central venous pressure (CVP) reflects cardiac filling pressure and is useful in assessing response to fluid therapy. Appropriate access site should be discussed with the surgeon in order to avoid using the 'flap donor site' for access. Femoral venous line is used if surgical access to the neck and chest is needed. Long lines placed from peripheral veins (e.g. antecubital fossa) are frequently poorly positioned and may not give accurate CVP readings.

Core temperature can be measured through the rectal route or by urinary catheters with built-in temperature measurement probe. Bladder temperature is preferred as rectal temperature frequently lags behind core temperature, especially with large fluid shifts[25]. Peripheral skin temperature is also measured to calculate the core to peripheral gradient in free flap transfer.

Positioning

Careful positioning is essential for the long length of operation to avoid well-recognized problems (e.g. pressure sores, nerve injury). Pressure points should be padded and the pulse oximeter probe should be moved frequently to prevent pressure necrosis. Almost all head and neck operations need supine positioning with the exception of latissimus dorsi and scapular flap surgery where the patient is turned intraoperatively to the lateral position for harvesting the flap. Head-up tilt and adjustment in the operating table are required to keep the limbs at the heart level which helps to decrease blood loss. Eyes are covered with eye shields and all pressure points should be padded. TED (thromboembolus deterrent) stockings and pneumatic compression boots should be used to reduce the risk of deep venous thrombosis.

Anaesthetic agents

Anaesthesia is usually maintained with a combination of remifentanil and a volatile agent. In animal models, isoflurane has been shown to be superior to halothane in maintaining flap perfusion[26]. This was attributed to maintenance of adequate cardiac output accompanied by mild vasodilation with isoflurane. Desflurane or sevoflurane is preferred if extubation is planned at the end of surgery, as both are haemodynamically stable with rapid offset of action.

Remifentanil analgesia provides intense analgesia with good intraoperative conditions. It also reduces the need for muscle relaxation and allows nerve monitoring or muscle twitch testing for isolation of nerves during neck dissection. The short half-life of 9 minutes enables titration of dose to match the surgical stimulation, during the operation which may vary from periods of minimal to intense stimulation[27]. It also enables rapid emergence and return of protective airway reflexes as well as having the advantage of a smooth transfer to an Intensive Therapy Unit (ITU) if indicated. It may be used in ITU to facilitate overnight 'light' sedation, minimizing inotrope requirements and allowing a quick wake up, extubation, and return of reflexes the following morning.

Total intravenous anaesthesia or target-controlled infusion with propofol or remifentanil can also be used. Nitrous oxide is best avoided in major resections with negative intravenous pressure in head-up tilt. Moreover, risk of postoperative nausea and vomiting and concerns regarding bone marrow suppression during prolonged surgery, do not justify its routine use, especially in the presence of suitable alternatives[28].

Surgery

Surgical management can be divided into two phases as the principal problems and management goals are very different for the two. The first phase involves resection of tumour, neck dissection, and harvest of the flap. This is followed by transplantation of flap and microvascular anastomosis. The main problems of phase 1 are intense stimulation and blood loss whereas maintenance of adequate blood pressure and flap perfusion are the main concerns in phase 2.

Resection of tumour and harvest of flap

During tumour resection significant blood loss may occur. The risk of bleeding is increased with previous radiotherapy, bilateral radical neck dissection, and craniofacial resection. Raising of large myocutaneous and some bone flaps, e.g. iliac crest, can also cause blood loss. With radial forearm and fibular flaps, blood loss is minimal as tourniquet is used.

Blood transfusion is reportedly required in 14–30% of head and neck cancer operations. In addition to the inherent risks, blood transfusion is independently associated with increased perioperative complications. An additional reason for avoiding blood transfusion in patients with cancer is its reported effect of immunosuppression with increased rate of recurrence. Specific to head and neck cancer, there are a small number of studies which looked at recurrence with allogenic blood transfusion. The results have been conflicting, primarily because of a range of variables that account for recurrence[29,30]. Despite this, the risks and cost of blood transfusion mandate that blood conservation strategies are used. We shall briefly examine the different methods that can be used to achieve this.

Hypotensive anaesthesia has been shown to improve the surgical field, decrease duration of surgery, and reduce blood loss (see Chapter 20). In the past, a wide range of hypotensive agents and anaesthetic drugs have been used to reduce blood pressure. Currently, remifentanil is the most commonly used agent in head and neck cancer surgery. Remifentanil infusion reduces neurohumoral stress response and provides an excellent operative field by controlled reduction of blood pressure without causing tachycardia. Its metabolism by tissue esterases and short context-sensitive half-life provides greater control and haemodynamic stability in the event of major haemorrhage

MAP is typically reduced by 20% of preoperative baseline pressure. Extreme caution should be exercised in patients with fixed stenosis, e.g. in coronary and carotid atherosclerosis, as blood flow distal to the stenosis may be compromised with the reduction in pressure. Deliberate hypotension should be avoided in uncorrected hypovolaemia and severe anaemia.

Additional methods that help to reduce blood loss are avoiding hypothermia, meticulous surgical technique, and use of ultrasonic harmonic scalpel (Table 16.5).

Venous drainage is improved by head-up tilt and adjusting the operating table so that the legs are at heart level.

Acute normovolaemic haemodilution has been shown to reduce the need for allogenic blood in major head and neck cancer surgery. Typically, after induction of anaesthesia 10 ml/kg of blood is withdrawn and stored in CPDA-1 buffer. This is transfused back to the

Table 16.5 Methods to reduce blood loss in head and neck cancer surgery

Anaesthetic factors	Surgical factors
Balanced anaesthesia	Meticulous surgical technique
Adequate analgesia	Harmonic ultrasonic scalpel
Avoid hypothermia, acidosis	Fibrin glue and sealants
Positioning 30° head up	Collagen and cellulose pads
Avoid extreme neck tilt, coughing	Infiltration of dilute adrenaline solution
Consider moderate-induced hypotension	
Consider acute normovolaemic haemodilution	

patient after surgical haemostasis is achieved. On a physiological basis, less red cell mass is lost per millilitre of blood lost during operation because of the dilutional effect. In addition, the whole blood that is returned to the patient has all the clotting products and platelets. Acute normovolaemic haemodilution should be considered where massive blood loss is expected[31,32].

Until recently, the consensus view on the use of cell salvage in cancer surgery was that the risk of viable cancer cell dissemination rendered its routine use too risky. In 2008 the National Institute for Health and Clinical Excellence (NICE) approved use of cell salvage in urological cancer surgery[33]. However, until further evidence is available of its safety in head and neck cancer, use of intraoperative cell salvage is probably best reserved for major blood loss in patients who refuse allogenic blood.

Reconstruction and microvascular anastomosis

Free flap microcirculatory perfusion

The principal goals of anaesthetic management for free flap transfer are to provide a full, hyperdynamic circulation with increased cardiac output, peripheral vasodilation, wide pulse pressure, and maintenance of normothermia to ensure optimum flap perfusion[34]. The evidence base in anaesthetic management of free flaps is limited because of the relatively low failure rate of vascularized free flap transfer. Much of what we know today is extrapolated from research on animal models.

Temperature regulation

The key to adequate flap perfusion is the maintenance of normothermia, especially during long operations with extensive exposure involving the flap donor and tumour site. Hypothermia has been shown to cause vasoconstriction, a rise in plasma viscosity, and increased platelet aggregation with resulting reduction in blood flow to the free flap[35].

Normothermia is maintained by active warming of intravenous fluids, using forced air warming systems, an under-heating mattress, humidification of anaesthetic gasses, low fresh gas flow rates, and raising ambient temperature.

Hypothermia must be avoided by minimizing exposure and starting active warming in the anaesthetic room at induction. This prevents the initial anaesthesia-related redistribution hypothermia by decreasing the core-to-periphery temperature gradient. Forced air warming is continued during the pre-incision period while invasive monitoring lines are being inserted and surface marking for surgery is carried out. The ambient theatre temperature is raised to around 22–24°C, a level sufficient to reduce patient heat loss, without being too uncomfortable for the theatre staff.

It is recommended that normothermia should be achieved prior to anastomosis and maintained for at least 48 hours postoperatively. Both the core and peripheral temperature should be monitored and the gradient should ideally be less than 1.5°C. A larger gradient indicates peripheral vasoconstriction.

Fluid therapy

Perioperative fluid management has a significant impact on outcome from free flap surgery. The insensible loss from the two exposed sites of surgery, i.e. donor and recipient site of the flap is often underestimated. Hypovolaemia with resulting vasoconstriction causes a reduction in flap perfusion. Fluid therapy is aimed at correcting hypovolaemia and reducing viscosity in order to improve microcirculatory flow (combined with haematocrit 0.30). Transfusion is required only if significant blood loss occurs during the resection and regular bedside haematocrit measurement may assist in this determination. Fluid management is aimed at keeping CVP 2–4 mmHg above baseline and urine output of 1–1.5 ml/kg/hour.

The role of hypervolaemic haemodilution is contentious[36]. There is no clinical evidence that this is beneficial despite the theoretical advantage of reduction in viscosity. On the contrary, there is some evidence that the resulting extravasation in flap tissue could be detrimental. Moreover, patients with ischaemic heart disease and left ventricular dysfunction may not tolerate hypervolaemic volume load. The resulting cardiac failure almost always guarantees flap failure.

The current knowledge base favours the use of colloids as large volumes of isotonic crystalloids predispose to interstitial oedema in the flap. The use of crystalloids is limited to replacement of insensible losses and preoperative deficit to minimize interstitial oedema. Hartmann's solution is preferred as fluids with high chloride content may lead to hyperchloraemic acidosis.

Colloids (starches or gelatine solutions) are used for volume expansion and haemodilution. Gelatin solutions remain in the intravascular compartment for a relatively short period, as compared to other colloids. There is some experimental evidence of beneficial effect of both tetrastarch and pentastarch on microcirculation. Starch solutions (Voluven or Haesteril) have been shown to reduce endothelial permeability and minimize reperfusion injury. The potential disadvantage is prolonged bleeding time in large doses and pruritus.

Dextran decreases platelet aggregation and adhesion and reduces platelet polymerization. Low-molecular-weight dextran (dextran 40 and 70) was routinely used after free flap transfer for its antithrombotic effect. Recent studies have shown that there is no benefit in terms of preventing microvascular thrombosis with prophylactic use of dextran[37]. Hypertonic saline has been used in severe flap oedema and after prolonged ischaemia time with variable success.

Table 16.6 gives a practical and logical regimen for fluid management in these cases.

Indicators of optimally filled circulation are increasing CVP trend, urine output greater than 1 ml/kg/hour,

Table 16.6 Guide to fluid management

Crystalloids
10–20 ml/kg to replace preoperative deficit
4–6 ml/kg/hour to replace insensible losses
Colloids
10–15 ml/kg for haemodilution
To replace blood loss
Blood
To maintain haematocrit at 30%

cardiovascular stability, and a narrow core to peripheral temperature gradient. Several recent studies have demonstrated the benefit of goal-directed fluid therapy over conventional fluid regimens. The titration of fluid administration to measured and dynamic physiological endpoints, such as stroke volume variation or cardiac output via the LiDCO system (LiDCO Ltd., Cambridge, United Kingdom), PiCCO system (Pulsion Medical Systems AG, Munich, Germany), or transoesophageal Doppler, may reduce morbidity, decrease length of stay, and improve gut function in surgical patients. Optimizing perioperative balance by calculating the variations in pulse pressure and stroke volume using LiDCO in patients undergoing free flap transfer is currently under investigation[38].

Rheology

The haematocrit is generally maintained at 30–35%. Haemodilution is accompanied with a marked increase in red cell velocity in the microcirculation. The product of haematocrit and erythrocyte velocity determines the erythrocyte flux, which reaches its maximum at this haematocrit. Consequently, the capacity to transfer oxygen is maximum at this level[39]. Extreme haemodilution should be avoided as it prolongs bleeding time and adversely affects oxygen-carrying capacity.

Vasoactive agents

Free flaps are different from pedicled flaps in that they are denervated with complete sympathectomy of all vessels, whereas the feeding artery and the draining vein, on which the flap vessels are anastomosed, have intact innervation. Our understanding of the exact effects of vasoactive agents on the blood vessels in free flaps is limited and based largely on animal experiments.

Theoretically using vasodilators to improve microvascular perfusion is an attractive option, but in practice the resultant reduction in MAP may adversely affect blood flow. Intravenous sodium nitroprusside has been shown to markedly reduce blood flow in free flaps[40]. There is some evidence that local intravascular injection of vasodilators such as papverine, verapamil and prostacyclin prevent vasospasm and improve flow. Topical vasodilators are routinely used by the surgeons during the operation to minimize vasospasm.

Inotropes are generally avoided in free flap surgery, despite there being little evidence to show that systemically administered inotropes reduce flap perfusion because of vasoconstriction. The exact effect of different inotropes on flap perfusion is uncertain. Interestingly, it has also been speculated that when the vessels in the flap are maximally constricted after handling and drop in temperature, an increase in mean arterial blood pressure with adrenaline may improve perfusion. The role of inotropes on flap flow is currently being investigated[38].

Shafik et al.[41] have shown that dobutamine increases cardiac index and flap blood flow in a small group of patients. This was accompanied by a decrease in systemic vascular resistance[41]. Milrinone has been shown to have no effect on flap flow, arterial spasm, or flap survival[42]. In animal models, vasopressors like systemic phenylephrine appear to reduce the blood flow[40].

In practice, small incremental doses of ephedrine or metaraminol are often used if required to correct hypotension intraoperatively and if an inotrope is required, it is logical on current evidence base to use dobutamine; however, it is essential that hypotension is addressed by optimizing cardiac preload through adequate fluid resuscitation to optimize flap flow before inotropes are commenced.

Analgesia

Intraoperatively remifentanil infusion provides excellent analgesia as part of a balanced anaesthetic technique. 0.15mg/kg of morphine may be given towards the end of the surgery for postoperative analgesia. Patient-controlled analgesia (PCA) containing morphine and regular paracetamol is usually adequate for most patients postoperatively. Non-steroidal anti-inflammatory drugs (NSAIDs) are generally avoided because of the risk of postoperative bleeding and haematoma. Pain in the head and neck region is surprisingly moderate and relatively easy to manage. In fact, majority of the pain after major head and neck surgery is from the flap donor and skin graft site. Amongst the commonly used flaps, severe postoperative pain is frequent in iliac crest bone flap.

Regional blocks

The role of epidural analgesia for donor site pain in flap surgery is contentious. Epidural anaesthesia reduces vasospasm and improves blood flow. However, in microvascular free flap transfer, because the flap is denervated, a chemical sympathectomy produced by an epidural may decrease blood flow. This is caused by reduction in mean arterial blood pressure and a steal phenomenon resulting from reflex vasoconstriction, which diverts blood away from the flap to normal tissues[43]. Animal studies have shown a reduction in blood flow in flaps with epidural analgesia especially with concurrent hypovolaemia.

However, regional analgesia has several advantages. These include reduction in the neuroendocrine stress response to surgery, reduced postoperative opioid requirement, reduced respiratory complications, reduction in deep vein thrombosis, and improved recovery. Interestingly, preliminary studies suggest that immunomodulation from better pain relief by regional anaesthesia may reduce recurrence after cancer surgery[44,45]. It remains to be seen whether further research in this field changes management of perioperative pain in cancer surgery.

We currently use epidural analgesia only for iliac crest flaps. The osteotomy of iliac bone and division of internal oblique, transversus abdominis, and iliacus muscles cause severe postoperative pain. Poor pain relief in the postoperative period is linked with chronic pain and gait problems. We use low thoracic (T10–11, T11–12) epidural for continuous infusion of bupivaciane 0.125% with fentanyl 2 mcg/ml in these patients. Some centres use multilumen catheters placed by the surgeon in the wound for continuous infusion of local anaesthetic. If epidural analgesia is used it is essential that hypovolaemia is avoided and vasopressors are used appropriately to correct hypotension, so that flap perfusion is not compromised.

Paravertebral block has been shown to be effective for latissimus dorsi flaps. Fibula donor site rarely causes significant pain and most patients can be controlled on day 3 with simple analgesics alone. Similarly, there is no clinical need for catheters for brachial plexus blockade in radial forearm free flaps as the pain responds well to paracetamol and morphine PCA.

Extubation

Extubation and any need for emergency re-intubation presents specific challenges in these patients. Patients undergoing limited resection and uncomplicated pedicle flap surgery may be extubated at the end of surgery. Extubation carries risk of laryngeal spasm, surge in blood pressure, or airway obstruction because of oedema and bleeding. Therefore, awake extubation in a semi-sitting position after recovery of neuromuscular function and normal breathing pattern is advisable to maximize airway protection and return of reflexes. Intravenous lidocaine or esmolol may be needed to suppress the surge in blood pressure on extubation. Prior to extubation, it is essential to examine the airway to detect oedema and bleeding, and to check for air leak on deflation of cuff. If the initial intubation was difficult, extubation over airway exchange or jet ventilation catheter should be considered to optimize oxygenation and facilitate re-intubation in case of loss of airway.

If the patient requires re-intubation in the immediate postoperative period, this may be challenging. Specific problems include difficult controlled ventilation and anticipated difficult intubation because of airway bleeding, flap or laryngeal oedema, limited mouth opening, or poor visualization of the larynx due to bulky intraoral flaps. In addition, attempts at laryngoscopy may cause damage to an intraoral free flap or its vascular pedicle leading to disruption of vascular supply. For these reasons awake fibreoptic intubation is the commonly preferred technique; this may be difficult if the patient is symptomatically short of breath or there is bleeding in the airway where the view may be poor and inhalational induction may also be considered. Each case is different and relative merits of preservation of airway reflexes and degree of anticipated difficulty in intubation needs to be considered. However, difficult intubation should be anticipated and planned for in the presence of the surgeon, if there is a chance of loss of the airway and need for emergency tracheostomy or cricothyroidotomy.

Postoperative care

The majority of patients undergoing major resection or free flap surgery are transferred to the intensive care unit for individual nursing care: monitoring and optimization of cardio respiratory function, care of tracheostomy, and management of free flap[46]. Patients are usually ventilated overnight to provide a still head in order to reduce the shear stress on the anastomosis. It is important that the patient's head is maintained in neutral position to avoid mechanical distortion of the vascular pedicle. Nursing in 30° head-up position helps to reduce airway oedema. Any pressure on the flap or its pedicle from tube ties, dressings, or elastic bands of the oxygen mask should be avoided.

In essence, postoperative management for free flap surgery involves continuation of all the measures taken

Table 16.7 Goals of postoperative management in free flap transfer

Normal blood pressure
Normothermia with core to peripheral gradient less than 1.5°C.
Haematocrit between 30–35%
Urine output greater than 1 ml/kg/hour
CVP 8–10 mmHg
Regular clinical inspection of flap
Continuous temperature measurement in flap
Low threshold for re-exploration

intraoperatively to ensure adequate flap perfusion, i.e. maintenance of normothermia, adequate filling with good postoperative analgesia. It is essential to avoid peripheral vasoconstriction caused by hypothermia, shivering, hypovolaemia, pain, and sympathetic stimulation (Table 16.7). Administration of fluids is aimed at maintaining a urine output between 1–1.5 ml/kg/hour. Conversely, caution is warranted to avoid overzealous fluid replacement which risks both fluid overload and flap oedema.

After the patient is awake, PCA with morphine and regular paracetamol is usually adequate for pain relief. In iliac crests flap, epidural or infusion through the wound catheter is commenced prior to stopping the sedation.

Intravenous antibiotics, antiemetics, and dexamethasone are continued for 48 hours.

Subcutaneous low-molecular-weight heparin is given for deep vein thrombosis prophylaxis. Low-molecular-weight heparin has also been shown to reduce anastomotic thrombosis and improve flap survival. In the absence of clinical proof of efficacy, aspirin and dextran are no longer used routinely following free flap surgery. Nutritional support through the fine bore nasogastric, percutaneous endoscopic gastrostomy (PEG) or jejunostomy is commenced as soon as possible. After reconstruction of oropharynx, videofluoroscopic study of oesophagus and assessment of swallowing is carried out at day 5 and oral intake is started if no abnormalities are seen. Chest physiotherapy is continued in the postoperative period to improve clearance of secretions. Patients are then transferred to the ward and tracheostomy decannulated, after the oedema has settled.

Monitoring of flap

Flap perfusion is monitored hourly for the first 3–5 days with decreasing frequency of monitoring thereafter, as free flaps rarely fail after that[47]. The clinical signs to assess are colour, turgor, capillary refill, and temperature gradient. Additional information on the condition of the flap can be obtained from percutaneous Doppler and dermal bleeding on pin prick.

Clinical evaluation is not possible in 'buried' free tissue transfers which have no visible external surface. Such transfers are commonly used for reconstruction of oropharynx and skull base. Regular nasal endoscopy is preferred in some head and neck units for free jejunum transfer. A small portion of buried flaps may be exteriorized to allow clinical monitoring. Implantable Dopplers and laser Doppler flow monitoring can also be used for monitoring buried flaps.

Clinical signs when present either singly or in combination, suggest a problem in perfusion. These include pale flap colour, reduction in flap temperature, loss of capillary refill, and loss of flap turgor, all of which indicate arterial insufficiency. Venous insufficiency, on the other hand, can result in a purple or blue hue in the flap, congestion, swelling, and rapid capillary refill in the initial stage followed by loss of capillary refill.

Simple measures like improving blood pressure, increasing fluid input, warming, and repositioning of external dressings may improve perfusion in an ischaemic flap. The threshold for triggering re-exploration of a flap for suspected arterial or venous thrombosis should be low as salvage rates are considerably higher with early identification and treatment.

Other specific surgery

Salivary gland surgery

Seventy per cent of all adult salivary gland tumours are seen in the parotid gland, 15% in the submandibular, and the remaining in sublingual and minor salivary glands. The only known predisposing factor is therapeutic external irradiation. Surgery remains the mainstay of initial definitive treatment for nearly all tumours of the major and minor salivary glands.

Only the specific features regarding anaesthetic management of salivary gland surgery will be discussed further. In parotid surgery, monitoring of the facial nerve is required to preserve the nerve. This is carried out by inserting two subdermal platinum electrodes in the upper and lower face which record facial muscle activity on stimulation. An audiovisual response is evoked on stimulation of the nerve.

If neuromuscular blocking agent is to be used to facilitate intubation a suitable dose should be administered so that full recovery takes place before monitoring begins. A remifentanil infusion reduces the need of subsequent doses of relaxants. Peripheral nerve monitoring (e.g. train of four) is essential to establish recovery of neuromuscular function, so that monitoring of nerve function can begin. A spontaneously breathing technique with reinforced laryngeal mask airway (LMA) has also been described for parotid surgery but the potential drawback is that the LMA is easily displaced during surgical manipulation and neck movement.

Limited mouth opening and trismus is seen if the parotid cancer involves temporomandibular joint. Direct laryngoscopy may be difficult if malignant lesions of the sublingual and submandibular gland invade the floor of mouth and fix the tongue.

Anaesthesia in patients with previous head and neck reconstruction
Presentation

Re-exploration in the immediate postoperative period following major head and neck surgery may be needed for several reasons, including salvage of an ischaemic flap, to control postoperative bleeding, and debridement of an infected flap. Airway management can be a challenge in these patients unless there is a tracheostomy *in situ* as discussed earlier[48,49].

Subsequent general anaesthesia may be required for insertion of osteointegrated implants, change of surgical obturator, panendoscopy for suspected recurrence, and contouring of flap. These patients present in an elective setting well after the original operation. As life expectancy improves with advances in management, it is foreseeable that many of these patients will undergo surgery for unrelated medical problems in the future.

Airway problems

In the immediate postoperative period, airway management is complicated by abnormal anatomy with severe distortion of the upper airway. In the initial postoperative period, oedema may be extensive from tissue handling, and reduced venous and lymphatic drainage. Moreover, inflamed and oedematous tissues in the postoperative period bleed on minimal trauma with instrumentation.

There are some specific technical difficulties in this group of patients. Postoperative pain and loss of supporting tissue may preclude tight mask seal for

Table 16.8 Sequelae of head and neck cancer treatment

Maxillectomy	Limited mouth opening secondary to fibrosis of pterygo-masseteric sling
Radiotherapy	Limited craniocervical extension Hard fixed tissues with minimal movement Trismus in osteoradionecrosis
Tongue, floor of mouth resection	Fixed immobile tongue Thick, woody, noncompliant tissue Limited mandibular space Difficult mask ventilation with increase in tongue to oropharynx ratio after reconstruction
Orpharynx reconstruction	Impaired swallowing Aspiration risk Difficult mask ventilation in bulky flaps
Bicoronal (bifrontal or bitemporal) flap	Temporalis contracture Pseudoankylosis of TMJ
Neck dissection	Damage to IX, X, XII nerves Impaired swallowing, aspiration risk Vocal cord palsy
Pedicled flap	Bulky flap Increased tongue: pharynx ratio Difficult mask ventilation
Craniofacial resection	Nasal route contraindicated Difficult mask seal

inhalational induction. Rarely, one may have a significant air leak on controlled ventilation, for example if an extensive maxillectomy has been performed. Awake fibreoptic intubation is technically challenging as identification of familiar anatomical structures may be difficult after reconstruction in the presence of oedema and blood[50]. It is also difficult to achieve adequate topical anaesthesia in the presence of excessive secretions. It is also worth noting that some recovery of sensory function does take place in free flaps following sensory re-innervation so topical anaesthesia of the flap tissue is also essential if awake intubation is planned.

Supraglottic devices (see Chapter 4) such as the intubating LMA (ILMA) and the i-gel, are essentially designed for a normal airway and a tight 'seat and seal' may not be achieved in the presence of severe airway distortion. Giraud and colleagues describe their inability to ventilate or view the glottic aperture by

fibrescope passed through an LMA, in patents who had received cervical radiotherapy because of distorted anatomy[51]. While video laryngoscopes and rigid intubating stylettes have been successfully used in patients with difficult airways, and may provide a useful addition to the practitioner's repertory of airway devices, there is limited evidence of their use in this setting[52]. Moreover, limited mouth opening may also preclude the use of ILMA and video laryngoscopes. Blind nasal intubation has two major limitations: infrequent success on first pass and increased risk of trauma with multiple attempts.

Table 16.8 lists potential problems that may be encountered after fibrosis and scarring following surgery[53–55]. When evaluating these patients, it is essential to consider the potential for such dynamic changes, even if initial airway management was straightforward.

Management

On airway examination the anaesthetist must be able to assess[56] difficulty in mask ventilation, aspiration risk, ability to ventilate using supraglottic devices, difficulty in awake fibreoptic intubation, and access for cricothyroidotomy and tracheostomy.

It is also crucial to detect impending obstruction because if the patient is rendered apnoeic, total obstruction can rapidly ensue.

A clear understanding of the problem and a calm, logical approach is essential in formulating a management plan. There should be a primary plan with clear and anticipated back-up plans in case the first plan encounters difficulties. This depends not only on anticipated problems, but also on the experience and training of the anaesthetist and the availability of equipment. Management of the airway should be a joint decision between the anaesthetist and surgeon in this situation.

Management depends on each individual case. The gold standard technique is usually that of an awake nasal endoscopy followed by awake fibreoptic intubation if possible. If potential loss of airway is anticipated, one approach is to insert a cricothyroid cannula for jet ventilation before the procedure, this serves as a back-up plan in case of failure. In some circumstances, tracheostomy under local anaesthesia may be the only option, particularly in the presence of significant narrowing of any part of the airway that cannot be navigated with a flexible scope or endotracheal tube, and with active bleeding in the upper airway, where the view on fibreoptic endoscopy is obscured.

In all cases where the balance of evidence suggests that an attempt at awake intubation or inhalational induction is justified, the personnel and equipment for an emergency surgical airway (in the form of rigid bronchoscopy and a double set-up) should be on standby. Injecting the soft tissue over the cricothyroid membrane with 1% lidocaine and 1:100 000 epinephrine will result in vasoconstriction and a much drier operative field if emergency cricothyroidotomy or awake tracheotomy becomes necessary.

If there is uncertainty about the ability to maintain the airway following induction of anaesthesia, pre-mptively placing a cricothyroid cannula, e.g. Ravussian jet ventilation catheter under local anaesthesia, should be considered[57]. Insertion of a transtracheal jet ventilation catheter prior to induction, under controlled circumstances, secures the ability to ventilate the lungs following induction. This allows safe, unhurried, and comfortable airway instrumentation and can be crucial for rescue ventilation in an emergency.

Craniofacial resection

Craniofacial resection for maxillofacial tumours extending into the anterior cranial fossa is done as a joint case by the neurosurgeons and maxillofacial surgeons. The intracranial part of the tumour is resected through a bicoronal incision or transnasal route.

A standard neuroanaesthetic is provided and the principal goals of anaesthetic management include: preservation of adequate cerebral perfusion pressure and oxygen delivery; avoidance of large and sudden swings in intracranial pressure; providing conditions that allow optimal surgical exposure with least brain retraction; and allowing rapid awakening of the patient, e.g. remifentanil–sevoflurane with invasive monitoring. Oral intubation is needed if a transnasal approach is used or excision of floor of anterior cranial fossa is planned. The extensive resections can cause significant bleeding. Other complications of skull–base surgery include cerebrospinal fluid (CSF) leak, neurological and ocular complications, vascular injury, and thrombosis. Broad-spectrum antibiotic cover is needed as the dura is breached and risk of contamination from sinuses, nasal and oral cavity is high. The defect is reconstructed by either pericranial, galeal, or free flaps. These flaps provide watertight separation of the intracranial space from the nasopharynx, preventing CSF leak and ascending infection.

The perioperative management of neurosurgical patients differs significantly from the management of patients with free flaps. In neurosurgical anaesthesia, vasodilation is avoided and fluid administration aims to maintain a slightly negative fluid balance. Diuretics and steroids may also be needed. The ideal perioperative conditions for free flaps are exactly the opposite and these may have to be compromised[58]. It is, therefore, important to appropriately select the ideal method for reconstruction and have an experienced microsurgical team.

Carotid blowout syndrome
Presentation

Carotid blowout syndrome (CBS) remains one of the most devastating complications of head and neck cancer and its treatment. The clinical severity of CBS ranges from threatened haemorrhage following asymptomatic exposure of the artery to small repeated bleeds and acute massive haemorrhage.

CBS is caused by invasion of the carotid artery by the tumour in advanced cancer or following infection in the surgical wound. This is more likely after wound dehiscence following radical neck dissection where the sternocleidomastoid muscle cover over the artery is removed. Radiotherapy by causing damage to vasa vasorum of the artery predisposes to CBS.

Treatment

Historically, treatment of CBS was emergency surgical ligation of the artery. This led to a high incidence of postoperative stroke and death as the patency of collateral circulation was not tested. In addition, operation on an unstable patient in an irradiated and often infected neck is difficult. Currently with advancement of endovascular techniques, stent insertion is the mainstay of treatment[59].

In the presence of advanced cancer with significant residual disease and where the prognosis is poor, palliative management should be considered. In potentially curable conditions, such as postoperative wound infection, management follows an ABC approach. The wound is packed with gauze, airway secured, and fluid resuscitation is started while interventional radiology treatment or surgical repair is carried out.

Conclusion

Treatment of patients with maxillofacial cancer present significant problems for the anaesthetist. An understanding of the anatomy and surgical techniques, operative conditions required, and postoperative complications and their management is essential.

Airway management may be challenging and require a primary management plan and appropriate back-up plans. Each individual patient presents their own problems and working in liaison with the surgeons and as part of a multidisciplinary team is essential to optimize outcome for these patients; this includes being part of the team to plan the specific treatment options for individual cases in assessing perioperative risk and survival with non-surgical techniques.

References

1. Cancer Research UK. Head and neck cancer statistics. Available online at http://info.cancerresearchuk.org/cancerstats/types/oral/incidence (accessed 15 April 2009).
2. Morton RP. (2008) Epidemiology of head and neck cancer. In Gleeson MJ, Jones NS. (eds) *Scott-Browns Otolaryngology, Head and Neck Surgery*. London: Edward Arnold, pp. 2343–51.
3. Gallimore A. (2002) Pathology of head and neck cancers. In Souhami RL, Tannock I, Hohenberger P, Horiot JC. (eds) *Oxford Textbook of Clinical Oncology*. Oxford: Oxford University Press, pp. 1292–301.
4. Shah JP, Gil Z. (2009) Current concepts in management of oral cancer – surgery. *Oral Oncol*, **45(4–5)**, 394–401.
5. British Association of Otolaryngologists Head and Neck Surgeons (2002) *Effective head and neck cancer management -third consensus document (2002)*. Available online at http://www.entuk.org/publications (accessed 05 June 2009).
6. Ferlito A, Rinaldo A, Robbins KT, *et al.* (2003) Changing concepts in the surgical management of the cervical node metastasis. *Oral Oncol*, **39**, 429–32.
7. Patel KN, Shah JP. (2005) Neck dissection: past, present and future. *Surg Oncol Clin N Am*, **14(3)**, 461–77.
8. Carroll WR, Esclamado RM. (2000) Ischaemia reperfusion injury in microvascular surgery. *Head Neck*, **22(7)**, 700–13.
9. Kerrigan CL, Scotland MA. (1993) Ischaemia reperfusion injury: a review. *Microsurgery*, **14(13)**, 165–75.
10. Siggurdsson GH, Thomson D. (1995) Anaesthesia and microvascular surgery: clinical practice and research. *Eur J Anaesthesiol*, **12(2)**, 101–22.
11. Macdonald DJ. (1985) Anaesthesia for microvascular surgery. A physiological approach *Br J Anaes*, **57(9)**, 904–12.
12. Martini J, Carpentier B, Intaglietta M, *et al.* (2006). Beneficial effects due to increasing blood and plasma viscosity. *Clin Hemorheol Microcirc*, **35(1-2)**, 51–7.
13. Supkis DE, Dougherty TB, Nguyen DT, *et al.* (1998) Anesthetic management of the patient undergoing head and neck cancer surgery. *Int Anesthesiol Clin*, **36(3)**, 21–9.
14. Ferrier MB, Spuesens EB, Le Cessie S. (2005) Comorbidity as a major risk factor for mortality and complications in head and neck surgery. *Arch Otolaryngol Head Neck Surg*, **131(1)**, 27–32.
15. Ozkan O, Ozgentas HE, Islamoglu K. (2005) Experiences with microsurgical tissue transfers in elderly patients. *Microsurgery*, **25(5)**, 390–5.
16. Watkinson JC. (2000) Complications. In Watkinson JC, Gaze MN, Wilson JA. (eds) *Head and Neck Surgery*. Oxford: Butterworth-Heinemann, pp. 83–99.
17. H Venn, Curran JE, Hayden PG. (2007) Anaesthesia and airway management for oral cancer and microvascular surgery. In: Booth PW, Schendel S, Hausamen JE. (eds) *Maxillofacial Surgery*. London: Churchill Livingstone, pp, 395–419.
18. Nadarajan SK, Clarke S, Mitchell V, *et al.* (2008) Anaesthesia for reconstruction of head and neck defects using microvascular tissue transfer. *CEPD*, **10(1)**, 17–23.
19. Castling B, Telfer M, Avery BS. (1994) Complications of tracheostomy in major head and neck cancer surgery; a retrospective study of 60 consecutive cases. *Br J Oral Maxillofac Surg* **32(1)**, 3–5.
20. Halfpenny W, McGurk M. (2000) Analysis of tracheostomy-associated morbidity after operations for head and neck cancer. *Br J Oral Maxillofac Surg*, **38(5)**, 509–12.
21. Sheng LS, Wang D, Fee W, *et al.* (2003) Airway management after maxillectomy: Routine tracheostomy is unnecessary. *Laryngoscope*, **113(6)**, 929–32.
22. Kruse-Lösler B, Langer E, Reich A, *et al.* (2005) Score system for elective tracheotomy in major head and neck tumour surgery. *Acta Anaesthesiol Scand*, **49(5)**, 654–9.
23. Scher N, Dobleman TJ, Panje WR. (1989) Endotracheal intubation as an alternative to tracheostomy after introral or orpharyngeal surgery. *Head Neck*, **11(6)**, 600–4.
24. Chandu A, Smith AC, Gebert R. (2000) Submental intubation: an alternative to short-term tracheostomy. *Anaesth Intensive Care*, **28(2)**, 193–5.
25. Torossian A. (2008) Thermal management during anaesthesia and thermoregulation for prevention of inadvertent perioperative hypothermia. *Best Pract Res Clin Anaesthesiol*, **22(4)**, 659–68.
26. Sigurdsson GH, Banic A, Wheatley AM, *et al.* (1994) Effects of halothane and isoflurane anaesthesia on microcirculatory blood flow in musculocutaneous flaps. *Br J Anaesth*, **73(6)**, 826–32.
27. Pushparaj S. Shetty, Hugo Boyce, *et al.* (2009) Anaesthesia for onco-plastic reconstructive surgery. *Current Anaes Crit Care*, **20(2)**, 18–21.
28. Myles PS, Leslie K, Silbert B, *et al.* (2004) A review of the risks and benefits of nitrous oxide in current anaesthetic practice. *Anaesth Intensive Care*, **32(2)**, 165–72.
29. Szakmany T, Dodd M, Dempsey GA. (2006) The influence of allogenic blood transfusion in patients having free-flap primary surgery for oral and oropharyngeal squamous cell carcinoma. *Br J Cancer*, **94(5)**, 647–53.
30. Taniguchi Y, Okura M. (2003) Prognostic significance of perioperative blood transfusion in oral cavity squamous cell carcinoma. *Head Neck*, **25(11)**, 931–6.
31. Habler O, Schwenzer K, Zimmer K, *et al.* (2004) Effects of standardized acute normovolemic hemodilution on intraoperative allogeneic blood transfusion in patients

undergoing major maxillofacial surgery. *Int J Oral Max-illofac Surg*, **33(5)**, 467–75.

32. Parkin IR, Chiu GA, Schwarz PA, *et al.* (2008) Acute perioperative normovolaemic haemodilution in major maxillofacial surgery. *Br J Oral Maxillofac Surg*, **46(5)**, 387–90.

33. National Institute for Health and Clinical Excellence. *Intraoperative cell salvage in prostatectomy and cystectomy overview.* Available online at http://www.nice.org.uk. (accessed 01 May 2009).

34. Quinlain J. (2006) Anaesthesia for reconstructive surgery. *Anaes Intensive Care Med*, **7(1)**, 31–5.

35. Awwad AM, White RJ, Webster MH, *et al.* (1983) The effect of temperature on blood flow in island and free skin flaps: an experimental study. *Br J Plast Surg*, **36(3)**, 373–82.

36. Sigurdsson GH. (1995) Perioperative fluid management in microvascular surgery. *J Reconstr Microsurg*, **11(1)**, 57–65.

37. Disa JJ, Polvora VP, Pusic AL. (2003) Dextran-related complications in head and neck microsurgery: do the benefits outweigh the risks? A prospective randomized analysis, *Br J Plast Surg*, **112(6)**, 1534–9.

38. Kely KA, Watt-Smith SR. (2009) Postoperative fluid balance in patients having operations on the head and neck. *Br J Oral Maxillofac Surg*, **47(3)**, 249.

39. Qiao Q, Zhou G, Chen GY, *et al.* (1996) Application of haemodilution in free flap transplantation. *Microsurgery*, **17(9)**, 487–90.

40. Banic A, Krejci V, Erni D, *et al.* (1999) Effects of sodium nitroprusside and phenylephrine on blood flow in free musculocutaneous flaps during general anesthesia. *Anesthesiology*, **90(1)**, 147–55.

41. Shafik, M. T.; Pugh, S., Raj, N. (2005) The effect of dobutamine on the blood flow of free flaps. *Anaesthesia*, **60(3)**, 310–11.

42. Jones SJ, Scott DA, Watson R. (2007) Milrinone does not improve free flap survival in microvascular surgery. *Anaesth Intensive Care*, **35(5)**, 720–5.

43. Erni D, Banic A, Signer C, *et al.* (1999) Effects of epidural anaesthesia on microcirculatory blood flow in free flaps in patients under general anaesthesia. *Eur J Anaesthesiol*, **16(10)**, 692–8.

44. Exadaktylos AE, Buggy DJ, Moriarty D, *et al.* (2006) Can anaesthetic technique for primary breast cancer surgery affect recurrence or metastasis? *Anesthesiology*, **105(4)**, 660–4.

45. Sessler DI. (2008) Does regional analgesia reduce the risk of cancer recurrence? A hypothesis. *Eur J Cancer Prev*, **17(3)**, 269–72.

46. Marsh M, Elliott S, Anand R, *et al.* (2009). Early post-operative care for free flap head & neck reconstructive surgery – a national survey of practice. *Br J Oral Maxillofac Surg*, **47(3)**, 182–5.

47. Khalid AG, Mitchell D. (2009). Postoperative monitoring of microsurgical free-tissue transfers for head and neck reconstruction: a systematic review of current technique. *Br J Oral Maxillofac Surg*, **47(6)**, 438–42.

48. Sulaiman L, Charters P. (2005) Survival after massive bleeding into the airway in a patient at risk from 'can't intubate, can't ventilate'. *Anaesthesia*, **60(12)**, 1231–4.

49. Williams AR, Burt N, Bailey M. (1998) Pharyngeal flap necrosis as a cause of airway obstruction during induction of anesthesia. *South Med J*, **91(11)**, 1047–9.

50. Koerner IP. (2005) Fibreoptic techniques. *Best Pract Res Clin Anaesth*, **19(4)**, 611–21.

51. Giraud O, Bourgain JL, Marandas P, *et al.* (1997) Limits of laryngeal mask airway in patients after cervical or oral radiotherapy. *Can J Anaesth*, **44(12)**, 1237–41.

52. Martin F, Buggy DJ. (2009) New airway equipment: opportunities for enhanced safety. *Br J Anaesth*, **102(6)**, 734–8.

53. Bonner S, Taylor M. (2000) Airway obstruction in head and neck surgery. *Anaesthesia*, **55(3)**, 290–1.

54. Burkle CM, Walsh MT, Pryor SG, *et al.* (2006) Severe postextubation laryngeal obstruction: the role of prior neck dissection and radiation. *Anesth Analg*, **102(7)**, 322–5.

55. Sanders B, Thorpe Y, Kallal R, *et al.* (1974) Pseudoankylosis of the mandible secondary to transbicoronal neurosurgical procedures. *J Oral Surg* **32**, 909–11.

56. Pearce A. (2005) Evaluation of the airway and preparation for difficulty. *Best Prac Res Clin Anaesth*, **19(4)**, 559–79.

57. James R. Boyce, Glenn E, *et al.* (2005). Preemptive vessel dilator cricothyrotomy aids in the management of upper airway obstruction. *Can J Anaesth*, **52(7)**, 765–69

58. Georgantopoulou A, Hodgkinson PD, Gerber CJ. (2003) Cranial-base surgery: a reconstructive algorithm. *Br J Plast Surg*, **56(1)**, 10–13.

59. Cohen J, Rad I. (2004) Contemporary management of carotid blowout. *Curr Opin Otolaryngol Head Neck*, **12(2)**, 1.

17

Adjuvant therapy for head and neck malignancy

Charles G. Kelly

Introduction

The non-surgical management of oral and oropharyngeal (OMF) tumours and head and neck cancer in general has changed over the last decade, with the development of new radiotherapy technology and techniques. Novel chemotherapy drugs, chemotherapy regimens, and the use of biological agents have also been introduced. These changes have altered the patterns of morbidity and side effects of non-surgical treatments both in the acute treatment phase and with long-term effects but most importantly has been the overall change in approach to the management of head and neck cancer, with much greater emphasis on organ preservation and post-treatment function. Presurgical adjuvant therapy is becoming increasingly common in the management of malignancy. This chapter describes the radio- and chemotherapeutic treatments for oral and maxillofacial malignancy and the consequences that are of most interest to the anaesthetist.

Multidisciplinary team meetings

The increasing use of these meetings, modelled on American tumour boards, try to ensure by consensus decision-making the best treatment plan for the patient under discussion, avoiding maverick decision-making, allowing for discussion from the evidence base (when it exists, which is not always the case in head and neck cancer), and allowing for multidisciplinary pretreatment assessment. These meetings can also be used as an audit tool, monitoring which treatments are decided on, and if these treatment decisions are carried out. As well as surgeons and oncologists, pathologists and radiologists are available for discussion of diagnosis and staging with other team members drawn from restorative dentistry, dietetics, speech and language, and clinical nurse specialists. Comorbidities, patient's past medical history, and degree of social support are also discussed and may contribute significantly to the final decision made for treatment. The meeting also helps optimize the patient's health status before treatment and allows for planning post-treatment rehabilitation. Common interventions include: assessing the need for percutaneous gastrostomy placement before treatment starts; encouraging smoking cessation with the prescription of nicotine substitutes; and referral for pretreatment dental evaluation and treatment.

One drawback of multidisciplinary team decision-making is that the patient is not a core member of the decision-making group, and is not included in the discussion until after a decision about what 'best treatment' is, has been made. This is being addressed, for example, it is now more common for a patient to meet previous patients who have gone through the same treatment plan, to discuss the treatment experience and rehabilitation.

When is radiotherapy and chemotherapy appropriate in oral and maxillofacial cancers?

Radiotherapy can be given as a primary treatment either alone or with chemotherapy, when surgery is thought to be less appropriate as the initial treatment because it gives less chance of cure, or would entail major cosmetic or functional loss.

Radiotherapy can also be given adjuvantly after surgery, to destroy any residual microscopic cancer cells remaining, and improve the chance of local control, especially if there has been intraoperative tumour spillage, close or positive surgical margins, multiple neck nodes present, or extra capsular spread from nodes. For patients with these factors giving a worse prognosis (which would include patients with cancers of the tongue, floor of mouth, or oropharynx, as these tumours subsites also carry a worse prognosis) chemotherapy would be added in the adjuvant setting.

Chemotherapy is being given more frequently in the neoadjuvant or induction setting, i.e. before the principal treatment modality. This is based on new work using drugs from the taxane family[1–3]. After induction chemotherapy, patients usually move on to concurrent chemoradiotherapy, but if induction chemotherapy fails to produce a significant response this may be an indication that concurrent chemoradiotherapy will also fail, and patients should abandon an attempt at organ conservation and will do better moving directly onto surgery.

There is some evidence that using neoadjuvant or induction chemotherapy may reduce the incidence of early metastatic spread[4].

Occasionally neo-adjuvant or induction radiotherapy with or without chemotherapy is used to downsize tumour or nodal masses, before surgery.

Both radiotherapy and chemotherapy can be used either concurrently or sequentially for managing recurrent or metastatic head and neck cancer.

Primary treatment for oral and maxillofacial tumours: non-surgical versus surgical

An initial important decision is whether the patient should have surgery with or without adjuvant radiotherapy or chemoradiotherapy afterwards, or primary radiotherapy, or, more commonly nowadays, chemoradiotherapy as the main form of treatment, with surgical salvage for any recurrence.

Several important studies have shown that it is possible to cure patients with head and neck cancer using chemoradiotherapy with both organ preservation and retention of organ function[5–7]. There is a surprisingly little evidence base in the literature for comparing these two approaches, but chemoradiotherapy is being used more where organ preservation is an aim of treatment. It is important to be able to maintain organ function as well as anatomical organ preservation, as preserving a non-functioning organ does not benefit the patient. Probably the most common clinical scenario in OMF practice, where organ preservation is considered, is in

oropharyngeal tumours, especially those affecting the base of the tongue where surgery may require laryngectomy with its functional and cosmetic loss.

Other advantages in using primary radiotherapy or chemoradiotherapy include producing better cosmesis, less post-treatment tissue loss and deformity, and without primary surgery, initiating chemoradiotherapy is not delayed. Elective radiotherapy can also be given to unilateral or bilateral neck lymph nodes. Recent advances in radiotherapy technology with linear accelerator intensity modulated radiotherapy (IMRT) or tomotherapy, coupled with the use of cervical node drainage level maps, allows for much more precise radiotherapy planning and the potential for decreased morbidity, but with the cost of much increased radiotherapy planning time.

Chemoradiotherapy should be more effective in a non-operated neck where no tumour cell spillage can have occurred, and where there are no postoperative areas of hypoxia producing radioresistance.

There is still dispute as to in which order elective neck dissection should take place, either before radiotherapy or chemoradiotherapy or 6–8 weeks after completing this treatment[8,9], but if radiotherapy or chemoradiotherapy is given first a proportion of patients will have a complete response, which can now be verified using positron emission tomography (PET) scanning, and they will be spared neck dissection. In patients with confirmed residual nodal disease at the end of radiotherapy, neck dissection performed during this window, 6–12 weeks after treatment, should not cause significantly greater morbidity.

Radiotherapy is not as effective as surgery for salvaging recurrent cancer, whereas surgery may salvage radiotherapy failures.

The disadvantages of using radiotherapy as initial treatment, instead of primary surgery, include: the absence of a pathological specimen giving information on completeness of excision; the longer treatment time for non-surgical treatments; and the acute and late morbidities associated with both radiotherapy and chemotherapy. Later surgery, after the immediate radiotherapy post-treatment window, may be more difficult in patients who have had radiotherapy, and more difficult again if patients had chemoradiotherapy, with fibrosis, loss of tissue planes, and poorer post-surgical healing. Delivering a second course of radiotherapy to previously irradiated tissue is usually compromised by the previous doses received by 'organs at risk' especially the spinal cord and brain stem in head and neck cancer.

Primary chemoradiotherapy is used less in oral cancers where laser-based surgery is used for organ conservation, for example, in lateral tongue tumours, or where close proximity or involvement of the mandible precludes the use of primary radiotherapy because of the accompanying risk of osteoradionecrosis which would require surgical intervention for sequestrum removal.

Methods of radiotherapy delivery

Radiotherapy can be delivered to a tumour in a variety of ways.

External beam radiotherapy

External beam radiotherapy (EBRT) is the most common method of giving radiotherapy, using photon beams from a conventional linear accelerator (Figure 17.1). Multiple beams can be directed at the centre of a tumour target and the beams can be manipulated using either alloy blocks or wedges to conform more to the tumour shape (hence 'conformal treatment'), and give as homogeneous coverage as possible across the tumour, and the least possible radiation dose to close radiosensitive structures, labelled 'organs at risk' (OAR), such as spinal cord or parotid gland (Figure 17.2).

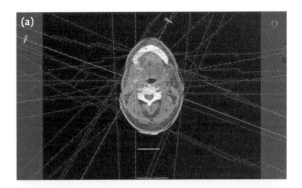

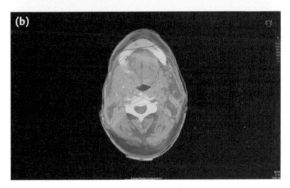

Figure 17.2 a This shows a typical conformal head and neck treatment plan using multiple linear accelerator beams summated giving maximum dose to a right oropharyngeal tumour and minimal spinal cord dose (courtesy of Mr Nick Willis). See also Plate 10. **b** Shows the high-dose area in colour wash (courtesy of Mr Nick Willis). See also Plate 11.

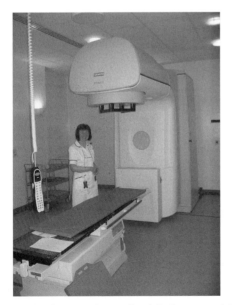

Figure 17.1 A linear accelerator for delivering external beam radiotherapy. The machine head can move 360° and the coach top rotates 360° and moves superiorly and inferiorly.

Brachytherapy

This means 'treatment at a short distance' and is achieved by directly inserting, under general anaesthetic, either live radioactive sources such as iridium wires or 'hairpins' into a tongue or floor of mouth cancer (Figure 17.3) using a relatively bulky introducer.

Under general anaesthetic a number of these introducers would be placed in line, within the substance of a tongue or floor of the mouth tumour, the hairpin then inserted and the introducer removed with the hairpin remaining *in situ* by sliding down the lateral gutters in the introducer. The hairpins are then stitched into place, the geometry of the implant reviewed, and the total exposure time calculated, usually 5–7 days for radical treatment. The stitches are then removed and the hairpins are removed using long forceps, and then returned to a radium safe. Removal does not usually

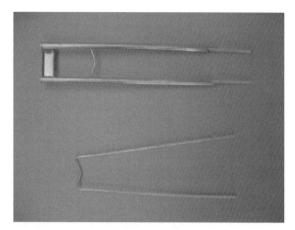

Figure 17.3 Radioactive iridium wire hairpin and second hairpin in introducer.

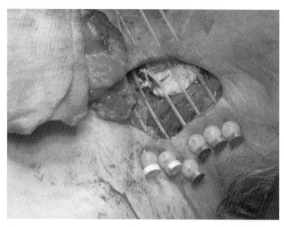

Figure 17.4 Brachytherapy after loading with silicon loading tubes in position.

require a general anaesthetic, unless there has been trauma to the tongue or soft tissues resulting in swelling, obscuring and preventing simple removal. Bleeding can be a risk after removal if the lingual artery has been punctured but this would usually present at insertion when the introducer was removed.

The introducer can cause unnecessary trauma, and uses live radioactive sources, exposing oncology and theatre staff to unnecessary radiation, and so now it is more common to use an after loading technique, where silicone holding tubes are inserted in theatre (Figure 17.4) into the volume to be treated, and these tubes are later connected to a delivery device such as a MicroSelectron (Figure 17.5), where a single radioactive source moves along the tubes and sits for a specified time, 'the dwell time', at predetermined positions to build up the dose required. For head and neck tumours, treatment usually lasts approximately 10 days with two treatments per day lasting 5–10 minutes per exposure with an intervening mandatory rest period to allow for normal tissue recovery.

Intensity-modulated radiotherapy and tomotherapy

These are important radiotherapy developments which have occurred over the last few years and will have major effects on head and neck radiotherapy in the future. The essential aim of IMRT is to have a very focused high-dose area covering the tumour with very rapid radiation falloff outside this area giving much lower doses to surrounding normal tissue, and a much sharper cut off of dose than was previously possible.

Tomotherapy is a form of IMRT using the High Art system machines produced by the TomoTherapy Corporation (Madison, WI, USA), but planning and volume defining is the same for all IMRT approaches.

The intensity of the beam can be altered, or 'modulated' by moving the linear accelerator machine head (Figure 17.1) around the patient while delivering treatment and using multileaf collimators, which consists of a series of metal leaves, set at 90° to beam

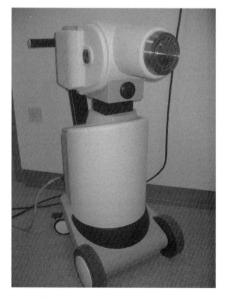

Figure 17.5 MicroSelectron brachytherapy delivery system. The silicon tubes in Figure 17.4 are connected up to the apertures seen at the end of the barrel of this machine.

direction, which can move in and out of the beam within the machine head, blocking parts of the beam, while it is moving around the patient. This allows differing amounts of dose to be built up within very small volumes giving a very complex three-dimensional distribution of radiation dose allowing for far greater conformity around the tumour and much less dose reaching nearby organs at risk.

Using IMRT techniques has already shown to reduce late xerostomia by reducing dose to at least one parotid gland during radiotherapy[10].These techniques also increase the amount of normal tissue receiving very low dose radiotherapy and there are concerns that the incidence of second, radiation-induced tumours, may increase in years to come.

Very precise volume planning radiotherapy delivery and beam quality assurance is essential when using IMRT techniques as the increased conformity around the tumour allows for much less geographical miss.

Radiotherapy dose and fractionation

In North America, conventional radiotherapy dose and fractionation is considered to be 70 Gray (Gy) given in 35 daily fractions at 2 Gy per fraction, treating 5 days a week for 7 consecutive weeks with no treatment breaks, save for weekends. Historically in the United Kingdom (UK), a wider range of radiotherapy regimens have been used, having developed empirically at different centres using regimens thought to be as effective and radiobiologically equivalent to the standard North American dose and fractionation. UK centres have and do use radical treatment regimens such as 66 Gy in 33 fractions over 6.5 weeks; 63 Gy in 30 fractions over 6 weeks, and 55 Gy in 20 fractions over 4 weeks, i.e. giving 2.75 Gy per day. These dose regimens may give differing acute and late morbidities and centres using relatively large dose/fraction regimens such as 55 Gy/20 fractions/4 weeks may reduce the volume being treated to reduce the acute radiation reaction.

These alterations in dose and fractionation have been based on radiobiological principles, in an attempt to improve outcomes. It is known that after 6 weeks of radiotherapy the tumour cell population remaining can enter a phase of 'accelerated repopulation' and some centres see it as important to complete all radiotherapy within 6 weeks. This can increase the acute radiation morbidity, but acute morbidity is usually reversible, unlike late radiation morbidity

changes which are usually the constraining factor on the total radiotherapy dose given.

Altered fractionation regimens

There has been interest in altering dose per fraction and fractionation schedules with the hope of improving outcome and survival. This has been done by using either accelerated or hyperfractionated schedules or a combination of both.

Accelerated fractionation

In accelerated fractionation, the overall treatment time is reduced therefore reducing the opportunity for cancer cells to repopulate. It is achieved by giving more than one fraction per day with a 6–8 hour gap to enable normal tissue repair.

Hyperfractionation

In hyperfractionation, the total dose is divided into a greater number of fractions than normal. If the total dose and overall time is kept to the same as with conventional treatment, then more than one fraction is given per day, but at a lower dose per fraction. As fraction size reduces there is a reduction in radiotherapy late effects, so if the total dose is kept the same then the patient should experience less late effects, or for the same level of late effect as with conventional treatment the total dose can be increased if a hyperfractionated schedule is used.

Often both accelerated and hyperfractionated scheduling is used together but in the CHART trial[11], while there was a significant benefit in using this approach in lung cancer, there was not a significant survival benefit for head and neck cancer patients.

'Concomitant boost' or 'simultaneously integrated boost' is another altered fractionation technique used more commonly in North America and Europe than in the UK (usually because of more limited radiotherapy resources in the UK), when during the last part of the radiotherapy course, an extra radiotherapy boost is given to a smaller volume within the initial volume, the boost being given as a second daily fraction after at least a 6-hour gap. This usually shortens overall treatment time.

These altered fractionation regimens usually cause more acute morbidity or 'early effects' for patients during and shortly after treatment and may impact on any anaesthetic or surgical procedure which has to be carried out during this time.

Radiotherapy and hypoxia

Tumours which contain hypoxic areas are more radioresistant and over the years attempts have been made to reduce hypoxia before and during radiotherapy, by either maintaining adequate haemoglobin levels or by the use of radiosensitizing drugs. It is important to try to maintain haemoglobin at 12 g/dl or above before and during radiotherapy. A trial has been conducted using erythropoietin to maintain adequate haemoglobin levels, but surprisingly those patients taking erythropoietin had worse outcomes than the control group[12].

Following the results of the DAHNCA studies in Denmark[13], nimorazole was introduced as a radio sensitizor and has now become the standard of care in Denmark for head and neck cancer patients receiving radiotherapy but its main side effect is nausea, to the extent that up to one-third of patients discontinue it. It is not in routine use in the UK.

There was also interest from the 1960s to the 1980s in the use of hyperbaric oxygen to try to overcome hypoxia but it has been difficult to overcome the practical obstacle of every radiotherapy department where head and neck cancer is treated, having its own hyperbaric oxygen unit. Also patients need to have radiotherapy immediately after completing the hyperbaric 'dive' as the tissues revert to normal oxygen pressure levels within a matter of minutes of leaving the hyperbaric chamber.

Chemotherapy

Chemotherapy alone is not curative in head and neck cancer but it can have both an additive tumouricidal and radiosensitizing effect with radiotherapy, so it is now used in chemoradiotherapy regimens for large primary tumours or where regional nodal disease is present (stage III or IVa). It is also used in smaller head and neck tumours, which are considered to have a worse prognosis, and that would include cancers of the tongue, floor of mouth and oropharynx. Occasionally chemotherapy is used before primary treatment to downsize a bulky tumour or to make fixed node masses mobile, and consequently more easily removed surgically, and for palliation in recurrent and metastatic cancers.

The use of chemotherapy with other local treatments in recent years was based on the 'Meta-analysis of chemotherapy in head and neck cancer (MACH-NC)'[14], based on data from over 10 000 patients. In

summary, there was a survival benefit of 8% in patients who received concurrent chemotherapy and no significant benefit from those receiving either induction or adjuvant chemotherapy. Single-agent platinum is now considered to be as useful as platinum and 5-fluorouracil (5-FU) in combination with less toxicity[15]. Consequently more single agent cisplatin is now used with radiotherapy and usually given every 3 weeks at the beginning, middle, and end of radiotherapy on days 1, 22, and 43 of radiotherapy, at $100mg/m^2$, although there are other regimens giving cisplatin weekly or even daily.

There had been some reports, using cisplatin intra-arterially, but this has not been shown to be beneficial and is not a practice found in the UK[16]. Since publication of the overview, studies have rekindled interest in the neo-adjuvant use of induction chemotherapy especially with the addition of a taxane in the chemotherapy regimen. Survival benefit has been demonstrated but with increased toxicity, and selecting patients who can tolerate these more intensive treatments is crucial, especially in this patient group who tend to be elderly and have multiple comorbidities.

Other studies are ongoing, and it is likely that induction chemotherapy using taxane-based drug combinations with concurrent chemoradiotherapy using either taxane and platinum combinations or platinum alone, will become the optimum regimen for selected fit younger patients[1].

In older patients with less physiological reserve, and more comorbidity, concurrent chemoradiotherapy with platinum-based regimens, if tolerated, will still be most appropriate treatment. For those patients who cannot tolerate cisplatin chemotherapy, for example, because of renal impairment, concurrent radiotherapy and use of a monoclonal antibody, epidermal growth factor receptor (EGFR) inhibitor, cetuximab is now being used.

There is some evidence for using chemotherapy with postsurgical adjuvant radiotherapy[17] for patients with poorer prognostic factors: large primary tumours, positive surgical margins, multiple positive neck nodes, or extra capsular spread. Primary cancers arising from the oral cavity or oropharynx would also be considered as being higher-risk tumours.

For recurrent and metastatic disease, palliative chemotherapy gives a 1-year survival of approximately 30% but there have been no large studies comparing this to palliative retreatment with radiotherapy or best supportive care. Here, chemotherapy is usually given in combination with the most common regimen being cisplatin 100mg/m^2 on day 1, and 5 fluorouracil 1000mg/m^2 on days 1–4 given via an infusion bottle. Again there is little evidence for survival benefit compared to single agent chemotherapy with cisplatin, but the response rate and toxicity are both increased.

Commonly used chemotherapy drugs in head and neck cancer and their toxicities

Chemotherapy agents commonly used include cisplatin (Table 17.1), carboplatin (Table 17.2), 5-FU (Table 17.3), methotrexate (Table 17.4), paclitaxel (Table 17.5) and docetaxel (Table 17.6).

Epidermal growth factor receptor inhibitors

These drugs are being introduced to head and neck cancer practice and currently going through clinical trials and the regulatory procedures required for use in the UK.

EGFR is known to be overexpressed in most head and neck cancers, and this overexpression has been shown to be linked to survival.

Table 17.1 Cisplatin

75–100 mg/m^2 IV three-weekly
Three cycles given concurrently with radiotherapy as radical treatment
Six cycles given for recurrent or metastatic disease without radiotherapy
Used in combination with 5-FU in both radical and palliative treatments
Can give renal toxicity, and its use may be precluded in patients with renal impairment
Glomerular filtration rate checked before starting use
Requires pre-and posthydration
Ototoxicity with high-frequency hearing loss possible
Neurotoxicity with peripheral neuropathy which can be permanent
Nausea and vomiting can be severe
Thrombosis is a rare complication
Less marrow toxicity than with carboplatin, nadir at 3 weeks
Biochemical hypomagnesaemia common

Table 17.2 Carboplatin

Dose given based on Calvert formula using glomerular filtration rate
Considered slightly less effective than equivalent cisplatin dose
Used more in a palliative setting where better toxicity profile is trade-off for diminished efficacy
Less renal toxicity, ototoxicity, nausea and vomiting, and peripheral neuropathy than cisplatin
Prehydration is not required therefore easier to use on an outpatient basis
More marrow toxicity

Cetuximab, a monoclonal antibody from this family of inhibitors, has seen most use in head and neck cancer and in a large trial has been shown to improve survival when used with radiotherapy[18]. Further trials are ongoing, looking at how effective cetuximab is when combined with chemoradiotherapy and how much increased toxicity is produced by the triple combination of biological agent and chemoradiotherapy. Patients using cetuximab are noted to have more marked radiation reaction but they can also develop an acniform rash outside the treatment area, which has been associated with being a surrogate marker for better response and outcome.

Other biological agents under trial at present are erlotinib and gefitinib which are defined as 'small molecule' tyrosine kinase inhibitors and do not act on cell membrane receptors, but block downstream pathways of EGFR.

Radiotherapy and radiochemotherapy morbidity

Radiotherapy has adverse effects on normal tissues as well as on cancer cells and the addition of chemotherapy to radiotherapy adds to this morbidity. These

Table 17.3 5-fluorouracil

Usually given in combination with either cisplatin of carboplatin as a 4-day infusion at 1000 mg/m^2 per day
Now used more for recurrent or metastatic disease
Main toxicities are mucositis and diarrhoea
Myelosuppression common and can give slight alopecia

Table 17.4 Methotrexate

One of the earliest chemotherapy agents used in head and neck cancer, now used in second-line or palliative regimens
Antimetabolite which acts as an antifolate by inhibiting dihydrofolate reductase which is crucial in folate metabolism
Most important toxicity is early myelosuppression at 7–10 days

Table 17.6 Docetaxel

A taxane, like paclitaxel developed from yew leaves
Commonest taxane used in head and neck cancer, especially in induction regimens
Can cause fluid retention starting with the ankles which then becomes generalized. This is due to increased capillary permeability and usually reversible by stopping treatment. Reduced by the use of prophylactic corticosteroids
Can also cause a hypersensitivity reaction

side effects may impinge on delivering anaesthesia if this is required during, immediately after, or even some years after a course of radiotherapy or chemoradiotherapy. Radiation effects are divided into 'early' and 'late' effects.

Early radiation effects

These effects cause the acute radiation reaction in head and neck cancer patients, and are inevitable with any radiotherapy given, other than at the lowest of palliative radiotherapy doses. The most common examples of these early effects would be acute intraoral mucositis and a skin reaction starting with erythaema. Acute effects are seen in tissues with a rapid cell turnover and are not seen immediately when beginning a course of radiotherapy but begin 1–2 weeks after starting treatment. This is the time period taken for oral mucosal replacement, so when mucosal cells damaged by radiotherapy, attempt mitosis, they die, are not replaced and the mucosa is denuded with an inflammatory reaction developing. More radio-resistant stem cells then initiate re-epithelialization.

While these acute effects are almost universal, they are usually reversible and self-limiting and most importantly, are usually not a criterion for limiting total radiotherapy dose given. A severe acute mucosal

Table 17.5 Paclitaxel

Acts by binding to microtubules, required for cell division, causing apoptosis
Can cause a severe neutropenia
Hypersensitivity in up to 3% of patients with flushing, bronchospasm, hypotension, usually with the first dose
Peripheral neuropathy can occur with higher dosages
Usually causes complete alopecia
Can cause a sinus bradycardia

reaction might require that the patient is temporarily rested from radiotherapy for a few days, and such a reaction is more likely if the patient is receiving chemoradiotherapy.

Acute effects usually settle within 3 weeks of completing radiotherapy, but again if chemoradiotherapy has been given, then the acute morbidity having been more intense, takes longer to settle.

Late radiation effects

These begin 3–6 months after radiotherapy has been completed and are thought to be due mainly to damage to the microvasculature and connective tissue changes caused by radiotherapy, repairing by fibrosis, and to any residual non-repairable parenchymal damage. These changes are in the main, what limits the total radiation dose given.

Later effects are now divided into consequential and true late effects.

Consequential late effects result from severe acute effects such as seen with the intense chemoradiotherapy regimens used for advanced head and neck tumours. An example of a consequential late effect would be dysphagia due to fibrosis of the pharyngeal constrictor muscles following a severe mucositis with chemoradiotherapy. Consequential late effects tend to follow on severe acute effects without a gap.

True late effects may appear months or even years after completing radiotherapy with no symptoms or signs in the intervening period after the acute side effects have settled. In head and neck cancer radiotherapy practice, the most devastating and important true late effect is radiation myelitis because of radiation overdose to the spinal cord. The radiation dose to, and length of spinal cord included in the radiation volume is recorded in the radiotherapy plan in the 'dose volume histogram' with the doses given to other organs at risk (OARs). These would include the optic nerves, optic chasm, doses to optic lens, parotid glands, and any areas of the brain and brainstem in the radiation treatment volume.

Management of radiotherapy morbidity

Morbidity from radiotherapy or chemoradiotherapy can be minimized by interventions before, during, and after radiotherapy treatment.

When choosing the most appropriate treatment for a patient with head and neck cancer, consideration must be given to the potential for early and late morbidity, noting factors that may contribute to more intense radiotherapy side effects; these would include a larger treatment volume, a higher total radiotherapy dose, a higher dose per fraction, a full radical radiotherapy course, whether chemotherapy is added to the radiotherapy course, the patient's age, comorbidities, and performance status, and the likelihood of useful functional organ preservation if radiotherapy or radiochemotherapy is the primary treatment.

Keeping the treatment volume to a minimum and the radiation dose to as low a level as required for adequate radical, i.e. potentially curative treatment, will help minimize radiotherapy side effects, but the intensity of radiation reactions can vary considerably in two patients having similar volumes treated with similar doses due to genetic differences in radiation responsiveness.

General challenges and interventions

Smoking

If a patient is still smoking before beginning radiotherapy they should be strongly encouraged to stop. As radiotherapy proceeds, continued smoking will exacerbate the developing mucositis[19] as well as making it less likely for the patient to discontinue smoking after treatment, thereby putting themselves at risk of developing a second smoking-related new primary cancer. There are now numerous aides available for giving up smoking, from nicotine patches to hypnosis to help patients.

Alcohol

Alcohol is not banned during radiotherapy but patients should be advised to dilute any alcohol taken and avoid spirits. If patients have an alcohol dependency this needs to be recognized and the patient supported through any voluntary or involuntary alcohol withdrawal triggered by starting treatment and a sudden cessation in alcohol intake. As alcohol is known to be synergistic with smoking in causing head and neck cancers, a radiotherapy treatment course with its associated morbidity, can be a useful opportunity to introduce alcohol reduction or cessation programmes.

Nutritional status and swallowing problems

Before radiotherapy treatment starts, dietetic and swallowing assessments should be carried out. If there has been significant weight loss or reduction in food intake, which can be due to an oral or oropharyngeal tumour mass itself, pain from the cancer or difficulty with chewing and swallowing, the patient may need oral supplements or consideration of the placement of a nasogastric tube or percutaneous endoscope gastrostomy (PEG) tube. This is more likely if the patient has had extensive surgery to the tongue or oropharynx, compromising the initiation of swallowing. It is also true if a large part of the tongue has been reconstructed but is not innervated. A nasogastric tube acts to some extent as a stent, helping to preserve some swallowing, but is obvious to all and can fall out relatively easily, requiring a hospital visit for replacement.

A PEG tube, although unobtrusive, requires an invasive procedure to insert it, carries some risk of peritonitis, and enables a patient to maintain nutritional status without swallowing at all, which may lead to complete stenosis of the pharynx, especially with modern intense chemoradiotherapy regimens[20], which appear to cause fibrosis to the constrictor muscles of the pharynx. It is therefore important, if there is no evidence of aspiration, to try to keep the patient swallowing naturally, if only with fluids, but doing this little and often, to give the best chance of retaining an intact swallowing mechanism. Aspiration into the trachea, which may occur in up to 60% of patients[21], needs to be excluded during and after radiotherapy. Such aspiration may be silent and requires formal assessment with the speech and language service using clinical assessment, fibre-optic endoscopic evaluation of swallowing (FEES) and video fluoroscopy, which is a modified barium swallow usually performed by the speech and language therapist and head and neck diagnostic radiologist. In endoscopic evaluation, fluids coloured with food dyes can be used to test swallowing function. From these investigations speech and language therapists can teach the patient to use exercises and techniques to compensate for their swallowing loss. If silent aspiration persists despite these exercise regimens for the pharyngeal musculature and training in 'active swallowing' manoeuvres, then long-term placement of a PEG tube may be required.

Established dysphagia due to pharyngeal or upper oesophageal stenosis[22] requires regular monitoring with bouginage as required and long-term rehabilitation[23,24].

In general, radiotherapy or chemoradiotherapy treatments, because of organ preservation, do not give problems with speech, as seen after extensive surgery, although xerostomia (dry mouth) may make public speaking, or speaking for a length of time more difficult.

Managing specific problems

Managing pain in head and neck cancer

In head and neck cancer, pain can be due to the primary tumour, related nerve infiltration, or other treatment side effects such as mucositis from chemoradiotherapy. It is also an important symptom of tumour recurrence. As with other symptoms a pain history is required with examination of the primary tumour for any potential causes of pain such as bony involvement, dental or soft tissue infection, and post-treatment tumour recurrence or osteoradionecrosis. A pain score chart is useful for continued monitoring. Imaging investigations would now start with a computed tomography (CT) scan, but an orthopantomogram (OPG) can still be useful for showing mandibular defects or tumour infiltration. Magnetic resonance imaging (MRI) is useful for soft tissue diagnosis especially at the base of the tongue and PET CT is being used more to diagnose recurrence.

If an obvious aetiology for pain is found to be from the primary tumour, mucositis, or dental infection then these causes need to be treated. In general the World Health Organization (WHO) analgesia ladder is followed, starting with non-opioid analgesics and adding non-steroidal anti-inflammatory agents relatively early on to reduce the discomfort of treatment mucositis. Weak opioids are then used such as codeine, but it is important to add a laxative, as these patients often have reduced oral intake and an increasingly low-fibre diet, dependent on liquid dietary supplements as they progress through radiotherapy. Tramadol has gained popularity in managing the discomfort of radiotherapy reactions.

Oral morphine suspension is widely used as pain worsens. It is cheap, can be made up in a variety of strengths, and can be titrated against the patient's symptoms. When a dose is reached that makes the patient pain-free, they can be transferred to a regular opiate regimen but retaining use of the opioid suspension for any breakthrough pain. Again, it is important to monitor for constipation. Opiate dependence is very rarely seen with head and neck cancer patients with genuine pain problems and opiates are used early and more freely than with other patient groups.

When pain control is not achieved with opiates, most oncologists would refer patients to local pain specialists in either anaesthesia (see Chapter 22) or palliative care, who have experience with tricyclic antidepressants, anticonvulsants, gabapentin, or ketamine which require careful titration. Occasionally in head and neck practice, there are indications for nerve blocks to relieve neuralgias due to direct nerve involvement by the primary tumour, radiotherapy damage to the nerve, or tumour recurrence where a neuralgia may be the only symptom representing recurrence for months before clinical or imaging signs become evident, although there is now some evidence that PET scanning can pickup recurrence earlier than CT or MRI alone[25].

Mucositis

Mucositis of the oral cavity and oropharynx is inevitable if the patient is given radiotherapy for radical treatment of head and neck cancers in these sites. It usually develops in the second or third week of treatment because the oral mucosa replaces itself approximately every 2 weeks. Its intensity depends on the number of factors including the size of the radiation volume, total radiation dose, dose per fraction, where a higher dose per fraction will give a more intense painful mucositis. If the patient is still smoking during treatment then the mucositis will be worse, and if chemotherapy is added to radiotherapy this will also exacerbate the radiation reaction. Some patients are genetically at risk of developing a more severe mucositis. Mucositis may continue to worsen in the first week or two after completing radiotherapy but has almost always settled by the time of the patient's 6-week follow-up visit.

Management of mucositis

Mucositis gives pain and can interfere with taste, chewing, and swallowing. Adequate pain relief as described earlier is essential and needs to be titrated against the patient's level of pain as this changes as radiotherapy progresses[26].

For local relief, topical anaesthetic agents such as 'lidocaine lollipops' using oral sponges infiltrated with lidocaine may allow meals to be taken orally. Regular oral toilet with mouthwashes helps to mechanically clear debris and prevent secondary infection and the use of fluoride toothpaste on a soft brush also aids oral hygiene.

Although secondary bacterial and fungal infection may have a role to play in the severity of the mucositis and patients immunity may be compromised by both poor nutritional status and concomitant chemotherapy (all the commonly used chemotherapeutic agents used in head and neck cancer can cause neutropenia, although this occurs less commonly with cisplatin) attempts to both treat and prevent mucositis with the prophylactic use of a variety of single agents and combinations of antifungals and antibiotics[27] have not been shown to improve mucositis or quality of life and no topical or systemic antibiotic regimen has come to the fore in managing mucositis.

Various other experimental strategies have been used in an attempt to reduce mucositis including using growth factors such as granulocyte macrophage colony stimulating factor (GM CSF) both topically[28], and by injection[29], and keratinocyte growth factor[30] also known as palifermin, but to date, these trials have been disappointing. Honey is being investigated at present[31].

Protecting the mucosa

Bland topical barrier gels such as Gelclair or Orabase may give some local pain relief and are undergoing trials.

Sucralfate which binds to ulcerated areas protectively coating the mucosa has not shown a proven outcome benefit in clinical trials[32], and although having its advocates is not used extensively in the UK.

Amifostine is a radioprotector given intravenously before daily radiotherapy which protects normal cells. Initial worries that it might protect tumour cells as well as normal tissues have been found to be untrue[33], but there's little convincing evidence of this drug improving outcomes in terms of reducing mucositis.

It is important to recognize specific fungal infections, and oral candidiasis can mimic a radiation mucositis, as well as infect it. Regular oral swabs during radiotherapy and prompt topical treatment with nystatin suspension or fluconazole tablets reduces discomfort for the patient.

Skin reaction and fibrosis

As with mucositis, the skin reaction seen in head and neck radiotherapy does not begin immediately with treatment but in the first 1–2 weeks. It starts with erythaema (grade 1) goes on to dry desquamation (grade 2), and in some cases it can go on to moist desquamation (grade 3), but nowadays it would be very unusual to see a grade 4 reaction with ulceration and necrosis. Pigmentation of the skin may accompany the acute skin reaction and take longer to subside, leaving some patients with some permanent pigmentation (Figure 17.6).

Management of the skin reaction

Patients should avoid wet shaving which increases trauma to the skin and are usually advised to avoid perfumed toiletries. As a skin reaction progresses, a bland aqueous cream can be used to avoid dryness. When radiotherapy has been completed, Flamazine ointment can be used, but if this is used when patients are receiving radiotherapy, as it contains silver, the photons in the radiation beam can interact with this metal causing superficial scattering of photons within the superficial layers of skin exacerbating the skin reaction.

Trismus

This develops some months after completing radiotherapy due to radiation-induced fibrosis affecting the jaw muscles and can have major implications for patients presenting for subsequent general anaesthesia (Figure 16.6). There is a wide variation in incidence[34,35] and one patient may develop marked trismus and

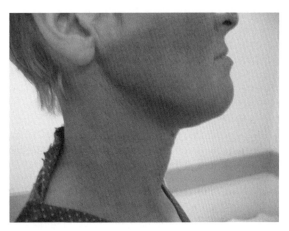

Figure 17.6 A pigmented radiotherapy skin reaction. See also Plate 12.

another, none, despite receiving the same radiotherapy dose, fractionation, and treatment volume.

Management of trismus

Trismus can be assessed simply by measuring the distance between the upper and lower incisors in millimetres. The condition is much more difficult to deal with if already established, so early intervention is crucial for best results. Patients who have compromised mouth opening from previous surgery or start developing this early on in radiotherapy are asked to start an exercise programme of opening and closing the mouth and are given a supply of wooden tongue depressors and asked to put a stack of these between the incisors, and to try to add two more tongue depressors on a daily basis. There are also commercial equivalents to tongue depressors available such as the 'Therabite' system[36]. Starting exercises once radiotherapy has been completed has less chance of success. Trismus can give problems with eating and speaking, but also reduces access to monitor the tumour site and may require future assessment to be by examination under anaesthesia.

Xerostomia and radiation caries

Xerostomia can be both an acute and late effect of radiotherapy. Salivary gland tissue is more radiosensitive than other mucosal and soft tissues of the head and neck and acute xerostomia often develops during radiotherapy, especially if both parotid glands are in the radiation volume. Late xerostomia, which may be permanent and decrease the quality of life[37], will result if salivary tissue remains in the radical treatment volume and receives a dose of more than 30 Gy in standard 2-Gy daily fractions. Xerostomia can also add to the impairment of the sense of taste. It also exacerbates swallowing difficulties especially with solid dry foods.

As well as reducing the amount of saliva, radiotherapy can change the biochemical composition, viscosity and pH of saliva. These changes contribute to the development of dental caries which characteristically occur at the gum margin (Figure 17.7), increasing the risk of teeth breaking off with any future procedures, such as intubation.

Management of xerostomia

This is difficult to manage when established, so prevention is especially important. New radiotherapy techniques have evolved where radiotherapy planning

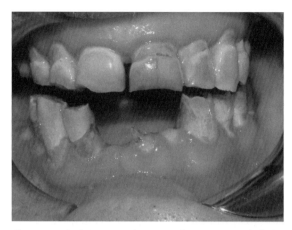

Figure 17.7 Radiation caries (courtesy of Dr Stewart Barclay). This shows extensive radiotherapy caries with the lower incisors having snapped off. See also Plate 13.

tries to spare at least one parotid gland, and as much normal mucosa containing the minor salivary glands. With IMRT and tomotherapy techniques, the parotid glands are delineated and considered as other 'organs at risk' with a radiation dose limit assigned to them of 24 Gy or less, reducing the risk of permanent xerostomia. This has been shown to improve quality of life[38].

Depending on tumour site, it may not be possible to shield adequate salivary tissue, and some patients benefit from oral pilocarpine tablets 5 mg, three times daily. Trials have shown benefit with increased saliva production[39,40] but this does not translate to a universal benefit for all patients, and most end up carrying water bottles because of both the lack of saliva production and its thicker viscosity. There are several brands of artificial saliva available and again some patients find these useful but many post-treatment patients report that do not last long enough in the mouth to be of practical use. A novel experimental approach that is being tried is to surgically transplant salivary glands out all the radiotherapy treatment field[41].

Loss of taste

This occurs when the taste buds on the tongue are included in the radiation field and is an early radiation effect. It may be exacerbated by xerostomia. As well as loss of taste, it can be altered with radiotherapy with some foods tasting 'metallic'. Recovery of taste can take months following radiotherapy, and for some patients it never returns to normal.

Osteoradionecrosis

This is a late radiotherapy effect which may occur years after radiotherapy treatment, after an episode of infection or trauma to the mandible (including dental extraction), where osteoblasts can be stimulated into attempting to repair the bone damage but instead, osteoblast cell death occurs because of the previous radiotherapy. The maxilla can also undergo osteoradionecrosis, but is much less likely site because of its better blood supply.

A similar condition to osteoradionecrosis has been described in the last few years in patients taking bisphosphonates, commonly used in breast and prostate cancer patients with bone metastases. Presentation of osteoradionecrosis can range from an asymptomatic area of exposed bone, to an infected, painful necrotic area with detached bony sequestra.

Because of the risk of radiation caries, subsequent infection and requirement of dental extraction with the risk of osteoradionecrosis, it is important to prevent the need for dental intervention for at least a year after radiotherapy to the jaw. Such patients are very prone to dental injury during airway instrumentation (see Chapter 12).

In our centre, restorative dental colleagues and dental hygienists attend the head and neck cancer clinic; patients who are going to have radiotherapy attend a preradiotherapy dental clinic 4 days later to enable any restorative dental treatment to begin before radiotherapy. Patients are also given advice on oral hygiene, the use of mouthwashes, protective oral gels and fluoride toothpaste. Patients are seen by a dental hygienist on a weekly basis during radiotherapy.

If osteoradionecrosis develops, then if limited it can be treated conservatively with bone penetrating antibiotics. If a larger area of mandible develops osteoradionecrosis or bony sequestra have developed, then surgery is indicated to remove the source of further infection and reconstruct the mandible. Hyperbaric oxygen 'dives' are also relatively widely used in an attempt to reoxygenate the relatively hypoxic bony tissue, despite a minimal evidence base. Patients usually have to travel to one of the national hyperbaric centres around the UK and spend several weeks having one or two 'dives' per day.

Thyroid dysfunction associated with radiotherapy

This is not uncommon and has been found in up to 40% of patients 5 years after completing radiotherapy[42],

but it has a much lower incidence in patients receiving radiotherapy to the oral cavity or oropharynx, when compared to head and neck cancer patients in general[43].

Carotid artery rupture

This is an uncommon occurrence after radiotherapy alone, and is more likely in patients who have tumour recurrence after neck dissection and adjuvant radiotherapy. This complication is almost always fatal, although there are documented survivors[44], who have usually been hospital in-patients with access to immediate resuscitation and surgery.

Depression and psychosocial morbidity

The acute and late physical morbidities from chemoradiotherapy are all too obvious in most patients receiving treatment for head and neck cancer, but the psychosocial morbidity can also be considerable, leading to patients becoming social recluses, refusing to eat in public or with family, or becoming unable to communicate with family, friends, and work colleagues.

Depression is not uncommon in head and neck cancer patients[45]. This can be because of surgical disfigurement and altered body image, pain, loss of function with speech and swallowing, anxiety about tumour recurrence, and radiotherapy and chemotherapy causing low mood. Patients developing head and neck cancers may have other psychological comorbidities such as alcohol and smoking dependence and poor social support. Facial disfigurement and compromised speech function can delay or prevent return to work giving financial anxieties. It is important that head and neck cancer patients have access to social benefits and support both during and after treatment.

Conclusion

The non-surgical management of oral and oropharyngeal (OMF) tumours include novel chemotherapy drugs, chemotherapy regimens, and the use of biological agents. These alter the patterns of morbidity and side effects. It is important to understand morbidity associated with radio- and chemotherapeutic treatments for oral and maxillofacial malignancy during surgical and anaesthetic care of the patients.

References

1. Lorch JH, Posner MR. Wirth LJ, Haddad RI. (2008) Induction chemotherapy in locally advanced head and neck cancer: a new standard of care? *Hematol Oncol Clin North Am*, **22(6)**, 1155–63, viii.

2. Posner MR, Hershock DM, Blajman CR. (2007) Cisplatin and fluorouracil alone or with docetaxel in head and neck cancer. *N Engl J Med*, **357(17)**, 1705–15.

3. Vermorken JB, Remenar E, van Herpen C, *et al.* (2007) Cisplatin, fluorouracil, and docetaxel in unresectable head and neck cancer. *N Engl J Med*, **357**, 1695.

4. Paccagnella A, Orlando A, Marchiori C, *et al.* (1994) Phase III trial of initial chemotherapy in stage III or IV head and neck cancers: a study by the Gruppo di Studio sui Tumori della Testa e del Collo. *J Natl Cancer Inst*, **86**, 265.

5. The Department of Veterans Affairs Laryngeal Cancer Study Group. (1991) Induction chemotherapy plus radiation compared with surgery plus radiation in patients with advanced laryngeal cancer. *N Engl J Med*, **324**, 1685.

6. Lefebvre J-L, Chevalier D, Luboinski B, *et al.* (1996) Larynx preservation in pyriform sinus cancer: preliminary results of a European Organization for Research and Treatment of Cancer phase III trial. EORTC Head and Neck Cancer Cooperative Group. *J Natl Cancer Inst*, **88**, 890.

7. Adelstein DJ, LeBlanc M. (2006) Does induction chemotherapy have a role in the management of locoregionally advanced squamous cell head and neck cancer? *J Clin Oncol*, **24**, 2624–8.

8. Jeong WJ, Jung EJ, Hah JH, *et al.* (2007) Preliminary results of pre-radiation neck dissection in head and neck cancer patients undergoing organ preservation treatment. *Acta Otolaryngol Suppl*, **558**, 121–7.

9. Brizel DM, Prosnitz RG, Hunter S. *et al.* (2004) Necessity for adjuvant neck dissection in setting of concurrent chemoradiation for advanced head-and-neck cancer. *Int J Radiat Oncol Biol Phys*, **58(5)**, 1418–23.

10. Daly ME, Lieskovsky Y, Pawlicki T, *et al.* (2007) Evaluation of patterns of failure and subjective salivary function in patients treated with intensity modulated radiotherapy for head and neck squamous cell carcinoma. *Head Neck*, **29**, 211–20.

11. Dische S, Saunders M, Barrett A. (1997) A randomised multicentre trial of CHART versus conventional radiotherapy in head and neck cancer. *Radiother Oncol*, **44(2)**, 123–36.

12. Henke M, Laszig R, Rube C, *et al.* (2003) Erythropoietin to treat head and neck cancer patients with anaemia undergoing radiotherapy: randomised, double-blind, placebo-controlled trial. *Lancet*, **362**, 1255–60.

13. Overgaard J, Eriksen JG, Nordsmark M. (2005) Plasma osteopontin, hypoxia, and response to the hypoxia sensitiser nimorazole in radiotherapy of head and neck cancer: results from the DAHANCA 5 randomised double-blind placebo-controlled trial. *Lancet Oncol*, **6(10)**, 757–64.

14. Pignon JP, Bourhis J, Domenge C, *et al.* (2000) Chemotherapy added to locoregional treatment for head and neck squamous-cell carcinoma: three meta-analyses of updated individual data. MACH-NC Collaborative Group. Meta-Analysis of Chemotherapy on Head and Neck Cancer. *Lancet*, **355**, 949–55.

15. Bourhis J, Le Maitre A, Baujat B, *et al.* (2007) Individual patients' data meta- analyses in head and neck cancer. *Curr Opin Oncol*, **19**, 188–94.

16. Kovacs AF. (2004) Intra-arterial induction high-dose chemotherapy with cisplatin for oral and oropharyngeal cancer: long-term results. *Br J Cancer*, **90(7)**, 1323–8.

17. Bachaud JM, Cohen-Jonathan E, Alzieu C, *et al.* (1996) Combined postoperative radiotherapy and weekly cisplatin infusion for locally advanced head and neck carcinoma: final report of a randomized trial. *Int J Radiat Oncol Biol Phys*, **36**, 999–1004.

18. Bonner JA, Harari PM, Giralt J, *et al.* (2006) Radiotherapy plus cetuximab for squamous-cell carcinoma of the head and neck. *N Engl J Med*, **354**, 567–78.

19. Porock D, Nikoletti S, Cameron F. (2004) The relationship between factors that impair wound healing and the severity of acute radiation skin and mucosal toxicities in head and neck cancer. *Cancer Nurs*, **27(1)**, 71–8.

20. Caudell JJ, Schaner PE, Meredith RF. (2009) Factors associated with long-term dysphagia after definitive radiotherapy for locally advanced head-and-neck cancer. *Int J Radiat Oncol Biol Phys*, **73(2)**, 410–15.

21. Nguyen NP, Frank C, Moltz CC. (2006) Aspiration rate following chemoradiation for head and neck cancer: an underreported occurrence. *Radiother Oncol*, **80(3)**, 302–6.

22. Nguyen NP, Smith HJ, Moltz CC, Frank C. (2008) Prevalence of pharyngeal and esophageal stenosis following radiation for head and neck cancer. *J Otolaryngol Head Neck Surg*, **37(2)**, 219–24.

23. Nguyen NP, Moltz CC, Frank C. (2004) Dysphagia following chemoradiation for locally advanced head and neck cancer. *Ann Oncol*, **15(3)**, 383–8.

24. Pauloski BR. (2008) Rehabilitation of dysphagia following head and neck cancer. *Phys Med Rehabil Clin N Am*, **19(4)**, 889–928.

25. Zimmer L, Snyderman C, Fukui M. (2005) The use of combined PET/CT for localizing recurrent head and neck cancer: the Pittsburgh experience. *Ear, Nose, Throat J*, **84(2)**, 104, 106, 108–10.

26. McIlroy P. (1996) Radiation mucositis: a new approach to prevention and treatment. *Eur J Cancer Care*, **5(3)**, 153–8.

27. El-Sayed S, Epstein J, Minish E. (2002) A pilot study evaluating the safety and microbiologic efficacy of an economically viable antimicrobial lozenge in patients with head and neck cancer receiving radiation therapy. *Head Neck*, **24(1)**, 6–15.

28. Sprinzl GM, Galvan O, de Vries A. (2001) Local application of granulocyte-macrophage colony stimulating factor (GM-CSF) for the treatment of oral mucositis. *Eur J Cancer*, **37(16)**, 2003–9.

29. McAleese JJ. Bishop KM. A'Hern R. Henk M (2006) Randomized phase II study of GM-CSF to reduce mucositis caused by accelerated radiotherapy of laryngeal cancer. *Br J Radiol*, **79(943)**, 608–13.

30. Borges L, Rex KL, Chen JN. (2006) A protective role for keratinocyte growth factor in a murine model of chemotherapy and radiotherapy-induced mucositis. *Int J Radiat Oncol Biol Phys*, **66(1)**, 254–62.

31. Rashad UM, Al-Gezawy SM, El-Gezawy E, Azzaz AN. (2009) Honey as topical prophylaxis against radio-chemotherapy-induced mucositis in head and neck cancer. *J Laryngol Otol*, **123(2)**, 223–8.

32. Lievens Y, Haustermans K, Van den Weyngaert D, *et al* (1998) Does sucralfate reduce the acute side-effects in head and neck cancer treated with radiotherapy? A double-blind randomized trial *Radiother Oncol*, **47**, 2, 149–53.

33. Brizel DM, Wasserman TH, Henke M, *et al.* (2000) Phase III randomized trial of amifostine as a radioprotector in head and neck cancer. *J Clin Oncol*, **18**, 3339–45.

34. Dijkstra PU, Kalk WW, Roodenburg JL. (2004) Trismus in head and neck oncology: a systematic review. *Oral Oncology*, **40(9)**, 879–89.

35. Dijkstra PU, Huisman PM, Roodenburg JL. (2006) Criteria for trismus in head and neck oncology. *Int J Oral Maxillofac Surg*, **35(4)**, 337–42.

36. Therabite information available online at <http://www.atosmedical.com/Products/Mouth_Jaw.aspx>

37. Dirix P, Nuyts S, Vander Poorten V, Delaere P, Van den Bogaert W. (2008) The influence of xerostomia after radiotherapy on quality of life: results of a questionnaire in head and neck cancer. *Supp Care Cancer*, **16(2)**, 171–9.

38. Eisbruch A, Ship JA, Dawson LA, *et al.* (2003) Salivary gland sparing and improved target irradiation by conformal and intensity modulated irradiation of head and neck cancer. *World J Surg*, **27(7)**, 832–7.

39. Johnson JT, Ferretti GA, Nethery WJ, *et al.* (1993) Oral pilocarpine for post-irradiation xerostomia in patients with head and neck cancer. *N Engl J Med*, **329**, 390–5.

40. Nyarady Z, Nemeth A, Ban A, *et al.* (2006) A randomized study to assess the effectiveness of orally administered pilocarpine during and after radiotherapy of head and neck cancer. *Anticancer Res*, **26(2B)**, 1557–62.

41. Kahn ST, Johnstone PA. (2005) Management of xerostomia related to radiotherapy for head and neck cancer. *Oncology*, **19(14)**, 1827–32; discussion 1832–4, 1837–9.

42. Turner SL, Tiver KW, Boyages SC. (1995) Thyroid dysfunction following radiotherapy for head and neck cancer. *Int J Radiat Oncol Biol Phys*, **31(2)**, 279–83.

43. Cetinayak O, Akman F, Kentli S, *et al.* (2008) Assessment of treatment-related thyroid dysfunction in patients with head and neck cancer. *Tumori*, **94(1)**, 19–23.

44. Porto DP, Adams GL, Foster C. (1986) Emergency management of carotid artery rupture. *Am J Otolaryngol*, **7(3)**, 213–17.

45. Chen AM, Jennelle RL, Grady V, *et al.* (2009) Prospective study of psychosocial distress among patients undergoing radiotherapy for head and neck cancer. *Int J Radiat Oncol Biol Phys*, **73(1)**, 187–93.

18

Anaesthesia for orthognathic surgery

Viki Mitchell

Introduction

Orthognathic surgery involves the manipulation of the facial skeleton: the maxilla, mandible, and dentoalveolar segments (the portion of the jaw supporting the teeth), these can all be surgically repositioned to treat malocclusion and deformity. The term orthognathic derives from the Greek words *orquos*, meaning to straighten, and *gnaqos*, which means jaws. Hence orthognathics is surgery to straighten the jaws.

The majority of patients are referred to the orthognathic team by an orthodontist because they have malocclusion which cannot be corrected by conservative measures (braces and appliances) alone. Abnormalities of dental alignment (the bite or occlusion) relate not only to the position of the teeth, they are intimately connected with the relative positions of the upper and lower jaw. Facial harmony depends on these relationships, but malocclusion does not only influence facial aesthetics, there are serious functional implications. Chewing, mastication, speech, temporomandibular joint (TMJ) function, the ability to nose-breathe, and the ability to maintain good oral hygiene may all be compromised. The correction of these functional elements underpins the rationale behind treatment.

A multidisciplinary team approach is standard, and treatment may take years to reach completion. An orthodontist is always involved if dental occlusion is at issue; the orthodontic workup generally starts a year or two before surgery and continues postoperatively. In addition, restorative dentists, dental hygienists, psychologists or psychiatrists, throat, nose and ear, plastic and neurosurgeons, speech therapists, specialist nurses, and audiologists may all contribute to planning and treatment[1–4].

Patient preparation and premedication

Preoperative evaluation

Most patients presenting for orthognathic surgery have abnormalities of dental occlusion which cannot be corrected with orthodontics alone. In all but the most extreme cases, surgery is delayed until late adolescence when bone growth is complete and the permanent teeth have all erupted, so most patients are in their teens or early twenties and have no significant medical comorbidities.

A minority have bony deficiencies secondary to cleft lips, cleft palates or craniofacial syndromic deformities such as Crouzon's or Apert's syndrome which may be associated with other significant medical abnormalities. Some have acquired skeletal anomalies or asymmetries, usually as a result of treatment of head and neck tumours in childhood or following trauma, and this group are much more likely to have challenging airways.

Preoperative planning for orthognathics often begins years before surgery and includes a full orthodontic workup, with imaging, dental impressions, and the construction of dental models (Figure 13.4). Model surgery is carried out to establish the feasibility of different treatment options and these models are used to generate wafers with impressions of the teeth on each surface. These interpositional occlusal wafers are important intraoperatively as they allow accurate repositioning of jaws to provide the desired occlusion. Presurgical orthodontics straightens the teeth and aligns the arches so that stable occlusion can be achieved postoperatively.

Anaesthetic input into the orthognathic or cranio-facial clinic helps to identify the more complex patients who may have a history of previous anaesthetic problems and significant medical comorbidities and those in whom perioperative airway management may not be straightforward. Teenagers are a distinct group who have their own set of psychosocial problems, which make them more challenging than children in many ways. In those with severe dentofacial abnormalities there is often a long history of unenjoyable hospital visits, and the usual fears and anxieties may be heightened. The opportunity to meet these patients early to provide information to help manage their expectations about the anaesthetic and to establish a rapport can be very helpful.

Immediate preoperative patient preparation and premedication

On the day of surgery, the preoperative visit is useful to prescribe sedative premedication if indicated and to establish guidelines for fasting. Postoperative analgesia can be discussed and the use of adjuncts such as ice packs, which help reduce pain and swelling, explained. It is helpful to warn patients if a lubricant ointment will be used to protect the eyes, as blurred vision postoperatively can cause considerable anxiety. An explanation about the numbness and loss of proprioception associated with local anaesthetic, a warning about a sore throat, and the benefits of an early oral intake help to manage patient expectations. A detailed anaesthetic and airway management plan should be devised in conjunction with the surgeon.

Maintenance of anaesthesia

Securing the airway

Nasal tubes are the mainstay of maxillofacial anaesthesia and the most versatile method of managing the airway in orthognathic surgery. The most common procedures are maxillary or mandibular osteotomies, or a combination of the two (the bimaxillary osteotomy). All these procedures use dental occlusion as a reference point for accurate fixation of the bony fragments. An oral tracheal tube is therefore contraindicated and a nasal tube is the usual method of securing the airway and providing optimal surgical access (Figure 18.1). If the surgical plan involves mid or upper facial work such as a nasal manipulation, if a bicoronal flap is planned, or if the nasal passages are occluded, submental intubation is preferable (Figure 18.2)[5]. On rare occasions,

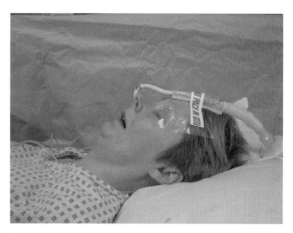

Figure 18.1 North polar nasotracheal tube and throat pack alert label.

when the airway is challenging and is likely to be further compromised for a significant period postoperatively, a tracheostomy may be necessary to provide secure airway control.

Preformed north-facing nasal tubes are ideal as they are stable once positioned and can be secured with strapping across the forehead which means that the bony contours and symmetry of the face are not obscured. Care must be taken to ensure that the tube lies passively and does not exert any traction on the nostril. This is particularly important for maxillary impaction as upward traction may cause distortion of the nasal septum and this may not be apparent until the patient is extubated and found to have a bent nose.

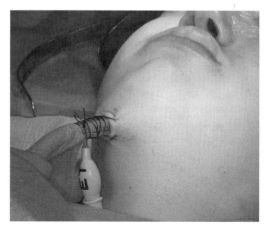

Figure 18.2 Submental tracheal tube. See also Plate 14.

Protecting the airway

A throat pack prevents soiling of the trachea with blood and debris and the passage of blood into the stomach. The pack should be inserted under direct vision avoiding excess bulk which can anteriorly displace the mandible, undesirable if chin or jaw surgery is taking place. The use of a pack must be recorded (Chapter 12) on the anaesthetic chart and a sticker on the tracheal tube to help ensure that it is removed at the end of surgery (Figure 18.1).

Suction under direct vision prior to extubation is important, to clear clots which may have formed in the mouth or behind the palate, the so-called coroner's clot. If the patient has had a mandibular osteotomy, it is very important not to apply forward traction to the mandible with a laryngoscope as it may displace the screws or plates which have been applied to the osteotomized segments.

Eye protection

The eyes are vulnerable during surgery. Eye pads may not be welcomed by the surgeon as they obscure the bony contours of the face and compromise the surgical field. A barrier ointment should be applied and further protection provided with the application of transparent eye tapes, Steri-Strips or surgical eye shields.

Antithrombotic prophylaxis

Venous thromboembolism is rare following orthognathic surgery[6] but it does occur, and standard prophylactic measures should be used.

Temperature regulation

Peripheral or rectal temperature probes avoid the difficulties of siting a probe in the nose. It is sensible to maintain normothermia to avoid shivering during emergence, which is both uncomfortable for the patient and increases their oxygen demands. It is easy to cause overheating during longer maxillofacial procedures as only the head and neck are exposed so it is essential to monitor the temperature.

Facilitating surgery

Optimizing the surgical field involves mutually satisfactory airway management and techniques to reduce blood loss. Bleeding at the saw insertion site obscures the bony cuts and makes a precise incision more

difficult during the osteotomy. There is always significant bleeding when the maxilla is down fractured during a Le Fort I and this will continue to some extent into the postoperative period. A head-up position to improve venous drainage, the use of adrenaline containing local anaesthetic or tumescent solutions to infiltrate the field prior to incision and moderate hypotension, are all helpful[7,8]. The antifibrinolytic, tranexamic acid, can be used prophylactically to reduce bleeding[9].

Extubation, emergence, and postoperative care

A smooth safe emergence is desirable. Coughing and agitation on emergence increase both arterial and venous pressure, and the risk of haematoma formation, suture disruption, and bleeding at the surgical site. Forceful coughing or mouth opening can disrupt mandibular fixation, and airway manoeuvres such as a jaw thrust or the application of a tight-fitting facemask may damage the surgical field. In general, there will be blood in the mouth at emergence even after meticulous oropharyngeal suction under direct vision, so it is safest to extubate patients awake with airway reflexes intact.

A remifentanil infusion can be used to provide an awake, cooperative patient who is tube-tolerant and in whom the cardiovascular responses to extubation are obtunded.

After some procedures, the tracheal tube can be exchanged for a laryngeal mask or supraglottic airway device before anaesthesia is lightened to provide a smooth emergence, but this technique is unsuitable following mandibular surgery when forceful mandibular manipulations are undesirable[10].

If the airway was challenging at the start of anaesthesia or if there is any uncertainty about the ability to reintubate or reoxygenate following extubation or in the immediate postoperative period, the tracheal tube should be removed over an airway exchange catheter. This can be left in place in the trachea, providing a conduit for oxygenation and reintubation should it be needed (Figure 18.3)[11–13].

Antiemesis

It is important to prevent postoperative nausea and vomiting in maxillofacial surgery. Vomiting is always distressing but is particularly so after surgery to the oral cavity. It is unpleasant for the patient and, since the

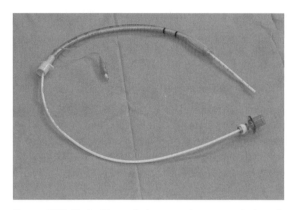

Figure 18.3 Cook Airway Exchange catheter passed through endotracheal tube. Reproduced courtesy of http://www. cookmedical.com.

forced involuntary muscular contraction of retching and vomiting raise the venous pressure, increasing the risk of bleeding and suture disruption, it should be avoided if possible.

Antiemetics with dexamethasone, a liberal preoperative fluid regimen, and encouragement to start oral fluids early after surgery are all helpful. There is a lower incidence of postoperative nausea and vomiting following total intravenous anaesthesia with propofol than after volatile anaesthesia[14].

Analgesia

In general, most orthognathic procedures are not very painful postoperatively. A combination of intraoperative local anaesthetic, simple analgesics, and morphine followed by regular paracetamol and a non-steroidal anti-inflammatory postoperatively is often sufficient. Oral medications should be prescribed in liquid or soluble form to make them easy to swallow. A patient-controlled analgesic (PCA) regimen is rarely necessary. Instructions to nurse the patient in a head-up or sitting position, the use of regular dexamethasone, and the application of ice packs reduce postoperative swelling and enhance patient comfort. Early resumption of oral fluid intake is also beneficial as it eases the sore throat and dry mouth which follows anaesthesia.

If supplemental oxygen is needed postoperatively humidification prevents drying and crusting of blood and secretions in the nose and the mouth.

Orthognathic surgical procedures

The commonest orthognathic procedures are Le Fort I maxillary osteotomy, bilateral sagittal split osteotomy of the mandible, and a combination of the above—the bimaxillary osteotomy, and genioplasty or osteotomy to the chin (Figure 18.4).

Le Fort I: maxillary osteotomy

A Le Fort I osteotomy involves complete mobilization of the maxilla which is then repositioned using the occlusal surface of the upper and lower teeth as a reference point, and stabilized with titanium screws and plates. An intraoral mucosal incision is made from the first molar tooth on one side to the same point on the other and a mucoperiosteal flap is raised. An oscillating saw is used to make the osteotomy cuts which extend from the lateral wall of the nose at the pyriform fossa into the pterygomaxillary fissure behind the posterior aspect of the maxilla. At the nasal floor, the septum is separated from the maxilla, the lateral nasal walls are osteotomized, and the inferior turbinates are trimmed if necessary. This allows down fracture of the maxilla which, although freely mobile, remains attached and viable by its soft tissue pedicle. The jaws are temporarily wired together over an interpositional acrylic wafer which has impressions of

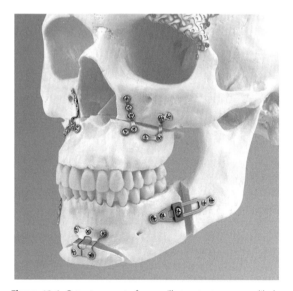

Figure 18.4 Osteotomy cuts for maxillary osteotomy, mandibular osteotomy, and genioplasty with plates in position. Reproduced courtesy of Synthes Ltd, Welwyn Garden City; http://www. synthes.com.

the teeth in perfect occlusion on each surface, and the maxilla is fixed in place using miniplates and screws.

The maxilla can be mobilized in any direction, forwards (advancement), upwards (impaction), downwards, backwards (setback), and it can be rotated. In some circumstances, a vertical maxillary split may be carried out to widen the upper dental arch or segmental osteotomy, dividing the maxilla into separate fragments which can be repositioned independently.

Postoperative rigid intermaxillary fixation (IMF) (jaw wiring) is rarely needed but light elastic traction attached to arch bars or orthodontic brackets is sometimes used to encourage correct final positioning[15]. Indications of Le Fort I: maxillary osteotomy are included in Table 18.1 and anaesthetic considerations in Table 18.2.

Mandibular osteotomy

The bilateral sagittal split mandibular ramus osteotomy (BSSO) is the most versatile and popular mandibular osteotomy. It allows forward or backward movement of the lower teeth and some rotation of the jaw is also possible.

The intraoral incision is made halfway down the vertical ramus of the mandible and extends as far as the last molar tooth. The neurovascular bundle is

---

Table 18.1 Indications of Le Fort I: maxillary osteotomy

- Maxillary-mandibular disproportion: jaw disproportion and malocclusion at the dentoalveolar level can be corrected in conjunction with presurgical orthodontics, and a Le Fort I maxillary osteotomy is often combined with mandibular surgery

- Late cleft palate surgery: after adolescence a maxillary advancement may be carried out to correct the significant midface hypoplasia which can occur after cleft closure

- Combined with high-level advance: Le Fort I and III osteotomies can be combined for midface advancements in patients with major craniofacial abnormalities

- Cranial base access: a LeFort I allows access to the nasopharynx, upper cervical spine, and cranial base

- Obstructive sleep apnoea

Table 18.2 Anaesthetic considerations during Le Fort I: maxillary osteotomy

- Patients are generally young adults without major comorbidities

- Nasal tube (or submental tube) necessary

- A passive tracheal tube position is important; it must not exert traction or pressure on the nose

- The nasal tube is vulnerable during osteotomy and can be punctured or transected[16]. It is advisable to use an airway exchange catheter if the tube needs to be changed intraoperatively

- Eye protection using viscous ointment +/- clear occlusive tapes is essential

- Bleeding following down fracture from the maxillary artery, pterygoid, and greater palatine veins can be significant

- Group and save preoperatively

- Throat pack mandatory

- Moderate hypotensive technique and head-up tilt helpful

- Meticulous oropharyngeal suction necessary prior to extubation

- Extubate awake

- Prophylactic antibiotics and dexamethasone are routine

- Fixation is stable and not especially painful. PCA is unnecessary

- Nurse sitting up to reduce swelling and bleeding

- If oxygen is needed postoperatively, humidification increases patient comfort as it prevents drying and crusting of blood in the nose

---

identified as it enters the mandibular canal and a horizontal osteotomy is made on the lingular surface with an oscillating saw. The vertical osteotomy cut is made on the buccal surface of the body of the mandible. The vertical and horizontal cuts are then joined with a sagittal osteotomy (parallel with the internal oblique line), the split is then completed using osteotomes, and the procedure repeated on the other side. The toothbearing portion of the mandible

Table 18.3 Anaesthetic considerations in mandibular osteotomy

- Patients are generally young adults without major comorbidities
- A nasal tube (or submental tube) is necessary as the surgeon needs to assess dental occlusion
- Eye protection is important, use viscous ointment and clear occlusive tapes
- Bleeding is rare but can be significant[17]
- Group and save preoperatively
- Throat pack mandatory
- Moderate hypotensive technique and head-up tilt advisable
- Meticulous oropharyngeal suction is necessary prior to extubation
- Mandibular position is partially dependant on soft tissue tone, hence reducing the depth of anaesthesia prior to definitive fixation may help the surgeon attain the optimal final position. A wake-up test can be carried out using a remifentanil infusion. The patient is allowed to regain consciousness during the procedure, prior to closure, so that the mandibular position can be assessed with near normal soft tissue tone[18]
- Avoid applying force to the mandible as it may disrupt fixation
- Direct laryngoscopy during at the end of surgery for removal of the throat pack and suctioning should be performed gently
- Avoid airway manoeuvres such as the jaw thrust
- Do not exchange tracheal tube for an LMA for emergence as forceful mouth opening is undesirable
- Aim for calm, controlled, awake extubation
- Postoperative bleeding is rare but can cause airway obstruction due to haematoma formation and swelling
- This procedure is not very painful. Small doses of intraoperative morphine combined with local anaesthetic, regular paracetamol, and a non-steroidal usually suffice; a PCA is not necessary
- Rigid IMF is rarely necessary. If it is used, the patient must be nursed in an high dependency unit with wirecutters immediately available. Light elastic traction attached to arch bars or orthodontic brackets which are sometimes used to encourage correct final positioning allow some mouth opening and special measures are unnecessary

is now mobile and can be repositioned using mini plates and screws or screws alone. An interpositional wafer is often used to permit accurate repositioning and may be left in place at the end of surgery. IMF may be necessary if the splits are considered unstable but is rarely used routinely. Anaesthetic considerations are included in Table 18.3.

Bimaxillary osteotomy

In many cases optimal correction of orthognathic deformities can only be achieved with surgery of both the mandible and maxilla—this is termed a bimaxillary osteotomy or bimax.

The maxillary osteotomy is performed first; an intermediate interpositional wafer (which has been generated using patient-specific dental models as part of the orthodontic workup) is placed between the upper and lower teeth. These are then wired together and the maxilla fixed in its new position, effectively using the original position of the lower teeth as a reference point. The IMF is released and the bilateral mandibular sagittal splits carried out. A second, 'final' wafer is used to reposition the mandible, so that this stage of the surgery uses the new position of the maxillary teeth as the reference point. Although a bimax takes longer than a single jaw osteotomy, the anaesthetic considerations are the same.

Genioplasty

The chin is critical to facial harmony. It influences the facial height, facial centre lines, and cosmetic appearance of the nose. Genioplasty can be used to augment or reduce chin size, to straighten an asymmetric face or to lengthen a short face. It can be carried out as a single procedure or combined with other osteotomies or soft tissue facial procedures.

After infiltration with adrenaline containing local anaesthetic solution, an intraoral incision is made behind the lower lip; the osteotomy is performed with an oscillating saw and the bony fragment repositioned using titanium screws. Anaesthetic considerations are included in Table 18.4.

Distraction osteogenesis

Distraction osteogenesis, a technique to generate bone and soft tissue, is gaining in popularity for the surgical correction of hypoplasias of the craniofacial skeleton. In the 1950s Gavril Ilizarov, a Russian orthopaedic surgeon, showed that osteogenesis could be induced if bone is expanded (distracted) along its long axis at the rate of 1 mm per day[19]. A corticotomy is used to fracture the bone into two segments which are gradually moved apart during the distraction phase. New bone forms along the vector of pull, avoiding the need for a bone graft, and offers the additional benefit of expansion of the overlying soft tissues, which are frequently deficient in these patients[20].

Distraction osteogenesis is used to augment a hypoplastic mandibular or maxillary alveolar ridge prior to dental implant insertion, distraction of the mandible to produce lengthening where there is

hypoplasia or deformity, and midface distraction for syndromic conditions associated with midface hypoplasia such as Crouzons and Aperts. The first two procedures involve a simple corticotomy to divide the bone and the fixation of the distractor plates to each of the two segments with screws. After a brief latent period, the distractor is adjusted via its external component to extend the gap gradually. Midface distraction is a much more complex, technically demanding, procedure, and is generally the preserve of specialist craniofacial centres (see Le Fort II and III osteotomies).

Dentoalveolar surgery

The alveolus is the part of the jaw that supports the teeth. Dentoalveolar surgery is concerned with management of the diseases of the teeth and the hard and soft tissues which support them.

Preprosthetic surgery and dental implants

This is a subspecialty of dentoalveolar surgery which involves the restoration of oral and facial form and function which has been lost through the loss of teeth and related bony structures. This may be as the result of extractions at an early age or following trauma, surgery or radiotherapy. Without reasonable dentition, normal speech, mastication, and swallowing are not possible, and there is soft tissue collapse so that both form and function suffer. If the teeth are removed or lost, bony resorption occurs, and the alveolar ridge

---

Table 18.4 Anaesthetic considerations during genioplasty

- The presenting population mainly consists of the anatomically normal patient who dislikes their chin because it is too large, too small, pointy or asymmetric. It also includes those with mandibular hypoplasia such as Treacher Collins and juvenile idiopathic arthritis (Still's disease), who may have challenging airways

- A nasal tracheal tube gives the best exposure and allows the surgeon to assess facial harmony when repositioning the chin

- The incision is inside the lower lip, therefore a throat pack is indicated

- The risk of significant intraoperative bleeding is minimal

- Avoid pressure on the chin with a facemask or a chin lift on emergence; a jaw thrust is not contraindicated. Extubation is best carried out awake; alternatively, the tracheal tube can be exchanged for a supraglottic airway

- This is not a painful procedure. Opiates are often unnecessary

- A genioplasty masks mandibular hypoplasia and may camouflage the predictors of difficult direct laryngoscopy as the length of the mandible is unchanged. It is important to tell the patient if they were difficult to intubate and to complete airway alert documentation so that subsequent anaesthetists are forewarned

becomes hypoplastic and will not provide adequate support for a denture.

The most widely used implant is the osseo-integrated implant, based on the discovery that titanium can be successfully fused into bone when osteoblasts grow on and into the rough surface of the implanted titanium. Osseo-integrated implants can be used either to provide anchor points for dentures or obturators or to allow construction of artificial teeth—they have the beneficial effect of stimulating bone growth. If there is insufficient bone to anchor a dental implant, bone grafting or distraction surgery are needed to augment the jaw prior to insertion.

Depending on their site and number, implants can be placed under local anaesthesia, with or without sedation, or under general anaesthesia. A sub-mucoperiosteal flap is raised, the bone is drilled, and the preliminary fixture inserted into the bone. A titanium healing cap (Figure 18.5) is screwed into the implant to prevent ingrowth of the oral mucosa and a period of months is allowed for integration. The second stage is much less invasive and can usually be carried out under local anaesthesia. The healing cap is removed and a prosthetic tooth moulded onto a titanium post is screwed into place.

Bone grafts

Bone grafts are used to augment bony deficiencies and may be carried out in isolation, in preparation for definitive surgical procedures, or as a component of other procedures. The common donor sites for bone grafts are the iliac crest, rib, maxilla, mandible, cranium, and tibial plateau. Corticocancellous bone can be used in blocks; particulate cancellous bone can be sandwiched into osteotomies or defects. A third form includes purely cortical grafts, primarily used to form a wall or strut in a defect that is simultaneously packed with particulate cancellous bone. Cortical grafts revascularize very slowly and have minimal to no cell survival. Cadaveric bone is occasionally used.

The morbidity associated with bone grafts is related to the donor site. Iliac crest grafts are painful and an epidural catheter can be left *in situ* to allow boluses or an infusion of local anaesthetic to be given for the first 24 hours.

High facial osteotomies: Le Fort II and III and facial advancement

Midfacial advancement[21] is indicated for patients with syndromic craniosynostosis and in severe developmental hypoplasia of the midface which can include cleft patients. In these patients, rigid internal fixation is an option but the degree of advancement required is often so great that restriction of the adjacent soft tissues may preclude stable advancement in one stage; distraction techniques are favoured as they allow gradual bone and soft tissue lengthening. These procedures are the preserve of specialist craniofacial centres and involve a multidisciplinary workup and treatment pathway[22,23].

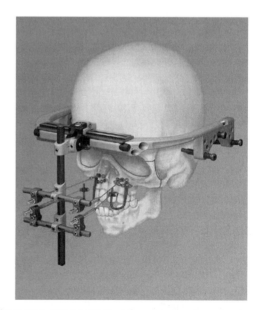

Figure 18.6 RED II external midface distractor. Reproduced courtesy of Synthes North America Ltd; http://products.synthes.com.

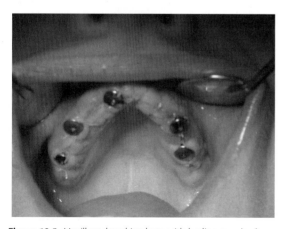

Figure 18.5 Maxillary dental implants with healing caps *in situ*.

The Le Fort II osteotomy is a procedure used in patients with midface hypoplasia in whom the maxilla and nose require movement together. Access is via incisions in the mouth, transconjunctival incisions behind the lower eyelids or lower eyelid (blepharoplasty). Access to the nose is via a bicoronal incision to raise the scalp.

The Le Fort III osteotomy is used to correct generalized midface hypoplasia which includes the malar complexes and the orbits. Osteotomies of the maxilla, nose, and zygomas allow the entire midface to be moved *en bloc* or in segments. The surgical approach is similar to the Le Fort II procedure[24]. If a distraction technique is used, a halo device is fixed on to the skull with pins, and distraction wires link titanium plates attached to the facial bones with the frame. These devices are designed to disarticulate with relative ease but do restrict access to the airway (Figure 18.6)[25]. Anaesthetic considerations are included in Table 18.5.

Temporomandibular joint surgery

The temporomandibular joint (TMJ) is a compound joint composed of the temporal bone, the condyle of the mandible, and the articular disc, contained within a tightly attached fibrous capsule and lined with a synovial membrane. The disc divides the joint into two compartments; the lower compartment permits hinge motion or rotation and the upper compartment permits sliding. It is a diarthrodial joint, a discontinuous articulation of two bones with the extent of movement dictated by associated muscles and ligaments. It is the

---

Table 18.5 Anaesthetic considerations for high facial osteotomies: Le Fort II and III and facial advancement

- Patients tend to be teenagers or young adults
- Craniofacial skeletal abnormalities may be associated with other syndromic abnormalities
- They may have sleep apnoea related to a small volume postnasal space. The airway may be improved postoperatively as the postnasal airspace is enlarged by midface advancement
- These are major and prolonged procedures
- A submental tracheal tube is often necessary—the nasal route is unavailable, and the oral route precludes an assessment of dental occlusion
- A throat pack is needed
- Significant intraoperative blood loss may occur
- Meticulous eye protection is needed
- Prophylactic antibiotics and dexamethasone are routine
- Distraction frames restrict access to the airway. The application of a facemask is difficult and rigid laryngoscopy is impossible with the frame in place. They can be disarticulated but a special screwdriver is required and the joints tend to become stiff with time[26]. A dedicated screwdriver and wirecutters should be available at the bedside in the postoperative period
- Patients may present for alteration of the frame to change the distraction vectors. This may be possible under sedation. Alternatively, the frame can be disarticulated prior to induction or a laryngeal mask can be used to manage the airway[27]. An awake, oral fibreoptic intubation is a reasonable alternative. A facemask technique with manual occlusion of the nostrils has also been described[28]
- Extubate awake: airway exchange catheter is a good option. It is well tolerated, allows administration of oxygen, and can be used as a conduit if reintubation is required
- Nurse sitting up to reduce swelling and bleeding
- If oxygen is needed postoperatively, humidification prevents drying and crusting of blood in the nose
- Regular analgesics are required during the postoperative period and the distraction phase as soft tissue stretching is painful

Table 18.6 Anaesthetic considerations during temporomandibular arthroscopy and arthrocentesis

- There is a correlation between TMJ dysfunction and stress and anxiety states; patients are often nervous
- There may be limitation of joint movement which can affect mouth opening
- The incision is extraoral but the surgeon will handle the oral cavity whilst manipulating the joint. The choice of airway management device should be discussed—a reinforced laryngeal mask airway may be acceptable provided there is good communication between surgeon and anaesthetist
- A throat pack is not necessary
- Use a viscous ointment to protect the eye—tapes interfere with the surgical field
- Muscle paralysis improves access to the joint space
- This is a painful procedure, and intravenous or intra-articular morphine is usually required in addition to paracetamol and NSAIDs. The surgeon may prefer not to use local anaesthesia as it causes facial paralysis

Table 18.7 Anaesthetic considerations during open meniscal surgery/arthrotomy

- Patient population as for TMJ arthroscopy
- Surgery is extraoral but a nasal tube is most convenient
- Good analgesia can be achieved with surgical infiltration of local anaesthetic and adrenaline; morphine may be required
- A smooth emergence and recovery is essential to protect the repair
- To avoid vigorous movement of the TMJ, aim for a smooth, controlled awake extubation
- Nurse head-up or sitting up and prescribe steroids and ice packs to reduce postoperative pain and swelling

most active joint in the body, moving up to 2000 times a day during talking, chewing, swallowing, yawning, and snoring[29].

There are two groups of patients with TMJ disorders: those with normal anatomy and abnormal function, and those with abnormal anatomy. The first group present with pain and clicking, the aetiology of which is incompletely understood but which may be triggered by abnormalities of occlusion which produce disharmonious joint movement and trigger muscle spasm. This is common, affecting over 10% of the population and representing the major cause of orofacial pain. These patients generally have a degree of trismus but this usually relaxes after induction of anaesthesia and they rarely present airway management issues. The second group of patients have anatomical derangements ranging from disc displacement, which causes symptoms but does not limit mouth opening, to ankylosis of the joint which prevents mouth opening[30].

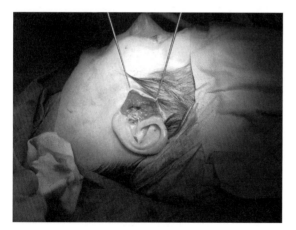

Figure 18.7 Exposure of temporomandibular joint by a preauricular incision.

Table 18.8 Anaesthetic considerations during coronoidectomy

- Patients likely to have mechanically restricted mouth opening which will not improve after induction
- Intraoral surgical route so nasal tube and throat pack necessary
- Mouth opening should be improved at the end of the procedure
- It is a painful procedure; morphine will be needed in addition to simple analgesics

Temporomandibular arthroscopy and arthrocentesis

An arthroscope is introduced into the joint and lavage carried out. Anaesthetic considerations are included in Table 18.6.

Open meniscal surgery/arthrotomy

TMJ symptoms caused by an abnormal articular disc may be treated with an open procedure in which the joint space is accessed via a preauricular incision (Figure 18.7). Anaesthetic considerations are included in Table 18.7.

Coronoidectomy

Excision of the coronoid process is sometimes performed for TMJ ankylosis. Anaesthetic considerations are included in Table 18.8.

Table 18.9 Anaesthetic considerations during temporomandibular joint replacement

- All patients have severely restricted mouth opening and a fibreoptic intubation is the airway management technique of choice
- They may be elderly or have conditions such as rheumatoid arthritis, so medical comorbidities are common[32]
- A nasal tracheal tube is necessary
- A throat pack is mandatory but may be difficult to insert as mouth opening is limited
- Use a viscous ointment to protect the eye; avoid tapes on the side of the surgery as the surgeon may want to see the eye
- Surgery is prolonged
- The surgeon may request moderate hypotension
- There is a risk of sudden, severe bleeding owing to the proximity of the carotid artery to the ankylosed joint
- Invasive arterial monitoring is advisable
- Mouth opening may be improved after surgery, but the joint is delicate and vigorous mouth opening or mandibular manipulation should be avoided
- Postoperative high dependency care is advisable for the first 24 hours
- This is a painful procedure; a PCA is required postoperatively

---

Temporomandibular joint replacement

TMJ replacement is reserved for severely deranged joints. The surgery is delicate and prolonged and generally only carried out in specialist centres[31]. Anaesthetic considerations are included in Table 18.9.

Conclusion

Orthognathic surgery necessitates a multidisciplinary team approach within which the anaesthetist has a pivotal role. Early communication with other members of the team and appropriate patient preparation is an important aspect of the anaesthetic care.

References

1. Riden K. (1998) *Key Topics in Oral and Maxillofacial Anaesthesia*. Oxford: BIOS Scientific Publishers Ltd.
2. Miloro M, Larsen P, Ghali GE, Waite P. (eds)(2004) *Peterson's Principles of Oral and Maxillofacial Surgery*, 2nd edn. Hamilton, Ontario: BC Decker.
3. Harris M, Hunt N. (eds)(2008) *Fundamentals of Orthognathic Surgery*, 2nd edn. London: Imperial College Press.
4. Reyneke JP. (ed.) (2003) *Essentials of Orthognathic Surgery*. Chicago: Quintessence Publishing Co Ltd.
5. Amin M, Dill-Russell P, Manisali M, Lee R, Sinton I. (2002) Facial fractures and submental tracheal intubation. *Anaesthesia*, **57(12)**, 1195–9.
6. Blackburn TK, Pritchard K, Richardson D. (2006) Symptomatic venous thromboembolism after orthognathic operations: An audit. *Br J Oral Maxillofac Surg*, **44(5)**, 389–92.
7. Precious DS, Splinter W, Bosco D. (1996) Induced hypotensive anesthesia for adolescent orthognathic surgery patients. *J Oral Maxillofac Surg*, **54(6)**, 680–3.
8. Choi WS, Samman N. (2008) Risks and benefits of deliberate hypotension in anaesthesia: a systematic review. *Int J Oral Maxillofac Surg*, **37(8)**, 687–703.
9. Choi WS, Irwin MG, Samman N. (2009) The effect of tranexamic acid on blood loss during orthognathic surgery: a randomized controlled trial. *J Oral Maxillofac Surg*, **67(1)**, 125–3
10. Nair I, Bailey PM. (1995) Use of the laryngeal mask for airway maintenance following tracheal extubation. *Anaesthesia*, **50(2)**, 174–5.
11. Mort TC. (2007) Continuous airway access for the difficult extubation: the efficacy of the airway exchange catheter. *Anesth Analg*, **105(5)**, 1357–62.
12. Biro P, Priebe HJ. (2007) Staged extubation strategy: is an airway exchange catheter the answer? *Anesth Analg*, **105(5)**, 1357–6.
13. Gray H. (2005) Extubation. In: Calder I, Pearce A (eds). *Core Topics in Airway Management*. Cambridge: Cambridge University Press, pp. 87–92.
14. Apfel CC, Kranke P, Katz MH *et al.* (2002) Volatile anaesthetics may be the main cause of early but not

delayed postoperative vomiting: a randomized controlled trial of factorial design. *Br J Anaesthesia*, **88(5)**, 659–68.

15. Van de Perre JPA, Stoelinga PJW, Blijdorp PA *et al.* (1996) Perioperative morbidity in maxillofacial orthopaedic surgery: a retrospective study. *J Cranio-Maxillofacial Surg*, **24(5)**, 263–70.

16. Hosseini Bidgoli SJ, Dumont L, Mattys M, Mardirosoff C, Damseaux P. (1999) A serious anaesthetic complication of a LeFort I osteotomy. *Eur J Anaesthesiol*, **16**, 201–3.

17. Teltzrow T, Kramer FJ, Schulze A, Baethge C, Brachvogel P. (2005) Perioperative complications following sagittal split osteotomy of the mandible. *J Cranio-Maxillofac Surg*, **33(5)**, 307–313.

18. Toro C, Robiony M, Costa F, Sembrionio S, Politi M. (2007) Conscious analgesia and sedation during orthognathic surgery, preliminary results of a method of preventing condylar displacement. *Br J Oral Maxillofac Surg*, **45(5)**, 378–81.

19. Ilizarov GA. (1971) Basic principles of transosseous compression and distraction osteosynthesis. *Ortop Travmatol Protez*, **32(11)**, 7–15.

20. McCarthy JG, Stelnicki EJ, Mehrara BJ, Longaker MT. (2001) Distraction osteogenesis of the craniofacial skeleton. *Plast Reconst Surg*, **107(7)**, 1812–27.

21. Gosain AK, Santoro TD, Havlik RJ, Cohen SR, Holmes RE. (2002) Midface distraction following Le Fort III and monobloc osteotomies: problems and solutions. *Plast Reconst Surg*, **109(6)**, 1797–808.

22. Greenberg AM, Prein J. (2002) *Craniomaxillofacial Reconstructive and Corrective Bone Surgery*. New York: Springer.

23. Samchukov ML, Cope JB, Cherkashin AM. (2001) *Craniofacial Distraction Osteogenesis*. St Louis: Mosby.

24. Jones K. (2002) In: Greenberg AM, Prein J. (eds) *Le Fort II and Le Fort III Osteotomies for Midface Reconstruction and Considerations for Internal Fixation in Craniomaxillofacial Reconstructive and Corrective Bone Surgery*. New York: Springer.

25. Nishimoto S, Oyama T, Shimizu F *et al.* (2004) Fronto-facial monobloc advancement with rigid external distraction (RED-II) system. *J Craniofac Surg*, **15(1)**, 54–9.

26. Figueroa AA, Polley JW, Ko E. (2001) Distraction osteogenesis for treatment of severe cleft maxillary deficiency with the RED technique. In: Samchukov ML, Cope JB, Cherkashin AM (eds) *Craniofacial Distraction Osteogenesis*. St Louis: Mosby.

27. Wong GB, Nargozian C, Padwa B. (2004) Anaesthetic concerns of external maxillary distraction osteogenesis. *J Craniofac Surg*, **15**, 78–81.

28. Tong J, Ahmed-Nusrath A, Smith J. (2007) External maxillary distraction: an alternative to awake fibreoptic intubation. *Br J Anaesth*, **99(2)**, 301.

29. Fletcher MC, Piecuch JF, Lieblich SE. (2004) Anatomy and pathophysiology of the temporomandibular joint. In: Miloro M, Larsen P, Ghali GE, Waite P (eds) *Peterson's Principles of Oral and Maxillofacial Surgery*, 2nd edn. Hamilton, Ontario: BC Decker.

30. Scrivani SJ, Keith DA, Kaban LB. (2008) Temporomandibular disorders. *N Engl J Med*, **359(25)**, 2693–705.

31. Guarda-Nardini L, Manfredini D, Ferronato G. (2008) Temporomandibular joint total replacement prosthesis: current knowledge and considerations for the future. *Int J Oral Maxillofac Surg*, **37(2)**, 103–10.

32. Kohjitani A, Miyawaki T, Kasuya K *et al.* (2002) Anesthetic management for advanced rheumatoid arthritis patients with acquired micrognathia undergoing temporomandibular joint replacement. *J Oral Maxillofac Surg*, **60(5)**, 559–66.

19

Anaesthesia for paediatric maxillofacial surgery

Ann Black and Senthil Nadarajan

Introduction

Probably the most common procedures undertaken by maxillofacial surgeons in children are either explorative dental procedures or soft tissue repair following facial trauma. Another large group of work is related to the primary and secondary management of children with cleft lip and palate. Maxillofacial surgeons work as part of a multidisciplinary team and services are configured in many different ways according to local arrangements. For example, primary cleft work is done in some areas by maxillofacial surgeons and in others exclusively by plastic surgeons. Similarly, craniosynostosis may be managed by maxillofacial, craniofacial, or neurosurgeons depending on local practice and expertise.

Whilst the principles involved in managing an anaesthetic in the older child are similar to adult practice, the expertise of the paediatric anaesthetist and the perioperative care of the paediatric nursing and medical teams are required in managing babies and young children.

The main groups of children who will need maxillofacial input are illustrated in Table 19.1.

Preoperative evaluation

Review of previous anaesthetic charts will reveal any previous difficulties on induction of anaesthesia, management of the airway, and complications on recovery. History of respiratory compromise such as presence of a significant pectus excavatum (an indicator of chronic airways obstruction), tachypnoea, tracheal tug, use of accessory muscles of respiration, or cyanosis have important anaesthetic implications. History of failure to establish adequate nasal breathing (choanal atresia), episodes of arterial oxygen desaturation related to airway obstruction, history of snoring, airway obstruction intermittently (especially during sleep), obstructive sleep apnoea (OSA), central apnoeas, preoperative oxygen requirement (especially note any recent increase), dependence on preoperative ventilation or continuous positive airway pressure (CPAP), history of feeding difficulties or failure to thrive should be elicited. In children with syndromic/dysmorphic features, the preoperative workup should include screening for the presence of coexisting congenital malformations, including cardiac defects.

Premedication

A preoperative visit enables the establishment of rapport with the child/parents, helps to allay anxiety, and gives the opportunity to discuss the anaesthetic plan. Midazolam is the mainstay of paediatric premedication. Whilst sedative premedication is contraindicated in a child with a precarious airway it is often useful in anxious children who do not have airway compromise. Sedative premedication is usually avoided in infants with cleft palate.

Anticholinergics such as atropine or glycopyrrolate are particularly useful if an advanced airway technique is to be used. By decreasing the airway secretions a gaseous induction is smoother and laryngospasm less likely. The view via the fibreoptic scope is better and clearance of secretions is much less of an issue. This is particularly so when using the smallest fibreoptic scope which does not have a suction channel.

Fasting requirements

Children are allowed to have clear fluids until 2 hours, breastfeeding until 4 hours, and formula feeds until 6 hours, prior to surgery[1].

Table 19.1 The main groups of children who will need maxillofacial input

Cleft lip and palate:
Primary and secondary surgery
Congenital abnormalities:
Crouzons
Aperts
Pfeiffers
Craniosynostosis
First arch abnormalities:
Pierre Robin
Treacher Collins
Goldenhar
Trauma:
Soft tissue or bony injuries
Caustic or thermal burns
Arteriovenous malformations:
Sturge–Weber
Tumours:
Benign or malignant
Infection:
Dental abscess
Septic arthritis of the temporomandibular joint
Atypical mycobacterium lymphadenitis
Inflammation:
Juvenile rheumatoid arthritis

Identification of the difficult airway

As an anaesthetist the main question is whether you expect to have difficulties in managing the airway or intubation in a syndromal child. Fortunately, it is very rare for the paediatric airway to be unexpectedly difficult to manage. Routine preoperative tests used in adult practice to identify the difficult airway (see Chapter 4), have not been validated in paediatric practice. However, there is usually plenty of warning that the anaesthetist may have difficulties with airway management and therefore preparation is possible.

Induction of anaesthesia

Inhalational anaesthesia remains the preferred technique of induction for management of the difficult pediatric airway[2,3]. Intravenous access is secured prior to intubation.

Managing difficult intubation in a child

Most difficult intubations in paediatrics are predictable as they are in syndromal children. Airway management

should be individualized based on careful history and physical examination of soft tissue and bony abnormalities in each child. There is an increasing range of specialized airway devices and equipment available for use in children. A selection of Straight, Macintosh, Miller, McCoy, and video laryngoscopes are available in a range of sizes[4,5]. Paediatric fibrescopes are available down to 2.2 mm in external diameter. However, the smallest scope with a working channel is 2.8 mm (Karl Storz, Germany) in external diameter, which can be used with a 3-mm tracheal tube[6].

Children will rarely tolerate awake fibreoptic intubation (FOI), so a technique that will work in the anaesthetized child is essential. There are two main issues to consider. Firstly, how to keep the child anaesthetized and monitored whilst doing the FOI and secondly, how to actually achieve the intubation. Laryngeal mask airway (LMA) in combination with a flexible fibrescope serves as an important tool in handling paediatric difficult airway and intubation. Use of a LMA allows anaesthesia to be maintained with a volatile agent, provides a conduit for tracheal intubation, and, most importantly, provides a secure airway during spontaneous ventilation until intubation is accomplished.

Choice of tracheal tubes in children

A wide selection of tracheal tubes has been designed for paediatric use. Surgical requirements tend to drive the choice of either an oral or a nasal tube. Uncuffed tubes are still the tube of choice for young children and are widely recognized as safe[7]. However, cuffed tracheal tubes, designed specifically for paediatrics, are available in all sizes and there is increasing interest in using these, though this remains controversial[8–10].

Use of throat packs

Most surgery on the airway will require use of a throat pack. It is used to provide a seal around the uncuffed tracheal tube, absorb blood and debris, and help stabilize the tracheal tube in the required position. This seemingly simple piece of equipment is fraught with potential for harm (see Chapter 12). Vigilance is required when a throat pack is used and the insertion and removal of the pack is carefully documented.

Antibiotic prophylaxis

Any intraoral/nasal surgery is associated with the risk of contamination with oral flora and broad-spectrum cover is required. Local practices dictate the choice of antibiotic prophylaxis used for surgery. Co-amoxiclav is a frequent choice if the child is not penicillin sensitive. When skin or bone grafting is planned, the infection risk is more likely to be due to *Staphylococcus aureus* and antibiotic prophylaxis is adjusted appropriately according to local guidelines. Antibiotic prophylaxis for children with cardiac lesions has been recently reviewed and the majority of conditions no longer require antibiotic prophylaxis[11,12].

Fluid management

For minor surgery perioperative fluids are not essential, however, there is good evidence that recovery is improved, and nausea and vomiting is less, if children are given fluids and are not required to drink until they are inclined to do so. Perioperative fluid management must be carefully managed, and it is divided into provision of a maintenance fluids and replacement fluids.

Maintenance fluids are given as isotonic crystalloid infusions. There has been much debate of the 'ideal' fluid to use in children as a maintenance solution. The suggested volumes are based on early work on the water needs of children undergoing surgery[13].

Volume required for maintenance:

- 4 ml/kg/hour (100 ml/kg/24 hours) for the first 10 kg body weight
- 2 ml/kg/hour (50 ml/kg/24 hours) for the second 10 kg
- 1 ml/kg/hour (25 ml/kg/24 hours) for each kg above 20.

Balanced isotonic salt solutions such as Hartmann's are satisfactory for perioperative use in most children; however, practice varies regarding the particular choice of fluids nationally and internationally. Recent guidelines have been published to inform and guide this discussion[14]. It is important to warm the fluids and monitor temperature to keep the child warm between 36–37°C.

Postoperative fluids are usually restricted to 50–75% of the estimated hourly maintenance volume. Children should be able to drink early after maxillofacial surgery and intravenous fluids are reserved for those who are unable to drink and those who have an intraoral repair should oral feeding if contraindicated. If postoperative fluids are required it is important to remember that replacement of surgical losses requires colloid or blood products and maintenance fluid requirement requires an infusion of either Hartmann's or 0.45% saline in 5% dextrose. If the child is not able to feed, then the blood glucose, urea, and electrolyte should be checked at least 1 hour after surgery, then every 4 hours and any abnormalities actively corrected.

Major maxillofacial surgery may result in both prolonged surgery and extensive blood loss and these are replaced with a mixture of blood products and colloid guided by the type and volume of measured and ongoing losses.

Regular point of care estimations of haemoglobin concentration and electrolyte measurements are essential to guide the choice of fluid. Protocols have been published which give clear guidelines for postoperative fluid replacement with the goal of maintaining a haemoglobin above 7 g/dl, ensuring satisfactory haemodynamics and be responsive to ongoing losses if present[15].

The compromised airway in the postoperative period

Children with craniofacial or mandibulofacial dysostosis are at high risk of postoperative respiratory compromise including obstructive sleep apnoea[16]. These patients may benefit from the insertion of a nasopharyngeal 'prong'. The prong fashioned from a paediatric tracheal tube is inserted at the end of the surgery, to keep the airway patent[17]. However, the use of a nasal tracheal tube should be avoided in any child who has had a pharyngoplasty. Prolonged surgery and excessive pressure exerted on the base of the tongue by the retractor may result in postoperative oedema causing potential airway obstruction[18]. A careful assessment of the airway and planning is essential prior to extubation. If stridor is present, nebulized adrenaline and a single bolus of intravenous dexamethasone are given and this is very effective in decreasing the risk of laryngeal oedema. Nursing these patients in head-up position helps in reducing oedema. In some cases, it may be necessary to intubate and ventilate them for a period of time.

Tracheostomy

A child who has a precarious airway preoperatively will be better able to thrive, grow, and be safe in the early postoperative period, if they have a tracheostomy. Early tracheostomy may be required in about 17–50% of infants with craniofacial dysostosis (e.g. Apert, Treacher Collins syndromes), having severe airway obstruction[19,20]. Successful decannulation of these children may take several years until midface advancement is complete[19].

A tracheostomy is sometimes essential in order to undertake major facial surgery safely. It is useful to remember that a tracheostomy can be done while the airway is being maintained with a tracheal tube, a LMA, a nasopharyngeal airway, or indeed a face mask. During the management of major paediatric facial surgery, the tracheostomy is kept until the series of operations is completed.

There is morbidity and mortality associated with tracheostomy, which can be early or late. Early complications include local trauma, bleeding, pneumothorax, pneumomediastinum, subcutaneous emphysema, and tube accidents such as accidental displacement or blockage of the tracheal tube. Late complications include tracheal stenosis, granulation formation, subglottic stenosis, and long-term speech damage[21].

Postoperative nausea and vomiting

Postoperative nausea and vomiting (PONV) is a common sequel. Some children, particularly those with known travel sickness are particularly prone to PONV and it is aggravated by blood being accidentally ingested postoperatively and by the use of opiates. PONV can be managed using the Association of Paediatric Anaesthetists (APA) guidelines which recommend a combination of ondansetron and dexamethazone prophylaxis[22].

Analgesia

Multimodal analgesia is routinely used. Most children will be satisfactorily managed with a combination of effective local anaesthetic, usually provided by the surgeon and paracetamol 15 mg/kg intravenously 6 hourly or 15–20 mg/kg rectally 6 hourly. Non-steroidal anti-inflammatory drugs (NSAIDs) are used if appropriate. NSAIDs (ibuprofen and diclofenac) have not been associated with an increased risk of perioperative bleeding in children[23]. However caution is exercised in surgical procedures with a high risk of bleeding.

Remifentanil is a predictable opioid that promotes rapid recovery and haemodynamic stability in paediatric anaesthesia. There are advantages for its use in neonates and infants due to their higher clearance of remifentanil[24]. If morphine is used, then it is usually given 40 minutes prior to the end of the procedure for optimal analgesia without compromising recovery[25].

Postoperatively, simple oral analgesics given in a regular dose regimen are very effective. Guidelines are available for dose regimens and balanced analgesia[26].

Local anaesthesia

Local anaesthetic given either as local infiltration or as specific nerve block is surprisingly effective. These include lidocaine 1% (maximum dose limited to 3 mg/kg), lidocaine 1% with adrenaline (1: 200 000 or 1: 80 000) up to a maximum dose limited to lidocaine 5 mg/kg and that of adrenaline limited to 5 mcg/kg or levobupivacaine 0.25% up to a maximum dose limited to 2.5 mg/kg (2 mg/kg in neonates).

Specific paediatric conditions requiring anaesthesia for maxillofacial surgery

Anaesthesia for cleft lip and palate

Cleft lip and palate are the commonest craniofacial anomalies[27]. Cleft lip occurs in 1 in 600 live births. Isolated cleft palate occurs in about 1 in 2000 live births. The clefts may be incomplete or complete involving lip, alveolus, hard and soft palate. The objective of correction of cleft lip/palate is to get a good cosmetic and functional outcome, which includes normal hearing and speech. A centralized care model, with eight to 15 regional centres and a multidisciplinary cleft team approach are recommended for improved outcome in these group of patients[27,28]. A child with a cleft will often need a planned series of operations spread over many years, depending on the severity of the condition. They also need the support of the wider cleft team comprising of maxillofacial, plastics, ear, nose, and throat (ENT), orthodontic surgeons, paediatrician, speech therapists, specialist nurses, educational support, and psychologists. Surgery is divided into primary and secondary cleft surgery.

Primary cleft surgery

Repair of cleft lip is done at 2–3 months of age in healthy infants and usually delayed until 60 weeks postconceptual age in premature infants. Neonatal repair of cleft lip is undertaken in some centres. Early repair may improve mother–infant interactions and maintain normal cognitive development of infants[29]. However, the potential for perioperative complications in the neonatal period must be carefully considered[30]. If surgery is done in the newborn, there is the

Table 19.2 Timing of cleft surgery

Timing of cleft procedures	Age
Lip closure ± anterior palate	0–3 months
Palate repair	9–12 months
Pharyngoplasty to correct velopharyngeal insufficiency	6–8 years
Alveolar bone graft (orthodontic treatment)	8–12 years
Maxillary/mandibular surgery	15–17 years

possibility that other congenital abnormalities will not yet have been detected and there is a risk that the neonate will revert to a transitional circulation perioperatively. In addition, closure of the lip and the anterior palate at the first operation, at about 3 months, results in better outcome in the long term.

Palate repair is considered at 9–12 months of age when the baby is starting to try to speak, this is timed to prevent delay in speech development. Infants with associated syndromes such as Pierre Robin, who have severe airway obstruction in the neonatal period are at high risk of postoperative hypoxaemia and will benefit from postponing the palate repair until the age of 12–18 months. Some units will delay surgery until a baby has reached 5 kg taking this as an indicator that the child is managing to thrive[30]. The timing of cleft surgery is in part determined by the child's age (Table 19.2).

Preoperative assessment

Whilst the majority of children with cleft lip and palate have no other abnormalities, this condition is associated with a wide variety of syndromal or dysmorphic features (Table 19.3). A more extensive cleft seems to be associated with a higher risk for associated malformations.

There is an increased prevalence of congenital heart disease in children with cleft palate[31]. Therefore it is important to perform a careful clinical examination, record preoperative oxygen saturation, and consider echocardiography.

Chronic rhinorrhoea is common in infants with cleft palate due to nasal regurgitation during feeds. If active infection is present, especially in children with a wide cleft, primary palate surgery is postponed to reduce perioperative respiratory complications[32].

The presence of a cleft palate can make sucking difficult so that breast- or bottle-feeding can be difficult to establish. Most infants will thrive with careful spoon or bottle-feeding using modified teats. Occasionally nasogastric feeding is necessary, for instance in infants with severe Pierre Robin sequence.

Partial upper airway obstruction is present in some infants with micrognathia especially during sleep. If uncorrected, resultant hypoxia may lead to right ventricular hypertrophy and, rarely, cor pulmonale[33]. Conservative measures like prone/lateral positioning are useful in mild cases and a range of surgical methods are used to relieve airway obstruction in severe cases[34].

Table 19.3 Common syndromes associated with cleft palate

Syndrome	Features	Anaesthetic considerations
Pierre Robin sequence	Micrognathia, cleft palate, glossoptosis; Feeding difficulties/ short stature present in 25%[35]; Congenital heart disease (20%): atrial septal defect, ventricular septal defect, patent ductus arteriosus[33]	Cor pulmonale due to chronic upper airway obstruction;[34] Difficult laryngoscopy and intubation; Airway improves with mandibular growth in 20% of cases
Velocardiofacial syndrome[36]	Pierre Robin sequence[35]; Developmental delay; Immune deficiency due to thymic hypoplasia	Sleep apnoea; Laryngomalacia (2%); Hypocalcaemia; Congenital heart disease
Stickler syndrome	Genetic connective tissue disorder[37]; Pierre Robin sequence (30%); Myopia/retinal detachment; Hearing difficulties	Mandibular and maxillary hypoplasia; Intubation difficulties during infancy
Treacher Collins syndrome	Maxilary, zygomatic, and mandibular hypoplasia; Retrognathia; Narrow nasopharynx; Basilar kyphosis[39]; Hearing difficulties	Obstructive sleep apnoea; Difficult mask ventilation and intubation; Often worsens with increasing age[40]
Goldenhar syndrome	Hemifacial microsomia; Micrognathia; Vertebral hypoplasia; Cardiac anomalies	Mask fit, laryngoscopy, and intubation difficult and often worsens with age; Important to evaluate for C1–C2 subluxation[41]

Occasionally babies will be oxygen dependent, or may need long-term nasal CPAP, usually because of a combination of partial airway obstruction and chronic lung disease. These children are particularly at risk of severe airway obstruction once the palate is closed. It is important to identify those patients prior to surgery so that they can be monitored and managed appropriately[42]. A small minority may need a temporary tracheostomy to cover the perioperative period[34].

In the healthy baby for a cleft lip repair, only a haemoglobin test is required; however, when palatal surgery is planned a group and save is also done. It is unusual for a child to actually require blood transfusion for closure of cleft palate.

Intraoperative management

- Monitoring: standard monitoring includes electrocardiogram, pulse oximetry, non-invasive blood pressure, temperature, end-tidal carbon dioxide, and agent monitoring

- Inhalational induction with sevoflurane is commonly employed and peripheral intravenous access is achieved at an appropriate depth of anaesthesia. Non-depolarizing neuromuscular blocking agent is used after confirmation of effective bag mask ventilation

- Tracheal intubation is straightforward in most of the infants[43]. If the cleft defect is wide, the laryngoscope blade tends to slip into the defect making intubation difficult. Packing the gap with gauze temporarily can avoid this occurrence and aid intubation

- Syndromal children, particularly those with significant micrognathia, can be difficult to intubate. A paraglossal approach using the straight blade improves the view and reduces tissue trauma[30,44,45]. However, advanced techniques may be required and paediatric fibreoptic scopes or video laryngoscopes must be available

- Orotracheal intubation is performed using a south-facing preformed RAE (Ring–Adair–Elwyn) tube and is fixed in the midline as this provides clear surgical access to the shared airway. A throat pack is used. Ventilation is controlled to achieve normocapnia

- As the airway is shared between the needs of the anaesthetic and surgical access, extra care is required. Once the child is positioned supine, with the neck extended, care is taken to confirm bilateral air entry, and check tidal volume and airway pressures. Inadvertent extubation or endobronchial intubation are potential risks during positioning and surgery[46]

- Analgesia: for isolated cleft lip repair, bilateral infraorbital block is a simple and effective mode of analgesia[47]. For palate repair, wound infiltration with local anaesthetic, paracetamol, intravenous morphine 0.05–0.1 mg/kg, and carefully titrated remifentanil infusion provides effective analgesia[48]

- Extubation: at the end of surgery, under direct vision, the pharyngeal pack is removed, and the airway checked to ensure that the airway is clear and that there is no active bleeding or increased swelling. Aim for a smooth emergence and an awake extubation

- Postoperative analgesia: regular oral paracetamol and as required oral morphine are prescribed. Diclofenac suppositories are given provided there is no evidence of bleeding and repeated after 12 hours. This provides good analgesia and reduces the need for opioids[49]. Extensive repair of the cleft palate results in significantly more pain postoperatively and a carefully titrated morphine infusion or nurse-controlled intravenous morphine can be very useful[50]. However, it is imperative to monitor the babies managed with these infusion regimens by a specialized paediatric pain service

- Postoperative complications include obstructive sleep apnoea and bleeding from the flap donor site[30]. Closure of the palate is an operation with a higher risk of postoperative hypoxaemia than other plastic surgical procedures[51], and it is particularly common in infants with Pierre Robin sequence or other congenital anomalies

- Patients with a potential for airway obstruction will benefit from a carefully positioned nasopharyngeal airway, which relieves the airway obstruction during the recovery period[51]

- Postoperative monitoring includes routine pulse rate, respiratory rate, arterial oxygen saturation and blood pressure measurements, and an apnoea monitor.

Secondary surgery for cleft lip and palate

A palatal fistula may occur as a late complication of palatal closure. These require re-operation and the general principles of management are the same as with primary palate closure.

Pharyngoplasty

Children with a repaired cleft lip and palate may have difficulties with the development of their speech. This usually presents in the 6–8-year age group and is identified when the child's speech is compromised so it is identified at school. Mostly the issue will be around a hypernasal speech brought about by impaired palatal function, velopharyngeal insufficiency (VPI). Children will be assessed by the speech therapist who is an integral part of the cleft team. Pharyngoplasty or palate re-repair may be recommended as this will tense up the palate and improve phonation so clarifying the speech. About 25% of children with cleft palate may need this procedure[52]. Palate re-repair has a lower morbidity and is more physiological than a pharyngoplasty or pharyngeal flap surgery[51,53].

Anaesthesia for pharyngoplasty

As the surgery is in the posterior pharynx a nasal tube is contraindicated. An oral RAE tube fixed in the midline is ideal. Use of a throat pack is essential. Local anaesthetic infiltrated into the palate is very effective. Simple analgesics are all that is required postoperatively. Following a pharyngoplasty the airway is not usually compromised and recovery is uneventful. Depending on the type of pharyngoplasty there may be little room for nasal escape of air post pharyngoplasty.

It is important to remember that any child who has had a pharyngoplasty has a reduced nasal airway and future use of a nasal tracheal tube should be avoided whenever possible so as to ensure the pharyngeal repair is not compromised. If a nasal tube is essential due to future surgical needs then a fibreoptic scope should be used to guide intubation.

Alveolar bone graft

Children with a cleft palate will have an incomplete dental arch. The size of the alveolar defect will depend on the initial extent of the cleft. As orthodontic techniques have improved, the procedure of grafting bone fragments to the alveolar cleft has become increasingly common. An alveolar bone graft (ABG) is done when the secondary teeth are established, at about 8–12 years of age.

A bone graft is taken either from the anterior iliac spine or from the tibia. The ABG provides a continuous maxillary arch, closes the oronasal fistula, and provides bony support for the teeth. If the cleft was bilateral it is usual to do an ABG to each side independently. The success rate for ABG is 81–90%[54,55].

Complications include failure of the graft, insufficient bony structure post ABG, pain at the donor site, and infection. Donor site complications are infrequent when the anterior iliac spine is the source of the bone graft. In contrast, bone grafts retrieved by trephining of the tibia can give rise to a number of serious complications. Tibial fractures are reported in up to 2.7% of patients having this approach causing significant disruption to the child's life[56].

Anaesthesia for alveolar bone graft

♦ Most children of this age are able to cooperate with anaesthesia and can choose their preferred method of induction

♦ Once asleep, the airway is generally easy to manage. An oral RAE tube is fixed in the midline, to accommodate use of a mouth gag (Figure 19.1). A throat pack is essential

♦ Blood loss is not significant

♦ Local infiltration of both the alveolus and the donor site is important and with this the need for postoperative opiates is decreased. Usually if effective local anaesthesia has been used simple analgesics such as paracetamol and ibuprofen are sufficient to manage postoperative pain with oral morphine kept as escape medication

♦ When a trephine needle has been used to collect the donor bone the resultant pain at the donor site is

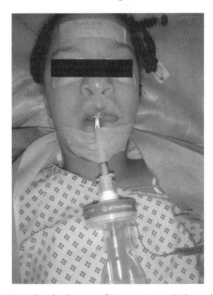

Figure 19.1 Alveolar bone grafting requires a RAE south-facing endotracheal tube and throat pack.

minimal. If a larger piece of bone has been harvested then pain at this site can be distressing. In this case use of a subcutaneous infusion of local anaesthetic is useful for the first 24–36 hours. For example, a 50-ml syringe of 0.25% levobupivacaine attached to a subcutaneously placed catheter and run at 2–4 ml/hour is effective

♦ Children having an ABG will stay in hospital for 1–2 nights; however, some centres have reported successful management of these patients as day-care patients with good outcomes[57].

Maxillary advancement and mandibular reduction

As the child grows, the discrepancy between the maxillary underdevelopment and the normal mandibular growth becomes more apparent. Surgically this requires a Le Fort I maxillary advancement and sometimes a mandibular osteotomy and reconfiguration. This is major surgery and is not undertaken until approximately 15 years of age when the bony development of the face has mostly been completed. The anaesthetic management of such cases is discussed in Chapter 18.

One important aspect is the postoperative care of children who have intermaxillary fixation (IMF). Any child in IMF without a tracheostomy should be nursed on an Intensive Care Unit (ICU) for the first postoperative night[58]. Should airway compromise occur, the IMF wires need to be cut to allow intubation. The position of each wire should be clearly documented and it is essential wire cutters are kept at the bedside at all times.

IMF is less commonly used now as interocclusive elastic bands placed between upper and lower jaws are satisfactory and can be fitted the day following surgery when the child has recovered from anaesthesia. This means that children can be managed on the routine maxillofacial ward rather than in an ICU.

Bimaxillary osteotomy

Depending on the airway assessment a fibreoptic technique may be required. A north-facing RAE or flexible nasotracheal tube is preferred. Care must be taken to fix the tracheal tube without exerting pressure on the nasal tip[59]. A combination of 15° head-up positioning and modest hypotension using remifentanil or inhalational agents may be helpful in reducing

bleeding, which can be significant. Damage to the tracheal tube can occur during the surgery[60]. Rarely, surgery may result in severe bradycardia[59,61].

Other major maxillofacial procedures

Temporomandibular joint ankylosis

Temporomandibular joint (TMJ) ankylosis usually presents in the young child with limited mouth opening (Figure 19.2), and who has feeding difficulties which result in the child failing to thrive. Common aetiology includes trauma, congenital diseases, septic arthritis, and juvenile rheumatoid arthritis. The resultant ankylosis at the TMJ can lead to failure of the mandible to grow leading to micrognathia. Surgical management involves releasing the TMJ and if there is micrognathia, mandibular augmentation either with a costochondral graft or by the use of a distraction device (Figure 19.3). Mandibular distraction has been shown to improve the airway and many children can subsequently manage without a tracheostomy[62].

Anaesthesia for TMJ ankylosis in these children can be challenging:

♦ Airway management: due to the minimal mouth opening it may not be possible to use either an oral airway or a LMA. Inhalational induction is favoured[2]. If the child's airway obstructs soon after

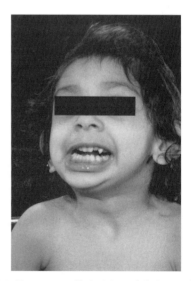

Figure 19.2 Temporomandibular joint ankylosis severely limiting mouth opening.

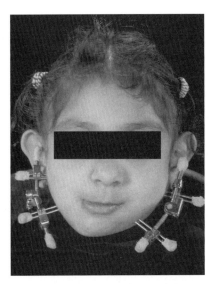

Figure 19.3 External distraction device for mandibular augmentation.

induction, placement of a nasopharyngeal airway early is effective in restoring an airway

◆ Tracheal intubation: intubation is achieved using a nasal fibreoptic technique. A cuffed tracheal tube should be used in one size less than predicted for the child. This allows a seal to be achieved with the cuff in a child in whom it is impossible to pack the throat due to limitation in mouth opening. Blind nasal intubation has also been reported as successful[63]

◆ Monitoring. in addition to routine monitoring an arterial line is used. This is for sampling and close monitoring of arterial pressure

◆ After the completion of surgery the mouth opening is restored and the child can be safely managed on the general ward

◆ Occasionally if the airway is particularly precarious, an elective tracheostomy is required to allow surgery and to ensure that the child is safe in the post-operative period.

Costochondral rib grafts

Costochondral grafts are used to augment the mandible as the presence of a joint interface allows ongoing growth in the grafted site and the augmented mandible will grow. Isolated pieces of rib are used as a simple graft to the jaw particularly if a part of the mandible has been removed due to benign or malignant tumour. The rib is joined to the mandible using plates and screws. When harvesting the graft, the surgeons will use a lateral incision in the anterolateral chest. If two ribs are needed, alternate ribs are used to minimize the risk of subsequent chest wall abnormality. Retrieval of these grafts is well tolerated. The risk that the pleura may be breached is managed by a 'bubble test' once the rib has been dissected out. The wound is filled with saline and a Valsalva manoeuvre performed to see if there is any leak of bubbles. If there is no breach of pleura a chest drain is not used. However, a post-operative chest X-ray is mandatory to confirm that there is no pneumothorax.

In addition to the routine analgesia for the facial surgery, the chest wound is infiltrated with a bolus of local anaesthetic. A surgically placed fine bore catheter, such as an epidural catheter, is placed in the sub-cutaneous space used to deliver continuous local anaesthetic using a syringe pump. Care is taken to ensure the dose of local anaesthetic is suitable for the size of the child. In practice a dose of 2–4 ml/hour of 0.25% levobupivacaine is sufficient when used in children above 20 kg.

Other donor sites for bone include the bone obtained from splitting pieces of skull during cranio-facial remodelling, and the anterior iliac crest.

Vascular malformations and tumours

An area affected with abnormal blood vessels always poses additional risks for anaesthesia. Sturge–Weber malformation is a capillary haemangioma affecting the face and deeper tissues including the brain. Oral tracheal tubes are preferred and bleeding anticipated if extraction is to be performed in an affected area. Facial tumours are rare. Biopsy is a minor procedure but excision can be challenging. The relevant factors are the same as discussed in the section on major surgery of the jaw.

Craniofacial procedures

Craniosynostosis results from premature fusion of one or more cranial sutures. Syndromic craniofacial dys-ostosis is a familial form of craniosynostosis in which there is sutural involvement of the cranium and the mid-face resulting in specific clinical features[64]. The common craniofacial conditions (Crouzon, Apert, and Pfeiffer) and the implications for anaesthesia are summarized in Table 19.4.

Reconstructive surgery of the cranium and the midface involves several sequentially phased proce-dures, which coincides with the craniofacial growth pattern and psychosocial development[64]. Maxillofacial

Table 19.4 Craniofacial synostoses

Syndrome	Important features	Implications for anaesthesia
Crouzons[65]	Bicoronal synostosis; Maxillary hypoplasia; Proptosis; Cervical fusion in 18%; Raised intracranial pressure; Chiari malformation[66]	Obstructive sleep apnoea; Poor mask fit and airway obstruction on induction; Tracheal intubation usually straightforward in primary surgery; Secondary surgery: potentially difficult laryngoscopy
Apert	Facial deformity is severe;[67] Hypertelorism (wide-set eyes); Maxillary hypoplasia; Choanal stenosis; Cervical fusion (C5–6)—68%	Similar to Crouzon; Primary mouth breather; airway obstruction if mouth is not open[40]; Tracheal intubation usually straightforward in primary surgery; Venous access: potentially difficult due to syndactyly
Pfeiffer[68]	Bicoronal and cranial base synostoses; Maxillary hypoplasia; Curved broad great toe and thumb; Cervical fusion-73% (C2–3)	Similar to Crouzon; Associated cardiovascular and tracheal anomalies; Chiari malformation, shunt-dependant hydrocephalus

surgeons have a major role with coordinated input from the neurosurgical, plastics, ENT, ophthalmologic, and orthodontic teams.

Frontocranial remodelling is undertaken in infancy (8–11 months) to expand the anterior cranial fossa, to allow brain growth and to protect the eyes (proptosis). Advancement of midface hypoplasia is undertaken in the young child between 4–6 years of age. Orthognathic surgery is undertaken in the young adult around 14–16 years of age.

Anaesthesia management
Multidisciplinary approach
Children for major craniofacial surgery are usually admitted for a week of formal preoperative assessment by a multidisciplinary team that includes anaesthetists, ENT, ophthalmologic, speech and language development, as well as the various surgical and nursing teams.

Long surgery

- Typically surgery will take 6–12 hours and has a potential to cause significant morbidity[3]

- Care with positioning is important, as surgical teams are usually large and access to the child during surgery is restricted

- Temperature control may be unpredictable. Core and peripheral temperature are monitored. Temperature control devices including heating blanket and fluid warmer are essential.

Potentially difficult airways

- Airway obstruction can occur at any time during the perioperative period and is an important

contributor of morbidity in this patient group[58]. Sleep studies are reviewed. The presence of OSA may indicate the need for a nasopharyngeal airway or a tracheostomy postoperatively

- Gaseous induction is preferred and spontaneous respiration is maintained until the anaesthetist is confident that bag and mask ventilation is effective. If the child's airway obstructs during induction, they will need an oral/nasal airway early

- Children with maxillary hypoplasia are less likely to be difficult to intubate than those with marked mandibular underdevelopment. Children who have significant limitation of neck mobility are more likely to be difficult to intubate

- The choice of tracheal tube will reflect the balance of surgical requirements and techniques available to the anaesthetist. It may not be possible to use a nasotracheal tube. A flexometallic tube is ideal and if used orally it can be fixed to the teeth with surgical wire. A throat pack is used

- A tracheostomy may be indicated. If this is likely then the child and family must be fully informed and made to understand the implications and postoperative course. Parents can gain the skills to manage their child's tracheostomy at home

- Children who have had correction of facial abnormalities can appear to have a normal airway. However it has been shown that this idea may be misleading and the anaesthetic airway management for these children may be even more difficult following corrective surgery[69]

- The majority of the patients may be extubated at the end of the surgery and managed in a high dependency unit. A small proportion of patients may require ventilatory support for a short period[15]

Raised intracranial pressure is a feature of some syndromes. If a ventriculoperitoneal shunt is present, it is checked to ensure that it is functioning well. If there is a substantial cranial component to the surgery then the potential for venous air embolism should be borne in mind.

Vascular access can be difficult, particularly as some syndromes are associated with limb abnormalities. For major surgery, in addition to good peripheral venous access, arterial and central venous lines are used. The central line is preferably placed in the femoral vein as this is further from the surgical site and less likely to be compromised during neck movement during surgery.

Managing blood loss and fluid balance in craniofacial surgery

Blood loss can be extensive. It is not unusual to replace one to two blood volumes[3]. About 20–50% of blood volume may be lost during craniosynostosis surgery[70]. Therefore, it is important to plan ahead, obtain full blood count (FBC), clotting screen, correct any abnormalities, and cross match blood preoperatively.

It is important to ensure good positioning, a head-up tilt, with no obstruction to venous drainage of the head and avoid any hypertension. Provided the intracranial pressure is normal, modest hypotensive anaesthesia is useful to reduce intraoperative blood loss.

Blood conservation strategies inclusive of preoperative erythropoietin administration and autologous blood donation have been successfully used to minimize the need for allogenic blood transfusion[71]. However these strategies are not widely available.

Assessment of blood loss is very difficult and reliance has to be based upon clinical parameters and regular point of care testing of haemoglobin and blood gases[15]. A dilutional coagulopathy must be treated early.

Intraoperative acute normovolaemic haemodilution and blood salvage have not been shown to be effective in decreasing the allogenic blood transfusion requirements[70–72]. Intraoperative fluids are made up of routine maintenance fluids and replacement of surgical losses.

Midface advancement

The aims are to improve the cosmetic appearance, dental occlusion, and the upper airway volume.

Osteotomy

Le Fort III osteotomy corrects moderate midface hypoplasia involving the nose, zygoma, and bony orbits and is performed in young adults when skeletal maturation is complete[73]. Recent advances include miniplate and screw fixation of osteotomy sites. This prevents the need for intermaxillary fixation and the associated problems[58]. Monobloc osteotomy is done to advance the orbits and the midface as one unit (Table 19.5). Facial bipartition osteotomy, done in hypertelorism, allows three-dimensional correction of maxilla and orbits at the same time[74]. This is major surgery associated with significant morbidity including substantial blood loss, postoperative intensive care, donor site morbidity, and occasionally, respiratory distress requiring tracheostomy[73,75].

Distraction osteogenesis

Recently, distraction osteogenesis, a technique of mechanically-induced growth of new bone and soft tissue, has been applied to midface advancement. This technique allows for greater mobilizations over a

Table 19.5 Phased craniofacial procedures for craniosynostosis[64]

Procedure	Anaesthetic implications
Single suture synostosis repair	Non-syndromic infant; short procedure
Multiple suture synostosis: Cranio-orbital decompression; Fronto-orbital remodeling; Posterior vault expansion	Infant; Syndromal craniosynostosis; Potential for massive haemorrhage; Prone position for posterior repair
Mid-face augmentation: osteotomy: Le Fort III Monobloc Facial bipartition[15]	Young child; Extensive procedure; Potentially difficult airway; Risk of accidental extubation; Potential for massive haemorrhage
Midface augmentation: Distraction osteogenesis and rigid extraction device (RED) Removal of distraction device	Young child; Staged procedures; Primary surgery—intubation usually uncomplicated; Presence of RED poses difficulty in airway management; Removal of vertical bar facilitates laryngoscopy and intubation

period of time, does not require bone grafting, and is associated with low operative and postoperative morbidity[73].

A second surgical procedure is required to remove the device. The presence of an external maxillary distraction device, although looking rather daunting does not pose as much difficulty as expected. The vertical bar can be removed to allow unobstructed direct laryngoscopy. It is important to train the personnel and have the appropriate screwdrivers and wire cutters to remove the vertical bar should a postoperative problem occur[76]. If a difficult direct laryngoscopy is anticipated, elective fibreoptic intubation is preferred for removal of maxillary distraction devices[69].

Postoperative management

Children are nursed in a high dependency unit postoperatively where general and neurosurgical observations can be made. Local swelling can be extensive and patients are nursed with their head elevated and given prophylactic dexamethasone. Analgesia is achieved with local infiltration, simple analgesics, and a postoperative morphine infusion. Postoperatively maintenance fluids are restricted to 75% of normal. Blood and colloid replacement (including fresh frozen plasma [FFP] and platelets) is targeted to maintain a haemoglobin concentration above 10 g/dl. Hypovolaemia is common and fluid management needs to be closely monitored.

Anaesthesia for minor oral and maxillofacial procedures

Anaesthesia for preoperative imaging

Imaging is very important in the planning phase of surgery. Careful assessment of the airway is key here. A baby can have computed tomography (CT) or magnetic resonance imaging (MRI) scans during normal sleep, but it is often difficult for children under about 8 years, or those who have learning difficulties to cooperate and remain still during these investigations. Sedation should be tried first as many children will be scanned successfully[77]; however, if the child's airway is precarious then sedation is contraindicated.

CT scans are quick but an MRI will take more than 45 minutes and the MRI scanner is an unfriendly environment. The child will need to be anaesthetized or sedated depending on their age and ability to cooperate, in order to acquire good quality images[78]. For those who need an anaesthetic, spontaneous respiration using a LMA is satisfactory in most children, even if they are syndromal. However, some children will have marked limitation of mouth opening and placement of LMA is not possible. These high-risk patients require tracheal intubation for an MRI scan.

Division of tongue tie

A short frenulum is sometimes a cause of compromised speech or feeding difficulty. Division of the tie is a procedure done mainly in infants. This is a quick procedure and does not usually require intubation. A LMA or use of a nasal mask is sufficient. The frenulum is first injected with local anaesthetic, a clip applied across it to leave an avascular crushed area, and this is cut. Feeding is established soon after surgery and simple oral analgesia is sufficient.

Surgical exploration of teeth

The maxillofacial team is required to manage dental extraction in children with cleft or craniofacial conditions and in those with unusual medical conditions. Teeth can be buried in unexpected places deep within the palate or in the cleft. Whilst the surgery can take much longer than simple extractions, the principles of management are the same: the provision of a stable, patent airway and minimal interference with the surgical field. A nasotracheal tube with throat pack is preferred. Contraindications to nasal intubation include history of epistaxis, coagulopathy, narrow nasal passages (e.g. previous cleft repair, first arch syndromes), previous pharyngoplasty, previous trauma to the nose, and a deviated septum. A flexible LMA can be used for some of these cases and indeed is very useful for minor surgery.

Dental blocks are avoided by some as there is a concern that children are more likely to bite their lip and also do not like the numb feeling associated with the block. Local infiltration is satisfactory and well tolerated.

Dental abscess

This is common in childhood and is secondary to dental infection. Trismus may be present but is unusual. If the infection has spread to the submasseteric area, then the resultant trismus may not relax on induction of anaesthesia and intubation will be difficult (see Chapter 11). A nasal fibreoptic intubation is the method of choice. In superficial infection, the trismus is more likely to relax on induction.

Hypertrophy of the gingiva

This is usually associated with use of phenytoin although can be associated with some rare syndromes such as juvenile hyaline fibromatosis. The soft tissue overgrowth can be so severe as to require gingivectomy. This is done with cautery to upper and lower gingivae so exposing the teeth. A nasal tracheal tube is required and intubation may be difficult due to poor access to the mouth. Fibreoptic intubation may be indicated[79]. The airway management is much improved following surgery. Postoperative pain can be severe and may require intravenous morphine.

Salivary gland surgery

Tumours of the salivary glands are rare in children. Chronic infection particularly related to chronic aspiration may lead to abscess formation but the most common reason for surgery is for excess drooling in a child with cerebral palsy. Children with excess drooling are premedicated with atropine or glycopyrolate. A nasal tube is preferred as it remains out of the surgical site. A throat pack is essential. Bleeding is not marked and simple analgesics and local infiltration is sufficient for postoperative pain management.

Tongue reduction

Macroglossia may be congenital as in Beckwith–Weidemann syndrome or acquired as in hypothyroidism. Macroglossia can cause airway obstruction and affect development of jaws. Laser tongue reduction has replaced 'excision with suturing' for macroglossia.

Airway management is based on the severity of macroglossia. Anaesthesia induction may result in early airway obstruction, which is relieved using an oral or nasopharyngeal airway. A nasotracheal tube is used[40]. Direct laryngoscopy is usually uneventful. However, fibreoptic techniques or occasionally tracheostomy may be required perioperatively[80]. Postoperative complications include bleeding and swelling of the tongue with potential for airway obstruction. Postoperative fluids will be required until oral feeding is established and careful use of intravenous morphine may be necessary for analgesia.

Trauma

Soft tissue facial trauma is a common indication for surgery. Aetiologies include road traffic accidents, falls, cycling, sporting injuries, or dental trauma. The possibility that an injury may be non-accidental should be kept in mind. If concerns are raised then local policies will guide the anaesthetist to liaise with the child protection lead, in their hospital[81].

Following head injuries or polytrauma, children will be managed on a paediatric ICU. Facial fractures are repaired once the acute head injury has been stabilized and any serious injuries treated. Lacerations will need urgent attention. Paediatric orbital fractures which present with bradycardia need urgent treatment as this indicates local entrapment of the inferior rectus muscle in the orbital floor fracture. Delayed treatment can result in permanent muscle and eye mobility problems. Reducing the local pressure will relieve the symptoms of the occulocardiac reflex. Anaesthetic implications are similar to that required for major facial surgery. Nasal tracheal tubes are preferred but not essential if contraindicated by the clinical situation.

Conclusion

Small children requiring anaesthesia for any surgery are challenging and risks are much greater in patients undergoing major reconstructive surgery. The expertise of the paediatric anaesthetist and the perioperative care of the paediatric nursing and medical teams are required in managing babies and young children.

References

1. Cook-Sather SD, Litman RS. (2006) Modern fasting guidelines in children. *Best Pract Res Clin Anaesthesiol*, **20**(3), 471–81.
2. Brooks P, Ree R, Rosen D, Ansermino M. (2005) Canadian pediatric anesthesiologists prefer inhalational anesthesia to manage difficult airways. *Can J Anaesth*, **52(3)**, 285–90.
3. Moylan S, Collee G, Mackersie A, Bingham R. (1993) Anaesthetic management in paediatric craniofacial surgery. A review of 126 cases. *Pediatri Anaesth*, **3(5)**, 275–81.
4. Kim JT, Na HS, Bae JY, *et al.* (2008) GlideScope (R) video laryngoscope: a randomized clinical trial in 203 paediatric patients. *Br J Anaesth*, **101(4)**, 531–4.
5. Crocker K, Black AE. (2009) Assessment and management of the predicted difficult airway in babies and children. *Anaesth Intens Care Med*, **10(4)**, 200–5.
6. Brambrink AM, Braun U. (2005) Airway management in infants and children. *Best Pract Res Clin Anaesthesiol*, **19**(4), 675–97.
7. Flynn PE, Black AE, Mitchell V. (2008) The use of cuffed tracheal tubes for paediatric tracheal intubation, a survey of specialist practice in the United Kingdom. *Eur J Anaesthesiol*, **25(8)**, 685–8.
8. James I. Cuffed tubes in children. *Paediatr Anaesth* 2001, **11(3)**, 259–63.
9. Weiss M, Dullenkopf A. (2007) Cuffed tracheal tubes in children: past, present and future. *Expert Rev Med Devices*, **4(1)**, 73–82.

10. Cox RG. (2005) Should cuffed endotracheal tubes be used routinely in children? *Can J Anaesth*, **52 (7)**, 669–74.

11. Wilson W, Taubert KA, Gewitz M, *et al.* (2007) Prevention of infective endocarditis: guidelines from the American Heart Association: a guideline from the American Heart Association Rheumatic Fever, Endocarditis, and Kawasaki Disease Committee, Council on Cardiovascular Disease in the Young, and the Council on Clinical Cardiology, Council on Cardiovascular Surgery and Anesthesia, and the Quality of Care and Outcomes Research Interdisciplinary Working Group. *Circulation*, **116(15)**, 1736–54.

12. Gould FK, Elliott TS,Foweraker J, *et al.* (2006) Guidelines for the prevention of endocarditis: report of the Working Party of the British Society for Antimicrobial Chemotherapy. *J Antimicrob Chemother*, **57(6)**, 1035–42.

13. Holliday MA, Segar WE. (1957) The maintenance need for water in parenteral fluid therapy. *Pediatrics*, **19(5)**, 823–32.

14. APAGBI. APA consensus guideline on perioperative fluid management in children. Available online at http://www.apagbi.org.uk/index.asp?PageID=6 (accessed 20 March, 2009).

15. Mallory S. (2008) Craniofacial and neurosurgery (2008) In: Bingham R, Lloyd-Thomas AR, Sury MRJ. (eds) *Hatch and Sumner's Textbook of Paediatric Anaesthesia*. London: Hodder Arnold, pp. 572–83.

16. Pijpers M, Poels PJ, Vaandrager JM, *et al.* (2004) Undiagnosed obstructive sleep apnea syndrome in children with syndromal craniofacial synostosis. *J Craniofac Surg*, **15 (4)**, 670–4.

17. Tweedie DJ, Skilbeck CJ, Lloyd-Thomas AR, Albert DM. (2007) The nasopharyngeal prong airway: an effective post-operative adjunct after adenotonsillectomy for obstructive sleep apnoea in children. *Int J Pediatr Otorhinolaryngol*, **71(4)**, 563–9.

18. Dell'Oste C, Savron F, Pelizzo G, Sarti A. (2004) Acute airway obstruction in an infant with Pierre Robin syndrome after palatoplasty. *Acta Anaesthesiol Scand*, **48(6)**, 787–9.

19. Sculerati N, Gottlieb MD, Zimbler MS, Chibbaro PD, McCarthy JG. (1998) Airway management in children with major craniofacial anomalies. *Laryngoscope*, **108(12)**, 1806–12.

20. Perkins JA, Sie KC, Milczuk H, Richardson MA. (1997) Airway management in children with craniofacial anomalies. *Cleft Palate Craniofac J*, **34(2)**, 135–40.

21. Kremer B, Botos-Kremer AI, Eckel HE, Schlondorff G. (2002) Indications, complications, and surgical techniques for pediatric tracheostomies – an update. *J Pediatr Surg*, **37 (11)**, 1556–62.

22. Carr AS, Courtman S, Holtby H, *et al.* APA Guidelines on the prevention of postoperative vomiting in children. Available online at <http://www.apagbi.org.uk/index.asp?PageID=221> (accessed 20 March, 2009).

23. Litalien C, Jacqz-Aigrain E. (2001) Risks and benefits of nonsteroidal anti-inflammatory drugs in children: a comparison with paracetamol. *Paediatr Drugs*, **3(11)**, 817–58.

24. Marsh DF, Hodkinson B. (2009) Remifentanil in paediatric anaesthetic practice. *Anaesthesia*, **64(3)**, 301–8.

25. Munoz HR, Guerrero ME, Brandes V, Cortinez LI. (2002) Effect of timing of morphine administration during remifentanil-based anaesthesia on early recovery from anaesthesia and postoperative pain. *Br J Anaesth*, **88(6)**, 814–18.

26. Howard R, Carter B, Curry J, *et al.* Association of Paediatric Anaesthetists: Good practice in postoperative and procedural pain. Available online at http://www.apagbi.org.uk/index.asp?PageID=6 (accessed 20 March, 2009).

27. CSAG. (1998) *Cleft lip and/or palate. Report of the Clinical Standards Advisory Group*. London: The Stationery Office.

28. Bearn D, Mildinhall S, Murphy T, *et al.* (2001) Cleft lip and palate care in the United Kingdom – the Clinical Standards Advisory Group (CSAG) Study. Part 4: outcome comparisons, training, and conclusions. *Cleft Palate Craniofac J*, **38(1)**, 38–43.

29. Murray L, Hentges F, Hill J, *et al.* (2008) The effect of cleft lip and palate, and the timing of lip repair on mother-infant interactions and infant development. *J Child Psychol Psychiatry*, **49(2)**, 115–123.

30. Ansermino M, Sury M. (2008) Plastic surgery. In: Bingham R, Lloyd-Thomas AR, Sury MRJ. (eds) *Hatch and Sumner's Textbook of Paediatric Anaesthesia*. London: Hodder Arnold, pp. 531–9.

31. Milerad J, Larson O, PhD D, Hagberg C, Ideberg M. (1997) Associated malformations in infants with cleft lip and palate: a prospective, population-based study. *Pediatrics*, **100(2 Pt 1)**, 180–6.

32. Takemura H, Yasumoto K, Toi T, Hosoyamada A. (2002) Correlation of cleft type with incidence of perioperative respiratory complications in infants with cleft lip and palate. *Paediatr Anaesth*, **12(7)**, 585–8.

33. Pearl W. (1982) Congenital heart disease in the Pierre Robin syndrome. *Pediatr Cardiol*, **2(4)**, 307–9.

34. Bull MJ, Givan DC, Sadove AM, Bixler D, Hearn D. (1990) Improved outcome in Pierre Robin sequence: effect of multidisciplinary evaluation and management. *Pediatrics*, **86(2)**, 294–301.

35. van den Elzen AP, Semmekrot BA, Bongers EM, Huygen PL, Marres HA. (2001) Diagnosis and treatment of the Pierre Robin sequence: results of a retrospective clinical study and review of the literature. *Eur J Pediatr*, **160(1)**, 47–53.

36. Yotsui-Tsuchimochi H, Higa K, Matsunaga M, Nitahara K, Shono S. (2006) Anesthetic management of a child with chromosome 22q11 deletion syndrome. *Paediatr Anaesth*, **16(4)**, 454–7.

37. Lansford M. (2008) Focus on the physical assessment of the infant with Stickler syndrome. *Adv Neonatal Care*, **8(6)**, 308–14.

38. Kucukyavuz Z, Ozkaynak O, Tuzuner AM, Kisnisci R. (2006) Difficulties in anesthetic management of patients with micrognathia: report of a patient with Stickler syndrome. *Oral Surg Oral Med Oral Pathol Oral Radiol Endod*, **102(6)**, e33–6.

39. Arvystas M, Shprintzen RJ. (1991) Craniofacial morphology in Treacher Collins syndrome. *Cleft Palate Craniofac J*, **28 (2)**, 226–30; discussion 230–1.

40. Nargozian C. (2004) The airway in patients with craniofacial abnormalities. *Paediatr Anaesth*, **14(1)**, 53–9.

41. Healey D, Letts M, Jarvis JG. (2002) Cervical spine instability in children with Goldenhar's syndrome. *Can J Surg*, **45(5)**, 341–4.

42. Antony AK, Sloan GM. (2002) Airway obstruction following palatoplasty: analysis of 247 consecutive operations. *Cleft Palate Craniofac J*, **39(2)**, 145–8.

43. Gunawardana RH. (1996) Difficult laryngoscopy in cleft lip and palate surgery. *Br J Anaesth*, **76(6)**, 757–9.

44. Sen I, Kumar S, Bhardwaj N, Wig J. (2009) A left paraglossal approach for oral intubation in children scheduled for bilateral orofacial cleft reconstruction surgery–a prospective observational study. *Paediatr Anaesth*, **19(2)**, 159–63.

45. Semjen F, Bordes M, Cros AM. (2008) Intubation of infants with Pierre Robin syndrome: the use of the paraglossal approach combined with a gum-elastic bougie in six consecutive cases. *Anaesthesia*, **63(2)**, 147–50.

46. Jordi Ritz EM, Von Ungern-Sternberg BS, Keller K, Frei FJ, Erb TO. (2008) The impact of head position on the cuff and tube tip position of preformed oral tracheal tubes in young children. *Anaesthesia*, **63(6)**, 604–9.

47. Rajamani A, Kamat V, Rajavel VP, Murthy J, Hussain SA. (2007) A comparison of bilateral infraorbital nerve block with intravenous fentanyl for analgesia following cleft lip repair in children. *Paediatr Anaesth*, **17(2)**, 133–9.

48. Steinmetz J, Holm-Knudsen R, Sorensen MK, Eriksen K, Rasmussen LS. (2007) Hemodynamic differences between propofol-remifentanil and sevoflurane anesthesia for repair of cleft lip and palate in infants. *Paediatr Anaesth*, **17(1)**, 32–7.

49. Sylaidis P, O'Neill TJ. (1998) Diclofenac analgesia following cleft palate surgery. *Cleft Palate Craniofac J*, **35(6)**, 544–5.

50. Sumpelmann R, Munte S. (2003) Postoperative analgesia in infants and children. *Curr Opin Anaesthesiol*, **16(3)**, 309–13.

51. Henriksson TG, Skoog VT. (2001) Identification of children at high anaesthetic risk at the time of primary palatoplasty. *Scand J Plast Reconstr Surg Hand Surg*, **35(2)**, 177–82.

52. Bicknell S, McFadden LR, Curran JB. (2002) Frequency of pharyngoplasty after primary repair of cleft palate. *J Can Dent Assoc*, **68 (11)**, 688–92.

53. Sommerlad BC, Mehendale FV, Birch MJ, Sell D, Hattee C, Harland K. (2002) Palate re-repair revisited. *Cleft Palate Craniofac J*, **39(3)**, 295–307.

54. Clarkson J, Paterson P, Thorburn G, *et al.* (2005) Alveolar bone grafting: achieving the organisational standards determined by CSAG, a baseline audit at the Birmingham Children's Hospital. *Ann R Coll Surg Engl*, **87(6)**, 461–5.

55. Bergland O, Semb G, Abyholm FE. (1986) Elimination of the residual alveolar cleft by secondary bone grafting and subsequent orthodontic treatment. *Cleft Palate J*, **23(3)**, 175–205.

56. Hughes CW, Revington PJ. (2002) The proximal tibia donor site in cleft alveolar bone grafting: experience of 75 consecutive cases. *J Craniomaxillofac Surg*, **30(1)**, 12–6; discussion 17.

57. Perry CW, Lowenstein A, Rothkopf DM. (2005) Ambulatory alveolar bone grafting. *Plast Reconstr Surg*, **116(3)**, 736–9; discussion 740.

58. Munro IR. (1988) Craniofacial surgery: airway problems and management. *Int Anesthesiol Clin*, **26(1)**, 72–8.

59. Rodrigo C. (2000) Anesthetic considerations for orthognathic surgery with evaluation of difficult intubation and technique for hypotensive anesthesia. *Anesth Prog*, **47(4)**, 151–6.

60. Bidgoli SJ, Dumont L, Mattys M, Mardirosoff C, Damseaux P. (1999) A serious anaesthetic complication of a Lefort I osteotomy. *Eur J Anaesthesiol*, **16(3)**, 201–3.

61. Campbell R, Rodrigo D, Cheung L. (1994) Asystole and bradycardia during maxillofacial surgery. *Anesth Prog*, **41(1)**, 13–16.

62. Steinbacher DM, Kaban LB, Troulis MJ. (2005) Mandibular advancement by distraction osteogenesis for tracheostomy-dependent children with severe micrognathia. *J Oral Maxillofac Surg*, **63(8)**, 1072–9.

63. Masood N, Abdullah S. (2005) Facilitated blind nasotracheal intubation in paralysed patients with temporomandibular joint ankylosis. *J Coll Physicians Surg Pak*, **15(1)**, 4–6.

64. Posnick JC, Ruiz RL. (2000) The craniofacial dysostosis syndromes: current surgical thinking and future directions. *Cleft Palate Craniofac J*, **37(5)**, 433.

65. Anderson PJ, Hall C, Evans RD, Harkness WJ, Hayward RD, Jones BM. (1997) The cervical spine in Crouzon syndrome. *Spine*, **22(4)**, 402–5.

66. Cinalli G, Spennato P, Sainte-Rose C, *et al.* (2005) Chiari malformation in craniosynostosis. *Childs Nerv Syst*, **21(10)**, 889–901.

67. Kreiborg S, Cohen MMJ. (1998) Is craniofacial morphology in Apert and Crouzon syndromes the same? *Acta Odontol Scand*, **56(6)**, 339–41.

68. Anderson PJ, Hall CM, Evans RD, Jones BM, Harkness W, Hayward RD. (1996) Cervical spine in Pfeiffer's syndrome. *J Craniofac Surg*, **7(4)**, 275–9.

69. Roche J, Frawley G, Heggie A. (2002) Difficult tracheal intubation induced by maxillary distraction devices in craniosynostosis syndromes. *Paediatr Anaesth*, **12(3)**, 227–34.

70. Wong ECC. (2004) Acute Normovolemic hemodilution: a critical evaluation of its safety and utility in pediatric patients. *Transfusion Alternatives in Transfusion Medicine*, **6(2)**, 10–21.

71. Velardi F, Di Chirico A, Di Rocco C, *et al.* (1998) "No Allogeneic Blood Transfusion" protocol for the surgical correction of craniosynostoses II. Clinical application. *Child's Nervous System*, **14(12)**, 732–9.

72. Deva AK, Hopper RA, Landecker A, Flores R, Weiner H, McCarthy JG. (2002) The Use of Intraoperative Autotransfusion during Cranial Vault Remodeling for Craniosynostosis. *Plastic and Reconstructive Surgery*, **109(1)**, 58.

73. Nout E, Cesteleyn LL, van der Wal KG, van Adrichem LN, Mathijssen IM, Wolvius EB. (2008) Advancement of the

midface, from conventional Le Fort III osteotomy to Le Fort III distraction: review of the literature. *Int J Oral Maxillofac Surg*, **37(9)**, 781–9.

74. Posnick JC. (1996) Monobloc and facial bipartition osteotomies: a step-by-step description of the surgical technique. *J Craniofac Surg*, **7(3)**, 229–50; discussion 251.

75. Mallory S, Yap LH, Jones BM, Bingham R. (2004) Anaesthetic management in facial bipartition surgery: the experience of one centre. *Anaesthesia*, **59(1)**, 44–51.

76. Wong GB, Nargozian C, Padwa BL. (2004) Anesthetic concerns of external maxillary distraction osteogenesis. *J Craniofac Surg*, **15(1)**, 78–81.

77. Scottish Intercollegiate Guidelines Network. (2008) SIGN Guideline 58: safe sedation of children undergoing diagnostic and therapeutic procedures. *Paediatr Anaesth*, **18(1)**, 11–12.

78. Sury M. (2008) Anaesthesia and sedation outside the operating theatres. In: Bingham R, Lloyd-Thomas AR, Sury MRJ. (eds) *Hatch and Sumner's Textbook of Paediatric Anaesthesia*. London: Hodder Arnold, pp. 659–70.

79. Seefelder C, Ko JH, Padwa BL. (2000) Fibreoptic intubation for massive gingival hyperplasia in juvenile hyaline fibromatosis. *Paediatric Anaesthesia*, **10(6)**, 682–4.

80. Kacker A, Honrado C, Martin D, Ward R. (2000) Tongue reduction in Beckwith–Weidemann Syndrome. *Int J Pediatr Otorhinolaryngol*, **53(1)**, 1–7.

81. Intercollegiate document. Child Protection and the Anaesthetist: Safeguarding Children in the Operating Theatre. Association of Paediatric Anaesthetists of Great Britain and Ireland, Royal College of Anaesthetists and RCPCH. Available online at <http://www.apagbi.org.uk/index.asp?PageID=6> (accessed 20 March, 2009).

20

Hypotensive anaesthesia

Andrew Jones

Introduction

The intentional lowering of systemic blood pressure during general anaesthesia in an attempt to minimize operative blood loss and improve the operating conditions has a selected role in anaesthesia for maxillofacial surgery. The safe application of deliberate hypotensive anaesthetic techniques is dependent on a comprehensive understanding of the physiology and pharmacology involved.

History

In his historical review of deliberate hypotension, G. Hale Enderby remarks on the lack of interest among anaesthetists in measuring blood pressure up to the 1950s[1]. Indeed, there is no mention of checking the anaesthetized patient's blood pressure in the chapter 'How to give an Anaesthetic' in the 1960 edition of *Anaesthetics for Medical Students*[2], although there is a brief discussion of profound hypotension[3]. In general, a high blood pressure as judged by palpating the pulse was thought desirable. However, as long ago as 1917 it had been noted that, although frequently contributing to the patient's death, haemorrhage did produce a dry neurosurgical field. In the 1940s and early 50s good operating conditions were produced by arteriotomy. This involved bleeding the patient of 1–2 litres of blood via an artery then optimistically reversing the process by replacing the blood intra-arterially. In 1951 Bilsland reported fatalities and complications due to ischaemia and irreversible haemorrhagic shock after arteriotomy, and the technique was abandoned[1].

Further progress in deliberate hypotension was made using vasodilating techniques. In 1948 Griffiths and Gillies used a high spinal technique. This was clearly not appropriate for head and neck operations, and a more controlled approach was developed using ganglion-blocking drugs with a head-up tilt. Early use of these agents featured unpredictable responses with extremes of no effect or unnecessarily prolonged hypotension. Magill introduced trimetaphan in 1953, which gave greater control when used in continuous infusion. Because of its ease of use it was widely employed, often by practitioners who were ignorant that they were committing the 'physiological trespass' described by Gillies[1]. By this he meant that hypotension, like muscle relaxation and controlled respiration, was the application of physiological deviations, previously thought to be incompatible with life, which were now reversibly applied to anaesthesia[4]. The first World Congress of Anaesthesiologists in 1956 produced a publication entitled *Safety in Hypotensive Anaesthesia* which emphasized the importance of understanding the pharmacology of hypotensive drugs and in particular close attention to dosage. The introduction of halothane in 1956 stimulated a new approach to hypotension[1]. The author remembers producing moderate hypotension by ventilating a curarized patient with halothane. In considering induced hypotension, care should be taken to distinguish between the heroic hypotension (sometimes as low as 'under 30 mmHg') used in the past[5], profound hypotension (systolic of 40–50 mmHg) used in the local resection of choroidal melanoma[6], and moderate hypotension (20% reduction) which may be applied to maxillofacial surgery[7].

Physiology

The physiological effects of profound hypotension depend on the technique employed to produce the fall in blood pressure. Broadly speaking, two techniques are employed in modern anaesthesia: vasodilatation, typically with a sodium nitroprusside infusion; or negatively inotropic, using β-blockade. β-blockade may also be used with vasodilating techniques to control reflex tachycardia.

Autoregulation controls vital organ bloodflow. When blood pressure is decreased below a certain level, bloodflow is no longer automatically controlled, but is dependent on flow to that organ. Consequently, if blood pressure is to be lowered below the threshold of autoregulation, adequate flow-related perfusion must be maintained. A vasodilating technique will achieve this except in the presence of a stenotic vessel, in which case a steal phenomenon by the vasodilated vessels may result in ischaemia in the territory of the stenotic vessel. The incidence of atheromatous stenosis increases with age.

The cerebral circulation

Cerebral bloodflow is subject to autoregulation between mean arterial pressures of 60 and 130 mmHg[8]. The minimum bloodflow to avoid cerebral hypoxia in normal conscious subjects is 30 ml/100 g/min (normal 50–60 ml/100 g/min). This corresponds to a mean arterial pressure of 35 mmHg. So cerebral perfusion may be compromised below a value of 60 mmHg systolic[8]. Reduction of cerebral metabolic rate may be protective if cerebral perfusion is reduced. Isoflurane reduces cerebral metabolic rate to a greater degree than enflurane or halothane [9].

In 1974 two cases of cerebral damage out of 15 patients were reported. In 1959 a series of 50 patients had one death due to cerebral thrombosis[10]. Some indications of cerebral damage have been reported after orthognathic surgery under general anaesthesia with hypotension. Raised cerebrospinal fluid adenylate kinase is a sensitive marker of brain cell damage. However, no difference was found in raised adenylate kinase levels and psychometric performance when patients subjected to hypotension were compared with a normotensive group[11]. In normotensive patients undergoing orthognathic surgery, adenylate kinase levels were elevated equally whether anaesthesia was maintained with propofol or isoflurane[12]. The cause of brain cell injury is unclear but is related more to anaesthesia and orthognathic surgery than hypotension.

Myocardial circulation

The coronary circulation is subject to autoregulation, but changes in resistance are less than in the cerebral circulation[13]. If hypotension is used it is essential that the myocardial oxygen supply is greater than oxygen demand. Oxygen demand depends on left ventricular wall tension, heart rate and contractility, and correlates well with heart rate[14]. Using a continuous infusion of sodium nitroprusside with trimetaphan, cardiac output increased with reducing blood pressure. If a β-blocker premedication was given, the cardiac output was maintained as the blood pressure fell[15]. β-blockade and peripheral vasodilatation should reduce cardiac work and hence myocardial oxygen demand, while the maintained cardiac output should ensure adequate myocardial perfusion. However, no pharmacological technique can maintain adequate perfusion in the presence of atheroma[14].

The balance between oxygen supply and demand is hard to measure in the clinical setting, so careful monitoring of the electrocardiogram ST segment is essential. Lead CMV5 is the most sensitive for revealing myocardial ischaemia[15]. Seven cases of myocardial ischaemia out of 1000 were reported in 1961 in a group of elderly patients undergoing prostatectomy[10].

Renal circulation

Renal bloodflow is determined by both extrinsic autonomic and hormonal regulation and autoregulation. Autoregulation takes place between mean arterial pressures of 80 and 180 mmHg. Urine flow ceases at 70 mmHg. There were no serious renal complications associated with hypotension in a 1961 series of 10 000 cases[10].

Splanchnic circulation

The splanchnic perfusion was studied during deliberate hypotension induced for orthognathic surgery. The effects of isoflurane and a combination of esmolol and glyceryl trinitrate were compared using gastric tonometry and plasma lactate. No compromise of splanchnic perfusion was found and overall organ perfusion was sufficient[16].

The main blood supply to the liver is from the portal vein, with a contribution from the hepatic artery and is not subject to autoregulation. Liver integrity as measured by serum α-glutathione S-transferase was transiently impaired after sodium nitroprusside-induced hypotension. Function returned to baseline during the first postoperative day[17]. However, another study concluded that controlled hypotension did not cause hepatocellular damage, although only 18 patients were studied[18].

Pulmonary circulation

Hypotension obtunds hypoxic vasoconstriction, increasing ventilation perfusion mismatch[10]. Physiological dead space increases during deliberate hypotension, an effect exaggerated by head-up posture. The inspired oxygen concentration should be increased to compensate, as should the minute ventilation.

Applications to maxillofacial surgery

Deliberate hypotension is said to reduce blood loss, improve the quality of the surgical field, and shorten operating time for orthognathic surgery, while being considered relatively safe[19]. Bleeding comes from the bony surfaces after mandibular and maxillary osteotomies. Severe bleeding may be caused by damage to vessels such as the descending palatine artery, sphenopalatine artery, pterygoid venous plexus, masseteric artery, and retromandibular vein[19]. Hypotension may be especially useful in bilateral maxillary osteotomies[20]. However, blood loss may be reduced in other ways. For instance use of aprotinin during simultaneous maxillary Le Fort 1 and mandibular sagittal split osteotomies, resulted in 52% less blood loss than controls[21].

Using several techniques, including acute normovolaemic haemodilution, cell saver, as well as moderate hypotension, is more effective than a single modality in reducing transfusion requirements[22]. Application of a simple protocol may reduce transfusion requirements[23]. The risk of blood transfusion can be reduced by autologous transfusion, possibly augmented by preoperative erythropoietin therapy[24].

Deliberate hypotensive anaesthetic techniques

Many agents have been used to produce deliberate hypotension, including glyceryl trinitrate, inhalational anaesthetics (including isoflurane), β-blockade, labetalol, nicardipine, adenosine, and prostaglandin E[7]. The author uses the following technique to allow the local resection of choroidal intraocular tumours, primarily melanomas, and similar techniques may be useful if deliberate hypotension is required in those undergoing maxillofacial surgery. For this procedure the blood pressure is reduced to 40 mmHg in the normotensive patient. This pressure produces a blood-free field during choroidal dissection. For maxillofacial surgery, a reduction in blood pressure of 20% will reduce blood loss[7].

At the preoperative visit the patient is assessed for possible contraindications to hypotension. In the author's practice, cerebrovascular and renovascular disease are absolute contraindications, and coronary artery disease is a strong relative contraindication. The patient with diabetes mellitus is difficult to assess for deliberate hypotension. The possible presence of autonomic neuropathy and small vessel vascular disease may cause problems even in apparently fit individuals.

Hypertension alone is not a contraindication. The blood pressure should be reduced in proportion to the normal systolic pressure. The author reduces the blood pressure to one-third of the patient's systolic blood pressure during surgery for choroidal malignant melanoma. Moderate hypotension for maxillofacial surgery should employ a similar but less severe pro rata reduction of 20%.

Once the decision has been made to use deliberate hypotension, this must be discussed with the patient. It should be explained that in return for the benefits of less blood loss and better operating conditions, the patient will undergo a small risk of adverse outcome. For choroidal surgery, a risk of 0.5% is quoted, but this is not based on actual adverse outcome[25]. The risk for moderate hypotension would be much less. The patient is asked to give informed consent to hypotension and the discussion should be documented.

Atenolol 50 mg is given on the night before and the morning of surgery, and may be accompanied by a sedative if required. β-blockade reduces bleeding owing to reflex tachycardia as the blood pressure is reduced. It will also have a useful hypotensive effect when combined with general anaesthesia, and this may be sufficient alone for moderate hypotension. Antithromboembolic treatment should also be given. Subcutaneous administration of dalteparin 2500 U should be considered and antiembolic stockings may prove very useful. The general anaesthetic technique should be suitable for the type of surgery to be performed. Isoflurane may be the most suitable volatile agent owing to its reduction in cerebral metabolic rate[9]. If a nasal endotracheal tube is used, care should be taken to avoid pressure on the tip of the nose as, because of lowered perfusion pressure, ischaemic necrosis may be caused[7].

If the degree of hypotension secondary to β-blockade and general anaesthesia is inadequate, an infusion of sodium nitroprusside, 50 mg dissolved in 5% dextrose 500 ml, is started. This is delivered via a volumetric pump and the rate is titrated to achieve the desired blood pressure. It is sensible to start the infusion at 5 ml/hour and observe the response. There is considerable variation between different individuals; 5 ml/hour may produce a dramatic fall in blood pressure in one patient, while over 100 ml/hour may be required in another. A maximum dose of 1.5 micrograms/kg/minute should not be exceeded[26]. If higher rates are used, cyanide toxicity may result, causing hypotension, tachycardia, and metabolic acidosis, eventually ending in death[7]. If the blood pressure goes lower than desired, slowing or temporarily stopping, the nitroprusside infusion results in an increase in blood pressure within a few minutes. If a more rapid rise is required, vasopressors such as ephedrine, metaraminol or phenylephrine are effective.

During profound hypotension, the following monitoring apparatus should be used: electrocardiogram, invasive arterial blood pressure, pulse oximetry, capnography, and a cerebral function monitor (Maynard CFAM4). The monitoring for moderate hypotension may not need to be so extensive, although such levels add reassurance. Unfortunately, it is not possible to monitor for spinal cord ischaemia, which is one of the more devastating complications of hypotension.

Recovery and postoperative care should be that needed for the particular surgical technique, with no special requirements for patients who have experienced deliberate hypotension.

Ethical considerations

In choosing to use deliberate hypotension, the anaesthetist has to not only perform a risk:benefit analysis, but present this to the patient in such a way that informed consent may be given.

Kerr published a series of 700 patients in whom the blood pressure was lowered to a systolic pressure of less than 50 mmHg without adverse effect to facilitate middle ear surgery[5]. Although reservations were expressed at the time[27], this paper was cited in an editorial in 1995 to illustrate the 'relative safety' of induced hypotension[28]. Unfortunately, a patient of Doctor Kerr's developed the profoundly disabling anterior spinal artery syndrome after profound hypotension for an operation in 1979. He was left with paraplegia and urinary and faecal incontinence. Legal proceedings were brought and the court found for the litigant.

The case of Hepworth v Kerr is of great importance to practitioners of profound hypotension. The court considered whether Doctor Kerr was justified in reducing patients' blood pressure to such low levels. Advice from an expert witness said that not only was this degree of hypotension not necessary, but was in fact contraindicated, as bleeding points could not be identified to allow haemostasis[25]. Hence there must be a clear indication for inducing hypotension, and the benefit from this must outweigh any risks, in the opinion of the patient.

The court also considered whether publication of a technique in a learned journal justified its use scientifically. Although Doctor Kerr had published a case series in the *British Journal of Anaesthesia*, he provided no scientific data and therefore had no scientific validity[25]. In addition, consideration was also given as to whether Doctor Kerr's patient was fit enough for a hypotensive anaesthetic. The patient was middle-aged, hypertensive, and a smoker. He was not warned that he might be at higher risk, and Doctor Kerr did not modify his technique in any way[25]. Most modern series investigating hypotensive anaesthesia in maxillofacial surgery recruit young, fit patients[29–32]. Caution should be exercised in using hypotensive anaesthesia in the elderly and in patients with significant comorbidity. If induced hypotension is indicated, the patient should be told that they are at higher risk than a fit patient.

Based on a review of the literature, it was felt that routine hypotension was justified for orthognathic surgery, because of reduction in blood loss and transfusion requirements and low morbidity. However, it was emphasized that careful patient selection and monitoring was mandatory[20].

Conclusion

The main benefit of deliberate hypotension in maxillofacial surgery is to reduce bleeding and to provide a better operative field. The technique should be used in conjunction with other methods of reducing homologous transfusion such as haemodilution, cell saver (in operations with no risk of contamination), and autologous transfusion. Although many small series show no morbidity associated with the technique in young healthy subjects, devastating complications such as death, myocardial infarction or paraplegia are unacceptable, however rare. The risk increases with development of atheromatous disease suggesting a relative contraindication in the elderly. However, it should always be borne in mind that a younger patient has longer to live with the consequences of a disabling complication. The old adage that hypotension should make an impossible operation possible may be a council of unattainable perfection, but should still be borne in mind in modern practice.

References

1. Enderby GEH. (1985) Historical review of the practice of deliberate hypotension. In: Enderby GEH (ed.) *Hypotensive Anaesthesia.* Edinburgh: Churchill Livingstone, pp. 75–91.

2. Ostlere G, Bryce Smith R. (1960) How to give an anaesthetic. In: *Anaesthetics for Medical Students.* London, J and A Churchill, pp. 110–111.

3. Ostlere G, Bryce Smith R. (1960) Controlled hypotension. In: *Anaesthetics for Medical Students.* London: J and A Churchill, p. 54.

4. Gillies J. (1951) Physiological trespass in anaesthesia. *Proc R Soc Med, Section of Anaesthetics,* **45(1),** 1–6.

5. Kerr AR. (1977) Anaesthesia with profound hypotension for middle ear surgery. *Br J Anaesth,* **49,** 447–52.

6. Singh AD. (2005) Uveal melanoma: resection techniques. In: Singh AD (ed.) *Ophthalmology Clinics of North America.* Saunders, pp. 119–200.

7. Rodrigo C. (1995) Induced hypotension during anesthesia, with special reference to orthognathic surgery. *Anesth Prog,* **42,** 41–8.

8. Enderby GEH. (1985). Cerebral Circulation. In: *Hypotensive Anaesthesia.,* Edinburgh: Churchill Livingstone, p. 30.

9. Oshima T, Karasawa F, Okazaki Y, Wada H and Satoh T. (2003) Effects of sevoflurane on cerebral blood flow and cerebral metabolic rate of oxygen in human beings: a comparison with isoflurane. *Eur J Anaesth,* **20:**7:543–547.

10. Lindop MJ (1975). Complications and morbidity of controlled hypotension. *Br J Anaesth,* **47,** 799–803.

11. Enlund M, Mentell O, Engstron C *et al.* (1996) Occurrence of adenylate kinase in cerebrospinal fluid after isoflurane anaesthesia and orthognathic surgery. *Upps J Med Sci,* **101 (1),** 7–111.

12. Enlund M, Mentell O, Flenninger A *et al.* (1998) Evidence of cerebral dysfunction associated with isoflurane or propofol based anaesthesia for orthognathic surgery, as assessed by biochemical and neuropsychological methods. *Upps J Med Sci,* **103(1),** 43–59.

13. Enderby GEH. (1985) Cardiac and cerebral complication of deliberate hypotension. In: *Hypotensive Anaesthesia.* Edinburgh: Churchill Livingstone, p. 257.

14. Enderby GEH (1985). Cardiac and Cerebral Complication of Deliberate Hypotension, In: *Hypotensive Anaesthesia.* Edinburgh: Churchill Livingstone, p. 256.

15. McClintick AJ, Plenderleith JL, Damato BE, Todd JG. Hypotensive anaesthesia for local resection of choroidal melanoma. Unpublished data

16. Andal D, Andal H, Hörauf K *et al.* (2001) The influence of deliberate hypotension on splanchnic perfusion balance with the use of either isoflurane or esmolol and nitroglycerine. *Anesth Analg,* **93,** 116–1120.

17. Suttner SW, Boldt J, Schmidt CC *et al.* (1999) The effects of sodium nitroprusside-induced hypotension on splanchnic perfusion and hepatocellular integrity. *Anesth Analg,* **89,** 1371.

18. Fukusaki M, Miyako M, Hara T *et al.* (1999) Effects of controlled hypotension with sevoflurane anaesthesia on hepatic function of surgical patients. *Euro J Anaesthesiol,* **16(2),** 111–16.

19. Krohner RG. (2003) Anesthetic considerations and techniques for oral and maxillofacial surgery. *Int Anesthesiol Clin,* **41(3),** 67–89.

20. Choi WS, Samman N. (2008) Risks and benefits of deliberate hypotension in anaesthesia: a systematic review. *Int J Oral Maxillofac Surg,* **37(8),** 687–703.

21. Stewart A, Newman L, Sneddon K *et al.* (2001) Aprotinin reduces blood loss and the need for transfusion in orthognathic surgery. *Br J Oral Maxillofac Surg,* **39(5),** 365–70.

22. Rohling RG, Haers PE, Zimmerman *et al.* (1998) Multimodal strategy for reduction of homologous transfusions in craniomaxillofacial surgery. *Int J Oral Maxillofac Surg,* **28(2),** 137–42.

23. Duncan C, Richardson D, May P *et al.* (2008) Reducing blood loss in synostosis surgery: the Liverpool experience. *J Craniofac Surg,* **19(5),** 1424–30.

24. Christopoulou M, Derartinian H, Hatzidimitriou G *et al.* (2001) Autologous blood transfusion in oral and maxillofacial surgery patients with the use of erythropoietin. *J Craniofac Surg,* **29(2),** 118–25.

25. Jones AG. (2002) Profound hypotension; ethical considerations. *Hosp Med,* **63(2),** 92–4.

26. *British National Formulary,* 58 2009 Chapter 2.5.1. On line bnf.org.

27. Donald JR. (1978) Profound hypotension for middle ear surgery. *Br J Anaesth,* **50,** 84–5.

28. Moss E. (1995) Cerebral blood flow during induced hypotension. *Br J Anaesth,* **74,** 6.

29. Praveen K, Narayan V, Muthesekhar MR *et al.* (2001) Hypotensive anaesthesia and blood loss in orthognathic surgery: a clinical study. *Br J Oral Maxillofac Surg,* **39(2),** 138–40.

30. Precious DS, Splinter W, Bosco D. (1996) Induced hypotensive anaesthesia for adolescent orthognathic surgery patients. *J Oral Maxillofac Surg,* **54(6),** 680–3.

31. Shepherd J. (2004) Hypotensive anaesthesia and blood loss in orthognathic surgery. Evidence based dentistry. Available online at nature.com

32. Yu CNF, Chow TK, Kwan ASK *et al.* (2000) Intraoperative blood loss and operating time in orthognathic surgery using induced hypotensive general anaesthesia: prospective study. *Hong Kong Medical Journal,* **6(3),** 307–11.

21

Anaesthesia for nasal and antral surgery

Sanjiv Sharma and Judith C. Wright

Introduction

Nasal and antral surgery are comon procedures usually performed under general anaesthesia. They often produce blood in the nasopharynx and protection of the airway is key. Many of these procedures are performed as day case surgery, and it is therefore important to use an anaesthetic technique that has minimal residual postoperative psychomotor effects. The aim of this chapter is to cover the principles of general anaesthesia for nasal and antral surgery, to mention briefly some of the local anaesthetic techniques used, and to discuss in more detail the techniques that are used for specific procedures.

General principles for anaesthesia for nasal and antral surgery

Preoperative assessment

In addition to routine preoperative assessment (Chapter 2), the following are of particular note; many patients presenting for nasal surgery have partially or totally obstructed nasal airways and it is important to assess airway patency carefully.

Nasal polyps have an association with allergy and sensitivity to non-steroidal anti-inflammatory drugs (NSAIDs), precipitating wheeze. Most patients will have taken these in the past and can tell you whether or not they can tolerate them. Patients with a persistent postnasal drip are more prone to developing chest complications.

The use of premedication drugs such as benzodiazepines can result in a prolonged recovery period. This is not desirable for two reasons. Firstly, the airway may be compromised and, secondly, many patients undergoing nasal and antral surgery are day case patients and, where possible, premedication drugs should be avoided.

The mainstay of most analgesic regimens for patients undergoing nasal/antral surgery is paracetamol and a non-steroidal. These are often given orally preoperatively as they are cheaper and, in the case of some of the NSAIDs, more effective given this way.

Patients will often require nasal packs and it is important to explain to them that they may wake up with packs in place and be unable to breathe through their nose[1].

Principles of general anaesthetic technique

Nasal and antral surgery will result in fluids, be they blood, mucus or pus, pooling in the nasopharynx. One of the main aims in protecting the airway is to prevent these fluids from entering the lungs. Although blood in itself is not particularly harmful to the lungs, blood clots can obstruct the airways and, when mixed with other fluids, cause infection. It is usual therefore to use a throat pack. There are a number of different packs available and some of these are more effective than others. Wet gauze packs have an advantage to some of the sponge packs available as the latter allow blood to run down the back of them and do not work as well. Documentation of throat pack insertion and removal both in the anaesthetic record and as part of the theatre check list is good practice and should ensure that the packs are not inadvertently left in place.

Traditionally patients undergoing these procedures were intubated, and this remains the technique of choice for many patients. In an adult a preformed cuffed RAE (Ring-Adair-Elwyn) tube (Figure 9.1) is used as it causes less obstruction of the surgical field and, once correctly placed, is more difficult to dislodge. RAE or South-facing endotracheal tubes are of a fixed length. They have a black line on them that should sit at the edge of the lips once in place. This is important as lack of attention to this detail can result in endobronchial intubation or displacement. Obese patients with 'short' necks are at particular risk of endobronchial intubation with an oral RAE tube due to the preformed angulation.

The laryngeal mask airway (LMA) is increasingly being used for airway management for nasal and paranasal surgical procedures. The LMA can protect the airway from blood, pus, and secretions when used with a throat pack, is easy to use, and results in fewer requirements for muscle relaxants. The LMA can be used in conjunction with a spontaneous respiration technique or positive pressure ventilation with low inflation pressures. It produces less coughing and facilitates a smoother recovery in the postoperative period. A patent airway is maintained until the patient is awake and has regained their laryngeal reflexes in the recovery period. The inability to protect against gastric content aspiration and easier dislodgement during surgery are amongst the main disadvantages of the LMA in nasal and antral surgery. Reinforced LMAs (Figure 4.8) are often chosen as they are more difficult to displace and can be taped away from the area of surgery.

Practically, the choice of anaesthetic technique usually comes down to the preference of the anaesthetist, the surgical access required, the surgeon's preference, and patient factors such as gastro-oesophageal reflux or a high body mass index where an endotracheal tube is indicated.

As previously discussed, nasal surgery involves sharing of the airway. The anaesthetist has limited access to the airway during surgery because of drapes, surgical instruments, and space constraints. There is an increased risk of accidental disconnections (partial or complete), partial obstruction of the airway because of kinking of tubes in the breathing circuit, and displacement of the endotracheal tube or laryngeal mask airway[2]. It is therefore good practice to check all connections, and tighten them accordingly prior to the placing of sterile drapes. A low threshold for suspecting airway disconnection is important. In case of accidental extubation of the airway, it is vital to remember to remove any throat packs before attempting to ventilate the patient with a mask airway.

Eye taping

Contamination of the eye with blood and other fluids may occur during nasal and antral surgery. However, as the surgeon may be operating close to the medial wall of the orbit it is important that they can see the medial aspect of the eye. Therefore ointment such as lacrilube combined with taping of the lateral aspect of the eye only will protect the eye without obscuring the surgeon's view.

The bloodless surgical field

Excess blood in the surgical field makes operating difficult. A clean and dry surgical field is important. A number of techniques may be used to minimize bleeding, including positioning in the head-up position, the use of vasoconstrictors, and hypotensive anaesthesia.

Posture

Placing the patient 30° head-up reduces venous congestion and may result in lower blood pressure in the arteries supplying the nose.

Vasoconstrictors

Various vasoconstrictor agents may be used as adjuncts to topical and infiltrative local anaesthesia in nasal surgery. The advantages of concomitant use of vasoconstrictor agents are decreased blood loss, reduced nasal mucosal congestion, and improved visualization owing to less bleeding in the operative field[2–9]. Vasoconstriction also slows the systemic absorption of local anaesthetic agents, leading to prolonged duration of action and reduced risk of toxicity.

Moffett's solution was described by Moffett in 1947; it contains 2 ml cocaine 8%, 1 ml adrenaline 1:1000, and 2 ml sodium bicarbonate[5,10]. This solution is dripped into the nostrils following insertion of a throat pack to prevent the solution from leaking into the nasopharynx. Acting as both a local anaesthetic and a vasoconstrictor it has largely been replaced, although other preparations of cocaine are still used.

Adrenaline, phenylepherine 0.5%, oxymetazoline, felypressin, and cocaine are all common vasoconstrictor agents used in nasal or paranasal sinuses surgery[4–7,10]. Adrenaline is used in combination with lidocaine and can also be used for infiltrative block. The common dilutions employed are 1:80 000, 1:100 000, and 1:200 000. It should be used with caution in patients with heart disease. The common side effects are tachycardia, sweating, and hypertension[6,8,10]. Profound hypotension has also been reported with its use. The use of adrenaline with halothane can lead to arrhythmias, although there is a much lower risk with newer volatile agents.

Cocaine is an ester local anaesthetic agent with vasoconstrictor activity[7,9–11]. It can be used as a topical agent in 4–10% strengths. Cocaine should never be injected. It should not be used in combination with solutions containing adrenaline as it can lead to cardiovascular instability. Serious adverse effects including arrhythmias, myocardial infarction, seizure, and death have been reported.

Deliberate hypotension

The risk of bleeding during nasal and paranasal sinus surgery is high because of the abundant vascularity of the nose. Intraoperative bleeding leads to reduced visibility in the surgical field, especially in the case of endoscopic surgical procedures.

The technique of deliberate hypotension (see Chapter 20) can be employed in nasal and paranasal surgery to reduce blood loss and improve the visibility of the surgical field[13–15]. The mean arterial pressure is targeted to between 50 and 65 mmHg. Invasive monitoring of blood pressure may be required with the use of β-blockers and vasodilator drugs. Elderly patients and those with pre-existing hypertension should have their blood pressure controlled to an appropriately higher target level. In all patients the fall in blood pressure should be proportionate to their normal blood pressure.

This technique is contraindicated in patients with vascular disease, especially ischaemic heart disease or cerebrovascular disease.

A wide range of pharmacological agents can be used peroperatively to produce deliberate hypotension. In practice, it is unusual to use antihypertensives, and judicious use of anaesthetic drugs such as remifentanil will usually control the blood pressure sufficiently. Although remifentanil is the most commonly used agent for this, magnesium has also been used successfully.

Deliberate hypotension is discussed in Chapter 20.

It is also important to recognize that a tachycardic patient will result in a more 'bloody' surgical field, and administering drugs that cause a tachycardia should be avoided during the surgery. For example, the intraoperative administration of the antiemetic cyclizine should be delayed until surgery has finished.

Analgesia

The NSAIDS, such as diclofenac or ibuprofen, and paracetamol can be given orally with a sip of water preoperatively or intravenously or as suppositories after induction of anaesthesia. These are useful adjuncts to anaesthesia and provide intraoperative and postoperative analgesia. Infiltration with local anaesthesia will reduce the immediate postoperative requirements for analgesia. Patients undergoing rhinoplasty will also usually require opiates, and fentanyl and morphine are the two most commonly used agents. Regular paracetamol and an NSAID, together with an opiate as rescue analgesia, provide good postoperative analgesia.

Antiemesis

Nasal and paranasal surgery is a risk factor for postoperative nausea and vomiting (PONV). Use of propofol-based anaesthetic techniques causes less PONV. The common antiemetics used are: antihistamines (cyclizine), antidopaminergic (prochlorperazine, phenothiazines) agents, antiserotonergics (ondansetron), and dexamethasone.

Emergence from anaesthesia and extubation

Secretions or blood in the airway can lead to coughing and laryngospasm. The patient should therefore be suctioned under direct vision after removal of the throat pack. Insertion and removal of the throat pack should be carefully documented. Blood can accumulate behind the soft palate which is not readily visible and it should be cleared with suction before extubation. If it is not cleared, the clot from blood pooled from surgery can be aspirated in the postoperative period, with fatal results (the coroner's clot).

Oral, maxillofacial, and ear, nose, and throat (ENT) theatres are often set up with the head end of the operating table distant to the anaesthetic machine. The table should be turned or the anaesthetic machine moved so that it is at the same end as the patient's head. Although there is some debate about whether to extubate patients deep or light, given that the patients often have nasal packs and blood in the airway, it is safer to extubate these patients awake and sitting up when they are able to protect their own airway. Where there are overriding reasons to extubate the patient in a deeper plane of anaesthesia, consideration should be given to inserting a Guedel airway prior to extubation. Children are often extubated in the left lateral position with the table tipped head down.

Local anaesthetic agents and nerve blocks for nasal surgery

Topical and infiltrative local anaesthetic techniques are used with intravenous sedation or general anaesthesia for nasal and paranasal sinus surgery. The local anaesthetic agents are available in various forms as liquids, sprays, gels, and ointments. The dose of local

Table 21.1 Common local anaesthetic agents in use in nasal and paranasal surgery

Local anaesthetic agent		Preparation (%)	Maximum total safe dose
Esters	Cocaine	Paste 1.2gms of 25%, or Moffetts (see below) Solutions 4–10%	1.5–2 mg/kg
	Procaine	0.25–0.50%	10 mg/kg
	Benzocaine	Up to 20%, as spray (also used as throat lozenge)	
Amides	Lidocaine	0.5–2% solution. Note dental syringes contain 2% lidocaine with 1:80,000 adrenaline	3 mg/kg. Up to 7 mg/kg with epinephrine
	Bupivacaine	0.25–0.5%	2 mg/kg

anaesthetic agent is dependent on the type and duration of surgical procedure, patient factors, and concomitant use of vasoconstrictor agents. The sensation of the nose is derived from the ophthalmic and maxillary divisions of the trigeminal nerve[4] (Chapter 6).

Classification of local anaesthetic drugs

Local anaesthetic agents are classified as either amides or esters (Table 21.1). Allergies are common to esters but are very rarely seen to the amides. Ester local anaesthetic agents are rapidly metabolized by plasma cholinesterase and toxicity is rare. Amide local anaesthetic agents are metabolized in the liver.

Topical anaesthesia

The total dose required for topical anaesthesia is usually less than that used for infiltration. There is no distortion of the tissue planes at the site of application. It can be used as an adjunct to general anaesthesia. Topical techniques include the application of cotton pledgets, the sequential layering of gauze soaked with local anaesthetic with vasoconstrictor, sprays or the application of paste topically.

Infiltrative local anaesthesia

Nerve blocks used for nasal surgery[2] are the infraorbital nerve block, maxillary nerve (Chapter 7), sphenopalatine ganglion block, and frontal nerve block. They may be used for the removal of small polyps, reduction of nasal fractures, and excision of small tumours.

Specific procedures

Foreign body in the nose

This is common in children. Unilateral discharge and nasal obstruction are usual features. There can be significant swelling and secretions, making it difficult to identify the foreign body.

Removal of foreign body in children

There is a risk of profuse bleeding in cases of unrecognized longstanding foreign bodies in the nose.

A local anaesthetic technique using a local anaesthetic plus vasoconstrictor spray can be used if the child is cooperative, but general anaesthesia is needed in the majority of children. A spontaneous respiration technique with a gas or propofol induction, LMA, nitrous oxide or air with volatile agent can be used safely. Removal of a nasal foreign body can be performed under local anaesthesia in adults. General anaesthesia may be required in less cooperative adults.

If there is a risk of a full stomach, then intravenous induction with rapid sequence induction (RSI) and securing of the airway with an endotracheal tube will be required.

Postsurgical nasal packing may be required for haemostasis. This may compromise oxygenation, and supplementary oxygen is occasionally required postoperatively.

Choanal atresia

Choanal atresia results from a failure of canalization of the bucconasal membrane. This is a rare anomaly that occurs at birth and is often associated with other congenital abnormalities. There is a 60% association with other congenital anomalies in cases of bilateral choanal atresia. Common associated anomalies, known by the acronym CHARGE, include colobama (C), congenital heart defects (H), atresia of choana (A), retarded growth (R), genital anomalies (G), and deafness (E)[16]. Diagnosis is confirmed by failure to pass a catheter through the nares into the nasopharynx.

Choanal atresia is commonly unilateral, although it can be bilateral, at which time it may become life-threatening. Immediate management involves the insertion of an orophayngeal airway, a McGovern's nipple or oral intubation as an emergency[17–19]. Puncture, dilatation, and stenting is the standard surgical treatment, but a nasal endoscopic surgical technique is now increasingly the treatment of choice[20].

Stenting is performed to prevent re-stenosis in the postoperative period, and stents may be required for 4–6 weeks.

Manipulation of nasal fractures

For optimal reduction of a nasal fracture, closed manipulation should be performed within a few hours of injury. However, it is rare for patients to present starved within this timeframe. There is subsequently associated swelling which takes around a week to subside. Manipulation of nasal fractures usually takes place within 10 days of the injury.

Anaesthetic technique

Preoxygenation and ventilation with a mask airway may be difficult because of an inability to maintain a good seal because of pain and swelling. Early use of a Guedel oral airway is recommended. A spontaneous breathing technique with insertion of an LMA to reduce contamination of the lungs with blood is usually used. Where significant bleeding is anticipated as a result of instrumentation, a throat pack should be inserted. Alternatively, where the nasal bones are being quickly manually manipulated, the procedure may be performed using total intravenous anaesthesia and intermittent mask/bag ventilation. The aim of anaesthetic technique is to provide short adequate anaesthesia and analgesia, allowing rapid recovery of the airway reflexes[21–27].

Fracture reduction can be performed under local anaesthetic technique with cocaine spray and pack plus infiltration with 2% lidocaine.

Incision and drainage of nasal septal haematomas

Nasal septal haematomas are the result of blood collecting under the perichondral layer. If left untreated, infection and abscess formation can result. Incision and drainage can be conducted in some cooperative adults; otherwise, general anaesthesia is indicated. The latter is necessary for children with nasal haematomas.

Epistaxis or nasal bleeding

The nose has an abundant blood supply. Epistaxis occurs commonly from the anterior part of nasal cavity. Little's area, or the Kiesselbach plexus, where branches from the internal carotid (ethmoid) and external carotid (facial and internal maxillary) form a rich plexus with the venous system, is a common source of epistaxis. Rarely, the source of bleeding is the posterior nasal cavity. Trauma is another common precipitating factor. Spontaneous nasal bleeds occur in patients with bleeding disorders, hypertension, or those on anticoagulants as well as during pregnancy.

The management of epistaxis includes airway protection, recognition and correction of hypovolaemia, and appropriate therapy after identification of the cause of bleeding[2,28]. A minor epistaxis may be controlled with pressure, local vasoconstrictors or cauterization. Major nose bleeds can require anterior packing of the nose or posterior packing of the nose with gauze or pneumatic catheters (Chapter 14). These have implications for anaesthesia as the patient is often anxious, uncomfortable, and must breathe through their mouth. This may compromise the airway and thus oxygenation of the patient.

Anaesthetic management

Persistent and severe nasal haemorrhage may necessitate surgical arterial ligation or embolization. Patients presenting for surgery to achieve haemostasis following an epistaxis may have lost significant amounts of blood. The true blood loss might be underestimated because of an unaccountable volume of swallowed blood in the case of posterior nasal cavity bleeding. There is always a risk of aspiration of fresh or swallowed blood. Assessment of hypovolaemia and adequate resuscitation with fluid or blood is needed before induction. Nasal packs and catheters can result in a poor fit for face masks and make access to the airway problematic. The larynx may be difficult to visualize due to blood, secretions, and swelling. Efficient suction is particularly important.

Crossmatched blood should be available. The patient should have a large bore cannula inserted if this has not already been done. An RSI should be performed and the trachea isolated with an endotracheal tube. Where a difficult airway/intubation is anticipated, inhalational induction in the left lateral/head-down position is an alternative. Once the airway has been secured and the bleeding controlled, a wide bore orogastric tube should be inserted to empty the stomach of swallowed blood. Extubation should be performed once the patient has fully recovered their laryngeal reflexes. Postoperatively, haemoglobin should be measured and the need for oxygen therapy assessed.

Nasal polypectomy

Nasal polyps are polypoidal sacs arising from the nasal mucosa and can totally obstruct the nasal airway. The pathogenesis is not completely understood but there is an association with asthma, cystic fibrosis, and recurrent sinusitis[28–33]. In asthmatic patients, nasal polyps tend to be more common in those with a sensitivity to NSAIDS. Therefore it is important to ask patients with nasal polyps about past use of NSAIDS as part of the preoperative assessment. Nasal polypectomy is usually performed as an endoscopic technique. The nasal airway may be completely obstructed and early use of a Guedel airway is recommended. Bleeding can be profuse and a throat pack should be inserted. Endotracheal intubation to protect the airway is preferred by many anaesthetists.

Septoplasty

Septoplasty involves the correction of a deviated nasal septum to create a patent airway. Although this procedure can be performed under local anaesthesia, endotracheal general anaesthesia is more common[28]. As the septum is a highly vascular structure, a throat pack should be inserted.

Rhinoplasty

This is a cosmetic procedure performed to correct deformity of the nose. Bone or cartilage graft may be used for reconstruction. The anaesthetic technique is similar to that employed for a septoplasty[28,33]. Topical and infiltration of vasoconstrictor agents decrease bleeding, and hypotensive anaesthesia, where appropriate, improves the surgical field. Packing of the nose is usually performed and a rigid shield is used for protection.

Turbinectomy

This procedure is usually performed as part of the treatment for hypertrophic or vasomotor rhinitis and it involves removal of a portion of the inferior or middle turbinates. Turbinectomy is also performed for excision of neoplasm of the turbinate. There is a risk of bleeding as this area is very vascular, so again the anaesthetic technique should include prevention of aspiration of blood.

Sinus surgery

Sinus surgery involves the removal of inflamed mucosa from the maxillary antrum. The sublabial approach is used but there is a risk of nerve damage leading to numb teeth. This operation can be performed under local anaesthesia, but the preferred method is general anaesthesia with an endotracheal tube.

Lasers, particularly the Nd:YAG laser, have a place in sinonasal surgery, and laser compatible anaesthetic equipment should be used. Specific lasers require additional patient protection e.g. eye pads and wet towels. Staff should all be appropriately trained and wearing appropriate eye protection. The use of lasers is discussed in Chapter 10.

Functional endoscopic sinus surgery

Functional endoscopic sinus surgery (FESS)[28–35] is performed in patients with paranasal sinus disease not responding to medical therapy. FESS is a minimally invasive surgical technique involving opening the sinus ostia under vision with a fibreoptic endoscope to restore mucociliary flow and normal sinus function. The aim of surgical therapy is to promote natural drainage and aeration of the sinuses. The use of image-guided endoscopy during surgery has reduced the risk of surgical complications[36]. The patient with sinus disease may have a triad of polyps, asthma, and aspirin sensitivity (Sampler's syndrome)[29].

A standard anaesthetic technique using a reinforced LMA or RAE endotracheal tube plus a throat pack is usual. Topical anaesthesia to decrease bleeding may be used (either 4% cocaine solution or 2% lidocaine with adrenaline spray). Alternatively, total intravenous anaesthetic techniques have the advantage of allowing greater control of the blood pressure. Where appropriate, deliberate hypotension provides a bloodless operative field.

Balloon sinusotomy

Balloon sinusotomy causes less scarring as compared to FESS. It involves dilatation of the ostium with a balloon catheter to restore normal drainage of paranasal sinuses. General anaesthesia is the preferred anaesthetic technique.

Sinonasal tumours

Sinonasal papilloma, nasopharyngeal angiofibroma, haemangioma, osteoma and rhinophyma are all benign nasal and paranasal sinus tumours which are resected surgically, commonly endoscopically. If endoscopic surgery is not feasible, an open surgical approach is used such as open rhinotomy or maxillectomy. The proximity of the lesions to the orbit and base of the skull makes surgery hazardous. Bleeding can be profuse.

Nasopharyngeal angiofibroma

Nasopharyngeal angiofibroma is an aggressive and vascular benign tumour[37]. Resection carries a risk of torrential bleeding as the blood supply is from the external carotid artery. Preoperative embolization 48–72 hours preoperatively reduces blood loss. Treatment is with either open surgical excision or endoscopically. Sinonasal malignancies are rare and account for only 3% of total head and neck malignancies. The surgical approach includes wide excision, lateral rhinotomy, midfacial degloving, and radical craniofacial resection procedures with flap repairs.

A detailed preoperative assessment paying particular attention to the airway is required for each patient. A senior anaesthetist who is competent in managing a difficult airway is essential. Patients may present with complete obstruction of the nasal airway and reconstruction involves multistep operative procedures. Good vascular access is essential and crossmatched blood should be available.

General anaesthesia with insertion of RAE endotracheal tube or flexometallic tube plus throat pack and an intermittent positive pressure ventilation (IPPV) technique is employed. Maintenance with inhalational agents or total intravenous anaesthesia (TIVA) technique with remifentanyl is common. If an inhalational technique is used, then desflurane with rapid onset and offset is preferred. Hypotensive anaesthesia may be beneficial provided there are no contraindications. Invasive monitoring is usually necessary, with the insertion of arterial and central venous pressure lines. Warm intravenous fluids and warming blankets should be used intraoperatively, and pressure areas should be meticulously padded. High dependency unit (HDU) or intensive care unit (ICU) admission may be required for postoperative management.

Conclusion

All nasal and antral surgery has the potential to cause soiling of the airway, and airway protection including intubation and throat pack insertion should be considered. Many of the procedures are conducted as day cases. Consequently, the anaesthetist has to consider techniques that facilitate early mobilization and allow the patient to be discharged several hours after anaesthesia and surgery.

References

1. Muluk NB, Apan A, Ozçakir S, Arikan OK, Koç C. (2008) Risk of respiratory distress in the patients who were applied nasal packing at the end of nasal surgery. *Auris Nasus Larynx*, **35**, 521–6.
2. Jones GW. (2007) Anaesthesia for ENT and maxillofacial surgery. In: Aitkenhead AR, Smith G, Rowbotham DJ (eds). *Textbook of Anaesthesia*, 5th edn. Edinburgh: Churchill Livingstone, Elsevier, pp. 574–7.
3. Roberts F. (2002) Ear, nose and throat surgery. In: Allman KG, Wilson IH (eds). *Oxford Handbook of Anaesthesia*. Oxford: Oxford University Press, pp. 523–6.
4. Mediscape, e-Medicine (2007) Anaesthesia, nose. <http://emedicine.medscape.com/otolaryngoly>
5. Lee YC, Wang CP. (2008) Cotton pledget method for nasal decongestive anesthesia prior to transnasal endoscopy. *Am J Gasteroenterol*, **103**, 3212–13.
6. Jage J. (1993) Circulatory effects of vasoconstrictors combined with local anesthetics. *Anesth Pain Control Dent*, **2** (2), 81–6.
7. Kameyama K, Watanabe S, Kano T, Kusukawa J. (2008) Effects of nasal application of an epinephrine and lidocaine mixture on the hemodynamics and nasal mucosa in oral and maxillofacial surgery. *J Oral Maxillofac Surg*, **66** (11), 226–32.
8. Pallasch TJ. (1998) Vasoconstrictors and the heart. *J Calif Dent Assoc*, **26**(9), 668–73.
9. Benjamin E, Wong DK, Choa D. (2004) 'Moffett's' solution: a review of the evidence and scientific basis for the topical preparation of the nose. *Clin Otolaryngol Allied Sci*, **29**(6), 582–7.
10. Wildsmith JAW. (2007) Local anaesthetic agents. In: Aitkenhead AR, Smith G, Rowbotham DJ (eds). *Textbook of Anaesthesia*, 5th edn. Edinburgh: Churchill Livingstone Elsevier, pp. 52–62.
11. Harper SJ, Jones, NS. (2006) Cocaine: what role does it have in current ENT practice? A review of the current literature. *J Laryngol Otol*, **120**(10), 808–11.
12. Rosenberg PH, Veering BT, Urmey WF. (2004) Maximum recommended doses of local anaesthetics: a multifactorial concept. *Reg Anesth Pain Med*, **29**(6), 564–75; discussion p. 524.
13. Cincikas D, Ivaskevicius J. (2003) Application of controlled arterial hypotension in endoscopic rhinosurgery. *Medicina*, **39**(9), 852–9.
14. Blackwell KE, Ross DA, Kapur, P, Calcaterra TC. (1993) Propofol for maintenance of general anesthesia: a technique to limit blood loss during endoscopic sinus surgery. *American Journal of Otolaryngology*, **14**(4), 262–6.
15. Manola M, De Luca E, Moscillo L, Mastella A. (2005) Using remifentanil and sufentanil in functional endoscopic sinus surgery to improve surgical conditions. *J Otorhinolargol*, **67**(2), 83–6.
16. Asher BF, Mcgill TJ, Kaplan L, Friedman EM, Healy GB. (1990) Airway complications in CHARGE association. *Arch Otolaryngol Head Neck Surg*, **116**(5), 594–5.

17. Rushman GB, Davies NJH, Catherman JN. (1999) Local anaesthetic agents. In: *Lee's Synopsis of Anaesthesia,'* 12th edn. Oxford: Butterworth–Heinemann, pp. 585–601.

18. Ballantyne JC, Harrison DFN. (1986) Nose and throat. In: *Rob & Smith's Operative Surgery: Nose and throat.* London: Butterworth, pp. 185–6.

19. Mediscape, e-Medicine (2007) Anaesthesia, Choanal atresia.<http://emedicine.medscape.com/otolaryngology>

20. Stankiewicz JA. (1990) The endoscopic repair of choanal atresia. *Otolaryngology—Head Neck Surg,* **103,** 931–7.

21. Mondin V, Rinaldo A, Ferlito A. (2005) Management of nasal bone fractures. *Am J Otolaryngol,* **26(3),** 181–5.

22. Khwaja S, Pahade AV, Luff D, Green MW, Green KM. (2007) Nasal fracture reduction: local versus general anaesthesia. *Rhinology,* **45(1),** 83–8.

23. Buck M. (1965) A method of local anaesthesia for the correction of simple fracture of the nose. *Br J Plast Surg,* **18 (4),** 363–8.

24. Demiraran Y, Ozturk O, Guclu E, Iskender A, Ergin MH, Tokmak A. (2008) Vasoconstriction and analgesic efficacy of locally infiltrated levobupivacaine for nasal surgery. *Anesth Analg,* **106(3),** 1008–11.

25. Jones TM, Nandapalan V. (1999) Manipulation of the fractured nose: a comparison of local infiltration anaesthesia and topical local anaesthesia. *Clin Otolaryngol Allied Sci,* **24(5),** 443–6.

26. Watson DJ, Parker, AJ, Slack RW, Griffiths, MV. (1988) Local versus general anaesthetic in the management of the fractured nose. *Clin Otolaryngol Allied Sci,* **13(6),** 491–4.

27. Newton CR, White PS. (1998) Nasal manipulation with intravenous sedation. Is it an acceptable and effective treatment? *Rhinology,* **36(3),** 114–16.

28. Roberts F. (2002) Ear, nose and throat surgery. In: Allman KG, Wilson IH (eds). *Oxford Handbook of Anaesthesia.* Oxford: Oxford University Press, pp. 535–6.

29. Alhaddad S. (1993) Anatomy of nasal wall. In: Levine HL, May M (eds). *Endoscopic Sinus Surgery.* New York: Theime, Medical Publishers INC, pp. 2–20.

30. Venkatraman G. (2006) Endoscopic sinus surgery. In: Lubin MF, Smith RB, Dodson TF, Spell NO, Walker HK (eds). *Medical Management of the Surgical Patient,* 4th edn. Pp. 757–8. Cambridge University Press, Cambridge, UK.

31. Dalziel K, Stein K, Round A, Garside R, Royle P. (2006) Endoscopic sinus surgery for the excision of nasal polyps: A systematic review of safety and effectiveness. *Am J Rhinol,* 20, 506–19.

32. Gross CW, Gurucharri MJ, Lazar RH, Long TE. (1989) Functional endonasal sinus surgery (FESS) in the pediatric age group. *Laryngoscope,* **99(3),** 272–5.

33. Nancymore P. (2003) Otorhinolaryngologic and head and neck surgery. In: *Berry's and Kohn's Operating Room Technique,'* 11th edn. Philadelphia: Mosby Elsevier, pp. 875–7.

34. Fornadley JA, Kennedy KS, Wilson JF, Galantich PT, Parker GS. (1992) Anesthetic choice for functional endoscopic sinus surgery. *Am J Rhinol,* **6(1),** 1–4.

35. Danielsen A, Gravningsbraten R, Olofsson J. (2003) Anaesthesia in endoscopic sinus surgery. *European Archives of Oto-rhino-laryngology,* **260(9),** 481–6.

36. Hornung DE. (2006) Nasal anatomy and the sense of monitoring of intra- operative visual evoked potentials during functional endoscopic sinus surgery (FESS) under general anaesthesia. *Otorhinolaryngol,* **63,** 1–22.

37. Jorissen M, Eloy P, Rombaux P, Bachert C, Daele J. (2005) Endoscopic sinus surgery for juvenile nasopharyngeal angiofibroma. *Acta Otorhinolaryngol Belg,* **54(2),** 201–19.

22

Orofacial pain

Tara Renton and Joanna Zakrzewska

Introduction

Orofacial pain is effectively pain within the trigeminal system. The trigeminal nerve supplies general sensory supply to face, scalp, and mouth (Chapter 6). A vast proportion of the sensory cortex represents the trigeminal input (over 40%). The trigeminal sensory region is very complex, incorporating the cranium, ears, eyes, sinuses, nose, pharynx, infratemporal fossa, jaw joint, teeth, jaws, salivary glands, oral mucosa, and skin. As many medical students are rarely exposed to ear, nose, and throat (ENT), otolaryngology, and dentistry, this region remains an enigma to most, with their singular experience of trigeminal pain being based on trigeminal neuralgia in relation to neurosurgical procedures.

Chronic orofacial pain syndromes represent a diagnostic challenge for any practitioner. Patients are frequently misdiagnosed or attribute their pain to a prior event such as a dental procedure, ENT problem or facial trauma. Psychiatric symptoms of depression and anxiety are prevalent in this population and compound the diagnostic conundrum. Treatment is less effective than in other pain syndromes, thus often requires a multidisciplinary approach to address the many facets of this pain syndrome[1].

Aetiology of facial pain

Facial pain can be associated with pathological conditions or disorders related to somatic and neurological structures[2]. There are a wide range of causes of orofacial pain and these have been divided into three broad categories by Hapak *et al.*[3]—musculoligamentous, dentoalveolar, and neurological and vascular. The commonest cause of orofacial pain is temporomandibular disorders, principally myofascial in nature[4]. As mechanisms underlying these pains begin to be identified, more accurate classifications which are

mechanism-based may come to be used. A major change in mechanism has been that burning mouth syndrome probably has a neuropathic cause using the newly defined definitions rather than being a pain due to psychological causes.

Incidence

Chronic orofacial pain is comparable with other pain conditions in the body, and accounts for between 20 and 25% of chronic pain conditions[4]. A 6-month prevalence of facial pain has been reported by between 1%[4] and 3%[5] of the population. In the study by Locker and Grushka[6], some pain or discomfort in the jaws, oral mucosa, or face had been experienced by less than 10% in the past 4 weeks. In 1980[7], Bonica estimated that 5–7 million Americans suffer from chronic pain in the face and mouth, and between 25 and 45% are affected at some time of life[4].

Most population-based studies have shown that women report more facial pain than men[4,8,9], with rates approximately twice as high among women compared to men[10]. In clinic populations the rates for women are even higher[1]. On the other hand, other studies have found no sex difference in the prevalences of orofacial pain[6,11].

Several studies have also shown variability in the prevalence across age groups. The age distribution of the facial pain population differs from that of the most usual pain conditions. In contrast to chest and back pain, for example, facial pain has been suggested to be less prevalent among older persons than younger ones[6,9]. Conversely, in 1993[4] Lipton *et al.* found the prevalence of facial pain to remain relatively constant across the age groups, while in a study in 2001[5] by Riley and Gilbert, no difference in prevalence was observed between the age groups of 45–64 years and older.

Diagnosis

The International Headache Society (IHS) has published diagnostic criteria for primary and secondary headaches as well as facial pain[12,13]. Criteria have also been published by the International Association for the Study of Pain (IASP), the American Academy of Orofacial Pain (AAOP), and the Research Diagnostic Criteria for Temporomandibular Disorders (RDCTMD)[14,15].

The impact of trigeminal pain must not be underestimated. Consequences include interruption with daily social function such as eating, drinking, speaking, kissing, applying make up, shaving, and sleeping[16,17]. Burning mouth syndrome has been reported to cause significant psychological impact in 70% of patients[6]. In temporomandibular disorders (TMD) pain, 29% patients report high disability resulting in unemployment[18,19]. A recent validated tool has been developed for the assessment of disability related to oral function (Oral Health Impact [OHIP 14])[20,21].

Classification of orofacial pain

The aim of this chapter is to address the causes of chronic orofacial pain (lasting >3 months). However, the most common causes of acute dental pain are due to trauma or infection of the dental pulp which contains the nerves and vessels supplying the tooth.

Dental disease of the hard tissues (caries of enamel, dentine, and cementum), and soft tissues and supporting bone (gingivitis/periodontitis) are recognized as the most common diseases to afflict the general population. These conditions are largely diagnosed and treated by dental practitioners by history, dental clinical examination, and radiographs.

By far the most common forms of oral pain are the acute form of pain that tend to last for short periods of time. These include toothache (dental pulpitis), gum pain (pericoronitis in 80% of the population), periapical periodontitis (owing to apical infection or post-endodontic therapy of high occlusal contact). Dentine sensitivity affects 40% of the adult population; dry socket is postsurgical intense pain that affects 10% of patients after extraction of their teeth. Other orofacial acute pain conditions include trauma or infection of the orofacial tissues[22].

Odontogenic pain

Odontogenic pain refers to pain initiating from the teeth or their supporting structures, the mucosa, gingivae, maxilla, mandible or periodontal membrane.

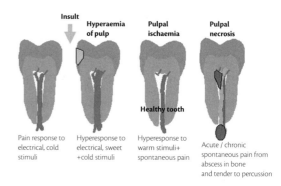

Figure 22.1 The stages and characteristics of dental pulpal pain. See also Plate 15.

Dental pulpitis ('toothache')

Dental pulpitis may be due to infection from dental caries close to the pulp, inflammation caused by chemical or thermal insult subsequent to dental treatment, and may be reversible or non-reversible. Once necrosis of the dental pulp has occurred, the infection spreads through the apex of the tooth into the surrounding bone and periodontal membrane, initiating a dental abscess. The different stages of infection have different clinical presentations (Figure 22.1). Typically the pain is described as aching or throbbing, initially worse following cold or sweet food or fluid intake.

The pulp becomes hyperaemic and self-strangulates within the confined pulpal chamber, resulting in irreversible pulpitis. This is characterized by sensitivity to warmth and heat, and less sensitivity to cold and sweet. The evoked pain is often neuralgic in nature—sharp and short-lasting. As the infection spreads periapically, the pain may be sharp following pressure applied to tooth cusps where the causal factor is a crack in the tooth. Ongoing pulpal inflammation usually leads to an acute abscess with very painful throbbing associated with swelling in the jaw, indicative of an acute infection (Chapter 11).

Exposed cementum or dentine

The tooth root surface, a thin layer of cementum overlaying dentine, is exposed from excessive and/or incorrect tooth brushing. There is tooth sensitivity from cold fluids and/or air, a reflection of a healthy pulp.

Pericoronitis

Pain commonly arises from the supporting gingivae and mucosa when infection arises from an erupting tooth (teething or pericoronitis). This is the most common cause for the removal of third molar teeth (wisdom teeth). The pain may be constant or intermittent, but is often evoked when biting down with opposing maxillary teeth. This elicits pain in the inflamed mucosa and gingivae surrounding the partially erupted tooth.

Apical pain

Premature contact

This is characterized by an initial sharp pain which becomes duller after a period. The pain is due to a recent tooth restoration that is 'high' compared with the normal occlusion when biting together.

Postendodontic surgery pain

This is severe aching pain following endodontic treatment such as root canal therapy or apicectomy. While the majority of patients improve over time (weeks), a few will develop a chronic neuropathic pain state (see below).

Alveolar osteitis

After extraction, the most common complication is a 'dry socket' which is a condition whereby the clot formation within the socket fails at 3–5 days; healing fails, resulting in an empty socket which traps food and debris. The resultant pain is caused by necrotic foodstuff aggravating bony nerve endings, causing intense pain following extractions. This is easily treated by irrigation of the socket and placement of a resorbable bacteriostatic dressing in the socket with additional reassurance for the patient. If the condition is poorly treated, the patient may develop osteomyelitis.

Maxillary sinusitis 'mimicking' toothache

Recurrent maxillary sinusitis may cause widespread pain in the maxillary teeth. The pain has a continuous aching quality and is usually made worse by bending forward. It can mimic the maxillary sinusitis-like symptoms in temporomandibular disease (TMD) (see below) or neuropathic pain. These dental conditions rarely present as chronic pain unless misdiagnosed.

Non-odontogenic facial pain

Non-odontogenic facial pain can be caused by inflammation due to tumour, infection, or trauma. Topographical classification is often applied to this complex region. Regions often presenting as orofacial pain complaints include the sinuses, salivary gland, ears, eyes, throat, mandibular and maxillary bone pathology.

Chronic orofacial pain

The various suggested classifications of chronic orofacial pain do conflict with each other. Several classifications of chronic orofacial pain have been presented and the authors will use the fourth classification for this chapter as it presents a pragmatic and clinically useful alternative[23](Figure 22.2).

Group 1: neurovascular (predominantly VI pain)[24–27]

This group includes migraine, cluster headache, cluster tic syndrome, tension-type headaches, medication overuse headaches, chronic daily headaches, temporal arteritis and short-lasting unilateral neuralgia with conjunctival irritation and tearing (SUNCT). However, one must exclude sinister headaches in patients >50 years old (tumour 1%), recent sudden onset, and subarachnoid haemorrhage (recent trauma or loss of consciousness).

Migraine

Migraines are perhaps the most studied of the headache syndromes. This is due in part to the high incidence and significant loss of productivity and limitation on quality of life suffered by those with the syndrome. It is estimated that 17% of women and 6% of men have migraine headaches. Onset is usually in the second or third decade. Migraines are characterized (Table 22.1) by headaches of moderate to severe intensity located unilaterally with a pulsating quality. Attacks last from 4 to 72 hours (2–48 hours in children <15 years old), and are aggravated by routine physical activities. To meet diagnostic criteria, there must be

Figure 22.2 Chart illustrating a suggested classification for chronic orofacial pain (from Woda *et al.* 2005 [23])

Trigeminal chronic pain		
Neurovascular	Neuropathic	Idiopathic
Tension HA; Migraine cluster HA; Giant cell arteritis; SUNCT	Trigeminal N; Typical / atypical PHN; Glosspharyngeal N; Post surgical N; Lingual inferior alveolar nerve injuries	Burning Mouth S TMJ pain Persistent idiopathic (ATFP / ATO)

Table 22.1 Characteristics of migraine

Five or more lifetime headache attacks lasting 4–72 hours each and symptom-free between attacks, moderate to severe pain, unilateral with or without aura visual signs

The female-to-male ratio is 3:1

It is unilateral but can be bilateral

The pain has a throbbing quality and feels as if it is associated with a pulse

Photophobia, phonophobia, and osmophobia are features of migraine, as is nausea

The pain worsens with exertion and improves with sleep

The patient may or may not experience aura

Pharmacological therapy includes abortive and preventative medications, depending on the frequency and severity of the headaches

Abortive agents include serotonin agonists, ergotamine, isometheptene, and anti-inflammatories. Preventative agents include antiepileptic drugs (AEDs), beta-blockers, calcium channel blockers, tricyclic antidepressants (TCAs), selective serotonin reuptake inhibitors (SSRIs), NeRIs(?), and angiotensin receptor blocking agents

---

nausea, vomiting, photophobia or phonophobia. Migraines may occur with or without aura. Migraine with aura is less common. Vision complaints are the most common manifestation of aura, but patients may experience paraesthesia, aphasia, nausea, and vomiting prior to the onset of headache. These findings are completely reversible and precede the headache by no more than 60 minutes.

Migraines seem to have a triggering event that precipitates a sterile inflammatory response around intracranial vessels that is mediated by the trigeminovascular system. Triggering factors may include stress, menses, pregnancy and oral contraceptive pills, infection in the head and neck, trauma or surgery, red wine, aged cheeses, vasodilating medications, strong odours, irregular diet or sleep, and bright sunlight or flickering lights. Recent studies have discovered serotonin receptor subtypes in the central nervous system that play significant roles in the neurological changes and intracranial blood vessel change. Newly available treatments such as sumatriptan target these receptors. Several other neuropeptides have been identified as proinflammatory and are believed to play a significant role in migraine development. It is hoped that further investigation will provide treatment alternatives with fewer side effects.

The treatment of migraine headaches may be approached using several strategies: aborting the attacks at their onset, controlling the pain once it is fully evolved, and reducing the frequency of attacks. Therapies aimed at aborting an attack should be started as soon as the premonitory or warning signs are noted. Abortive therapy has been revolutionized with the introduction of 5-hydroxytryptamine (5-HT) receptor agonists. These include sumatriptan (Imitrex), available in oral, subcutaneous injection or nasal spray forms, naratriptan (Amerge), rizatriptan (Maxalt), and zolmitriptan (Zomig), all of which are available in oral preparations. These medications have allowed the migraine sufferer to treat attacks several times a month quickly and effectively with minimal side effects. Other medications used to abort headaches include ergotamine tartrate administered sublingually, or in combination with caffeine by mouth. Dihydroergotamine 45 is administered in a nasal spray. Butorphanol is a mixed narcotic agonist/antagonist available by nasal spray. It does have potential for abuse and chronic use is contraindicated. Midrin is an orally administered compound of acetaminophen, isometheptene mucate, a sympathomimetic amine, and dichloralphenazone, a mild sedative. It has a low side effect profile and may be used until relief is attained. Many NSAIDs have been shown to be effective in migraine headaches. The short-rise time, short-acting medications such as naproxen, ketorolac, ibuprofen, and choline magnesium trisalicylate have the greatest usefulness. Lidocaine administered intranasally in 4% spray, either singly or in combination with nasal decongestants, has been shown to be effective, although of short duration. Intravenous lidocaine with diphenhydramine may also be effective.

If abortive therapy fails, management should be aimed at reducing the intensity of the pain and controlling associated symptoms such as nausea and vomiting. It is desirable to avoid opiates for the treatment of migraine.

Patients experiencing two or more attacks per month should be started on a prophylactic regimen. Appropriate first steps are to limit the activities or factors that trigger the headaches. This may be effective by itself, but medical prophylaxis is often needed as well. Multiple antidepressant medications have been shown to be effective in the prevention of migraine headache. These include amitriptyline, nortriptyline, doxepin, trazodone, imipramine, and desipramine. The newer SSRIs, including Prozac and Zoloft, have not been shown to be effective in migraine therapy.

Bellergal, a low dose sustained relief ergotamine, may be useful in preventing attacks. NSAIDs have some usefulness in the prevention of attacks as well as the treatment of the acute headache. Beta-blockers, specifically propranolol, nadolol, atenolol, timolol, and pindolol, have been used with some success but are contraindicated in patients with depression, asthma, or diabetes. Calcium channel blockers (verapamil, nifedipine, and nimodipine) have shown some effectiveness in preventing migraine attacks as well.

Fifty-one per cent of migraine sufferers obtained complete prophylaxis for an average of 4.1 months' duration after the injection of botulinum toxin type A (BOTOX) into the facial and scalp musculature. An additional 38% obtained a partial response for an average of 2.7 months. The investigators also reported a 70% complete response rate among patients treated acutely for migraine headache within 1–2 hours post-treatment. These results hold promise for a novel treatment modality for the migraine sufferer.

Needless to say, the treatment of migraine can be a time-consuming and frustrating proposition. Lifestyle changes with the avoidance of the triggering event must be stressed to the patient. Medication changes should be adequately evaluated before dismissed as ineffective, and all medications should be started one at a time at the lowest dose. It is often necessary to combine medications for acute pain or abortive therapy with those used for prophylaxis; however, some interactions do occur and this should be done with caution. The reader is referred to the manufacturers' data regarding recommended dosages, contraindications, and complete list of interactions and side effects for all the medications listed.

Cluster headaches (5%)

Cluster headache (CH) is characterized (Table 22.2) by intensely severe pain (sometimes termed *suicide headache*) with boring or burning qualities located unilaterally in the orbital, supraorbital, or temporal area. Attacks last from 15 to 180 minutes. The headache is associated with at least one symptom of autonomic hyperactivity: conjunctival injection, lacrimation, nasal congestion, rhinorrhoea, forehead and facial sweating, miosis, ptosis, or eyelid oedema. Attacks occur from one to every two days and range up to eight headaches per day. At least five such attacks must occur to meet the diagnostic criteria. Nausea and vomiting is uncommon and there is no aura. Onset is usually in the second to fifth decades. Cluster headache is the

Table 22.2 Characteristics of cluster headaches

Male:female ratio 4:1 to 20:1/30 years +
The onset of pain is sudden
Unilateral orbital, supraorbital or temporal
Severe episodic pain lasting 15–180 minutes
Episodes last 30–180 minutes
Up to eight times a day to every other day for a period of 2–12 weeks
The pain is characterized as severe, boring, and burning
It awakens the patient from sleep and does not improve with rest. Many individuals pace and may injure themselves because of the pain severity
Associated symptoms include ipsilateral conjunctival injection, tearing, and nasal congestion
The male:female ratio is 6:1
Abortive treatment includes oxygen (8–15 l), sumatriptan injections, and/or dihydroergotamine
Preventative treatment includes verapamil, lithium, divalproex sodium, and topiramate (Rozen, 2006)

only headache syndrome with a male preponderance. It is associated with alcohol use and intolerance, and during an active phase or 'cluster', alcohol may precipitate an attack.

There are both episodic and chronic types. Episodic CH has periods of activity alternating with periods of inactivity. Active periods vary in frequency from two or more per year, to one every two or more years, and tend to occur in regular intervals. The duration of active periods ranges from 7 days to a year. In chronic forms, the remission phases last <14 days while the prolonged ones are absent for at least 1 year.

Treatment is aimed at preventing an attack during a cluster. Once an effective therapy is discovered, it is continued for 6–8 weeks and then gradually tapered. Options for treatment include calcium channel blockers (nifedipine, nimodipine, and verapamil), low dose daily ergotamine (Bellergal), and lithium carbonate (especially in chronic forms of CH). Methysergide has been found to be effective but use is limited to 4 months as prolonged continuous use may cause retroperitoneal fibrosis. Trials with valproic acid are ongoing. Some have used antihistamines, both H_1 and H_2, blockers with limited success. The role of steroids is controversial, but they are frequently used in prophylaxis during an active period.

Some treatments have been found to be effective in the acute treatment of an attack. Oxygen inhalation, 6–10 litres per minute administered by face mask, seems to be particularly effective in young patients with attacks primarily at night. 5-HT receptor agonists are effective in shortening an attack if given at the first indication of pain. Intranasal lidocaine (either 4% topical or 2% viscous) administered at the posterior aspect of the inferior turbinate, effecting a sphenopalatine block, may be effective in terminating an acute attack.

Tension-type headaches

Tension-type headache (TTH) is the most common type of headache. It occurs in 69% of men and 88% of women over a lifetime, and the annual prevalence is 63% in men and 88% in women. TTH can be further be distinguished as 'episodic' TTH (ETTH) or 'chronic' TTH (CTTH). The distinction is made largely on frequency of occurrence (<15 days a month for ETTH and >15 days a month for CTTH). The diagnostic criteria that distinguish TTH from other headache syndromes are largely related to the quality, intensity, location, and duration of the pain. Headaches last from 30 minutes to 7 days. They are often described as pressing or tightening (non-pulsating) in quality. The intensity is mild to moderate, and may limit but not prohibit activities. Its location may be bilateral or variable. There is no aggravation with physical activity, nausea and vomiting is rare, and photophobia or phonophobia may occur, though not simultaneously.

Patients who acknowledge the role of stress in the aetiology of their headaches, especially those with ETTH, are frequently well managed by biofeedback and stress reduction techniques. Posture correction and physical exercises should be prescribed as indicated. Patients with bruxism may benefit from a dental splint. For patients with ETTH, medications may be avoided, but when needed, the patient may do well with low dose benzodiazepines or amitriptyline once daily in a short course spanning several weeks. Pharmaceuticals are more likely to be necessary in the patient with CTTH. Abortive medications include aspirin, acetaminophen, aspirin/ caffeine/butalbital or phenacetin combinations or short half-life NSAIDs. Preventive medications include daily antidepressants, muscle relaxants, and long half-life NSAIDs. Opiates and benzodiazepines may be effective, but prolonged use is contraindicated. Daily NSAID use should be limited to less than 1 week. The treatment regimen employed must be individualized based upon the triggering factors elucidated in the history and physical exam findings.

Table 22.3 Characteristics of tension-type headache

Highest socioeconomic impact, affecting 30–78% of the population

At least 10 episodes, occurring less than 1 day a month on average

Infrequent episodes lasting from 30 minutes to 7 days

Typically bilateral

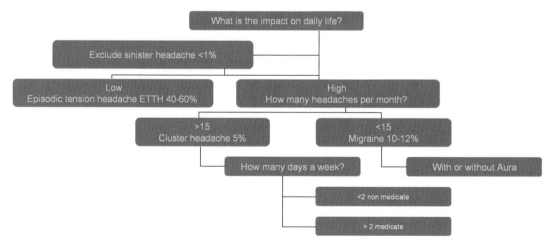

Figure 22.3 A simple algorithm for the differentiation of common causes of headache.

A simple algorithm has been developed, enabling the practitioner to differentiate between the common headache variants (Figure 22.3), and the migraine in primary care (MIPCA) questionnaire provides a useful three-question differential[27].

Jabs and jolts syndrome, primary stabbing headache, or ice-pick headache

♦ Head pain occurs as a single stab or a series of stabs

♦ The pain is exclusive or predominantly felt in the distribution of VI

♦ Stabs last for up to a few seconds and recur with irregular frequency ranging from one to many per day

♦ No other accompanying symptoms are noted, and it cannot be attributed to another disorder

♦ This syndrome is refractory to medical treatment (Pareja, 1996).

Chronic daily headache and medication overuse headaches (30–78%)

Chronic daily headache (CDH) is described as headache occurring at least 6 days a week for a period of at least 6 months. The pain is usually present throughout the day with little time spent pain-free. The head pain is typically bilateral, frontal or occipital, non-throbbing and moderately severe. The syndrome is associated with the overuse and abuse of many common over-the-counter pain medications (aspirin, acetaminophen, ibuprofen, etc.), barbiturates, and opioid analgesics. A careful history will reveal an increasing need for medications and the emergence of a chronic headache that is qualitatively distinct from the headache for which it was originally taken. This led to the idea of CDH being a 'transformed migraine'.

The treatment centres on the withdrawal of the causative medication. To be successful, several points should be followed: these include that the patient must understand the syndrome, the offending medication should be tapered over 10 days and be completely ceased for a minimum of 2 months, the substitution of other agents that may perpetuate the disorder must be avoided (antidepressant medications prescribed at gradually increasing dosages aid in withdrawal of the offending medication), adjuvant therapy such as physical therapy or biofeedback should be employed, and, in refractory cases, consultation with a neurologist with inpatient management may be required to ensure

complete abstinence from the medication and to control withdrawal symptoms.

Withdrawal symptoms may be prominent, usually occurring in the first 4 days, but sometimes occurring up to 3 weeks after cessation of the causative medication. These include nervousness, restlessness, increased headaches, nausea and vomiting, insomnia, diarrhoea, and tremor.

Short-lasting unilateral neuralgia with conjunctival irritation and tearing (SUNCT)

This is possibly a variation of the cluster tic syndrome. It is characterized by brief (15–120 seconds) bursts of pain in the eyes, temple, or face. The pain is usually unilateral and is described as burning, stabbing, or electric. It occurs frequently in a 24-hour period (>100 episodes). Neck movements can trigger the pain[28–30].

SUNCT syndrome is refractory to medical therapy[31] but there is increasing evidence for treatment with lamotrigine[32].

Temporal arteritis

Temporal arteritis is characterized by daily headaches of moderate to severe intensity, scalp sensitivity, fatigue, and various non-specific complaints with a general sense of illness. Ninety-five per cent of patients are over 60 years old. The pain is usually unilateral, although some cases of bilateral or occipital pain do occur. Pain may also be felt in the tongue and is a continuous ache with superimposed sharp, shooting head pains. The pain is similar to and may be confused with that of CH, but CH tends to occur in younger patients. The two may also be distinguished on physical exam, when dilated and tortuous scalp arteries are noted. The erythrocyte sedimentation rate (ESR) is markedly elevated in temporal arteritis[33].

Definitive diagnosis is made by artery biopsy from the region of the pain, although negative biopsy may be caused by the spotty nature of the disease and does rule out the diagnosis. High dose steroid therapy usually precipitates a dramatic decrease in head pain. Failure to respond to steroid therapy with a negative biopsy should call the diagnosis into question. If the diagnosis seems likely based on history and physical examination, steroids should be started immediately to avoid vision loss, the most common complication of the disorder, occurring in 30% of untreated cases. The biopsy remains positive for 7–10 days from starting steroid therapy. Steroids may be tapered to an every other day maintenance schedule when the pain resolves and ESR normalizes. The disease is usually active for 1–2 years, during which time steroids should be continued to prevent vision loss.

Group 2: neuralgia

This group includes trigeminal neuralgia (typical or atypical), postherpetic neuralgia, glossopharyngeal neuralgia, post-traumatic V neuralgia, and other peripheral neuropathies affecting the trigeminal system (diabetes mellitus, human immunodeficiency virus (HIV), chemotherapy, and multiple sclerosis (MS)).

Trigeminal neuralgia (typical or atypical)

Typical trigeminal neuralgia is characterized by severe bursts of lancinating pain in one or more branches of the trigeminal nerve. Bursts are quick, repetitive, electric shock-like sensations with paroxysmal pain attacks lasting from a few seconds to less than 2 minutes. The pain is severe and distributed along one or more of the branches of the trigeminal nerve with a sudden, sharp, intense stabbing or burning quality. Between attacks the patient is completely asymptomatic without gross neurological defects. The pain may be precipitated from trigger areas or with certain daily activities such as eating, talking, washing the face or brushing the teeth. Attacks are the same in an individual patient. If there is no specific trigger zone or the pain lasts longer than seconds, then atypical trigeminal neuralgia may be diagnosed. Structural causes of facial pain should be excluded. The syndrome is most common in patients over 50 years. The course may fluctuate over many years, and remissions of months or years are not uncommon[34,35].

Aetiology

The cause in 60–88% of cases is vascular compression of the trigeminal ganglion leading to demyelination and hence 'short-circuiting' of A-b fibres with A-d and C-fibres. In a smaller group of patients, trigeminal neuralgia is symptomatic due to tumours, arteriovenous malformations (A-V) and MS. Recently, international guidelines on trigeminal neuralgia have been published[34,35].

Features

The presence of trigeminal sensory deficits, bilateral involvement, and abnormal trigeminal reflexes may indicate the presence of symptomatic trigeminal neuralgia due to tumours, A-V malformations and MS. Younger age of onset, involvement of the first division, and unresponsiveness to treatment do not correlate consistently with symptomatic trigeminal neuralgia. Abnormal trigeminal reflexes are associated with an increased risk of symptomatic trigeminal neuralgia and should be considered useful in distinguishing symptomatic trigeminal neuralgia from classic trigeminal neuralgia. Routine head imaging identifies structural causes in up to 15% of patients.

Treatment

The first-line treatments of choice are anticonvulsant medication. Carbamazepine remains the gold standard drug but there is now evidence that oxcarbazepine is equally effective and has improved tolerability, although full randomized controlled trials (RCT) have not been published. Baclofen and lamotrigine may be considered useful. More recently, a RCT using Consolidated Standards of Reporting Trials (CONSORT) guidelines reported that gabapentin, together with weekly injections of ropivacain into the trigger area number, yielded a number needed to treat of 2.4 (50% reduction of pain) at 4 weeks[36]. There is only limited data to help patients decide when to have surgery but often the factors used are refractoriness to medical therapy and loss of tolerability. Surgery such as microvascular decompression or radiofrequency gangliolysis offer good results although there is associated long-term morbidity of facial paraesthesia that can be a major complaint among patients.

A wide variety of surgical techniques are available. Gasserian ganglion percutaneous techniques, gamma knife, and microvascular decompression are all options. Microvascular decompression may be considered over other surgical techniques to provide the longest duration of pain freedom, but it is the most invasive procedure. Results from gamma knife therapy, although non-invasive, show nerve damage, and sensory loss can sometimes develop 6 months after the procedure has been performed. It can be bothersome in 5% of patients and there are patients who have developed anaesthesia dolorosa[37]. The role of surgery versus pharmacotherapy in the management of trigeminal neuralgia in patients with MS remains uncertain.

A decision analysis study done with 156 patients with trigeminal neuralgia showed that surgical techniques narrowly offer the highest chance of maximizing patient quality of life. However, surgery is not right for everyone, and patients should be informed about their full range of choices[38]. Patients are keen to remain informed about trigeminal neuralgia as shown by their attendance at conferences[39] and the demand for specific printed patient-orientated information[40,41].

Postherpetic neuralgia

In patients over 50 years of age there is a 60% incidence of developing postherpetic pain[42]. Herpetic skin eruption is caused by the reactivation of latent varicella zoster virus from the sensory nerve ganglia. The reactivated virus is carried via the axons distally to the skin where it produces a painful rash with crusting vesicles in a dermatomal distribution. The trigeminal nerve is the second most commonly affected after nerves in the thoracic region. Ramsay Hunt syndrome occurs when herpes zoster infection of the geniculate ganglion causes earache and facial palsy.

Pain that persists 2 or more months after the acute eruption is known as postherpetic neuralgia. The pain is neuropathic in nature, severe, and it is associated with allodynia and hyperalgesia, most commonly affecting the I distribution of the trigeminal nerve[43]. High doses of antivirals, steroids, and amitriptyline are often used for the acute eruption in otherwise healthy individuals. Antivirals, NSAIDs, and opiates are often used in immunocompromised patients. More recently, there is evidence that topical 5% lidocaine patches (Versatis) worn alternatively every 12 hours are very effective[44].

Glossopharyngeal neuralgia

Glossopharyngeal neuralgia is characterized by pain attacks similar to those in trigeminal neuralgia, but is located unilaterally in the distribution of the glossopharyngeal nerve. Pain is most common in the posterior pharynx, soft palate, base of tongue, ear, mastoid or side of the head. Swallowing, yawning, coughing or phonation may trigger the pain. Management is similar to that for trigeminal neuralgia[45].

Post-traumatic trigeminal neuopathic pain

Traumatic injuries to the lingual and inferior alveolar nerves may induce a pain syndrome owing to the development of a neuroma. The diagnosis of post-traumatic neuopathic pain is based upon a history of surgery or trauma temporally correlated with the development of the characteristic neuritic pain. Age, poor wound closure, infections, foreign material in the wound, haematoma, skull fracture, diabetes mellitus or peripheral neuropathy elsewhere in the body predispose to neuroma development. The pains commonly persist 2–6 months after the injury and can be permanent[46,47]. Medical therapy is similar to that used in neuropathic pain conditions depending on the patients' symptoms. In a recent survey of 220 iatrogenic trigeminal nerve injuries related to dental treatment, 95% of patients presented with pain. This highlights the problems related to postsurgical neuropathy aggravated by the fact that many patients may not have been warned at all about nerve injury or told that they would risk numbness[48].

Group 3: idiopathic

This group includes preauricular pain related to the TMJ, burning mouth syndrome (BMS), and persistent idiopathic facial pain.

Temporomandibular disorders (TMD)

TMD pain is characterized by focal tenderness to one or both TMJs and is usually aggravated by chewing, talking, and jaw movement. The quality of the pain is similar to that of persistent idiopathic facial pain (PIFP); that is, dull, aching, crushing, or burning. The treatment for temporomandibular disorder (TMD) is often directed either at the articular joint itself or at fatigue of the temporalis muscles. There are three main categories of temporomandibular-related pain: myogenic or functional, arthritides, and derangement.

TMDs include a heterogeneous group of processes, all with a similar clinical presentation. Common symptoms of TMD include temporal headache, earache, facial pain, limited jaw opening or joint noise. The majority of TMDs originate spontaneously, with only 40% able to recall a specific event, usually trauma, preceding the onset of pain. This suggests that there is a significant role of emotional and psychological factors in the aetiology of spontaneously occurring TMD[49]. As a result of relatively recent advances in the understanding of the pathogenesis of TMD, they may be further classified as internal derangements, degenerative joint disease (DJD), and myofascial pain[50,51].

The Nuprin Pain Report showed that the major health complaint in the USA was pain (88%)[52]. In the same US population, recurrent or persistent orofacial pain, excluding 'toothache', has been estimated to occur in 6–12% of people, with a similar figure of 5% of the population in the Netherlands. The variability in the US figures is probably related to the respective investigators adopting different diagnostic criteria in achieving a firm diagnosis of TMD[53]. Other names ascribed to this condition include: Costen's syndrome, temporomandibular joint dysfunction, and craniomandibular disorder. TMD is characterized by a complex of signs and symptoms, with orofacial pain as a main symptom.

TMD is the most common orofacial pain disorder but its prevalence varies between studies owing to age-related differences in the groups analysed[54]. One survey reported the prevalence of TMD symptoms or signs in 70–80% of young adults. TMD is commoner in women in the 18–35-year age group. In this group, TMD is usually of limited duration (days to weeks) and it is often recurrent because 'stress' is a prime causal factor. Nearly 2% of the population seeks treatment for their symptoms. However, it should be noted that TMD occurs in another targeted age group (45–60 years); patients referred to a medical multidisciplinary pain centre reported chronic 'persistent' pain, in contrast to 'recurrent' pain[55,56]. No definitive reason has been established for 'persistent' pain, although there is compelling evidence to indicate that one cause is muscle spasm secondary to neuropathic orofacial pain, and thus, the consequent development of a TMD[57,58].

Pain that truly originates in the TMJ is rare and is characterized by tenderness to palpation of the condyle and pain with joint movement. Internal derangements are characterized by anterior and medial displacement of the articular disk. This produces a 'click' as the disk is suddenly reduced within the joint during mouth opening or closing. This clicking may be benign, with minimal clinical symptoms or discomfort. When symptomatic, pain occurs just before or during the click and the joint is mildly tender to palpation. Patients may have limited mouth opening as a result of attempts to avoid pain. TMD dysfunction or derangement has a similar presentation, with pain at joint movement and crepitus over the joint. The painful stage usually lasts less than 1 year[59]. Long-standing DJD causes flattening of the condyle and osteophyte formation, making it easily recognizable radiographically. The vast majority of patients (60–70%) have combined muscle and joint pain, with muscle pain dominating the clinical picture[60]. These patients usually have tenderness to palpation of the muscles of mastication.

Diagnosis

Many patients with orofacial pain expect to have imaging studies done and yet this can result in more problems. Wiese et al.[61], in a very carefully controlled study on patients with TMD, showed that degenerative changes of the TMJ were not correlated to pain but rather to increasing age, female gender, and coarse crepitus in all movements of the TMJ[28].

A variety of psychological questionnaires have been used to assess the psychosocial profile of patients with TMD. Although patients with joint pain had more impairment of jaw function, no significant differences in depression, in somatization or psychological factors were noted. Given that psychosocial profiles do not relate to the type of TMD pain, the use of psychological interventions cannot be based on site of pain[62].

Treatment

From a meta-analysis of the literature, it has been estimated that 15% of those with TMD may require some form of treatment[63]. Only those patients who have moderate or severe signs and symptoms of TMD and seek help should be actively managed. The rest can be reassured. Biopsychosocial treatment instituted early in those patients predicted to become chronic sufferers is both symptomatically and economically effective[64]. Self-care has always been important in managing TMD[65]. Mulet et al.[64], in a RCT, showed that self-care, supplemented by Rocabado's exercises, did not improve outcomes; both groups thus benefited potentially.

The European Academy of Craniomandibular Disorders has published guidelines on TMD management for dentists[12], stressing the importance of providing adequate information and counselling. Despite a lack of robust data, they are, however, advocates of the early use of occlusal splints. Although still in common use, there is no evidence to support irreversible occlusal rehabilitation. There is limited evidence that physiotherapy may be beneficial. Dentists have been warned against the use of prosthetic reconstructions or orthodontic treatments as a means of preventing or treating TMD[66]. The tension suppression system (NTI-tss) device is an anterior bite stop which has been proposed as a useful device in patients with TMD. A recent systematic review suggests it may be useful in some patients who are bruxists, clenchers, and for acute cases of TMD, but patients need to be compliant[67].

There are numerous studies on the effect of low-level laser therapy in the treatment of TMD. The study designs have been of poor quality, not RCTs and they do not comply with CONSORT guidelines. One recent study of good quality concluded that there is currently insufficient evidence for the use of low-level laser therapy in pain relief of TMD[68].

A recent small RCT study shows that acupuncture can be effective in TMD but only in the 7 days post-therapy[69]. A RCT pilot study of traditional Chinese medicine and naturopathic medicine comparing specialty care in 160 women suggests that there may be some evidence for its efficacy when compared to self-care.

NSAIDs and physical therapy are the mainstays of treatment for TMD. Similar to tension headache, biofeedback and trigger point injection may be beneficial. Benzodiazepines are useful for muscle pain, but chronic use may lead to dependence and tolerance. Muscle relaxants are of little benefit. In chronic muscle pain, antidepressants may be more useful than analgesics or anxiolytics. Tricyclic antidepressants (TCA) are useful in those patients with sleep disturbance,[70] or SSRIs may be used for patients intolerant of TCA. To date, there is no evidence for occlusal adjustment, bite guards or surgical intervention for treating TMDs. There are four Cochrane reviews highlighting the insufficient evidence for management of TMDs[71–75]. Bessa – Norgueira et al [75] have also assessed these systematic reviews from a methodological standpoint.

Burning mouth syndrome

Burning mouth syndrome (BMS), glossodynia or stomatodynia is defined as a chronic, idiopathic oral mucosal pain or discomfort in which no clinical lesions or systemic disease are identified[76]. Clinical evidence (clinicalevidence.bmj.com) maintains a regularly updated article on management of BMS and there is also a Cochrane Systematic Review on this topic[77].

There is a predilection for the condition for women in the menopausal to postmenopausal age group. The prevalence varies from 0.5 to 15% in this targeted group. Afflicted patients report a constant burning sensation. The preferred site for the pain is the anterior portion of the tongue, although the anterior portion of the hard palate and the labial mucosa of the lip region are other common sites of pain.

There are increasing numbers of studies to suggest that this condition is not caused by psychological factors alone but may be a form of neuropathic pain which then results in psychological effects. Studies have noted that not only do patients have a sensation of burring in their mouths but there are often changes in taste and salivation. Eliav et al.[78], using patients with BMS and controls with a symptom of burning mouth which could be attributed to other causes, showed that BMS showed dysfunction of their chorda tympani and therefore this could account for these abnormal taste

sensations as well as tingling sensations. Of the RCTs it would appear that clonazepam used topically may be helpful as well as cognitive behaviour therapy[76]. In the last 2 years a well designed RCT reporting under CONSORT methodology showed that *Hypericum perforatum* (a form of St John's wort) did not result in a positive response[79]. There is increasing evidence that BMS is caused by a peripheral neuropathy[80], the cause of which remains unknown.

Persistent idiopathic facial pain (PIFP)

The term atypical facial pain was first introduced by Frazier and Russell in 1924. It has since been renamed persistent idiopathic facial pain (PIFP). PIFP refers to pain along the territory of the trigeminal nerve that does not fit the classic presentation of other cranial neuralgias[12]. The duration of pain is usually long, lasting most of the day (if not continuous). Pain is unilateral and without autonomic signs or symptoms. It is described as a severe ache, crushing or burning sensation. Upon examination and workup no abnormality is noted.

Definition

According to the International Association for the Study of Pain (IASP), chronic facial pain refers to symptoms which have been present for at least 6 months. 'Atypical' pain is a diagnosis of exclusion after other conditions have been considered and eliminated (i.e. it is idiopathic), and is characterized by chronic, constant pain in the absence of any apparent cause in the face or brain. Many information sources suggest that all 'unexplained' facial pains are termed atypical facial pain but this is not the case. Categories of idiopathic facial pain conditions include neuropathic pain due to sensory nerve damage, chronic regional pain syndrome (CRPS) from sympathetic nerve damage and atypical facial pain[81].

Atypical odontalgia, or phantom tooth pain, is a variation of atypical facial pain where intense discomfort is centred around a tooth or group of teeth with no obvious dental or oral disease.

Epidemiology

PIFP is more common in women than in men; most patients attending a facial pain clinic are women aged between 30 and 50 years. Although any area of the face can be involved, the most commonly affected area is the maxillary region. In the majority of patients there is no disease or other cause found. In a few patients the symptoms represent serious disease.

In a small number of patients the pain may be one consequence of significant psychological or psychiatric disease[82].

Clinical presentation

PIFP has a very variable presentation. Often it is characterized by continuous, daily pain of variable intensity. Typically, the pain is deep and poorly localized, is described as dull and aching, and does not waken the patient from sleep. At onset the pain may be confined to a limited area on one side of the face, while later it may spread to involve a larger area. PIFP is a diagnosis of exclusion for pain not meeting the diagnostic criteria of other facial pain syndromes. Mongini et al[50] refers to the term atypical facial pain as outdated and includes its description in psychogenic facial pain. Indeed, the description of the pain may be inconsistent with bilateral pain that often changes locations over weeks to months. The pain is not triggered and is not electrical in quality. Intensity fluctuates but the patient is rarely pain-free. Pain is typically located in the face and seldom spreads to the cranium in contradistinction to tension headache[9,83]. It is more common in women aged 30–50 years old. Between 60 and 70% of these patients have significant psychiatric findings, usually depression, somatization or adjustment disorders, therefore psychiatric evaluation is indicated. Treatment is with antidepressants, beginning with low dose amitriptyline at bedtime and increasing the dose until pain and sleep are improved[84].

Accurate figures are difficult to obtain because of the lack of agreement on classification criteria[12]. Estimated incidence is 1 case per 100 000 population, although this number may be underestimated[82]. PIFP affects both sexes approximately equally, but more women than men seek medical care[82]. The disorder mainly affects adults and is rare in children[82].

PIFP is essentially a diagnosis of exclusion. Daily or near-daily headaches are a widespread problem in clinical practice[82]. According to population-based data from the United States, Europe, and Asia, chronic daily headache affects a large number (approximately 4–5% of the population) of patients[12].

Importantly, PIFP must be distinguished from various other chronic daily headache syndromes, including hemicrania continua[84], TMD, migraine, chronic cluster headache, SUNCT, TN, and many others[12]. A careful history and physical examination, including a dental consultation, laboratory studies, and imaging studies, may be necessary to rule out occult pathology. Underlying pathology such as malignancy, vasculitis, infection, and central or peripheral demyelination may manifest early as neuralgia, and, not until focal neurological deficits, imaging abnormalities, or laboratory abnormalities are discovered, does the diagnosis become evident. Rare cases of referred pain must also be considered.

Atypical odontalgia (AO) is characterized by continuous, dull, aching, or burning pain of moderate intensity in apparently normal teeth or endodontically treated teeth and occasionally in extraction sites. AO is not usually affected by testing the tooth and surrounding tissues with cold, heat or electrical stimuli. The pain remains constant despite repeated dental treatment, even extractions in the region, often rendering patients with persistent pain but whole quadrants stripped of dentition. Moreover, the toothache characteristics frequently remain unchanged for months or years, contributing to the differentiation of AO from pulpal dental pain. Occasionally, the pain may spread to adjacent teeth, especially after extraction of the painful tooth. These patients are defined as having pain in a tooth or tooth region in which no clinical or radiological findings can be detected.

Several studies have been conducted to define this group more clearly. AO patients have more comorbid pain conditions, higher scores for depression and somatization, significant limitation in jaw function, and lower scores on quality of life measures when compared with controls[85]. When compared to patients with TMD, AO patients were more likely to describe their pain as aching, find rest relieving but cold and heat aggravating. Over 80% relate the onset of their pain to dental treatment. Both groups show worsening of symptoms on chewing, but more patients with TMD have other chronic pain[86]. These patients have somatosensory abnormalities, suggesting that generalized sensitization of the nociceptive mechanism may be occurring[87]. The relationship with previous surgical intervention infers that this condition may, in some cases, be partial postsurgical neuropathy of the superior alveolar nerves.

The lack of RCTs makes evidenced-based care in AO difficult[88]. One of the major problems with this condition is convincing the patient, and informing their dentist, that there are no dental causes for their pain, so avoiding unnecessary irreversible invasive dental treatment. AO patients are often diagnosed late[87] and therefore need a multidisciplinary approach. In her recent review, Baad-Hansen[88] presents a sensible progressive approach to managing AO, beginning with topical lidocaine or capscasian, then TCAs. Penultimately, the drugs used in neuropathic pain are gabapaentin and pregablin, and finally tramadol or oxycodone.

Medical care

Medical treatment of PIFP is usually less satisfactory than medical treatment for other facial pain syndromes[88,89]. Medications used to treat PIFP include antidepressants, anticonvulsants, substance P depletion agents, topical anaesthetics, N-methyl-D-aspartate (NMDA) antagonists, and opiate medications. Of these classes of medications, anticonvulsants and antidepressants appear to be the most effective. The neuropathic component of pain responds well to anticonvulsants and antidepressants. Pharmacotherapeutic knowledge is paramount in the treatment of this refractory pain syndrome. A multimechanistic approach, using modulation of both ascending and descending pain pathways, is frequently necessary. The goal of therapy is to manage the pain effectively with the fewest adverse medication effects. Anticonvulsants and antidepressants are the mainstays of medication treatment. Alternative therapies such as acupuncture and neuromuscular re-education have been tried and should be considered as part of a comprehensive treatment plan. Psychiatric treatment is important in the overall management of a patient with chronic pain. A holistic approach as for many other chronic pains is needed. Available data on alternative treatments are limited.

Surgical care

Details of neurosurgical interventions are beyond the scope of this review. Analgesic surgery should be considered at a centre well versed in these procedures[88,90].

Consultations

Psychometric testing may be of benefit in the evaluation and treatment of patients with headache and facial pain. Many tests have been applied, but probably the most widely used is the Minnesota multiple personality inventory (MMPI). While especially useful in the evaluation of chronic headache and facial pain patients, a thorough discussion of psychometric testing is beyond the scope of this discussion and is mentioned here only for completeness. Consultation with a dentist may be of benefit. All treatments should be provided in cooperation with the patient's primary care physician.

Future novel treatments in development include several phase three trials assessing specific pain receptor and channel blocking agents for neuropathic pain. Several studies have reported upregulation of peripheral TRPV receptor and sodium channel receptor expression in the human trigeminal system[91,92].

Recent recognition of genetic factors contributing to nociception, pain behaviour, and suffering may also lay the foundations for future strategies for improved treatment of patients with chronic pain. Of the 3.16 billion base pairs comprising the 23 pairs of chromosomes, the Human Genome Project has sequenced about 2.8 billion base pairs to date. Only 3% of the human genome actually codes for proteins, and about 15% of the non-coding DNA in humans is conserved (has functional importance). It is estimated that there are approximately 25 000 genes in the human genome and it is as yet unknown how many genes are involved in pain mediation, perception, and behavioural response. To date, gene coding for TRPV1 channel is associated with altered pain responses[93], and sodium ion channels coded by an SCN9A mutation was found in a Pakistani family with an inability to experience pain[94]. Catechol-O-methyltransferase and the cytochrome P450 variant allele *CYP3A5* have been linked with pain behaviour attributed to dopamine metabolism which defined how patients coped with their pain experience[95].

The ability to evaluate the phenotype and genotype of the patient with pain may enable to clinician to provide specific and tailor-made treatment in the future.

Conclusion

Chronic orofacial pain continues to present a diagnostic challenge for many practitioners. Patients are frequently misdiagnosed and they suffer from psychiatric symptoms of depression and anxiety. Treatment is less effective than in other pain syndromes and a multidisciplinary approach treatment is desirable.

References

1. Madland G, Feinmann C. (2000) Chronic facial pain: a multidisciplinary problem. *J Neurol Neurosurg Psychiatry*, **71(6)**, 716–19.
2. Okeson JP. (2008) The classification of orofacial pains. *Oral Maxillofac Surg Clin North Am*, **20(2)**, 133–44.
3. Hapak L, Gordon A, Locker D, Shandling M, Mock D, Tenenbaum HC. (1994) Differentiation between musculoligamentous, dentoalveolar, and neurologically based craniofacial pain with a diagnostic questionnaire. *J Orofac Pain*, **8(4)**, 357–68.

4. Lipton JA, Ship JA, Larach-Robinson D. (1993) Estimated prevalence and distribution of reported orofacial pain in the United States. *J Am Dent Assoc*, **124(10)**, 115–21.

5. Riley JL 3rd, Gilbert GH. (2001) Orofacial pain symptoms: an interaction between age and sex. *Pain*, **90(3)**, 245–56.

6. Locker D, Grushka M. (1987) The impact of dental and facial pain. *J Dent Res*, **66**, 1414–17.

7. Bonica JJ. (1980) Pain: introduction. *Res Pub Assoc Res Nerv Ment Dis*, **58**, 1–17.

8. Von Korff M, Simon G. (1996) The relationship between pain and depression. *Br J Psych*, Suppl. 30, 101–8.

9. Aggarwal VR, McBeth J, Zakrzewska JM, Macfarlane GJ. (2008) Unexplained orofacial pain—is an early diagnosis possible? *Br Dent J*, **205(3)**, E6–1.

10. Dao TT, LeResche L. (2000) Gender differences in pain. *J Orofac Pain*, **14(3)**, 169–84; discussion 184–95.

11. Aggarwal VR, McBeth J, Lunt M, Zakrzewska JM, Macfarlane GJ. (2007) Development and validation of classification criteria for idiopathic orofacial pain for use in population-based studies. *J Orofac Pain*, **21(3)**, 203–15.

12. Benoliel R, Birman N, Eliav E, Sharav Y. (2008) The International Classification of Headache Disorders: accurate diagnosis of orofacial pain? *Cephalalgia*, **28(7)**, 752–62.

13. Zebenholzer K, Wober C, Vigl M, Wessely P, Wober-Bingol C. (2006) Facial pain and the second edition of the international classification of headache disorders. *Headache*, **46(2)**, 259–63.

14. Türp JC, Hugger A, Nilges P *et al.* (2006). Schmerz. International Association for the Study of Pain (IASP) Recommendations for the standardized evaluation and classification of painful temporomandibular disorders: an update. *International Association for the Study of Pain (IASP)* **20(6)**, 481–9.

15. De Boever JA, Nilner M, Orthlieb JD, Steenks MH. (2008) Recommendations by the EACD for examination, diagnosis, and management of patients with temporomandibular disorders and orofacial pain by the general dental practitioner. *J Orofac Pain*, **22(3)**, 268–78.

16. Aggarwal VR, McBeth J, Zakrzewska JM, Lunt M, Macfarlane GJ. (2008) Are reports of mechanical dysfunction in chronic oro-facial pain related to somatisation? A population based study. *Eur J Pain*, **12(4)**, 501–7.

17. Bertoli E, de Leeuw R, Schmidt JE, Okeson JP, Carlson CR. (2007) Prevalence and impact of post-traumatic stress disorder symptoms in patients with masticatory muscle or temporomandibular joint pain: differences and similarities. *J Orofac Pain*, **21(2)**, 107–19.

18. Dworkin SF, Burgess JA. (1987) Orofacial pain of psychogenic origin: current concepts and classification. *J Am Dent Assoc*, **115(4)**, 565–71.

19. Wong MC, McMillan AS, Zheng J, Lam CL. (2008) The consequences of orofacial pain symptoms: a population-based study in Hong Kong. *Community Dent Oral Epidemiol*, **36(5)**, 417–24.

20. John MT, Reissmann DR, Schierz O, Allen F. (2008) No significant retest effects in oral health-related quality of life assessment using the Oral Health Impact Profile. *Acta Odontol Scand*, **66(3)**, 135–8.

21. Wolf E, Birgerstam P, Nilner M, Petersson K. (2008) Nonspecific chronic orofacial pain: studying patient experiences and perspectives with a qualitative approach. *J Orofac Pain*, **22(4)**, 349–58.

22. Renton T. (2008) An update on pain. *Br Dent J*, **204(6)**, 335–8.

23. Woda A, Tubert-Jeannin S, Bouhassira D *et al.* (2005) Towards a new taxonomy of idiopathic orofacial pain. *Pain*, **116(3)**, 396–406.

24. Dieleman JP, Kerklaan J, Huygen FJ, Bouma PA, Sturkenboom MC. (2008) Incidence rates and treatment of neuropathic pain conditions in the general population. *Pain*, **137(3)**, 681–8.

25. Hall GC, Carroll D, Parry D, McQuay HJ. (2006) Epidemiology and treatment of neuropathic pain: The UK primary care perspective. *Pain*, **122(1-2)**, 156–62.

26. Schwaiger J, Kiechl S, Seppi K *et al.* (2009) Prevalence of primary headaches and cranial neuralgias in men and women aged 55–94 years (Bruneck Study). *Cephalalgia*, **29 (2)**, 179–87.

27. Dowson AJ, Lipscombe S, Sender J, Rees T, Watson D. (2008) New guidelines for the management of migraine in primary care. MIPCA Migraine Guidelines Development Group. Migraine In Primary Care Advisors. *Curr Med Res Opin*, **18(7)**, 414–39.

28. Titlic M, Jukic I, Tonkic A *et al.* (2008) Lamotrigine in the treatment of pain syndromes and neuropathic pain. *Bratisl Lek Listy*, **109(9)**, 421–4.

29. Williams MH, Broadley SA. (2008) SUNCT and SUNA: clinical features and medical treatment. *J Clin Neurosci*, **15(5)**, 526–34. Epub 2008 Mar 5.

30. Lenaerts ME. (2008) Update on the therapy of the trigeminal autonomic cephalalgias. *Curr Treat Options Neurol*, **10(1)**, 30–5.

31. Pareja JA, Kruszewski P, Sjaastad O. (1997) SUNCT syndrome. Diagnosis morbi. Shortlasting unilateral neuraligiform headache attacks, with conjunctival injection, tearing and rhinorrhoea. *Neurologia Suppl*, **5**, 66–72.

32. Balasubramaniam R, Klasser GD, Delcanho R. (2008) Trigeminal autonomic cephalalgias: a review and implications for dentistry. *J Am Dent Assoc*, **139(12)**, 1616–24.

33. Affolter B, Thalhammer C, Aschwanden M, Glatz K, Tyndall A, Daikeler T. (2009) Difficult diagnosis and assessment of disease activity in giant cell arteritis: a report on two patients. *Scand J Rheumatol*, **5**, 1–2.

34. Cruccu G, Gronseth G, Alksne J *et al.* (2008) American Academy of Neurology Society; European Federation of Neurological Society. AAN-EFNS guidelines on trigeminal neuralgia management. *Eur J Neurol*, **15(10)**, 1013–28.

35. Gronseth G, Cruccu G, Alksne JI *et al.* (2008) Practice parameter: the diagnostic evaluation and treatment of trigeminal neuralgia (an evidence-based review): report of the Quality Standards Subcommittee of the American Academy of Neurology and the European Federation of Neurological Societies. *Neurology*, **71(15)**, 1183–90.

36. Lemos L, Flores S, Oliveira P, Almeida A. (2008) Gabapentin supplemented with ropivacain block of trigger points improves pain control and quality of life in trigeminal neuralgia patients when compared with gabapentin alone. *Clin J Pain*, **24(1)**, 64–75.

37. Little AS, Shetter AG, Shetter ME, Bay C, Rogers CL. (2008) Long-term pain response and quality of life in patients with typical trigeminal neuralgia treated with gamma knife stereotactic radiosurgery. *Neurosurgery*, **63(5)**, 915–23.

38. Spatz AL, Zakrzewska JM, Kay EJ. (2007) Decision analysis of medical and surgical treatments for trigeminal neuralgia: how patient evaluations of benefits and risks affect the utility of treatment decisions. *Pain*, **131(3)**, 302–10.

39. Zakrzewska JM, Jorns TP, Spatz A. (2009) Patient led conferences—who attends, are their expectations met and do they vary in three different countries? *Eur J Pain*, **13(5)**, 486–91. Epub 2008 Jul 24.

40. Zakrzewska JM. (2006) *Insights: facts and stories behind trigeminal neuralgia*. Gainesville: Trigeminal Neuralgia Association.

41. Zakrzewska JM, Linskey ME. (2009) Trigeminal neuralgia. *Clin Evid*. Available online: http://clinicalevidence.bmj.com (accessed 12 March, pii, 1207)

42. Closmann JJ, Fielding CG, Pogrel MA. (2008) Prevention and management of trigeminal herpes zoster and postherpetic neuralgia. *Gen Dent*, **56(6)**, 563–6; quiz 567–8, 591–2.

43. Volpi A. (2007) Severe complications of herpes zoster. *Herpes* (Suppl), **2**, 35–9.

44. Baron R, Mayoral V, Leijon G *et al.* (2009) Efficacy and safety of 5% lidocaine (lignocaine) medicated plaster in comparison with pregabalin in patients with postherpetic neuralgia and diabetic polyneuropathy: interim analysis from an open-label, two-stage adaptive, randomized, controlled trial. *Clin Drug Investig*, **29(4)**, 231–41.

45. Teixeira MJ, de Siqueira SR, Bor-Seng-Shu E. (2008) Glossopharyngeal neuralgia: neurosurgical treatment and differential diagnosis. *Acta Neurochir (Wien)*, **150(5)**, 471–5; discussion 475. Epub 2008 Feb 4.

46. Benoliel R, Eliav E. (2008) Neuropathic orofacial pain. *Oral Maxillofac Surg Clin North Am*, **20(2)**, 237–54, vii.

47. Hillerup S. (2008) Iatrogenic injury to the inferior alveolar nerve: etiology, signs and symptoms, and observations on recovery. *Int J Oral Maxillofac Surg*, **37(8)**, 704–9. Epub 2008 May 23.

48. Renton T, Thexton A, Crean SJ, Hankins M. (2006) Simplifying the assessment of the recovery from surgical injury to the lingual nerve. *Br Dent J*, **200(10)**, 569–73.

49. Afari N, Wen Y, Buchwald D, Goldberg J, Plesh O. (2008) Are post-traumatic stress disorder symptoms and temporomandibular pain associated? Findings from a community-based twin registry. *J Orofac Pain*, **22(1)**, 41–9.

50. Mongini F, Ciccone G, Ceccarelli M, Baldi I, Ferrero L. (2007) Muscle tenderness in different types of facial pain and its relation to anxiety and depression: A cross-sectional study on 649 patients. *Pain*, **131(1–2)**, 106–11.

51. Von KM, Dunn KM. (2008) Chronic pain reconsidered. *Pain*, **138(2)**, 267–76.

52. Isong U, Gansky SA, Plesh O. (2008) Temporomandibular joint and muscle disorder-type pain in U.S. adults: the National Health Interview Survey. *J Orofac Pain*, **22(4)**, 317–22.

53. Nilsson IM, List T, Drangsholt M. (2007) Incidence and temporal patterns of temporomandibular disorder pain among Swedish adolescents. *J Orofac Pain*, **21(2)**, 127–32.

54. LeResche L, Mancl LA, Drangsholt MT, Huang G, Von KM. (2007) Predictors of onset of facial pain and temporomandibular disorders in early adolescence. *Pain*, **129(3)**, 269–78.

55. Glaros AG, Urban D, Locke J. (2007) Headache and temporomandibular disorders: evidence for diagnostic and behavioural overlap. *Cephalalgia*, **27(6)**, 542–9.

56. Balasubramaniam R, de LR, Zhu H, Nickerson RB, Okeson JP, Carlson CR. (2007) Prevalence of temporomandibular disorders in fibromyalgia and failed back syndrome patients: a blinded prospective comparison study. *Oral Surg Oral Med Oral Pathol Oral Radiol Endod*, **104(2)**, 204–16.

57. Wiesinger B, Malker H, Englund E, Wanman A. (2007) Back pain in relation to musculoskeletal disorders in the jaw-face: a matched case-control study. *Pain*, **131(3)**, 311–19.

58. Svensson P, Jadidi F, Arima T, Baad-Hansen L, Sessle BJ. (2008) Relationships between craniofacial pain and bruxism. *J Oral Rehabil*, **35(7)**, 524–47.

59. Glaros AG, Williams K, Lausten L. (2008) Diurnal variation in pain reports in temporomandibular disorder patients and control subjects. *J Orofac Pain*, **22(2)**, 115–21.

60. Glaros AG, Owais Z, Lausten L. (2007) Reduction in parafunctional activity: a potential mechanism for the effectiveness of splint therapy. *J Oral Rehabil*, **34(2)**, 97–104.

61. Wiese M, Svensson P, Bakke M *et al.* (2008) Association between temporomandibular joint symptoms, signs, and clinical diagnosis using the RDC/TMD and radiographic findings in temporomandibular joint tomograms. *J Orofac Pain*, **22(3)**, 239–51.

62. Reissmann DR, John MT, Wassell RW, Hinz A. (2008) Psychosocial profiles of diagnostic subgroups of temporomandibular disorder patients. *Eur J Oral Sci*, **116(3)**, 237–44.

63. Al-Jundi MA, John MT, Setz JM, Szentpetery A, Kuss O. (2008) Meta-analysis of treatment need for temporomandibular disorders in adult nonpatients. *J Orofac Pain*, **22(2)**, 97–107.

64. Stowell AW, Gatchel RJ, Wildenstein L. (2007) Cost-effectiveness of treatments for temporomandibular disorders: biopsychosocial intervention versus treatment as usual. *J Am Dent Assoc*, **138(2)**, 202–8.

65. Riley JL III, Myers CD, Currie TP *et al.* (2007) Self-care behaviors associated with myofascial temporomandibular disorder pain. *J Orofac Pain*, **21(3)**, 194–202.

66. Mulet M, Decker KL, Look JO, Lenton PA, Schiffman EL. (2007) A randomized clinical trial assessing the efficacy of

adding 6 × 6 exercises to self-care for the treatment of masticatory myofascial pain. *J Orofac Pain*, **21(4)**, 318–28.

67. Stapelmann H, Turp JC. (2008) The NTI-tss device for the therapy of bruxism, temporomandibular disorders, and headache—where do we stand? A qualitative systematic review of the literature. *BMC Oral Health*, **8**, 22.

68. Emshoff R, Bosch R, Pumpel E, Schoning H, Strobl H. (2008) Low-level laser therapy for treatment of temporomandibular joint pain: a double-blind and placebo-controlled trial. *Oral Surg Oral Med Oral Pathol Oral Radiol Endod*, 105(4), 452–6.

69. Smith P, Mosscrop D, Davies S, Sloan P, Al-Ani Z. (2007) The efficacy of acupuncture in the treatment of temporomandibular joint myofascial pain: a randomised controlled trial. *J Dent*, **35(3)**, 259–67.

70. Ritenbaugh C, Hammerschlag R, Calabrese C *et al.* (2008) A pilot whole systems clinical trial of traditional Chinese medicine and naturopathic medicine for the treatment of temporomandibular disorders. *J Altern Complement Med*, **14(5)**, 475–87.

71. Hampton T. (2008) Improvements needed in management of temporomandibular joint disorders. *JAMA*, **299(10)**, 1119–21.

72. Koh H, Robinson PG. (2004) Occlusal adjustment for treating and preventing temporomandibular joint disorders. *J Oral Rehabil*, **31(4)**, 287–92.

73. Al-Ani MZ. (2004) Stabilisation splint therapy for temporomandibular pain dysfunction syndrome. *Evid Based Dent*, **5(3)**, 65–6.

74. Koh H, Robinson PG. (2004) Occlusal adjustment for treating and preventing temporomandibular joint disorders. *J Oral Rehabil*, **31(4)**, 287–92.

75. Bessa-Nogueira RV, Vasconcelos BC, Niederman R. (2008) The methodological quality of systematic reviews comparing temporomandibular joint disorder surgical and non-surgical treatment. *BMC Oral Health*, **26**, 8:27.

76. Patton LL, Siegel MA, Benoliel R, De Laat A. (2007) Management of burning mouth syndrome: systematic review and management recommendations. *Oral Surg Oral Med Oral Pathol Oral Radiol Endod*, **103** (Suppl.), S39.e1–13.

77. Zakrzewska JM, Forssell H, Glenny AM. (2005) Interventions for the treatment of burning mouth syndrome. *Cochrane Database Syst Rev*, **1**, CD002779.

78. Eliav E, Kamran B, Schaham R, Czerninski R, Gracely RH, Benoliel R. (2007) Evidence of chorda tympani dysfunction in patients with burning mouth syndrome. *J Am Dent Assoc*, **138(5)**, 628–33.

79. Sardella A, Lodi G, Demarosi F *et al.* (2008) *Hypericum perforatum* extract in burning mouth syndrome: a randomized placebo-controlled study. *J Oral Pathol Med*, **37(7)**, 395–401.

80. Yilmaz Z, Renton T, Yiangou Y *et al.* (2007) Burning mouth syndrome as a trigeminal small fibre neuropathy:

Increased heat and capsaicin receptor TRPV1 in nerve fibres correlates with pain score. *J Clin Neuroscience*, **14**, 864–71.

81. Zakrzewska JM, Harrison SD. (2002) Assessment and management of orofacial pain. In: Zakrzewska JM (ed.) *Series on Pain Research and Clinical Management*. London: Elsevier, pp. 103–115.

82. Evans RW, Agostoni E. (2006) Persistent idiopathic facial pain. *Headache*, **46(8)**, 1298–300.

83. Volcy M, Rapoport AM, Tepper SJ, Sheftell FD, Bigal ME. (2006) Persistent idiopathic facial pain responsive to topiramate. *Cephalalgia*, **26(4)**, 489–91.

84. Abrahamsen R, Baad-Hansen L, Svensson P. (2008) Hypnosis in the management of persistent idiopathic orofacial pain—clinical and psychosocial findings. *Pain*, **136(1–2)**, 44–52.

85. List T, Leijon G, Helkimo M *et al.* (2007) Clinical findings and psychosocial factors in patients with atypical odontalgia: a case-control study. *J Orofac Pain*, **21(2)**, 89–98.

86. Baad-Hansen L, Leijon G, Svensson P, List T. (2008) Comparison of clinical findings and psychosocial factors in patients with atypical odontalgia and temporomandibular disorders. *J Orofac Pain*, **22(1)**, 7–14.

87. List T, Leijon G, Svensson P. (2008) Somatosensory abnormalities in atypical odontalgia: A case-control study. *Pain*, **139(2)**, 333–41.

88. Baad-Hansen L. (2008) Atypical odontalgia—pathophysiology and clinical management. *J Oral Rehabil*, **35(1)**, 1–11.

89. Ogütcen-Toller M, Uzun E, Incesu L. (2004) Clinical and magnetic resonance imaging evaluation of facial pain. *Oral Surg Oral Med Oral Pathol Oral Radiol Endod*, **97(5)**, 652–8.

90. Rozen TD. (2002) Interventional treatment for cluster headache: a review of the options. *Curr Pain Headache Rep*, **6(1)**, 57–64.

91. Renton T, Yiangou Y, McGurk M *et al.* (2003) Presence of VR1 and P2X3 sodium channels in tooth pulp. *J Orofacial Pain*, **17**, 245–50.

92. Renton T, Yiangou Y, Tate S, Bountra C, Anand P. (2005) Sodium channel Nav1.8 immunoreactivity in painful human dental pulp. *BMC Oral Health*, **5(1)**, 5.

93. Fertleman CR, Baker MD, Parker KA *et al.* (2006) SCN9A mutations in paroxysmal extreme pain disorder: allelic variants underlie distinct channel defects and phenotypes. *Neuron*, **52(5)**, 767–74.

94. Kim H, Mittal DP, Iadarola MJ, Dionne RA. (2006) TRPV1 Genetic predictors for acute experimental cold and heat pain sensitivity in humans. *J Med Genet*, **43(8)**, e40.

95. Diatchenko L, Slade GD, Nackley AG *et al.* (2005) Genetic basis for individual variations in pain perception and the development of a chronic pain condition. *Hum Mol Genet*, **14(1)**, 135–43. Epub 2004.

23

Sleep apnoea

Chris Dodds

Introduction

Sleep disorders that are affected by problems related to the upper airway have been recognized for at least the past 50 years. The impact that patient characteristics such as facial morphology, dynamic changes in airway tone with sleep state, and surgical procedures on the head and neck have on the incidence or risk of obstructive sleep apnoea (OSA) is still being identified. This growing understanding does inform the surgical treatment options being considered and will have an, often significant, influence on outcome.

OSA is characterized by repetitive episodes of upper airway obstruction that occur during sleep, usually associated with a reduction in blood oxygen saturation[1].

The underlying pathophysiology of OSA is an essential element in assessing the predisposition of a given patient to OSA either before surgery or afterwards. The improvement in airway control and chemoreceptor sensitivity following effective treatment is vital for safe anaesthesia, but if the treatment is mechanical, e.g. by continuous positive airway pressure (CPAP) devices, these must be available at all times during the peri-operative period or an alternative airway such as a tracheostomy must be considered.

A brief outline of the physiology of sleep

There are three phases or states of life. These are the familiar wakefulness and the two sleep phases (non-REM and REM sleep). Of these, only non-REM sleep mirrors the traditional textbook teaching of how we control our breathing, based on the central chemoreceptors, especially those for carbon dioxide. In both wakefulness and REM sleep this basic drive is modulated by downward traffic from the higher centres, such as the cortex.

Non-REM is the 'essential' component of sleep and occurs preferentially early in a sleep cycle. It is during this phase that the majority of restorative processes take place, such as the release of endogenous anabolic hormones. It is classically described as having several stages of increasing 'depth', with depth in this case being a marker for how much stimulation is necessary to wake the subject. Stage 1 is the lightest sleep stage and most of us recognize this as drowsiness. It is true sleep, but short-term memory processing is still active. If awoken, the subject can 'replay' what has happened: 'I woke because a door slammed shut'. Once the second stage is entered, this short-term memory is deleted. This is why we cannot say precisely when we went to sleep. The final stage of non-REM—slow wave sleep (SWS)—is the most important stage, as mentioned above (current definitions include both stages 3 and 4 of SWS as one single stage) (Figure 23.1).

REM sleep is an active state, in many aspects identical to wakefulness. There is often dreaming, but in the majority of people (unlike some other mammals) there is hyperpolarization of the motor neurons from C5 downwards leading to motor paralysis. This protective mechanism is occasionally breached and then we see patients who act out their dreams. During both wakefulness and REM sleep, the pattern of breathing reflects the content of mentation. If we dream we are swimming underwater we go apnoeic, if running up a hill, tachypnoeic, and if we dream we have chest pain, that is real angina.

Sleep phase changes in control of ventilation

The normal wakeful response to hypoxia is to increase the rate of breathing as the PaO_2 falls. As pure hypoxia is unusual, this response is normally hidden in the response to hypercarbia. It is the response to

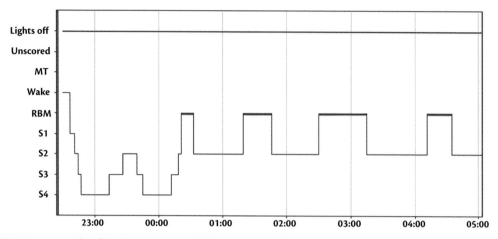

Figure 23.1 A summary plot of the sleep stages recorded during an overnight study in a normal subject. The 'essential' slow wave sleep predominates in the early phases of sleep whereas REM, marked as solid bold lines occurs later.

hypercarbia that drives normal ventilation. This is seen initially as a rise in tidal volume (altering the ratio between dead space and perfused lung tissue) but later there is also a rise in respiratory frequency.

Both of these reflex responses are attenuated during sleep, gradually during non-REM sleep but markedly during REM sleep. Indeed, some authors have described an almost zero response to rising $PaCO_2$ during REM. It is these vital reflexes that are affected in patients with OSA. Only after prolonged effective treatment do they return *towards* normal.

Sleep-disordered breathing

Ask the majority of doctors how we breathe in and they will answer 'by activating the diaphragm via the phrenic nerves and by the use of the intercostal muscles'. What actually happens is different when we are awake from when we are asleep.

During wakefulness, as the inspiration is initiated there is a sequential process of activation of the pharyngeal musculature, so increasing tone to keep the upper airway open against the physical effects of the large negative pressure created once the diaphragm and intercostals are activated.

The pressure necessary to initiate fluid flow in a tube has to overcome inertia as well as resistance. The upper airway acts as a 'Starling resistor' where the negative pressure within the lumen has to be balanced against the external (in this case, atmospheric) pressure. Collapse is prevented by this initial increase in pharyngeal tone. Once bulk flow occurs, the pressure needed to

maintain flow is less and the activation ramps down. (The fall in airway resistance in the lower airways is less important to our considerations.)

Expiration is normally a passive process and minimal upper airway tone is necessary.

During sleep, indeed from the very onset of stage 1 non-REM sleep, there is a decrease in tone of the pharyngeal constrictors. The mechanics of inspiration remain the same but there is now a progressive narrowing of the entire upper airway as the balance of forces maintaining the airway move towards closure. At a certain point the velocity of the airflow, and pressure necessary to generate this, can lead to turbulence and vibration of the *entire* upper airway—snoring.

If the airway is further compromised, by fatty loading of the airway or tumour for instance, then narrowing progresses and the snoring gets louder until there is a collapse of the airway and complete obstruction. At this stage the crescendo snoring suddenly stops and the silence of apnoea ensues.

Once airway collapse occurs, further inspiratory effort simply keeps the airway shut. The basal metabolism continues to utilize oxygen but only the oxygen remaining in the vital capacity of the lungs is available. The longer the apnoeic episode lasts, the lower the oxygen saturation will fall (mirroring the curve of the oxygen dissociation curve). Eventually the effort of trying to breathe in (not the degree of hypoxia) leads to a brief arousal from sleep and rescue of the upper airway by an increase in tone. This arousal is too fast (about 5 seconds) for patient awareness because this takes at least 30 seconds of arousal to occur. These microarousals do fragment deep sleep and are the cause of the daytime sleepiness seen in patients with severe OSA.

The physical consequences of these repetitive desaturations (Table 23.1) include respiratory, cardiac, and neurological changes, some of which are reversible while others are not.

Respiratory effects of OSA

The normal control process to match ventilation to perfusion in the lungs includes the matching of bloodflow to individual perfused alveolae according to the PO_2 in the alveoli. Falls in alveolar PO_2 lead to a hypoxic pulmonary vasoconstriction that effectively diverts the bloodflow to the alveolae with normal PO_2. If the entire respiratory system becomes hypoxic, such as during complete airway obstruction, there is a dramatic increase in pulmonary arterial resistance leading to acute pulmonary hypertension. Values of 120 mmHg are not unusual in young patients.

The effort of trying to inspire against a closed upper airway leads to profound intrathoracic negative pressures. These may precipitate oesophagogastric regurgitation and airway contamination. The brainstem mechanism for triggering arousal and resolution of the apnoea is the imbalance between effort and airflow, not the degree of hypoxia.

Table 23.1 Some of the immediate and delayed consequences of OSA in adults

Immediate	Delayed
Hypoxia	Hypersomnia
Pulmonary hypertension	Pulmonary hypertension
Bradycardia	Right heart failure
Hypercarbia	Memory failure-failing executive function
High levels of catecholamines	Night sweats
Brainstem arousal—sleep disruption	Nocturia
	Reduced hypoxic drive
	Reduced hypercarbic drive
	Systemic hypertension
	Mood disorders-aggression
	Sleep-related accidents

One measure of severity of OSA is the number of obstructions/desaturations recorded averaged over the night. This is the apnoea/hypopnoea index (AHI). Initially it was defined as the number of falls in saturation >4% (twice the operating error of the pulse oximeters of that time) per hour occurring more than five times per hour (an arbitrary number without evidence). As severe OSA has an AHI often exceeding 60/hour, the actual numerical value is seen as indicative rather than diagnostic. However, treatment should eliminate these apnoeas completely. Spurious claims of success using a standard of 'more than a 50% reduction in AHI' were common in the early surgical literature.

Once there is a cessation of ventilation, clearly the rate of metabolism will determine how fast oxygen is utilized. The more recumbent the patient and the more obese they are, the greater will be the reduction in vital capacity and the faster the fall in oxygen concentration/saturation. Equally, the recovery from a profound fall in oxygen will also depend on effective ventilation and, where there are marked V/Q abnormalities such as are present in these patients, return to a normal level of oxygenation may not occur. This leads to a prolonged hypoxic state and may lead to a compensatory increase in haemoglobin concentrations.

One anaesthetic contributory factor is the use of neostigmine in patients who have partially recovered from neuromuscular blockade, as this reduces upper airway tone and can precipitate airway obstruction in these patients. This does not appear to occur with the novel reversal agents currently being introduced into anaesthetic practice[2].

Cardiac effects of OSA

As oxygen desaturation occurs there is a bradycardia induced, in a similar manner to the diving reflex, which is followed by a tachycardia on resolution of the hypoxia. This tachycardia is also associated with a rapid onset of systemic hypertension owing to the catecholamine release triggered by the arousal. These repetitive 'pulses' of hypertension are thought to exacerbate existing hypertension, and may precipitate it in other patients. The marked hypertension and tachycardia are clearly hazardous in the presence of underlying ischaemic heart disease.

The pulmonary vascular effects of the profound hypoxic vasoconstriction lead to pulmonary hypertension and right heart strain.

The degree of hypoxia in OSA may be severe and this can cause significant cardiac dysrhythmias. At oxygen saturations of about 70%, conduction is affected and, at 60% or below, episodes of asystole lasting more than 10 seconds or ventricular tachycardia/fibrillation may occur.

Neurological effects of OSA

The repetitive pattern of respiratory obstruction leading to arousal fragments the deep stages of sleep. These arousals are too fast for the patient to be aware of and are known as microarousals. They have to be differentiated from the normal tendency to wake from very light sleep every 1–1.5 hours, which has no impact on daytime performance. The frequency of microarousals determines the degree of sleep deprivation. The patient with severe OSA will fall asleep in any situation where extreme concentration is not needed. What is more dangerous is that they have 'microsleeps' as a mirror effect of the microarousals. These are 3–5-second episodes of true sleep that occur without the patient being aware of even feeling sleepy. This is the cause for the 20-fold increase in serious road accidents in these patients, for instance.

The cumulative physiological effects of obstruction (hypercarbia and hypoxia) are not completely resolved during the short periods of hyperventilation that occur on arousal. The central chemoreceptors reset as a result of this and the more severe the OSA, the more insensitive these reflexes become. This predisposes these patients to profound hypoventilation if sedated, and to very poor protective responses if their airway is compromised during recovery from anaesthesia or sedation. Exquisite sensitivity to opiates has caused deaths in the past.

Sleep deprivation has profound effects at both psychological and physiological levels. Executive decision-making fails, as does concentration. Irritability and aggressive behaviour develop. It is not uncommon for these effects to cause unemployment and marital disharmony. The fragmentation of the deep SWS in non-REM phases prevents normal hormone production via the hypothalamic–pituitary axis. The most striking effect in children is the reduction in growth hormone.

The effect of right heart strain and repetitive arousal leads to nocturia in many patients.

Anatomical effects of OSA

The airway is a dynamic structure and remodelling of the airway occurs if there is marked OSA in children. This leads to the 'adenoidal' facies recognized in children who have had severe tonsillar disease, where there is narrowing of the mid-face and a downwards rotation of the palate, leading the normal soft palate to extend into the lower pharynx.

The airway in snorers, and more markedly in patients with OSA, becomes oedematous. This resolves on treatment with CPAP over a period of about 10 days.

Making the diagnosis

As with many conditions in medicine, the first part of making a diagnosis is to realize that the disease actually exists and look for it.

History

The problem with sleep disorders in general is that the patient is asleep! This sounds facile but presents real difficulties if they are interviewed in isolation. Whenever there is a suggestion of a sleep disorder, a witness is necessary. Equally, there are fundamental differences between paediatric and adult presentations, history, and findings.

The adult patient can usually identify that they are becoming more sleepy through the day although, as this is a gradual, insidious process, they may not recognize the significance or degree of their sleepiness. There is usually a considerable delay between the development of OSA and diagnosis, often of the order of 5 years. It is important to go back a considerable time in their past to pick this up. The most common screening questionnaire is the Epworth eight-question scale[3], which has been validated for most major languages. The maximum score is 24 and upper limit of normal is 10. Most would feel that a score of >12 is significant and above 15 indicates a serious risk to driving.

The Epworth sleepiness scale

How likely are you to doze off or fall asleep in the following situations, in contrast to feeling just tired? This refers to your usual way of life in recent times. Even if you have not done some of these things recently, try to work out how they would have affected you. Use the following scale to choose the most appropriate number for each situation:

0 No chance of dozing

1 Slight chance of dozing

2 Moderate chance of dozing

3 High chance of dozing.

Situations:

1) Sitting and reading

2) Watching TV

3) Sitting inactive in a public place (e.g. theatre or a meeting)

4) As a passenger in a car for an hour without a break

5) Lying down to rest in the afternoon when circumstances permit

6) Sitting and talking to someone

7) Sitting quietly after lunch without alcohol

8) In a car, while stopped for a few minutes in traffic.

There are other complaints that also relate to the sleep deprivation caused by frequent arousals. These may include failing concentration, changed mood with a more aggressive and irritable tendency, poor decision-making and memory. A job history showing a slowing in progression or frequent work-related accidents should raise suspicions.

Social aspects of life are more difficult to elicit, but marital problems are very common as the snoring gets louder and louder. They may admit to restricting their driving and sporting activities as they become more sleepy and exhausted.

Weight gain is a common association, but about 20% of patients are not obese. These non-obese patients tend to be younger and their early presentation reflects potential airway dysfunction. Many identify that they wake through the night with nocturia or night sweats.

Check the collar size; men with a >16-inch collar are more likely to get OSA than those with smaller neck sizes. If they don't know their collar size, then measure it!

Hypersomnolence is not a feature of paediatric OSA. Children may present with a recurrence of enuresis[4], hyperactivity, and poor attention. They may fail at school, or display behavioural problems[5,6] at a preschool age. This array of symptoms in a child who has an identified craniofacial abnormality should prompt a specialist sleep review. Nationally, specialist paediatric sleep services are limited, and referral pathways should be identified for services that include children as part of their case mix.

Witness statement

The history elicited from a witness (either a spouse, partner, parent or friend) is invaluable. Even patients who live alone go on holiday, socialize, and work with others who can provide a commentary on their nocturnal breathing patterns. Whilst it will be a proxy report, it is still valuable.

There are several aspects to cover.

- The first is to confirm if the patient snores. If they do—is it position-dependent, is it continuous, have they always snored, does anything make it worse (such as alcohol or nasal obstruction with hayfever or colds), has it got worse with weight gain?

- *Do they stop breathing?* This is the most important question to ask, as the answer, especially in children, is highly predictive

- Have there been mood changes, have they lost their jobs because of falling performance or falling asleep at work? Do they 'nod off' when being talked to, or seem to go blank/vague for a few seconds?

- Have they fallen asleep when driving, or at work?

- In children the presentation is mostly behavioural and may be missed if the question on snoring and stopping breathing is omitted.

Examination

Adults are more likely to be obese and middle-aged if the cause is laxity of the pharyngeal area, and younger and thinner if there are underlying morphological or alcohol problems. Talking to the witness may be enough distraction for the patient to display excessive sleepiness, as can a careful observation in the waiting area before being seen. It is pathological to sleep in outpatients or a preadmission clinic.

Listening to the patient's speech often identifies the rasping pharyngeal nature of phonation.

Close attention should be paid to the facial and mandibular features, looking for many of the features linked to difficult airway management, such as a narrow face and mandible or a high arched palate. Inspection of the mouth, dentition, and pharynx often confirms the severity of the snoring by the oedematous nature of the oral mucosa. Many patients with severe sleep apnoea have a limited gag reflex and will tolerate extensive instrumentation of the airway with ease.

Florid cases will demonstrate the respiratory and cardiovascular changes of right heart failure, and an 'overlap' syndrome of respiratory failure and frank 'Pickwickian' features will be obvious in severe cases.

Investigations

No single investigation can be used to diagnose OSA. This is especially true in children.

Overnight pulse oximetry

This is probably the commonest investigation (Figure 23.2) in adults and is one of the most valuable. It does not replace the need for a comprehensive history and can be unreliable if the patient is disturbed by the probe. This is usually performed as a domiciliary procedure and the data downloaded and reviewed subsequently. If the history is positive and the oximetry is normal, believe the history and repeat the investigation.

One caveat—the elderly have an increasing incidence of episodic desaturations that is not clinically significant. The number of episodes of obstruction increases with age but has no survival impact. They are usually only considered for active treatment if there is evidence of sleepiness or other restrictions to everyday living.

Respiratory pattern

The measurement of thoracic and abdominal movement gives very clear information about the pattern of breathing (Figure 23.3a). Central apnoea is seen as complete loss of respiratory effort (movement). Hypopnoea is defined as a 50% reduction in amplitude

of both signals from the baseline lasting more than 10 seconds. Obstructive episodes demonstrate the paradox seen in anaesthetized patients with upper airway obstruction. The abdominal and thoracic signals become out of phase (Figure 23.3b).

One pattern that has caused some confusion is the mixed apnoea seen in many patients. This is simply where an obstructive episode leads to arousal. This triggers hyperventilation because of the raised PCO_2 (itself a consequence of sleep-induced downregulation of central chemoreceptors and apnoea). Once sleep returns, so does the reduced hypercarbic ventilatory response and a relative hypocarbic apnoea occurs. As the CO_2 rises, ventilation starts, but with a collapsible airway that is soon closed by increasing effort. The waveform produced is paradoxical ventilation, arousal, apnoea, gradually increasing ventilation leading to paradoxical ventilation, and so on.

Ambulatory respiratory studies

More complex multivariable studies include pulse oximetry and respiratory pattern, but may also include

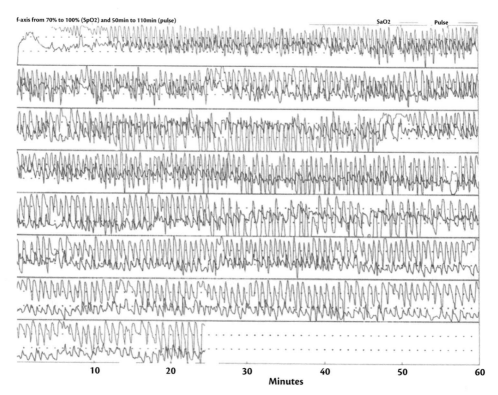

Figure 23.2 Oximeter trace from a patient with severe OSA. Each plot is 1 hour long and includes oxygen saturation (scale 100–70%) and heart rate (scale 60–140 bpm). The severe and repetitive falls in saturation can clearly be seen, often falling to below 70%.

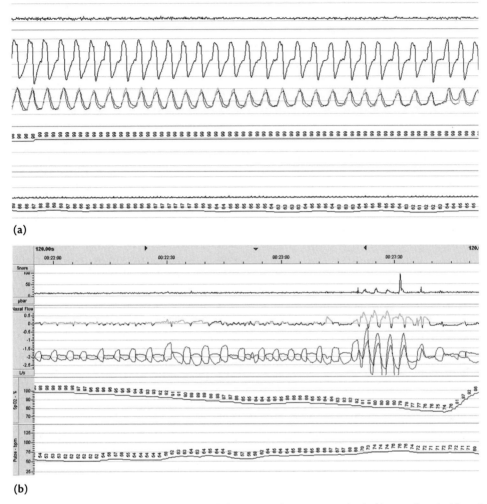

(a)

(b)

Figure 23.3 See also Plate 16 for full colour version. **a** A sample from a normal respiratory study. The blue waveform is airflow, the red is rib cage movement, and the green is abdominal movement. Both red and green traces are in phase, indicating normal respiratory effort. Oxygen saturation is below with the values inserted, and the heart rate trace is the lowest on the printout. **b** This sample is using the same montage as normal (Figure 23.3a), but paradoxical movements of rib cage and abdominal wall and absent airflow show complete obstruction. There is a gasping resolution with large tidal airflow and normalization of ventilation. The characteristic delay between the obstructive event and the fall in oxygen saturation is clearly seen.

position sensors, microphones to record snoring, ECG, EMG, and limited EEG. These are often used in the diagnosis of borderline or complex cases or where there is limited access to a formal sleep centre. They are valuable for making a secure diagnosis of OSA and for guiding treatment[7].

Polysomnography (PSG)

This has been referred to, inaccurately, as the 'gold standard' for sleep investigations. It is only possible in a custom-built sleep laboratory where the ambient conditions (sound, temperature, humidity, and lighting) can be controlled. The physiological data include formal EEG (8–32 channels), EMG (ocular, submental and pretibial), ECG, position, sound, infrared video, airflow, and respiratory pattern[8]. This is recorded, often on two nights, and delivers several gigabytes of information. The majority are automatically scored but must be manually reviewed by a skilled and experienced senior technician.

Paediatric studies

Neonates presenting with congenital airway or pulmonary problems require customized PSG monitoring and assessment by experienced paediatric sleep specialists. Respiratory paradox is common and can reflect the flexibility of their chest walls rather than obstruction. Changes in their control of breathing should be assessed, as this will inform analgesic regimens if surgery is necessary.

Paediatric studies are necessary on children suspected of having OSA or complex airway problems. They require high resolution continuous video surveillance as well as multichannel recordings. The changes in respiratory control with maturation have to be understood, which is why all such studies should be manually reviewed by an expert technician in concert with a skilled paediatric sleep physician. These are rare resources and are not necessary for most children who snore.

Conditions that increase the risk of suffering from OSA

A history of snoring is a clear indication that the patient has a narrow, collapsing airway. The younger the patient the more significant is this finding. Anything that leads to a restricted airway at any site may lead to airway narrowing during inspiration and, potentially, airway closure. It is useful to describe these conditions as those that directly affect the airway and those with a more indirect effect.

Direct

Primary anatomical variations

These result in a narrowing of the airway and can be either bony anomalies or of the soft tissue. They may be congenital or acquired. The acquired may be pathological, traumatic or even a direct result of planned surgery. The major congenital craniofacial abnormalities (Chapter 19), such as Pierre–Robin sequence or Treacher–Collins, may present with life-threatening airway obstruction, especially when sleeping. Treatment at this age usually requires tracheotomy rather than non-invasive pressure support.

Less pronounced micrognathia may still lead to a reduction in the dimensions of the lower part of the upper airway. This may not be directly troublesome but will predispose the child to OSA if there is soft tissue enlargement within the airway, such as adenoidal or tonsillar hypertrophy.

There are other conditions that are associated with soft tissue enlargement that may precipitate OSA despite an otherwise normal bony structure. The macroglossia associated with Down's syndrome is relatively common[9,10], whilst adenoidal and tonsillar hypertrophy is often seen in the much rarer mucopolysaccharidosis syndromes[11]. A high level of suspicion is necessary to identify these children early.

A history from any parent of a child who snores and stops breathing is pathognomonic of paediatric sleep apnoea.

Indirect

Neuromuscular and neurological conditions may precipitate sleep-related breathing disorders. The coordination necessary to maintain ventilation, especially during sleep, is easily eroded as conduction pathways are damaged or disordered. Both central and obstructive apnoeas may occur and ventilatory support at night may be necessary.

Surgical causes

The surgical treatment of some congenital abnormalities has an unpredictable effect on the airway. Cleft lip and palate repair is associated with alterations in the patency of the upper airway, often transformed from a wide open to a narrow oedematous one initially. This is a well recognized complication and was reported in early literature as a cause of postoperative mortality.

More complex midface and mandibular corrective surgery will be unpredictable in effect and requires close observation during the early postoperative period, especially overnight. Mandibular recession after adolescence is another procedure with similar risks[12].

Tumours affecting the upper airway, whether benign such as cystic hygromas or more sinister such as the lymphomas or other malignancies[13,14], can all compromise an otherwise normal airway. They may do so during sleep before any symptoms are identified when awake. Equally, effective treatment will resolve these nocturnal symptoms first. Rare presentations of oral haemangiomas have been reported with severe OSA requiring CPAP until effective treatment returns the airway to normal.

It is important to remember that there is a high incidence of OSA in patients following perioral radiotherapy (Chapter 17), and any increase in sleepiness or reports of worsening snoring should be followed up. Any lymphoedema of the neck or face may also precipitate sleep apnoea.

Medical causes

The most common medical causes are obesity and hypothyroidism. It is also common following a CVA, in end-stage renal failure, and in eclampsia of pregnancy. Diabetes is being recognized as a common precursor, and the endocrine disorders are another frequent cause of OSA. Acromegaly[15] is frequently associated with airway problems due to the macroglossia but, whilst CPAP treatment may be effective, it cannot be used if trans-sphenoidal pituitary surgery is undertaken.

Trauma

Facial trauma (see Chapter 14) should raise two questions. Did the accident occur because of OSA or will it cause it (or both)?

If the trauma was due to a road traffic accident involving only one vehicle, especially between 2 and 4 am, a sleep-related cause must be assumed, and OSA is the likeliest culprit. The implications for airway control and anaesthesia are described above, but a combination of sedation and opiate analgesia are extremely hazardous in these (usually untreated and undiagnosed) OSA patients.

If there is no obvious sleep-related cause, the injury should be assessed for airway compromise. The close relationship of the upper airway to major vasculature, cervical spine and nerves, facial skeleton, and endocrine structures mean that any injury in this area may compromise breathing, especially during sleep.

If the patient is assessed or proves to have a difficult airway to manage, OSA must be considered. Referral for sleep investigations should follow once the immediate surgical and anaesthetic management is satisfactory[16].

Treatment of OSA

Medical causes for OSA should be sought and treated wherever possible. These include obesity, hypothyroidism, acromegaly, severe renal failure, and diabetes mellitus. Bariatric surgery does improve OSA where there is successful weight loss, and effective renal support or transplantation will improve those in renal failure.

The close relationship between acute stroke[17–19] and congestive cardiac failure[20] with OSA means that a high index of suspicion should be maintained if such medically compromised patients are considered for surgery.

In adults

There is only one effective surgical and one effective mechanical treatment. All other treatments may be considered as worthy of consideration *only* if the primary treatments fail. They are surgical tracheostomy and nasal CPAP.

Surgical tracheostomy

Surgical tracheostomy has a long established record and is the only treatment that bypasses the affected part of the (upper) airway. Unfortunately, caring for, and coping with, a permanent tracheostomy limits its acceptance in adults. However, it remains a mainstay of neonatal care, especially if there are complex facial and airway problems.

CPAP

CPAP was developed in the mid 1980s by Colin Sullivan in Australia and has become the gold standard treatment of OSA. The application of a low positive pressure through a nasal or full face mask prevents airway collapse and maintains the airway throughout sleep. The effects are dramatic, both physiologically and clinically. Patients are returned to normal vigilance and their pattern of breathing returns to normal. Control reflexes recover over a period of 2–4 weeks, as does airway oedema.

Compliance with CPAP varies from 60 to 95%; it is very dependent on the support given in the first stage of initiation. There are several types of device and many different interfaces to connect the patient. The standard fixed pressure device is suitable for almost all patients, but variable performance devices are better tolerated by some patients. Where there is underlying chest disease, the high expiratory resistance through fixed performance machines may lead to CO_2 retention and hypoventilation. Bilevel devices are necessary in these patients—BiPAP (bilevel positive airway pressure).

The sleep unit will titrate the pressure generated by the CPAP/BiPAP machine to be optimal for that patient. *It is imperative that this preset pressure is accepted and not adjusted.* Patients on CPAP will know to bring their machines into hospital with them, and they must be used at night and in recovery after surgery. If the patient is admitted as an emergency, it is unlikely that their machine will be available, nor the pressures known. Some units issue their patients with identity bracelets but not all do this. If such a patient is admitted, contact the sleep unit to borrow a CPAP machine. Most are preset to 10 cmH_2O and this will provide a degree of support to all patients. Some are capable of automatic titration but most will be preset. The maximum possible pressure (20 cmH$_2$O) is rarely used even in morbidly obese patients.

Surgical considerations in patients treated with CPAP

If planned surgery will include the upper airway, the bony structures around it, or may alter the neuro-muscular function, then the impact this has on the ability to deliver CPAP must be considered. If there is a risk of losing the ability to use CPAP, the patient should be protected by a surgical airway for the immediate perioperative period.

In children

Adenotonsillectomy is the most common airway procedure used to treat paediatric OSA and has long-term benefits in both symptomatic and morphological aspects[21]. Where there are identified structural problems, surgical correction is likely to improve the OSA[22] but, as these are rarely encountered, they are best managed in specialist units.

Rescue surgery

CPAP therapy has variable long-term compliance, and several surgical procedures have been suggested either to provide a definitive treatment or to improve compliance with the CPAP[23–26]. As upper airway collapse is usually multisite, staged procedures with adequate follow-up between them is essential.

Conclusion

Sleep apnoea is common, is usually undiagnosed, and will require active investigation by all involved in head and neck surgery at all ages. If 'skeletal' procedures are being planned, assessment[27] of the possible impact on the airway is recommended.

References

1. Obstructive Sleep Apnea. (2001) *The International Classification of Sleep Disorders (revised); diagnostic and coding manual American Academy of Sleep Medicine*, p. 52. isbn 0–9657220–1–5.
2. Eikermann M, Zaremba S, Malhotra A *et al.* (2008) Neostigmine but not sugammadex impairs upper airway dilator muscle activity and breathing. *Br J Anaesth*, **101(3)**, 344–9.
3. John MW. (1991) A new method for measuring daytime sleepiness: the Epworth sleepiness scale. *Sleep*, **14(6)**, 540 –5.
4. Basha S, Bialowas C, Ende K, Szeremeta W. (2005) Effectiveness of adenotonsillectomy in the resolution of nocturnal enuresis secondary to obstructive sleep apnea. *Laryngoscope*, **115(6)**, 1101–3.
5. Garetz SL. (2008) Behavior, cognition, and quality of life after adenotonsillectomy for pediatric sleep-disordered breathing: summary of the literature. *Otolaryngol Head Neck Surg*, **138**(1 Suppl.), S19–S26.
6. Baldassari CM, Mitchell RB, Schubert C, Rudnick EF. (2008) Pediatric obstructive sleep apnea and quality of life: a meta-analysis. *Otolaryngol Head Neck Surg*, **138(3)**, 265–73.
7. Patel MR, Davidson TM. (2007) Home sleep testing in the diagnosis and treatment of sleep disordered breathing. *Otolaryngol Clin North Am*, **40(4)**, 761–84.
8. Thakkar K, Yao M. (2007) Diagnostic studies in obstructive sleep apnea. *Otolaryngol Clin North Am*, **40(4)**, 785–805.
9. Shott S. R, Amin R, Chini B *et al.* (2006). Obstructive sleep apnea: Should all children with Down syndrome be tested? *Arch Otolaryngol Head Neck Surg*, **132(4)**, 432–6.
10. Merrell JA, Shott SR. (2007) OSAS in Down syndrome: T&A versus T&A plus lateral pharyngoplasty. *Int J Pediatr Otorhinolaryngol*, **71(8)**, 1197 –1203.
11. Yeung AH, Cowan MJ, Horn B *et al.* (2009) Airway management in children with mucopolysaccharidoses. *Arch Otolaryngol Head Neck Surg*, **135(1)**, 73 –9.
12. Ramesh BV, Vinod N, Murugesan K. (2005) Pharyngeal airway changes following mandibular setback surgery. *Indian J Dent Res*, **16(4)**, 147–50.
13. Payne RJ, Hier MP, Kost KM *et al.* (2005) High prevalence of obstructive sleep apnea among patients with head and neck cancer. *J Otolaryngol*, **34(5)**, 304–11.
14. Nesse W, Hoekema A, Stegenga B *et al.* (2006) Prevalence of obstructive sleep apnoea following head and neck cancer treatment: a cross-sectional study. *Oral Oncol*, **42(1)**, 108–14.
15. Chanson P, Salenave S. (2008) Acromegaly. *Orphanet J Rare Dis*, **3**, 17.
16. Chung F, Yegneswaran B, Herrera F *et al.* (2008) Patients with difficult intubation may need referral to sleep clinics. *Anesth Analg*, **107(3)**, 915–20.
17. Bonnin-Vilaplana M, Arboix A, Parra O *et al.* (2009) Sleep-related breathing disorders in acute lacunar stroke. *J Neurol*, Jul 22 (e-publication).
18. Martinez-Garcia MA, Soler-Cataluna JJ, Ejarque-Martinez L *et al.* (2009) Continuous positive airway pressure treatment reduces mortality in patients with ischemic stroke and obstructive sleep apnea: a 5-year follow-up study. *Am J Respir Crit Care Med*, **180(1)**, 36–41.
19. Portela PC, Fumado JC, Garcia HQ *et al.* (2009) Sleep-disordered breathing and acute stroke. *Cerebrovasc Dis*, **27** (Suppl. 1), 104–110.
20. Paulino A, Damy T, Margarit L *et al.* (2009) Prevalence of sleep-disordered breathing in a 316-patient French cohort of stable congestive heart failure. *Arch Cardiovasc Dis*, **102** (3), 169–75.
21. Zettergren-Wijk L, Forsberg CM, Linder-Aronson S. (2006) Changes in dentofacial morphology after adeno-/ tonsillectomy in young children with obstructive sleep apnoea—a 5-year follow-up study. *Eur J Orthod*, **28(4)**, 319–26.

22. Lin SY, Halbower AC, Tunkel DE *et al.* (2006) Relief of upper airway obstruction with mandibular distraction surgery: Long-term quantitative results in young children. *Arch Otolaryngol Head Neck Surg*, **132(4)**, 437–41.

23. Colin WB. (2004) Comprehensive reconstructive surgery for obstructive sleep apnea. *J Ky Med Assoc*, **102(4)**, 154–62.

24. Souter MA, Stevenson S, Sparks B *et al.* (2004) Upper airway surgery benefits patients with obstructive sleep apnoea who cannot tolerate nasal continuous positive airway pressure. *J Laryngol Otol*, **118(4)**, 270–4.

25. Chandrashekariah R, Shaman Z, Auckley D. (2008) Impact of upper airway surgery on CPAP compliance in difficult-to-manage obstructive sleep apnea. *Arch Otolaryngol Head Neck Surg*, **134(9)**, 926–30.

26. Kezirian E, Goldberg AN. (2006) Hypopharyngeal surgery in obstructive sleep apnea: an evidence-based medicine review. *Arch Otolaryngol Head Neck Surg*, **132(2)**, 206–13.

27. Lye KW. (2008) Effect of orthognathic surgery on the posterior airway space (PAS). *Ann Acad Med Singapore*, **37(8)**, 677–82.

24

Postoperative nursing considerations for the maxillofacial surgical patient

Lindsay Garcia

Introduction

Approximately 7000 cases of head and neck cancer will present every year in the United Kingdom. Over 50% will present with oral cavity and pharyngeal lesions, predominantly in the elderly population, many of whom smoke heavily and are alcohol dependent[1]. Oral cancers are primarily treated by surgery and, where indicated, subsequent adjuvant radiotherapy. The choice of treatment is dependant on factors related to the tumour, patient, and organizational structure[2].

In general, patients are now older, sicker, and more dependant than in previous decades. The incidence of coexisting morbidity is also higher. Complex therapies and investigations previously unavailable or deemed too risky are now commonplace due to developments in nursing, medical, surgical, and anaesthetic care[3] with inherent consequences and warrant consideration in the postoperative period. Consequently it is important to establish which patients may develop postoperative complications of their disease or treatment by identifying those vulnerable individuals[3]. The 'National Confidential Enquiry into Patient Outcome and Death' published in 2001 demonstrated how audit can be used to assist the learning process and advance practice in highlighting many consistent challenges to good patient perioperative care[4].

Fortunately, for most patients recovery from anaesthesia and surgery is uneventful and without mishap. However, for some, recovery can be accompanied by life-threatening complications[5]. Good surgical care starts on admission with the provision of preoperative education to reduce the inherent physical risks of surgery[6]. Patients, who present with cancers of the head and neck, can have important underlying health problems reflecting high-risk behaviour such as heavy smoking and alcohol consumption. The resulting comorbidities complicate management, as fitness to undergo therapy can be a key issue in determining the options for treatment[7].

Perioperative complications are unexpected potentially devastating events that have serious consequences for the maxillofacial surgical patient[8]. Postoperative complications delay the patient's return to normal life and function and significantly increase the morbidity and mortality of this patient population[9].

The performance of complex surgical procedures on a patient population with multiple comorbidities should be preceded by an accurate perioperative assessment, the main objective of which is to predict and possibly reduce the risk of medical and surgical complications[2].This predominantly relies upon thorough, accurate preoperative assessment to identify potential risks for surgical complications and to prepare for, and possibly prevent, their eventuality[8]. Patients presenting for oral and maxillofacial surgery pose complex perioperative problems. For example, aggressive surgical resection followed by soft tissue and osseous reconstruction[10] carries a 20–50% incidence of postoperative complications[11]. Factors which make patients susceptible to postoperative complications are multifactorial but include advancing age, emergency surgery, pre-existing disease, rebleeding after surgery, large blood transfusions, and patients having to return to critical care units from general wards[3].

Grant and colleagues[2] evaluated the role of APACHE II (Acute Physiology and Chronic Health Evaluation) score as a predictive tool of immediate surgical complications following major head and neck cancer surgery. Excluding flap failure, they found a significant association between an increasing APACHE II score and the occurrence of immediate surgical complications associated with free tissue compromise and other immediate surgical complications. Prolonged radical maxillofacial surgery leads to extensive tissue injury resulting in the release of inflammatory mediators and consequent physiological derangement. An elevated APACHE II score would be an indicator of extensive tissue trauma and may serve as a marker for an increased likelihood of perioperative complications. Alternatively, the occurrence of a perioperative surgical complication, such as an ischaemic free flap, may itself cause physiological derangement and thus an elevated APACHE II[2].

Unfortunately, postoperative physiological monitoring and recording of observations are often incomplete and abnormal results are often not recognized or treated appropriately. Knowledge levels of the basic principles of care for the at-risk patient have been reported as surprisingly low[12].

Perioperative and postoperative management of the patient includes periodic assessment and monitoring of respiratory and cardiovascular function, neuromuscular function, mental status, temperature, pain, nausea and vomiting, drainage, bleeding, and urine output[13]. Acute illness can lead to physiological deterioration that may progress to organ failure and ultimately cardiorespiratory arrest. With early recognition and appropriate treatment, such abnormal physiology is potentially reversible, often requiring only simple measures to support the airway, breathing, and circulation[14].

When nursing an acutely ill or postoperative maxillofacial patient at risk of deterioration, it is vital to undertake a complete thorough initial assessment of the patient and subsequent frequent reassessments. These are made easier if the assessment scheme is simplified and if every member of the healthcare team uses the same systematic approach. This reduces the likelihood of mistakes or misunderstanding and ensures the whole team is working towards a common goal[3]. Immediate assessment, monitoring, and treatment using the airway, breathing, and circulation approach is advocated. Regular assessment is important in order to evaluate the effect of any intervention as patients may continue to deteriorate despite

treatment[3]. There are several aspects of the postoperative care of oral and maxillofacial patients that merit discussion.

Airway compromise

Most oral and maxillofacial surgical procedures have the potential to compromise the airway and particular attention must be paid at all times to the maintenance of a patent airway[15]. Following the surgical procedure a decision will be made regarding the appropriateness of extubation. Patients who have severe masticator space infections or acute facial trauma may have to be left intubated and on a ventilator after their surgical procedure, especially if a tracheostomy is not performed. The patients most at risk of airway compromise include those who have had mandibular resections, neck dissections, uvulopalatoplasty, maxillomandibular fixation, and temporomandibular joint (TMJ) arthroscopic procedures. Following the last listed procedure and prior to extubation, the oropharynx should be examined for swelling on the lateral aspects of the pharyngeal walls. Fluid used to irrigate the TMJ preoperatively can cause extracapsular extravasation leading to partial or complete closure of the airway[16]. Patients who are electively ventilated following oral and maxillofacial surgery should only be extubated when the risk of airway compromise has passed (Table 24.1).

Swelling of the oropharyngeal soft tissues and the floor of the mouth requires careful management of the airway. The swelling may not manifest fully until 12 hours postoperatively and may continue to increase for 48 hours after surgery. Swelling tends to be in the upper airway and not around the laryngeal inlet. Prophylactic dexamethasone is used routinely to minimize swelling of the upper airway in elective cases[17].

Similarly, unilateral radical neck dissection may result in swelling of the lower face and neck on the

Table 24.1 Common criteria for extubation following oral and maxillofacial surgery

Patient can follow and obey verbal commands
No active bleeding from the oral surgical site or drains
No evidence of haematoma adjacent to airway or trachea
No evidence of gross oedema of the tongue
No evidence of excessive of thick secretions in the oropharynx
Sustaining head lift or hand grip for 5 seconds
Evidence of good respiratory effort (respiratory rate of less than 24 breaths/minute and a tidal volume of greater than 5 ml/kg)
Maintaining an oxygen saturation of greater than 95%[15]

ipsilateral side. The oedema reaches a maximum at 1 week and progressively decreases in a few weeks. Bilateral radical neck dissection performed simultaneously with ligation or resection of both internal jugular veins can also result in facial oedema, cerebral oedema, or both. Facial oedema commonly appears in patients with previous irradiation and can lead to chemosis. If bilateral radical neck dissection is required, preserving one external jugular vein can lessen this complication. Staging the neck dissections 4 to 6 weeks apart may also be beneficial[17].

The primary objective in the immediate postoperative period is to maintain pulmonary ventilation and thus prevent hypoxia and hypercapnea. Both can occur if the airway is obstructed and ventilation is reduced. Airway obstruction can be life threatening, partial, or complete, and occur at any level of the respiratory tract from the mouth to the trachea. Recognition of airway obstruction can be achieved by the familiar look, listen, and feel technique.

A talking patient has a patent airway. When there is a complete airway obstruction there are no breath sounds at the mouth or the nose. Paradoxical chest and abdominal movements and the use of accessory muscles of respiration may be evident. Central cyanosis is a very late sign of airway obstruction. In partial airway obstruction air entry is diminished and often noisy. Certain noises[3] such as gurgling (fluid in the mouth or upper airway), snoring (partial pharyngeal obstruction by the tongue), crowing (laryngeal spasm), inspiratory stridor (croaking respirations indicating partial upper airway obstruction), and expiratory wheeze (noisy musical sound caused by turbulent flow of air through narrowed bronchi and bronchioles, more pronounced on expiration), will assist in localizing the level of obstruction[18]. Airway obstruction, left unmanaged, may lead to hypoxia and ultimately death. Principles of basic and advanced airway management skills should be applied in the postoperative maxillofacial patient[3].

Following surgery in the oral and maxillofacial region, airway obstruction may be due to swelling caused by the procedure. When this is deemed likely, an elective tracheostomy is performed to minimize the risk of postoperative airway obstruction[17] (see Chapter 5). Such patients must return to a critical care area or a specialist ward environment competent to deal with tracheostomies[19]. Routine care of an established tracheostomy is a basic ward nursing skill, but unfamiliarity with tracheostomies and the simple rules governing their routine care often leads to anxiety for both patient and carer. Assiduous routine care is not difficult and will avoid almost all emergencies.

The majority of non-traumatized patients who have oral or maxillofacial procedures are at low risk for postoperative respiratory complications, but they still require extensive monitoring during the immediate postoperative period[15].

Ventilatory compromise

Regular assessment of airway patency, respiratory rate and pattern, depth of respiration, symmetry of chest movement, use of accessory muscles, colour of patient and oxygen saturation should be done during emergence and recovery[13,20]. Alterations in respiratory rate are an early and sensitive indicator of a patient's deterioration. Rising respiratory rates are an ominous sign[18]. The rate may slow down appropriately in response to treatment; however, where the underlying problem has not been corrected slowing rates may be indicative of impending respiratory arrest and therefore must be considered in context[18].

Assessment and monitoring of respiratory function during postoperative recovery is a fundamental nursing skill. Measuring oxygen saturation by pulse oximetry has become standard care for all postanaesthetic patients. The rapid detection of low oxygen levels or hypoxaemia is critical to optimize patient outcome[20-22].

It is important to appreciate that various factors can contribute to poor signals from the pulse oximeter and potentially inaccurate readings that could affect ongoing management. These include reduced tissue perfusion, poor peripheral circulation, hypothermia (shivering), poor sensor adherence to the skin, patient movement, and signal dropout problems amongst others[23]. Strong light can affect the photo detector of the probe and cause low oximeter readings[24]. It must also be remembered that oxygen saturation does not provide any information about the adequacy of ventilation. Whilst of great value, pulse oximetry is only an adjunct to the basic clinical nursing observations of the patient's respiratory rate, rhythm, depth, and use of accessory muscles.

Conditions such as hypovolaemia and underlying pulmonary or cardiac disease can affect oxygen transport and thus reduce oxygen saturation[22]. If the patient is unable to meet the body's demand for increased oxygenation in the postoperative period, respiratory failure can occur. This can be assessed by arterial blood gas analysis of pH, partial pressure of oxygen and carbon dioxide, and non-invasive techniques such as end-tidal carbon dioxide monitoring[25].

Respiratory complications

The aetiology of postoperative respiratory complications in maxillofacial patients is multifactorial and ideally those at most risk will have been identified preoperatively[26,27]. Keeping the bed-head elevated assists breathing and the management of oral secretions. Inadequate respiratory drive after routine oral and maxillofacial surgery is often drug related. Ongoing sedation, incomplete reversal of neuromuscular blockade, and pain predispose to hypoventilation. The degree of sedation should be assessed continually by observing the patient's spontaneous awakening, maintenance of the airway when not stimulated, and the ability to follow simple commands[5]. Any patient given a specific antagonist for excessive sedation or hypoventilation such as nalaxone or flumazenil, should be transferred to an appropriate clinical area where more intensive nursing observation can take place. Hypoventilation can reoccur because the half-life of the antagonist is shorter than most opioids or benzodiazepines and their effectiveness diminishes after 60 minutes[15].

Hypoxia and hypoxaemia

Hypoxia in oral and maxillofacial surgery patients is a major concern in the early postoperative period and its incidence is high[15]. An estimated 8% of adults have haemoglobin saturation levels below 90% in the initial stages of postanaesthesia[15]. Adequate oxygenation is dependent on the condition of the lungs, haemoglobin concentration, cardiac output, and oxygen saturation[26]. Pain and shivering can increase oxygen requirements whilst hypotension, hypovolaemia, and severe anaemia can all reduce oxygen availability. Anaesthesia is associated with a mismatch of ventilation and perfusion (V/Q) which can result in atelectasis, a common cause of postoperative hypoxia[28]. Signs and symptoms of hypoxia/hypoxaemia in the postoperative periods are increased respiratory and heart rate, decreased lung expansion, laboured breathing, pallor, or central cyanosis.

Hypoventilation has numerous causes including central nervous system depression, pain, suboptimal positioning, alveolar impairment, and a thick short neck. The body compensates for mild hypoxia by increasing heart and respiratory rates but often attempts at compensation become inadequate. Irreversible damage to major organs of the body can result if left uncorrected[26].

The British Thoracic Society guidelines remind us that oxygen is a treatment for hypoxaemia, not breathlessness. If breathing spontaneously, the patient should receive 15 litres of oxygen through a high concentration oxygen mask with a non-rebreathing reservoir bag during the acute phase of their illness.

Oxygen therapy

All oral and maxillofacial patients require supplemental oxygen for a brief period in the immediate postoperative period but some high-risk patients require oxygen for a longer period. Smokers, patients who have pre-existing pulmonary disease, elderly patients, patients who are morbidly obese, and individuals who have ischaemic heart disease, are all at increase risk of hypoxaemia. Supplemental oxygen should be given postoperatively until they are re-warmed, haemodynamically stable, fully awake, able to sit up and are pain free[29]. Periodic episodes of nocturnal hypoxia, often recurring for up to 72 hours, have been reported following major surgery and anaesthesia. Any swelling around the airway after major oral and maxillofacial surgery may exacerbate these hypoxic episodes in the immediate postoperative period[15].

Oxygen should be prescribed to achieve a target saturation of 94–98% for most acutely ill patients. For those with known hypercapnic respiratory failure a target saturation of 88–92% should be achieved. Oxygen delivery devices and flow rates should be adjusted to keep the saturation at target range and signed for on the drug chart on each drug round[30]. If a patient is transferred back to the ward on oxygen therapy and is not on the target saturation system, the need for ongoing oxygen therapy should be reviewed as soon as possible. If oxygen therapy is to be continued, it should be prescribed using the target saturation scheme unless there is an alternative time-limited instruction. Effective communication is essential.

Postoperative patients should have their oxygen prescribed by the anaesthetist responsible for the case. The instructions should be documented on the anaesthetic record as well as prescribed on the patient's drug chart. The instructions and prescription should be adhered to unless there is a change in the patient's condition. In this situation the doctor reviewing the prescription of oxygen should document clearly in the patients' medical records the reason for this change.

Postoperative aspiration pneumonitis

Aspiration in maxillofacial patients may occur perioperatively because of decreased or absent throat reflexes. Factors which affect postoperative swallowing function after oral and maxillofacial surgery include resections of the base of the tongue, age under 60 years, the type of reconstructive surgery performed, and any history of adjunct radiation therapy.

Gastric juices are highly acidic and very irritating to the lung parenchyma, potentially causing a chemical pneumonitis. Hypoxia results from oedema formation, alveoli collapse, and ventilation perfusion mismatch. Most aspirate is irrigative, but can be infectious if nasopharyngeal or gastric florae are involved[26]. Preoperative administration of antacid or H2 blockers and insertion of a nasogastric tube before induction of anaesthesia can reduce the risk of aspiration pneumonitis[26].

Mild postoperative aspiration may pass unnoticed other than an irritable cough or chest infection. The signs and symptoms of a significant aspiration can include central cyanosis, dyspnoea, gasping, and tachycardia. Without prompt and effective treatment gastric aspiration could cause lung collapse, consolidation, and cardiac instability[8]. Treatment should be instituted immediately by removal of as much aspirate as possible and limiting the spread of what is left in the lung. Continuous monitoring of the respiratory and cardiovascular systems is necessary and prophylactic antibiotics should be considered depending on the circumstances[26].

Normal oropharyngeal swallowing requires coordinated actions of structures of the oral cavity, pharynx, larynx, and upper oesophagus without refluxing into the nasopharynx or penetrating the laryngeal airway. Some or all of these structures and their functions can be temporarily or permanently altered from the surgical management of tumours of the oral cavity and oropharynx. Smith et al.[32] concluded that early swallowing in patients undergoing oral cavity and oropharyngeal resection with free flap construction is significantly affected by a history of radiation therapy and surgical extirpation of more than 50% of the tongue base. Patients with either of these factors are more likely to have difficulty with aspiration during the first 3 months of the postoperative period. It is recommended that patients with these risk factors should be considered candidates for perioperative gastrostomy placement.

During oral and maxillofacial surgical resection for malignancy, the challenge faced is to achieve complete resection margins whilst preserving a functional swallowing mechanism so avoiding postoperative dysphagia and aspiration. Several reconstructive techniques are used to repair tongue defects. Small defects can usually be closed primarily without significant functional loss and with minimal dysphagia. When more than 50% of the tongue base is resected, free flap reconstruction may provide the best swallowing outcomes[33,34] (see Chapter 16). Even with the best reconstructive techniques, significant dysphagia is reported to affect 12–69% of patients with head and neck cancer, 6–9 months after treatment[35]. Severe dysphagia can lead to malnutrition, aspiration pneumonia, and even death[36,37]. Staff nursing such patients should be fully cognisant of this risk.

Laryngospasm and bronchospasm

Laryngospasm is a partial or complete closure of the vocal cords precipitated by local irritation of the vocal cords from gastric contents, blood, secretions, and endotracheal tubes. It is important to perform effective oropharyngeal suction after oral and maxillofacial surgery, particularly in the immediate postoperative period. Laryngospam can occur at any time. Signs and symptoms of laryngospasm include wheezing, stridor, reduced compliance, central cyanosis, and respiratory obstruction[26]. Treatment includes 100% oxygenation with or without applied continuous positive expiratory pressure (CPAP), reassurance, anaesthesia, and tracheal intubation depending on the circumstances. Nebulized saline or epinephrine (1 in 1000) can also be beneficial and may obviate the need for reintubation.

Bronchospasm is smooth muscle contraction that causes narrowing of the lumen in the bronchi and bronchioles. Smokers, patients with asthma or infective or chronic pulmonary disease, and those who aspirate, are more susceptible to bronchospasm. Oxygenation can deteriorate and carbon dioxide elimination hindered because of reduced or possibly absent airflow. Bronchodilators can cause dysrhythmias and are therefore administered with caution with appropriate haemodynamic monitoring. Patients may also be unresponsive to bronchodilators because of a disruption in acid–base balance[26].

Pneumonia

Risk factors for postoperative pneumonia include age, chronic lung disease, and chest surgery. Mechanically ventilated patients are at increased risk because of alterations in normal defence mechanisms such as cough, as are those patients who have had surgery affecting the cough reflex or the cilia lining the respiratory cells. Patients may aspirate microorganisms from the oropharynx[38]. Postoperative physiotherapy and antibiotics as appropriate should be provided for those patients deemed to be at risk.

Venous thromboembolism

Venous thromboembolism (VTE) is the formation of a blood clot in a vein which may dislodge from its site of origin leading to an embolism. Most thrombi occur in the deep veins of the legs and are termed deep vein thrombosis (DVT). Dislodged thrombi may travel to the lungs where a pulmonary embolism (PE) can be fatal[39]. Thrombi can also cause long-term morbidity due to venous insufficiency and post-thrombotic syndrome potentially leading to venous ulceration.

The risk of DVT in all postoperative patients not given prophylaxis is 25% to 30%, increasing to 70% following some specific procedures.

Fortuitously, the incidence of DVT and PE after major oral and maxillofacial surgery is very low. In a study of 130 maxillofacial units over a 5-year period, 64% reported no cases of DVT, and 68% no cases of PE. The study estimates the incidence of VTE as a complication associated with all oral and maxillofacial surgical procedures under general anaesthesia to be from 0.00035% to 0.06%[40].

Risk factors for VTE are numerous and multifactorial and include malignancy, respiratory or heart failure, atrial fibrillation, acute medical illness, obesity, smoking, age over 60 years, travel for more than 3 hours approximately 4 weeks before or after surgery, family history of VTE, use of oral contraceptives or hormonal therapy, immobility, and others[39]. If the patient is sedentary in bed for a prolonged period of time, blood flow to the lower extremities may be decreased by more than 50% resulting in intraoperative venous stasis. Venous thromboembolism is of particular concern in the immediate postoperative phase of surgical intervention[8].

Patients at risk for DVT are classified into three groups: low, moderate, and high risk. For patients at high risk for VTE anticoagulation should be instituted as a preventative measure throughout the perioperative period[41,42]. The use of other modalities such as antiembolism stockings or an intermittent pneumatic compression devices have been proven effective. Those most at risk may merit placement of a vena cava filter[26]. Thromboprophylaxis in patients undergoing major surgery saves lives and reduces healthcare costs. Even though the incidence in oral and maxillofacial patients is low, most patients have identifiable risk factors such as malignancy or trauma. Using the appropriate preventative methods the incidence of VTE and the postphlebitic syndrome can be reduced[41].

There are two foci addressed when looking at DVT prophylaxis: venous stasis and coagulation defects. Venous stasis is treated with intermittent pneumatic compression devices, elastic stockings, and early ambulation in the recovery process[39,43]. Anticoagulation is the mainstay of DVT treatment. The purpose of anticoagulation is to prevent formation of a new thrombus, prevent pulmonary embolism, and allow autogenous circulating thrombolysis to occur[44]. The newest modality for treating DVT is low-molecular-weight heparin[8]. When compared to heparin, low-molecular-weight heparin has many advantages which include longer half-life and 90% bioavailability when injected subcutaneously. The complication profile is also significantly less in relation to thrombocytopenia, recurrent thromboembolism, major bleeding, and mortality. It is also more convenient and cost-effective on account of the single daily dose and absence of the need to monitor its action[44].

Circulatory compromise

Because of the body's physiological response to stress and the inherent risk of haemorrhage and shock with organ hypoperfusion, regular postoperative nursing observations are the cornerstone of safe surgical practice[45,46]. Routine monitoring of pulse, blood pressure, electrocardiogram, capillary refill time, urine output, and temperature should be done during emergence and in the immediate postoperative recovery period[13]—the frequency and duration of any of the observations being determined by the patient's health status and the surgery undertaken.

Hypotension

Postoperative hypotension should be carefully evaluated. Bleeding from the surgical site must always be excluded. If left untreated, or a delay occurs in instituting effective treatment, the patient's condition can rapidly deteriorate and organ failure supervenes. In this respect the brain, heart, and kidney are the most vulnerable organs particularly in the elderly with pre-existing artherosclerotic disease. The most common causes of hypotension in the oral and maxillofacial patient are intravascular volume depletion and excessive peripheral vasodilatation on rewarming in the immediate postoperative period[43]. Other causes of postoperative hypotension include excessive pre-anaesthetic medication, opiate analgesia, sudden changes in patient position, circulatory abnormalities, cerebral or pulmonary embolism, myocardial infarction or ischaemia, anaphylaxis, and hypoxia[46].

It is essential that the hypotensive patient is adequately and closely monitored. The minimum monitoring required includes respiratory rate, non-invasive blood pressure, heart rate, temperature, oxygen saturations, inspired oxygen (FiO2), conscious level, fluid balance and hourly urine output. Observations should be recorded and trends over time reviewed as well as absolute values[18]. Pallor, central cyanosis, clammy skin, cold peripheries, and altered consciousness are ominous signs[46].

The majority of postoperative hypotensive patients require restoration of their circulating blood volume either as a result of volume depletion or to compensate for peripheral vasodilatation. The goal of any treatment is to restore adequate perfusion to the major organ systems. Measures such as providing oxygen and rapid intravenous infusion to increase blood volume should be instituted promptly. Fluid should be titrated in accordance with clinical response and nursing observations.

The primary goal of volume resuscitation is the restoration of oxygen uptake into the vital organs to sustain aerobic metabolism. The major determinants of oxygen uptake are cardiac output and haemoglobin. Blood products do not preferentially enhance blood flow as a result of their increased viscosity. Therefore crystalloid fluid and colloid should be the initial management strategy for volume resuscitation[47]. Ultimately the clinical indicators that are readily observable determine the end parameters of volume resuscitation. A favourable clinical response includes adequate blood pressure and heart rate, urine output of greater than 1 ml/kg/hour and adequate oxygen saturation[47]. In certain situations, where the patient's normal physiological mechanisms have been altered, vasopressors may be considered once the patient has received adequate volume replacement. Vasopressors are designed to cause vasoconstriction of arterioles and veins while promoting myocardial contraction.

Hypertension

The most common reason for postoperative hypertension is a preoperative history of hypertension, fluid overload, pain, gastric or bladder distension[15]. Treatment is aimed at identifying and treating the cause and prevention. Hypertension usually occurs as a result of withdrawal of a long-term hypertensive regimen. The patient should be instructed to continue any antihypertensive therapy right up to the day of surgery. An exception may be angiotensin-converting enzyme (ACE) inhibitors which some anaesthetists prefer to omit on the morning of surgery. Any chronic antihypertensive therapy should be reinstituted as early as possible in the postoperative period. In the case of a hypertensive emergency, or if the patient cannot resume normal oral intake after oral and maxillofacial surgery, parenteral antihypertensive therapy is indicated[43].

A labile blood pressure in the perioperative period might be indicative of undiagnosed hypertension. Severe persistent and uncorrected hypertension can lead to myocardial and cerebral ischaemia

Fluid imbalance

In health, fluid balance is regulated by autoregulatory homeostatic mechanisms. Optimal fluid balance is essential for the normal functioning of all bodily systems[48]. In ill-health, or following surgery there is disturbance to this homeostasis, which the extrinsic or negative feedback mechanism of fluid and electrolyte balance attempt to redress[20].

Postoperative monitoring of the fluid balance following major surgery is essential. Fluid input and output should be closely monitored at least hourly and a cumulative fluid balance recorded. Monitoring patients for signs of fluid loss or gain should also be undertaken. It is important to be aware of the patient's fluid status, current therapies, and to anticipate changes in urine and electrolyte output. Daily measurement of serum sodium, potassium, urea, and creatinine together with 24-hour urine volume are necessary to assess fluid and electrolyte balance[49]. Current fluid balance should be evaluated taking into consideration the preceding day's fluid intake and electrolyte measurements. This will help evaluate the patient's response to fluid administration and will guide the ongoing fluid regimen[49].

Oliguria

Oliguria is common during the immediate postoperative period[17]. This may be a result of the surgical stress response or fluid and blood loss. Insufficient postoperative analgesia also can precipitate acute urinary retention because of the hormonal effects of the stress response[15]. In addition, general anaesthesia causes a decrease in renal blood flow and glomerular filtration rate[15]. The postsurgical effect is temporary and should not last more than 24 hours. The commonest cause of patients who cannot, or have no desire to urinate after 2 to 3 hours postoperatively, is hypovolaemia[15,50]. Renal function and urine production is dependant on an adequate blood flow and perfusion to normally functioning kidneys in the absence of outflow obstruction[18]. In adults, an adequate urine output averages 0.5–1 ml/kg/hour. Urine output of less than 0.5 ml/kg/hour for more than 2 consecutive hours may be indicative of acute renal failure (ARF)[15]. Early recognition, diagnosis, and treatment can reverse potential renal failure which would dramatically increase morbidity and mortality. Indwelling urinary catheters should always be checked for patency when presented with a declining or suddenly absent urine output.

Postoperative oliguria can be categorized as pre renal failure, post renal failure, or acute intrinsic renal failure[18]. Patients with normal kidney function may develop acute renal failure because of reduced renal perfusion, commonly caused by hypovolaemia, dehydration, shock, and sepsis (see Chapter 11). For optimum postoperative renal function, patients need to be haemodynamically stable with a near preoperative baseline blood pressure. If resuscitation is adequate and perfusion is restored promptly, this type of acute renal failure is entirely reversible[18]. Postrenal failure is caused by obstruction to the flow of urine that could be due to a blocked or misplaced catheter, renal calculi, enlarged prostate gland and trauma[18]. Acute intrinsic renal failure refers to the impairment of renal function despite correction of haemodynamic and obstructive factors[15]. Causes include nephrotoxins, glomerular disease, nephritis, rhabdomyolosis renal vascular disease[18], and medications.

The therapeutic goal in oliguria is to prevent the development of acute renal failure by early recognition of the problem and aggressive management of the precipitating cause. Poor perfusion is the commonest cause of renal impairment. Hypovolaemia should be corrected before considering any other treatment options in the postoperative patient with poor urine output[18]. Recent investigations and blood results should be reviewed, with particular attention to the trends of urea, creatinine, and potassium values.

Non-steroidal anti-inflammatory drugs (NSAIDs) can decrease urine output temporarily for a few hours after administration and should not be given to patients who are oliguric, hypotensive, or hypovolaemic. NSAIDs and the selective cyclooxgenases cause prerenal ARF by blocking prostaglandin production, which also alters local glomerular arteriolar perfusion. Patients who have pre-existing renal disease are at greater risk[51].

Temperature imbalance

Hypothermia

Hypothermia is defined as a body temperature less than 36° Celsius (C). Sixty per cent of patients are hypothermic following anaesthesia[52]. The anaesthetized patient with a temperature less than 36°C will recover from anaesthesia more slowly than a warm patient. Ideally the patient should have a body temperature above 36°C before the induction of anaesthesia. Patients lose heat during prolonged surgery and may remain cold thereafter unless active rewarming measures are instituted[15]. Preventative measures to minimize heat loss during and after surgery include maintaining an adequate environmental temperature, providing warm blankets, and minimizing exposure by adequately covering the patient. The use of humidifiers, fluid warmers, and forced air devices should also be considered[53] for any oral and maxillofacial surgery lasting longer than 1 hour to minimize postoperative hypothermia.

Hypothermia causes vasoconstriction, shivering, increased oxygen demand, increased cardiac afterload, discomfort, and exacerbates pain[15]. Shivering may be induced in patients with temperatures less than 36°C. The muscle movements from shivering produce heat, utilize glucose to produce carbon dioxide, and can increase oxygen consumption from 135% to 486% of basal values[15]. Oxygen therapy should be initiated, maintained postoperatively, and its effect constantly evaluated in the postoperative period[52]. Vasoconstriction caused by hypothermia can cause intravascular volume loss and contribute to a fluid shift from the extracellular space. Rewarming causes vasodilation, and the patient may require large amounts of fluid to avoid hypovolaemia[52]. Hypothermia also decreases platelet activity and increases fibrinogen. These two factors combined increase the tendency for postoperative bleeding[52].

Hyperthermia

The postoperative patient's temperature may be elevated as a result of an infectious process, sepsis, or rarely malignant hyperthermia[52], the latter being beyond the scope of this chapter. Postoperative hyperthermia should be categorized into hyperthermia within 48 hours of surgery and hyperthermia occurring after 48 hours[15]. Hyperthermia in the first 48 hours postoperatively is invariably caused by atelectasis. Measures to prevent this include deep breathing, physiotherapy, early ambulation, intermittent positive airway pressure breathing, and adequate pain control. Beyond 48 hours wound infection, urinary tract infection, pneumonia, and infection at transcutaneous catheter sites[15] should all be excluded. The first three being the most frequent[36]. Both peripheral and central intravenous cannulae and intra-arterial lines should be inspected several times a day for signs of sepsis, erythaema, or swelling and the findings documented. If of concern, the line should be removed immediately and the tip set for microbiological culture[54].

Fever can be a response to infection or trauma such as surgery. Sepsis is the systemic inflammatory response resulting from infection. Health professionals must always be alert to a medical cause of sepsis in a surgical patient. The mechanisms and principles of management are the same in both of the above groups. One major difference is that sepsis is commonly a consequence of an operation and is far more likely to be reversible by correcting the source than a medical source of sepsis[54]. It is important to inspect the drains for both quantity of the fluid loss and its consistency. The material should be sent for microbiological culture[54] and blood cultures performed as indicated. Systemic inflammatory response syndrome (SIRS) is the febrile response that occurs after surgery. Sepsis and SIRs in the oral and maxillofacial patient is discussed in Chapter 11.

Wound care

Wounding or injury unleashes a tightly choreographed array of cellular, physiological, biochemical, and molecular processes directed toward restoring the integrity and functional capacity of the damaged tissue. A variety of local and systematic factors can hinder the healing process of orofacial tissue restitution that can adversely affect outcomes[55]. Although attention invariably focuses on local wound care, consideration of systemic factors is important. An understanding of the continuum provides a framework for developing the skills required to care for wounds and facilitate healing[55].

Considerations of wound care are dependant on which part of the maxillofacial structure is involved

and the type of wound whether it be incisions, grafts, or flaps. Because of the variety of surgical procedures that are performed in the oral and maxillofacial region each procedure has its unique wound care requirements[15].

Factors associated with impaired healing can be grouped under local and systematic. Local factors include the presence of foreign bodies, tissue maceration, wound ischaemia, and increased bioburden. Systematic factors include malnutrition, coexisting disease, and advanced age[55]. As people age, the healing process occurs more slowly. The major components of the healing response in aging skin or mucosa are deficient or damaged with progressive injuries[56]. The regional vascular support may be subjected to extrinsic deterioration and systemic disease decompensation resulting in poor perfusion capability[55]. In addition, elderly patients have a greater incidence of chronic conditions including cardiovascular and pulmonary disease and diabetes. Systematic disease frequently compounds the deterioration in the regional vascular support and the restricted tissue perfusion can impair healing. In elderly patients undergoing maxillofacial surgery pre-emptive steps to prevent complicated healing include minimizing extensive stripping of the periosteal and soft tissue envelope[55].

The effects of therapeutic radiation are permanent and related directly to the dose delivered[57] (see Chapter 17). There is an increased incidence of a complicated healing process after surgery or traumatic injury in irradiated tissue. The irradiated site is often relatively hypoxic and as a result, wound dehiscence common and wounds heal slowly or incompletely. Ulceration and colonization by opportunistic bacteria can occur. If patients cannot mount an effective inflammatory response progressive necrosis of the tissues may follow. Healing can be achieved only by excising all non-vital tissue and covering with a well vascularized skin flap[55].

Current wound management focuses on three principles: control or elimination of causative factors, systemic support to reduce existing cofactors, and maintaining a physiologic wound environment. Traditional passive ways of treating wounds have been superseded by approaches that enhance healing beyond its normal maximal inherent rate through the use of growth factors, extracellular matrix components, living skin equivalents, and bioabsorbable collogen scaffolds[55].

The basic principles of wound closure are important in the head, face, and neck where the goal is a mechanically sound wound closure and a cosmetically acceptable scar. All wounds should be rendered as clean as possible, debriding them of non-viable tissue or foreign bodies. Copious saline irrigation may be used to dilute bacterial and other particulate contaminants. Ragged wound margins must be revised[55].

General principles of nursing postoperative wounds are the minimization of bacterial colonization of the wound during the early healing period, the prevention of trauma to the wound and immobilization of the wound edges. In general, facial incisions show no negative effect on healing from exposure. To minimize scarring the early removal of sutures as soon as the wound is robust should be considered. Suture marks must be avoided meticulously. An accumulation of blood or serum around a suture as it passes out of the skin may cause a small stitch abscess so it is important the sutures are cleansed frequently and blood is not allowed to coagulate around them[15].

Intraoral wounds present many challenges because of the need to ingest liquids and solids of a diverse texture and temperature. There is also the presence of a diversity of indigenous oral microorganisms that may cause opportunistic infections (Table 11.1). The primary goal of intraoral wound care is to provide optimal conditions for the natural reparative processes of the wound to proceed. Mouth care and cleanliness is essential to good healing as a clean wound heals better and faster. The need for antibiotics for intraoral wounds is a clinical decision made on the basis of the type of surgery, its potential to become infected, the immune status of the patient, and the health of their organ systems[15].

Skin flap loss

Surgery with and without radiation therapy remains the current standard of care in the treatment of the majority of oral cancers[58]. Microvascular flap reconstruction has proved to be very reliable for repairing defects in the oral cavity and the oropharynx (see Table 16.3). The incidence of flap failure is low, primary wound healing high[59,60], and it facilitates an acceptable aesthetic result in restoring bony and soft tissue contours[60,62,63]. Failure rates are reported between 2–8% with a re-exploration rate of 6–14%[63,64].

Early recognition of vascular compromise in free tissue transfers is essential if re-exploration and salvage of the flap is to be successful[62]. Any risk factors should be made aware to the health professionals nursing the patient in the immediate postoperative period who should remain extra vigilant, particularly within the first 72 hours. The flap should be regularly inspected and the findings documented. The monitoring of, and the physiological parameters necessary to maintain oral and maxillofacial skin flap viability in the postoperative period, is discussed in detail in Chapter 16.

Salivary fistula

Salivary fistula occurs more frequently when a patient has previously had adjuvant radiation therapy and the oral cavity, pharynx, or cervical oesophagus has been opened in association with the neck dissection. The fistula usually appears within 4–5 days postoperatively although they may occur after an interval of up to 2–3 weeks in patients with a history of preoperative irradiation. Fistula may range from a small leak that is well managed by conservative measures, to a large leak that involves infection of the whole neck with flap necrosis. These patients require postoperative enteral or parenteral feeding, controlled exteriorization of the fistula, and local wound care before closure of local skin or myocutaneous flaps formation[17].

Haematoma

A haematoma is a collection of blood, and can occur anywhere where bleeding occurs. The use of suction drains to avoid accumulation of blood under the skin flap and to prevent the formation of haematoma is common practice. Some surgeons use a floppy moderately compressive dressing in addition to the suctioning system. The disadvantage is that compressive dressings leave the flaps unavailable for nursing inspection, which is the best way to watch for the formation of a haematoma. A haematoma is usually evident in the first few hours after the operation. Sudden bleeding in the postoperative period indicates that an untied vessel has opened or that a ligature has slipped from the vessel. Blood under the flap accumulates rapidly.

The treatment of a haematoma comprises re-exploration and opening and elevating the neck flaps and evacuating the haematoma. If the haematoma is recognized and treated early, no adverse consequences occur. However, if the haematoma is found late, airway compromise, infection, or flap necrosis may occur[17]. Early diagnosis is critical and meticulous nursing care and observation in the postoperative period should address this.

Donor site complications

Postoperative nursing observations should also include any flap donor site. The well nursed donor site has few associated complications as it is usually not diseased and undergoes one procedure instead of the comparable two, resection and reconstruction at the recipient site. The donor site is also free from the challenges of respiration, mastication, deglutination, and salivation posed by the upper aerodigestive tract.

Free flap donor site complications usually improve with conservative nursing management and standard wound care. The most common complications are partial split thickness skin graft loss and sensory defects[65]. The role of regional analgesia in providing pain relief at the flap donor site is discussed in Chapter 16.

Wound infection

The incidence of postoperative wound infection following oral and maxillofacial surgery depends on the type of surgery, length of surgery, quality of postoperative nursing care, advanced tumour mass, and the use and timing of prophylactic antibiotics. Additional factors include obesity, diabetes, anaemia, malnutrition, therapeutic steroids, irradiated tissue, chemotherapy, preoperative bronchitis, and prolonged postoperative ventilation[38].

The clinical diagnosis of wound infection is usually made on the basis of presenting signs such as induration, pus, pain, erythaema, a purulent discharge, or heat around the incision[54,55]. Infection can be confirmed by a wound culture greater than 105 organisms per gram of tissue[66].

All wounds, and in particular oral cavity wounds, are contaminated and progression to frank infection can be visualized as a set of scales. The beneficial effects of local wound care and host immunocompetence tip the scale in the direction of healing. Opposing factors include the quantity and nature of the infecting microorganisms and the presence of any potentiating factors such as haematoma, necrotic tissue, and foreign bodies[55]. Other factors that may allow the wound infection continuum to advance after oral surgery include continued tissue trauma from prostheses, avascular bone chips in fractures, or osteotomies and implanted biomaterials[55].

Postoperatively wounds should be inspected on a daily basis. If there is evidence of discharge, metal clips or sutures should be removed aseptically. Poor healing may be the first marker of a lower grade infection. Although wound infections start as localized infections, they do form part of the group of soft tissue infections responsible for 5–10% of all causes of severe sepsis[54]. Wound infection is unlikely when radical neck dissection is performed alone. However radical neck dissection involving the opening of the aerodigestive tract as part of a composite resection or laryngectomy increases the potential for wound infection markedly.

If a wound infection develops, the flap should be opened, cultured, the pus evacuated, and the wound irrigated and necrotic tissue should be carefully debrided. Local wound care with frequent dressing changes, control of any salivary fistula and irrigation of the wound is important. Once the infection is under control and the necrotic tissue removed, healthy granulation tissue should appear[17]. Major resections with the placement of flaps and or grafts require antibiotic prophylaxis[67,68]. A postoperative course is indicated especially if drains are placed and reconstruction of the floor of the mouth is performed[69].

Antimicrobial considerations

Chemotherapeutic management of the microbial milieu that impacts patients undergoing surgery is profoundly important in surgery involving the head and neck region. The region is a repository for a diverse population of microbes which stand ready to invade the underlying structures once the barriers have been infiltrated[69].

Nosocomial infections are a concern in the care of the maxillofacial surgical patient and contribute significantly to patient morbidity and mortality. Pneumonia, urinary tract infections, blood-borne infections, and wound infections are the most commonly seen nosocomial infections[69].

The microbial flora in patients undergoing oral and maxillofacial surgery is intrinsic to that site and is usually considered non-pathogenic. The presence of this intrinsic population of microbes serves several purposes, including decreasing and preventing colonization and invasion of other pathological organisms. The function helps provide a secure and effective defence at the mucosal surface thereby enabling normal local host resistance to infection[69].

The more common organisms that are implicated in infections are Gram-positive cocci and anaerobic Gram-negative rods. For surgery that involves grafts or flaps taken from the lower regions of the body, aerobic

Gram-negative bacilli may also be involved[69]. Factors influencing the pathogenicity of these microbes include saliva, diet, changes in the local micro-environment, and the presence of other microorganisms. Changes in the pH, temperature, flow, and dietary content of the saliva influence the number and type of microorganisms present in the oral cavity and surrounding tissues, which affect how the body responds to infection. Infections may arise when a change occurs in the intrinsic microbial flora.

The mortality rates associated with severe sepsis and septic shock are estimated at 36 800 deaths per year in the United Kingdom alone[70]. The reasons for this high mortality rate are multifactorial[71] and include an increasing elderly population, increase in comorbidities, increasing number of immunocompromised patients, increase in the use of invasive procedures and catheterization, and a lack of early recognition of the problem. Early identification and the speed and appropriateness of treatment administered in the early development of the syndrome is highly likely to influence outcome[70,72,73]. The early administration of antibiotics is crucial. Each hour of delay in administering antibiotics following the recognition of septic shock has been shown to increase mortality by 7.6%[74]. The presentation and management of sepsis is discussed in detail in Chapter 11.

Chylous fistula

Chylous fistula is evident in the postoperative period in approximately 1–2% of patients who undergo neck dissection procedures. Chyle can be identified by the appearance of a milky clouded fluid in the haemovac drains. Chyle accumulation under the flap can cause redness and swelling of the flap with induration of the surrounding tissues. The leak, if minimal, is usually controlled by aspiration and pressure dressings. When the drainage is in excess of 500 ml and conservative management has failed, ligation of the thoracic duct offers the only remedial cure[17].

Nutritional support

Nutritional support in the oral and maxillofacial surgical and critically ill patient has been recognized as one of the critical components in perioperative nursing care. Several studies have delineated the association between degrees of nutritional deficit and poor outcomes in the surgical patient[75]. Malnourished surgical patients have increased risk of morbidity and mortality and can compromise the function of many organs, including the heart, lungs, kidneys, and gastrointestinal tract[76] as well as contributing to a longer hospital stays, higher readmission rates, and healthcare costs[77]. Immune function and muscle strength also are impaired leaving these patients more vulnerable to infection, delayed wound healing, and to a protracted surgical recovery[77].

Major maxillofacial surgery or trauma generates a systemic neuroendocrine stress response characterized by a hypermetabolic catabolic state with increased protein and energy requirements. A redistribution of macronutrients from the labile reserves of adipose tissue and skeletal muscle to more metabolically active tissues, such as the liver, bone, and visceral organs occurs. This response can lead to the onset of protein calorie malnutrition. The rate of development of malnutrition after major surgery is a function of pre-existing nutritional status and degree of hypermetabolism[78].

The goal of nutritional support is to prevent morbidity or mortality by attenuating the induced hypermetabolic response, reduces the rate of infectious complications and maintains the integrity of the gut mucosa[79]. Advanced age, major injury, including maxillofacial surgery, or the presence of comorbidities can markedly deplete the patient's nutritional reserve. Early feeding in such patients is desirable[78].

Postoperatively, it is important to resume enteral feeding as soon as possible. If there are difficulties with swallowing or oropharyngeal wounds, a feeding tube can be an alternative conduit. Total parenteral nutrition may be necessary if the gastrointestinal system must be bypassed[55]. Enteral feeding is often required in many patients after treatment of oral cavity and oropharyngeal cancer[80]. Some studies advocate prophylactic gastrostomy tubes in patients undergoing treatment for head and neck cancers[34,81]. However, enteral feeding is not without its disadvantages. Gillespie and colleagues[82] reported that patients who had been without oral intake for more than 2 weeks had worse swallowing outcomes, possibly owing to swallowing deconditioning, atrophy of pharyngeal musculature, or increased pharyngeal fibrosis. Other studies have reported a substantially decreased quality of life in patients with head and neck cancer receiving enteral feed[82,83].

It would be advantageous to avoid enteral feeding in patients who are able to swallow safely. The difficulty lies in the ability to predict which patients would benefit from a gastrostomy tube placement after free flap reconstruction of oral cavity and oropharyngeal defects[32].

Nausea and vomiting

Postoperative nausea and vomiting (PONV) is a common, distressful, and debilitating occurrence affecting up to 35% patients, many of whom recall it as the most distressing part of their anaesthetic and surgical experience[84]. Surgical factors affecting postoperative nausea and vomiting include surgical site and duration of procedure. Certain patient-specific factors adversely affect the incidence of PONV. These include age, gender, smoking, positive history and motion sickness[44], nitrous oxide, anticholinesterases, and opioids. The last listed are associated with a 4-fold increase in PONV. Inadequate analgesia is another contributory factor. NSAIDs, regional anaesthesia, and liberal infiltration of local anaesthesia all contribute to a decreased need for postoperative opioids, thus reducing the prevalence of PONV. Propofol used for maintenance of anaesthesia has been shown to decrease the incidence of PONV[44].

Patients undergoing surgery of the head and neck or intraoral procedures also may be at higher risk for PONV. Ingestion of blood during and after intraoral or nasal surgery causes vomiting which may raise venous and arterial blood pressure, which in turn may cause bleeding from the surgical sites. The use of a throat pack prevents ingestion of blood although good evidence for their role in minimizing PONV is lacking[17].

Before administering antiemetics it is important to consider if any of the patient's current medication is the precipitant, if it is secondary to swallowed blood, or if an existing nasogastic tube is blocked[15].

The American Society of Anesthesiologists' guidelines[13] recommend that prophylactic antiemetics should be administered to prevent and treat nausea and vomiting. Prophylaxis improves patient comfort and satisfaction, reduces cost and time to discharge[8]. The guidance also recommends that nausea and vomiting be assessed periodically during the emergence and postoperatively, though the literature was insufficient to indicate whether assessment was associated with fewer complications.

Conclusion

Complications occurring in the perioperative period in the oral and maxillofacial surgical process can significantly increase morbidity and mortality and at the very least contribute to a slower return to normal life. The APACHE II score, which is routinely measured in patients on critical care units, may have a predictive value as regards postoperative morbidity and mortality following major maxillofacial oncological surgery by raising awareness of those patients with comorbidities most at risk.

All postoperative complications are not necessarily preventable but by assiduous and meticulous postoperative nursing care, constant assessment, continuous monitoring and early detection of physiological changes, the healthcare team will be alerted to what could ultimately become a major complication in a prompt and timely manner. Early detection, diagnosis, and management may make the treatment of postoperative complications a seamless process.

References

1. Cancer Registration Statistics. (2001) National Statistics Online. Available online at http://www.statistics.gov (accessed 26 May 2009)
2. Grant CA, Dempsey GA, Lowe D, Brown JS, Vaughan ED, Rogers SN. (2007) APACHE II scoring for the prediction of immediate surgical complications in head and neck cancer patients. *Plastic Reconstruc Surg* 119(6), 1751–8.
3. Smith G. (2003) *Acute Life-Threatening Events Recognition and Treatment*, 2nd edn. University of Portsmouth: Learning Media Development.
4. National Confidential Enquiry into Patient Outcome and Death. (2001) *Changing the way that we operate*. London: NCEPOD.
5. Barone CP, Pablo CS, Barone GW. (2004) Postanaesthetic care in the critical care unit. *Crit Care Nurse* 24, 38–45.
6. Hughes S. (2002) The effects of giving patients preoperative information. *Nurs Stand* 16, 33–7.
7. National Institute for Clinical Excellence (2004). *Guidance on Cancer Services: Improving Outcomes in Head and Neck Cancers. The Manual*. Available online at http://www.nice.org.uk (accessed 26 May 2009)
8. Wadlund DL. (2006) Prevention, recognition and management of nursing complications in the intraoperative and postoperative surgical patient. *Nurs Clin N Am*, 41(2), 173–92.
9. Leaper DJ, Peel ALG. (2003) *Handbook of Postoperative Complications*. Oxford: Oxford University Press.
10. Forastiere A. Koch KW. Trotti A. (2001) Head and neck cancer. *N Engl J Med*, 345, 1890–1900.
11. De Melo, GM, Ribeiro KC, Kowalski LP. (2001). Risk factors for postoperative complications in oral cancer and their prognostic implications. *Arch Otolaryngol Head Neck Surg*, 127, 828–33.
12. Smith GB, Poplett N. (2002) Knowledge of aspects of acute care in trainee doctors. *Postgrad Med J*, 78, 335–8.
13. The American Society of Anesthesiologists. (2002). Practice guidelines for postanaestheic care: Report of the

American Society of Anesthesiologists Task Force on postoperative care. *Anesthesiology*, **96**, 742–52

14. McGloin H, Adam SK, Singer M. (1999) Unexpected deaths and referrals to intensive care of patients on general wards. Are some cases potentially unavoidable? *J Roy Coll Phys Lond*, **33**, 255–9.

15. Ogle OE. (2006) Postoperative care of the oral and maxilliofacial surgery patients. *Oral Maxilliofac Surg Clin N Am*, **18**, 49–58.

16. Handler BH, Levin LM. (1993) Postobstructive pulmonary oedema as a sequela to temporomanibular joint arthroscopy – a case report. *J Oral Maxilliofac Surg*, **51**, 315–17.

17. March AR, Pinedo JT. (2007) Radical neck dissection. eMedicine Otolaryngology and Facial Plastic Surgery. Available online at http://emedicine.medscape.com/article/849895 (accessed 26 May 2009).

18. Northwest Critical Care Network (2009) *Acute illness management. Greater Manchester Critical Care Skills Institute.* Available online at http://www.gmcriticalcareskillsinstitute.org.uk (accessed 26 May 2009).

19. The Intensive Care Society. (2008) *Standards for the care of adult patients with a temporary tracheostomy. Standards and guidelines.* London: The Council of the Intensive care Society.

20. Blaylock V, Brinkman M, Carver S, *et al.* (2008) Comparison of finger and forehead oximetry sensors in postanaesthesia care patients. *J Perianaesth Nurs* **23**, 379–86.

21. St. John, R. (2006) Airway and ventilatory management. In: Chulay M, Burns S. (eds) *AACN Essentials of Critical Care Nursing.* New York: McGraw, Hill, pp. 26

22. Clancy J, McVicar A. (2002) *Physiology and Anatomy: A Homeostatic Approach*, 2nd edn. London: Arnold. pp. 44.

23. Durban C, Rostow S. (2002) More reliable oximetry reduces the frequency of arterial blood gas analyses and hastens oxygen weaning. A prospective randomized trial of the clinical impact of a new technology. *Crit Care Med*, **30**, 1735–40.

24. Anderson I. (2003) *Care of the Critically Ill Surgical Patient*, 2nd edn. London: Arnold. pp. 18

25. Capovilla J. (2000) Noninvasive blood gas monitoring. *Crit Care Nurs Q* **23**, 79–86.

26. Phillips N. (2004) *Potential Postoperative Complications*, 10th edn. St, Louis, MO: Mosby, pp. 126

27. Trayner E, Celli BR. (2001) Postoperative pulmonary complications. *Med Clin N Am*, **85**, 1129–39.

28. Xue FS, Huang YG, Tong SY. (1996) A comparative study of early hypoxaemia in infants, children and adults undergoing elective plastic surgery. *Anaesthesia*, **83**, 709–15.

29. Xue FS, Li BW, Zhang GS. (1999) The influence of surgical sites on early post operative hypoxaemia in adults undergoing elective surgery. *Anesth Analg*, **88**, 213–19.

30. British Thoracic Society (2008) *Guideline for Emergency Oxygen Use in Adult Patients.* Available online at http://www.brit-thoracic.org.uk (accessed 26 May 2009).

31. Torrance C, Serginson E. (2000) *Surgical Patient.* London: Balliere, Tindall, pp. 38

32. Smith JE, Suh JD, Erman MA, Nabili V, Chhetri DK, Blackwell KE. (2008) Risk factors predicting aspiration after free flap reconstruction of oral cavity and oropharyngeal defects. *Arch Otolaryngol Head Neck Surg*, **134**, 1205–8.

33. Haughey BH, Taylor SM, Fuller D. (2002) Fasciocutaneous flap reconstruction of the tongue and floor of the mouth: outcomes and techniques. *Arch Otolaryngol Head Neck Surg*, **128**, 1388–95.

34. Hsiao HT, Leu YS, Lin CC. (2002) Primary closure versus radial forearm flap reconstruction after hemiglossectomy: functional assessment of swallowing and speech. *Ann Plast Surg* **49**, 612–16.

35. Nguyen NP, Moltz CC, Frank C. (2006) Evolution of chronic dysphagia following treatment of head and neck cancer. *Oral Oncol*, **42**, 374–80.

36. Mekhail TM, Adelstein DJ, Rybicki LA, Larto MA, Saxton JP, Lavertu P. (2001) Enteral nutrition during the treatment of head and neck carcinoma: Is a percutaneous gastrostomy tube preferable to nasogastric tube? *Cancer*, **91**, 1785–90.

37. Eisbruch A, Lyden T, Bradford CA. (2002) Objective assessment of swallowing dysfunction and aspiration after radiation concurrent with chemotherapy for head and neck cancer. *Int J Radiat Oncol Biol Phys*, **53**, 23–8.

38. Perlino CA. (2001) Postoperative fever. *Med Clin N Am*, **85**, 1129–39.

39. National Institute for Health and Clinical Excellence (2007). *Venous thromboembolism: Reducing the risk of venous thromboembolism (deep vein thrombosis and pulmonary embolism) in inpatients undergoing surgery.* NICE clinical guideline 46. Available online at http://www.nice.org.uk/CG046 (accessed 26 May 2009).

40. Lowry JC. (1995) Thromboembolic disease and thromboprophylaxis in oral and maxilliofacial surgery: experience and practice. *Br J Oral Maxilliofac Surg*, **33**, 101–6.

41. Geerts WH, Heit JA, Clagett GP. (2001) Prevention of thromboembolism. *Chest*, **119**, 132s–75s.

42. Sorathia D. Naik-Tolani, S. Gulrajani R. (2006) Prevention of venous thromboembolism. *Oral Maxilliofac Surg Clin N Am*, **18**, 95–105.

43. Evans D, Read K. (2001) Graduated compression stockings for the prevention of postoperative venous thromboembolism. *Best Prac*, **5.2**, 1–6.

44. Sparks SR, Bergin J. (2004) Deep vein thrombosis. In: Phillips N. (ed) *Berry & Kohn's Operating Room Technique*, 10th edn. St. Louis, MO: Mosby, pp. 955

45. Hughes E. (2004) Principles of postoperative care. *Nurs Stand*, **19**, 43–51.

46. Hodgetts T, Ineson N, Shaikh L. (2004) In-hospital cardiac arrest: Treatment guidelines. Available online at http://www.metproject.org.uk (accessed 26 May 2009).

47. Weitz HH. (2001) postoperative cardiac complications. *Med Clin N Am*, **85**, 1141–54.

48. Watcha MF. (2002) Postoperative nausea and vomiting. *Anaesthesiol Clin N Am*, **20**, 471–84.

49. Giannakopoulos H, Carrasco L, Alabakoff J, Quinn PD. (2006) Fluid and electrolyte management and blood product usage. *Oral Maxilliofac Surg Clin N Am*, **18**, 7–17.

50. Tortora GJ, Grabowski SR. (2003) *Principles of Anatomy and Physiology*, 10th edn. New York: John Wiley & Sons, pp. 1018

51. Jevon P. (2007) *Treating the Critically Ill Patient*. Oxford: Blackwell, Publishing, Oxford, pp. 135

52. Thadhani R, Pascual M, Bonventre JV. (1996) Medical progress: acute renal failure. *N Engl J Med*, **334**, 1448–52.

53. Griffin M.R. Yared A. Ray W.A. (2000) Nonsteroidal anti-inflamatory drugs and acute renal failure. *Am J Epidemiol*, **151**, 488–96.

54. Rothrock JC. (2003) *Alexander's Care of the Patient in Surgery*, 12th edn. St. Louis, MO: Mosby, p. 192

55. Leaper DJ, Peel ALG. (2003) *Handbook of Postoperative Complications*. Oxford: Oxford University Press. p. 34

56. Nutbeam T, Laver K. (2007) *Survive Sepsis: the official training programme of the Surviving Sepsis Campaign*, 1st edn. Birmingham: Good Hope Hospital.

57. Shetty V, Shwartz HC. (2006) Wound healing and perioperative care. *Oral Maxilliofac Surg Clin N Am*, **18**, 107–113.

58. Reed MJ, Koike T, Puolakkainen P. (2003) Wound repair in aging. A review. *Methods Mol Med*, **78**, 217–37.

59. Tibbs MK. (1997) Wound healing following radiation therapy. *Radiotherapy Oncology*, **42**, 99–106.

60. Funk GF, Karnell LH, Robinson RA, Zhen WK, Trask DK, Hoffman HT. (2002) Presentation, treatment, and outcome of oral cavity cancer: a National Cancer Database Report. *Head Neck*, **24**, 165–80.

61. Suh JD, Abemayor EA, Sercarz JS, Calcaterra TC, Rawnsley JD, Blackwell KE. (2004) Analysis of outcome of complications in 400 cases of microvascularhead and neck reconstruction. *Arch Otolaryngol Head Neck Surg*, **130**, 962–6.

62. Abemayor E, Blackwell KE. (2000) reconstruction of soft tissue defects in the oral cavity and oropharynx. *Arch Otolaryngol Head Neck Surg*, **126**, 909–12.

63. Roumanas ED, Garrett N, Blackwell KE. (2006) Masticatory and swallowing threshold performances with conventional and implant supported prostheses after mandibular fibula free flap construction. *J Prosth Dent*, **96**, 289–97.

64. Whitaker IS, Gultati V, Ross GL, Menon A, Ong TK. (2007) Variations in the postoperative management of free tissue transfers to the head and neck in the United Kingdom. *Br J Oral Maxilliofac Surg*, **45**, 16–18.

65. Rogers SN, Kenyon P, Lowe D. (2005) The relation between health related quality of, life, past medical history and American Society of Anaesthesiologists' ASA grade in patients having primary operations for oral and oropharyngeal cancer. *Br J Oral Maxilliofac Surg*, **43**, 134–43.

66. Rosenthal EL, Dixon SF. (2003) Free flap complications: when is, enough, enough? *Otolaryngol Head Neck Surg*, **11**, 236–9.

67. Funk GF, Karnell LH, Whitehead S. (2002) Free tissue transfer versus prediced flap cost in head and neck cancer. *Otolaryngol Head Neck Surg*, **127**, 205–12.

68. Bowler PG. (2003) The 105 bacterial growth guideline: reassessing its clinical relevance in wound healing. *Ost Wound Manag*, **49**, 44–53.

69. Penel N, Fournier C, Roussel-Delvallez, M. (2004) Prognostic significance of wound infections following major head and neck cancer surgery: an open non-comparative prospective study. *Support Care Cancer*, **12**, 634–9.

70. Rodrigo JP, Surez C, Bernaldez R. (2004) Efficicy of piperacillin-tazobactam in the treatment of surgical wound infection after clean-contaminated head and neck oncologic surgery. *Head Neck*, **26**, 823–8.

71. Doonquah L, Doonquah L. (2006) Infection, host, resistance, and antimicrobial management of the surgical patient. *Oral Maxilliofac Surg Clin N Am*, **18**, 173–84.

74. Otero RM. (2006) Early goal directed therapy in severe sepsis and septic shock revisited. *Chest*, **130**, 1579–95.

75. Robson W, Daniels R. (2008) The sepsis six: helping patients to survive sepsis. *Br J Nurs*, **17**, 16–21.

76. López-Hellin, J, Baena-Fustegueras, JA, Shwartz Riera, S. (2002) Usefulness of short lived proteins as nutritional indicators in surgical patients. *Clin Nutr*, **21**, 119–25.

77. Allison SP. (2000) Malnutrition, disease, and, outcome. *Nutrition*, **16**, 590–3.

78. Huckleberry Y. (2004) Nutritional support and the surgical patient. *Am J Health Syst Pharm*, **61**, 671–82.

79. Fang JC, Chirag DN. (2006) Nutritional aspects of care. *Oral Maxilliofac Surg Clin N Am*, **18**, 115–30.

80. Lewis SJ, Egger M, Sylvester PA. (2001) Early enteral feeding versus nil by mouth: systematic review and meta-analysis of controlled trials. *BMJ*, **323**, 773–6.

81. Scolapio JS, Spangler PR, Romano MM, McLaughlin MP, Salassa JR. (2001) Prophylactic placement of gastrostomy feeding tubes before radiotherapy in patients with head and neck cancers: is it worthwhile? *J Clin Gastroenterol*, **33**, 215–17.

82. Gillespie MB, Brodsky MB, Day TA, Lee FS, Martin-Harris, B. (2004) Swallowing related quality of life after head and neck cancer treatment. *Laryngoscope*, **114**, 1362–7.

83. Cheng SS, Terrell JE, Bradford CR. (2006) Variables associated with feeding tube placement in head and neck cancer. *Arch Otolaryngol Head Neck Surg*, **132**, 655–61.

84. Tramer MR. (2001) A rational approach to the control of postoperative nausea and vomiting: evidence from systematic reviews. Part I. Efficacy and harm of antiemetic interventions and methodological issues. *Acta Anaesthesiol Scand*, **45**, 4–13.

Index

Page numbers in *italics* indicate illustrations; those in **bold** indicate tables.

ABC(DEF) primary survey 190, 191–2
abducent nerve 82
accessory nerve (cranial XI) 85–6
N-acetylcystine 197
acute respiratory distress syndrome (ARDS) 147
adenotonsillectomy 308
adjuvant therapy, for head and neck malignancy 225–39
adrenaline (epinephrine)
    as additive to local anaesthetic 133
    high concentrations 91, 97, 100
    in nasal and antral surgery 276
    prefilled cartridges 91, 101
advance decisions 32, 33
aesthetic surgery
    demand for 131
    laser techniques 136–41
    patient profile 132
    preoperative anaesthetic considerations 133–4
    psychological issues 132
age, as risk factor 14
    see also elderly patients
airway
    accidental disconnections 276
    anatomy *50*
    assessment 35–7
    in burn patients 191, 195–7, 200
    choice 124–5, 254
    difficult 35–48, 122, 220–1
    infection 145–6
    injuries 178
    maintaining 44–6
    obstruction 115, 212, 313
    in orthognathic surgery 241–2
    in paediatric patients 121, 254, 262
    postoperative compromise 312–13
    preoperative assessment 183, 211–12

surgical 44, 46, 49–63
    thermal damage 195–7
airway management
    emergency 178–80
    in head and neck cancer 213–14
    for oral and maxillofacial surgery 38–40
    outpatient vs inpatient 46
    in paediatric patients 121, 254
    in patients with learning disabilities 122
    in patients with previous surgery 220–2
Akinosi–Vazirani method 95–6, 99
alcohol
    abuse **105**, 207, 211, 212, 233
    and cluster headache 287
    during radiotherapy 233
    intoxication in burn patients 191
allergy
    to benzodiazepines 107, 109
    to local anaesthetics 100, 132
alternative therapies, in TMD pain 292–3
alveolar bone 168
    graft 259–60
alveolar osteitis 285
ambulatory respiratory studies 304–5
amifostine 235
AMPLE history 192
anaemia 18–19, **104**
anaesthesia
    for aesthetic surgery 131–41
    for burn excision and grafting 200–2
    for burn patients 201
    coining of term 3
    for craniofacial surgery 262–3
    for dental surgery 119–30
    elective or semi-urgent 183
    for emergency tracheostomy 61–2
    for facial laser procedures 140
    failure 97–8
    for head and neck surgery 207–24
    hypotensive techniques *see* hypotensive anaesthesia
    maintenance 184–5

for maxillofacial trauma 177–87
    as medical specialism 8
    for minor procedures 264–5
    for nasal and antral surgery 275–82
    for orthognathic surgery 241–52
    for paediatric maxillofacial surgery 253–68
    in patients with previous surgery 220–2
    for pharyngoplasty 259
    for preoperative imaging 264
    for tumour resection and reconstruction 211–14
anaesthetists, in dental surgery 120
analgesia
    after dental surgery 127
    after orthognathic surgery 244
    in head and neck surgery 218
    in nasal and antral surgery 277
    for paediatric patients 256, 258
    World Health Organization (WHO) ladder 234
anatomical variations 98, 156, 306
    see also syndromic craniofacial abnormalities
angina **104**
Angle's classification 156
animal bites 185
ansa cervicalis 88
    upper root 86
anterior ethmoidal nerve 75, 80
anterior middle superior alveolar nerve block 93–4
anterior superior alveolar nerve block 93
anterograde amnesia 109
antibiotic prophylaxis
    in infective endocarditis 122, 148–9
    in maxillofacial surgery 148–9
    in paediatric patients 254–5
anticholinergics, premedication 253
anticonvulsants, for trigeminal neuralgia 290

antiemesis 243–4, 276
see also postoperative nausea and vomiting
antihypertensive drugs 12
antimicrobial therapy 144, 321–2
antiplatelet agents 12
antipsychotics **105**
antithrombotic prophylaxis 243
antral surgery 275
anxiolysis 109, 123–4
anxious/phobic patients 103, 111, 112, 120
signs and symptoms of anxiety **104**
treatment planning 105–6
APACHE II score 312, 323
Apert's syndrome *see* syndromic craniofacial abnormalities
apical pain 285
asphyxiation anaesthesia 2
aspiration pneumonitis 315
aspirin 12, 16, 154, 219, 288, 289
sensitivity 280
asthma 14, **104**
atropine 253
auricular branch of the vagus nerve 85
auriculotemporal nerve 66, *66*, 69

balloon sinusotomy 280
Beckwith–Weidemann syndrome 265
Bennett shift 36
benzodiazepines 106–7, 114
beta-blockade 27, 269, 270
bicarbonate
as additive to local anaesthetic 132–3
in smoke injury 197–8
Bigelow, Henry J. 3
bilateral sagittal split mandibular ramus osteotomy (BSSO) 245–6
bimaxillary osteotomy 246, 260
biofeedback 287, 289, 293
birthmarks, removal 141
bisphosphonates 237
bleeding disorders, preoperative assessment 19–20
bleeding/blood loss
in burn patients 200
from maxillofacial trauma 180
in nasal and antral surgery 276, 277
risk 19
blepharoplasty, anaesthetic considerations 134
blood conservation
in craniofacial surgery 263
in maxillofacial surgery 271
in orthognathic surgery 243
strategies 215, **216**
blood pressure
historical aspects 269
monitoring 192, 202
see also hypotensive anaesthesia

blood transfusion 19, 198, 200, 215, 271, 272, 311
blow out fracture 174–5
blunt trauma *see* maxillofacial trauma, blunt
body mass index 109, 121
Bolam test of negligence 28, 29
bone grafts 248
donor sites 259–60, 261
Boott, Francis 3
botox injections 141
Boyle's machine 7, 8, 113
brachial plexus 88–9
brachycardia, reflex 184–5
brachytherapy 227–8
brain, anatomical protection 167, 171, 177, *178*
breathing, in burn patients 191
breathing disorders *see* respiratory disorders
breathing tubes, extendable 45
bronchospasm 315
brow lift, anaesthetic considerations 134
buccal branch of facial nerve 76–7
buccal branch of mandibular nerve 66, 69
buccal infiltration technique 91, 99
buccal nerve 66, 78
burn patients
long-term management 202–3
monitoring 192, 201–2
other injuries 190
physical examination 192
psychological care 202
Burn Unit, referral and transfer 192, **193**
burning mouth syndrome 283, 284, 293
burns
early debridement 199–200
epidemiology 189–90
treatment 192

CAD/CAM modelling 166, *167*
calcium channel blockers 18, **286**, 287
Caldwell's view 169
capacity *see* competence
capnography, in burn patients 202
carbon dioxide, asphyxiation anaesthesia 2
carbon monoxide, toxicity 194–5
cardiac arrhythmias 126
cardiac disorders
infective endocarditis 148
medical management 16
in patients with learning disabilities 122
preoperative assessment 14–18
cardiac function, non-invasive tests **15**

cardiac output monitoring 202
cardiac risk stratification 15–16
cardiorespiratory disease, severe **105**
carotid blowout syndrome (carotid artery rupture) 222, 237
carotid branches of the glossopharyngeal nerve 84
causation 29
cavernous sinus thrombosis 145
cell salvage, in cancer surgery 216
central venous pressure 147
cerebral circulation, autoregulation 270
cerebral haematoma 177
cerebrospinal fluid leaks 182–3
cervical nerve 77
cervical plexus 87–8
cervical spine
control/stabilization 178, 191
injuries/suspected injuries 43, 47, 177, 178, 180
cervical sympathetic trunk 86–7
cetuximab 231
CHARGE syndrome 278
cheeks, sensory innervation 78
chemoradiotherapy 226, 227, 231–3
chemotherapy 226, 230–1
children *see* paediatric patients
chin, aesthetic considerations 246–7
chloroform, 19th-century use 4, 5
choanal atresia 278–9
chorda tympani branch of the facial nerve 70
chronic airways disease **104**
chronic obstructive pulmonary disease (COPD) 14, 314
chylous fistula 322
ciliary ganglion 82
circulatory compromise
in burn patients 191
postoperative 316–17
circulatory support, in odontogenic infection 147
civil law 27
cleft lip/palate 241, 253, **254**
surgery 248, 256–8, 306
Clover, Joseph 5–6
cocaine 7, 134, 276–7
Coleman, Alfred 5
Colton, Gardner Quincy 2, 5
combustion, toxic products 197
common law 27
communication problems 122, 123
comorbidities
in cancer patients 212–13
in head and neck cancer 311
in odontogenic infection 144, 146
in paediatric patients 121
competence, and consent 30–2
compressed gas cylinders 5
cone beam CT 165, *175*, 176

conscious sedation 103–17
  clinical procedure 109–10
  complications 114–16
  definition 103
  discharge procedures 110
  for facial aesthetic procedures 133
  failure 116, 121
  paediatric patients 114, 115
  patient instructions **106**
  venous access 109
consent
  for conscious sedation 106, 109
  forms 29
  for general anaesthesia 122–3
  for hypotensive anaesthesia 271
  legal aspects 29–34
continuous positive airway pressure
    (CPAP), and obstructive sleep
    apnoea 307–8
continuous venovenous
    haemofiltration 148
coronary revascularization 16
coroner's clot 243
coronoidectomy 250, 251
cosmetic surgery *see* aesthetic surgery
costochondral rib grafts 261
court of protection 34
craniofacial anatomy 65, 166–7
  abnormal 156
craniofacial dysjunction 171
craniofacial dysostosis 256
craniofacial procedures 261–4
craniofacial resection, for maxillofacial
    tumours 222
craniosynostosis 253, 261
  phased procedures **263**
cricothyroid membrane, anatomy
    49, *50*
cricothyroidotomy kits 53
criminal law 27
Crouzon's syndrome *see* syndromic
    craniofacial abnormalities
CT
  cone beam 165, *175*, 176
  for facial fractures 171–2, *175*
  techniques 165, *166*
curare 8
cyanide toxicity 195
cyclizine 127

Davy, Humphry 1–2
day case surgery 18, 35, 43, 46, 123,
    126, 275, 281
  see also outpatient procedures
daytime sleepiness 301, 302
decannulation 60
decayed, missing, or filled teeth
    (DMFT) scores 120
deep temporal nerves 69
deep vein thrombosis (DVT) 316
dental abscess 144, 146, 147, 264

dental anaesthesia
  choice 126
  fatalities 9
  history 1–10
  personnel 120
  postoperative complications 127–8
  risks 9
  safety 119
  standards 119, 120
dental anatomy 151–2, 167–8
dental caries
  in drug abusers 155
  microbiology 144
  in paediatric patients 121
  predisposition to dental injury 153,
    154, 158
  prevalence 143, 144, 284
  radiation-related 236, 237
dental cysts 144
dental damage *see* dental injury
dental examination, in anxious/phobic
    patients 105
dental history 105, 120
dental imaging, specialist area 165
dental implants 170, 248
dental injury
  classification 157, 158
  during anaesthesia 151, 167, 237
  immediate management 158–9
  predisposing factors 153–4
  prevention 157–9
  protective strategies 152
dental nomenclature 151, 168, *169*
dental pain, acute 284
dental panoramic tomogram (DPT)
    165, *166*
dental prostheses
  damage during anaesthesia 156–7,
    159, 167
  imaging 170
dental pulpitis ('toothache') 284
dental surgery
  anaesthesia 119–30
  in anxious/phobic patients 103
  in paediatric patients with cleft or
    craniofacial conditions 264
  patient positioning 124
dental/oral disorders
  and anaesthesia-related injury 153–4
  epidemiology 144
  pathophysiology 143–4
dentists, training in anaesthesia 6–7, 9
dentoalveolar surgery 247–8
dentoalveolar trauma, imaging 170
depression
  in head and neck cancer
    patients 237
  in patients with orofacial pain 283,
    287, 292, 294
dermabrasion 136
desflurane 214
dexamethasone 127, 128, 244, 256
dexmeditomodine 39

diabetes
  contraindication for beta-blockers 287
  contraindication for free flap
    transfer 211
  and hypertension 17
  neuropathy 290, 291
  and obstructive sleep apnoea 307
  predisposition to dental injury 154
  predisposition to dental/gingival
    disease 20
  predispostion to aspiration 18
  preoperative assessment **13**, 20, 271
  risk factor for ischaemic heart
    disease 15, 16
  sedation **104**
  and wound care 319, 321
diclofenac 127
diffusion hypoxia 112–13
digastric nerve 75
digestive tract *see* gastrointestinal tract
disinhibition, under sedation 115
distraction osteogenesis 247, 263–4
diuretics 13
docetaxel **232**
dog bites 185
donor site, pain/complications 218,
    248, 259–60, 321
Down's syndrome 122, 306
drug abuse/misuse
  and conscious sedation **105**
  high risk patients 148
  and periodontal disease 155
drug intoxication, in burn
    patients 191
dural tears 182–3
dysphagia 233–4, 315

Eisenmenger's syndrome 122
elderly patients
  burns 190
  midazolam sedation 110
  preoperative assessment 22–3
  risk of dental injury 155–6
  sedation 104–5
electrical nerve stimulator 47
electrocardiogram, in burn patients
    192, 202
Emergency Management of Severe
    Burns (EMBS) course 189
emotional problems *see* psychiatric
    problems
enamel microfractures 151
endocarditis, infective 122, 148–9
endodontic surgery, postoperative
    pain 285
endotracheal intubation
  direct laryngoscopy 35
  historical aspects 7–8
  indication 124
  oral, in emergency situation 178
endotracheal tube tree 45

enteral feeding, postoperative
    resumption 322
epidermal growth factor receptor
    inhibitors 231
epidural analgesia
    for donor site pain 218, 248
    see also regional anaesthesia
epilepsy **104**, 108, 112, 121, 200
epinephrine see adrenaline
epistaxis 19, 161, 279–80
Epworth sleepiness scale 302–3
ergotamine 286, 287
escharotomy 191, 192
ether, early use 1, 2–3
ethical considerations
    in hypotensive anaesthesia 272
    see also consent
ethyl chloride 7
Evans, T. W. 5
external beam radiotherapy
    (EBRT) 227
external nasal nerve 66, 67
extraoral approach
    in regional anaesthesia 93
    to the mandibular nerve 94
extubation
    accidental 45, 184, 258, **263**, 276
    after head and neck resections 218–19
    after open meniscal surgery/
      arthrotomy 250
    after rhinoplasty 135
    appropriateness 312
    in burn patients 198, **199**
    and choice of anaesthetic agents
      215, 243
    criteria **312**
    injuries 152
    in nasal and antral surgery 277
    in orthognathic surgery 243
    in paediatric patients 258
    in patients with sepsis 147
    strategies 185
eye
    injuries during surgery 162
    injuries in road traffic accidents 177
    protection during surgery 243, 276

face
    aesthetic procedures 131
    anatomy see craniofacial anatomy
    burns 189–205
    disfigurement 177, 202, 237
    innervation 65–7
    laser resurfacing 140
facelift, surgical 135
facial fractures
    aetiology 177
    and airway obstruction 47
    bleeding 180
    postoperative care 185
    tracheostomy 178–9
    types 170–2

facial nerve (cranial VII)
    anatomy 47, 65, 75–7
    branches 75–7
    monitoring 220
facial oedema 312–13
facial pain see orofacial pain
facial skeleton
    bony buttresses 167
    imaging 169
facial trauma see maxillofacial trauma
fasting
    in paediatric patients 121, 124, 253
    preoperative 18, 61, 242
fentanyl 108, 112, 126, 218, 277
fibreoptic bronchoscopy, flexible 40
fibreoptic devices, emergency airways
    178, 179
fibreoptic endoscopic evaluation of
    swallowing (FEES) 233
fibreoptic intubation
    asleep 61
    awake 61, 147, 203, 213, 214, 219,
      221, 222, 254
fibrosis, in head and neck
    radiotherapy 235
First World War, influence on
    anaesthesia 7
flamazine ointment 235
flaps
    coronal 183, *184*
    free 210–11
    harvesting 215–16
    loss 320
    microcirculatory perfusion 216,
      217–18
    pedicled 209–10
    perfusion monitoring 219–20
floor of the mouth, sensory
    innervation 79
flow-related perfusion 270
fluid balance 263, 317
fluid management 216–17, 255
fluid resuscitation 191–2
flumazenil 107, 111, 114, 115, 314
5-fluorouracil 230, **231**
foreign body
    inhalation 168, 170
    in the nose 278
fractionation regimens 229
frontal nerve 75
frontal sinuses, imaging 170
frontocranial remodelling 262
Frost, Eben 2
functional endoscopic sinus
    surgery 280
fungal infections 235

GABA (gamma-aminobutyric acid)
    system 106
ganglionic branches, from the maxillary
    nerve 71

gas, nasal delivery 5
gaseous toxins, systemic 194
gastrointestinal disorders 18, 122
gastro-oesophageal reflux disease 124
general anaesthesia
    avoidance 9
    clinical setting 123
    and dental injuries 151–64
    in dentistry 119–30
    equipment and drugs 123
    for facial aesthetic procedures 131–2,
      133–4
    GDC guidance 119
    indications 120–1
    referral 120
    repeat attendance 120
genioplasty *244*, 246–7
gingivae
    contusions 159
    hypertrophy 154, 265
    innervation 77
    pain 284–5
gingivitis 20, 143, 144, 153, **155**, 284
Glasgow Coma Score 179
glossopharyngeal nerve (cranial IX)
    79, 84
glossopharyngeal neuralgia 291
glycaemic control 148
glycopyrrolate 253
Goldenhar syndrome **257**
Goldman, Victor 9
Gow–Gates method 96, 99
great auricular nerve 67, 83
greater (anterior) palatine nerve 73,
    79, 81
    block 94
Guedel airway 277, 279, 280
Guerin fracture 171
gunshot wounds 177, *179*, 180, 185–6

haematological disorders
    preoperative assessment 18–20
    see also bleeding disorders
haematoma
    and airway comprompise 38, 50
    in bleeding disorders 19
    caused by laryngoscopy 159
    cerebral 177
    in facial trauma 47, 171, 179, 180, 291
    postoperative 218, 243, 246, 320
    septal 174, 279
    sign of vascular injury 178
haemodilution, in flap perfusion
    216–17
haemothorax 191
Hagen–Poiseuille law 211
halothane
    and cardiac arrhythmias 126
    hepatitis 201
    historical aspects 9, 269
    vs other volatile agents 126, 201, 215,
     270, 276

Halstead approach 95
head and neck, innervation 65–89
head and neck cancer
    adjuvant therapy 225–39
    airway management 46–7, 213–14
    airway obstruction 211–12
    analgesia 218
    anatomical distribution *208*
    comorbidities 212–13, 311
    extubation 218–19
    histopathology **208**
    management options 207–11
    non-surgical vs surgical treatment
        226–7
    oromaxillofacial tumours 176
    pain management 234
    pathology 207
    postoperative care 219–20, 311–12
    preoperative assessment 22
    radiotherapy and chemotherapy
        225–6
    risk of OSA 306
    staging 207, **209**
    surgical management 208–11
    treatment, sequelae **221**
head and neck injuries, assessment and
    triage 177–8
head and neck innervation,
    variability 89
head and neck surgery
    access and monitoring 214
    airway management 46–7
    anaesthetic agents 214
    microvascular anastomosis 216
    patient positioning 214
    postoperative analgesia 218
    postoperative care 219–20
    reconstruction following tumour
        resection 209–11
    tracheostomy 214
    tumour resection/flap harvesting
        215–16
head wrap *45*
headaches
    chronic 289, 294
    cluster 287–8
    diagnostic algorithm *288*, 289
    stabbing 289
    tension-type 288–9
    see also migraine
healing, impaired 319
heart failure 16–17, **104**
    see also cardiac disorders
hemifacial paresis 100
heparin 13, **19**, 197, 219, 316
hepatic disease *see* liver disorders
Hepworth *v* Kerr 272
herpes infection, reactivation 100
herpes zoster infection 291
Hewitt, Sir Frederic 6–7
hiccups 116
Hickman, Henry Hill 2
history-taking, importance 14

hoarseness
    in airway injury 47, 178, 196
    in inhalational injury 193
    postoperative 159–60
    recent changes 212
Holmes, Oliver Wendell 3
human papilloma virus 207
hyaluronidase, as additive to local
    anaesthetic 133
5-hydroxytryptamine receptor agonists
    286, 288
hyperactivity 124
hypertension
    postoperative 317
    preoperative assessment 17
    and sedation **104**
    see also blood pressure
hyperthermia, postoperative 318–19
hypoglossal nerve (cranial XII) 86
    branches from the cervical plexus 88
hypotension
    caused by sedative drugs 116
    contraindications 271
    deliberate 269
    historical aspects 269
    postoperative 316–17
hypotensive anaesthesia 269–73, 277
hypothermia 191, 318
hypothyroidism, and obstructive sleep
    apnoea 307
hypoxaemia, postoperative 314
hypoxia 194, 230, 314

imaging
    oral and maxillofacial 165–76
    in pain management 234
    under anaesthesia 264
incisive nerve, block 96–7
incisors, vulnerable to damage 152–3
independent mental capacity advocates
    (IMCAs) 33–4, 123
induction
    asleep 213
    inhalational 61, 62, **106**, 201, 219,
        220–1, 222, 253, 254, 258, 260,
        262, 278, 279
    intramuscular 126
    intravenous 60, 61, 134, 135, 140
    intravenous vs gaseous 126
    nitrous oxide 5, 108
    in paediatric patients 253, 254, 258,
        259, 260, 262
    personnel 179
    rapid sequence 180, **199**, 201, 278
    soft tissue injuries 160
induction chemotherapy 226, 230, **232**
infections
    airway compromise 145–6
    and anaesthesia 143–9
    and imaging 176
    intracranial 171
    noscomial 321

odontogenic 144–7
oral cavity 143
transmission 148
infective endocarditis *see* endocarditis,
    infective
inferior alveolar and lingual nerve
    block 94–6
inferior alveolar nerve 70, 77–8
inferior cervical ganglion 87
infiltration anaesthesia 91
inflammation 98, 99
information, and consent 29–30
infraorbital nerve 66–7, *66*, 72, 81
    block 93
infratrochlear nerve 66, 67, 75
inhalational anaesthesia
    in paediatric patients 254
    see also induction, inhalational
inhalational injury 189–90, 192–5,
    197–9, **198**
inhalational sedation **106**, 112–14
injection pain 99
injection problems, with
    midazolam 115
inotropes 17, 21, 192, 215, 218
intensity modulated radiotherapy
    (IMRT) 226, 228–9
intensive care therapy, for burns 199
intermaxillary fixation, postoperative
    care 260
intermittent positive pressure
    ventilation (IPPV) 111
internal carotid plexus 87
intracranial effects, of local
    anaesthesia 99
intracranial injuries 179
intracranial pressure 184, 222, **262**, 263
intraligamentary anaesthesia 97
intranasal sedation 111, 114
intraocular tumours, local
    resection 271
intraoperative intermaxillary fixation
    (IMF) 183
intraoral anaesthesia, specialized
    techniques 97
intraosseous anaesthesia 97, *98*
intrapulpal anaesthesia 97, *98*
intravascular injection, inadvertent 99
intravenous anaesthesia 8, 184
    see also total intravenous anaesthesia
intubation
    asleep 41
    awake 39, 40
    emergency room procedures 179–80
    in facial trauma 183–5
    failed 49
    oral 38
    in paediatric patients 254
    retrograde 44, 47
    in smoke inhalation 198
    submental 184, *185*
    in thermal oropharyngeal injury 196

iridium 227, *228*
ischaemic heart disease 15
  see also cardiac disorders
isoflurane 214, 215, 270, 271

jabs and jolts syndrome 289
jet ventilation 51, 179, 219, 221, 222
Johnson, Bernard 8

ketamine 126, 234
Koller, Carl 7

lacrimal nerve *66*, 67, 74–5
  branch *66*
lactose intolerance 121
Laplace's law 211
larygeal angle 35–6
laryngeal mask airway
  in dental/oral procedures 125
  flexible 42–3
  introduction 9
  in nasal and paranasal surgery 276
  in paediatric patients 254, 264
  in percutaneous tracheostomy 56
  in rhinoplasty 135
  use in emergency 179
laryngeal trauma 47, 178, 180
laryngoscopy
  dental or soft tissue trauma 152–3
  direct 35, 36, 37, 38
  video-assisted 43–4
laryngospasm 315
larynx, mobility 37
laser techniques
  in aesthetic surgery 136–41
  postoperative pain 140
  safety aspects 138–9
  in sinonasal surgery 280
lasting power of attorney 32–3, 34
lateral facial view 169
laughing gas *see* nitrous oxide
Le Fort fractures 47, 171–2
Le Fort I osteotomy 244–5, 260
Le Fort II osteotomy 248–9
Le Fort III osteotomy 248–9, 263–4
left recurrent laryngeal nerve 85
lesser occipital nerve 83
lesser petrosal nerve 84
lesser (posterior) palatine nerve 73, 79
levobupivacaine 256, 260, 261
lidocaine
  in awake procedures 39, 222
  historical aspects 7, 8, 9
  infiltration 91
  for injection pain 108
  in laser techniqes 140
  nerve damage 100
  pharmacology 132, **278**
  topical 39, 40, 99

lignocaine *see* lidocaine
lingual branches of the
    glossopharyngeal nerve 84
lingual infiltration technique 91, 99
lingual nerve 69–70, 79
  block 94–6
  damage 100
liposuction of face 135
lips
  anaesthetic related injuries 159
  sensory innervation 78
Liston, Robert 3
Little's area 161, 279
liver disorders 21–2, **105**
living wills *see* advance decisions
local anaesthesia
  for awake intubation 39
  complications 97–101
  during general anaesthesia 91
  for facial aesthetic procedures 131,
    132–3
  historical aspects 7
  for nasal and antral surgery 277–8
  for paediatric patients 256
local anaesthetics, chemical/
    pharmacological properties 132–3
Long, Crawford Williamson 2
long buccal nerve block 97
Ludwig's angina 145, 146
lungs, 'smoke' injury 197–9

McConnell, William 8
Macintosh, Professor Sir R. R. 8
McKesson, E. I. 8
macroglossia 159, 160, 265, 306
Magill, Ivan 7
major tranquillizers **105**
Mallampati classification 37–8
malocclusion 156, 241, 250
mandible
  movements 36
  trauma 175–6
mandibular distraction 260, *261*
mandibular fractures 183, 185
mandibular hypoplasia 247
mandibular nerve 65, 77
  anatomy 67, *68*
  branches 68–70
  cutaneous branches *66*
  regional anaesthetic techniques 94–7
mandibular osteotomy 242, 243, *244*,
    245–6
mandibular reduction 260
mask ventilation 35
masseteric nerve 68
mastoid air cells 167
maxillary advancement *see* Le Fort I
    osteotomy
maxillary division of the trigeminal
    nerve, blocks **92**

maxillary molar nerve block 93
maxillary nerve 65, 71–3, 80, 82
  cutaneous branches 66–7
  regional anaesthetic techniques 92–4
maxillary osteotomy *see* Le Fort I
    osteotomy
maxillary sinusitis 144, 285
maxillofacial anatomy *see* craniofacial
    anatomy
maxillofacial local anaesthesia,
    complications 97–101
maxillofacial surgery
  antibiotic prophylaxis 148–9
  in high risk patients 148
  hypotensive techniques *see*
    hypotensive anaesthesia
  paediatric 253–68
  postoperative nursing 311–25
  risk of OSA 306
maxillofacial trauma
  aetiology 177
  airway problems 47, 179
  anaesthesia 177–87
  blunt 180
  fracture repair 183
  and obstructive sleep apnoea 307
  in paediatric patients 265
  penetrating 180–1
  preoperative assessment 23
Mayfair Gas Company 8
mediastinitis 145
medical history, prior to sedation
    103–4
medication
  continuing or stopping 12
  and dental disease 154–5
  overuse headaches 289
meningeal branch(es)
  of the hypoglossal nerve 86
  of the mandibular nerve 68
  of the vagus nerve 85
meningeal nerve 71
Mental Capacity Act 2005 27, 30–2,
    34, 123
mental nerve *66*
  block 96–7
methadone 148, 155
methohexitone 9
methotrexate 231, **232**
microarousals 301, 302
microcirculation, physiology 211
micrognathia 22, 257, 258, 260,
    261, 306
midazolam
  anterograde amnesia 107, 109
  contraindications 109
  intravenous 103, **106**, 108–10
  with opioid 111–12
  oral/intranasal 111, 114
  for paediatric patients 114, 115, 253
  paradoxical effects 115
  prolonged recovery 115–16

respiratory depression 106, 111, 112, 115
for sedation **104**, **106**, 108–10, 111, 114
titration regime 110
middle cervical ganglion 87
midfacial advancement 248, 263–4
migraine 285–7
migraine in primary care (MIPCA) questionnaire 289
Minnesota Multiphasic Personality Inventory (MMPI) 295
mivacurium 126
Moffett's solution 134, 276
Morton, William 2–3
mouth opening, limited *213*, 219, 220, 221, **221**, 236, 260
mouthguards 159
movement disorders **104**
MRI 165, 169
mucosa, protecting 235
mucosal atomization device (MAD) 111
mucositis 234–5
multidisciplinary team management 22, 202, 208, 225, 241, 248, 253, 256, 262, 283, 292, 294
muscle relaxants
benzidiazepines 107
for burn patients 201
in facial surgery 135, 220
in general anaesthesia 62
historical 8
for intubation 126
non-depolarizing 27, 201
reduced requirement 276
in temporomandibular disorders 293
in tension-type headaches 288
in tracheostomy 56, 60
muscles of facial expression 65, 75
muscular branches of the hypoglossal nerve 86
mylohyoid nerve 70
myocardial circulation, hypotension 270

naloxone (Narcan) 108
nasal airways 42, 275
nasal bleeding *see* epistaxis
nasal cavity, innervation 80
nasal endoscopy, awake 212, 221
nasal fractures 174, 177, 279
nasal intubation
advantages and disadvantages **184**
allows surgical access 38, 125
blind 40–1
contraindications 264
in orthognathic surgery 242
nasal packs 275
nasal polyps 161, 162, 275, 280
nasal reconstruction, historical 131
nasal septal haematomas 174, 279

nasal surgery 275
nasociliary nerve 75
nasoethmoidal injury 174
naso-maxillary buttress 167
nasopalatine nerve 73, 79, 81
block 94
nasopharyngeal angiofibroma 281
nasopharyngeal 'prong' 255
nasotracheal intubation, associated injuries 161–2
National Health Service (NHS), introduction 8
nausea and vomiting *see* postoperative nausea and vomiting
nebulizer regimens 197
neck
contractures 203
dissection 226, 312–13
innervation 83–9
penetrating injuries 180–1, **182**
necrotizing ulcerative gingivitis (Vincent's angina, trench mouth) 144
needle cricothyroid puncture 49–53
needle-phobic patient 111, 112
negligence 27–9
nerve blocks
for awake intubation 40
for nasal surgery 277–8
see also regional anaesthesia
nerve damage, after regional block 100
nerve to the lateral pterygoid muscle 69
nerve to the medial pterygoid muscle 68
nervus intermedius 75
neuralgia 290–1
neuromuscular blockade 47
neurosurgical patients, perioperative management 222
next of kin, consulting 32
nimorazole 230
nitroprusside infusion 271–2
nitrous oxide
avoidance in head and neck surgery 215
in conscious sedation 103, 108
in gaseous induction 126
historical aspects 2, 5
in inhalational sedation **106**, 112–14
pollution **106**, 114
non-steroidal anti-inflammatory drugs (NSAIDs)
decrease need for opioids 323
in facial trauma 183, 185
as gastrointestinal disorders 18
for headache 286, 287, 288
in immunocompromised patients 291
in nasal and antral surgery 277
and oliguria 318
risk of bleeding 218, 256
sensitivity 275, 280

in temporomandibular dysfunction 293
use in paediatric patients 256
noradrenaline (norepinephrine) 147
nose, innervation 134
nursing care, postoperative 311–25
nutrition, for critically ill patients 148
nutritional status
in cancer patients 212–13
and radiotherapy 233–4
nutritional support, postoperative 322

obesity 38
and dental disease 121
difficult airway 38
and obstructive sleep apnoea 301, 303, 307, 308
in patients with learning disability 122
and poor dental health 121, 144
risk factor for aspiration 18
risk factor for hypoxaemia 314
risk factor for respiratory disorders 14
risk factor for venous thromboembolism 316
risk factor for wound infection 321
and tracheostomy 53, 54, 59
obstructive sleep apnoea
anatomical effects 302
cardiac effects 301–2
diagnosis 302–3
and facial trauma 307
following perioral radiotherapy 306
increased risk 306–7
investigations 303–6
neurological effects 302
paediatric 303, 308
in paediatric patients 253, 255, 258
respiratory effects 301
as risk factor 14
occipitomental 30° view 169
oculomotor nerve (cranial III) 81
odontalgia, atypical 294–5
oedema, secondary 185
oesophageal injury 181
olfactory nerves (cranial I) 80
oliguria, postoperative 317–18
ondansetron 127, 256, 277
operating table, rotation 45
ophthalmic assessment 181–2
ophthalmic nerve
anatomy 65, 74
branches 67, 74–5
opiates/opioids
for burn patients 201
in conscious sedation 108, 111–12
in dental surgery 126
in head and neck cancer 234
in nasal and antral surgery 276
for paediatric patients 256
tolerance 148

optic nerve (cranial II) 82
oral cancer, prevalence 207
oral cavity
    evaluation 37–8
    infection 143
oral and maxillofacial anatomy
    see craniofacial anatomy
oral and maxillofacial cancer see head
    and neck cancer
oral and maxillofacial surgery, regional
    anaesthetic techniques 91–101
oral musculature, innervation 79, **80**
oral soft tissue injuries, anaesthetic
    related 159–61
orbital floor fracture 174–5
orbital nerves 72–3, 81
orbital repairs, pain control 185
organ preservation, in cancer
    treatment 226
orodental tissues, innervation 77
orofacial pain 283–98
    aetiology 283
    chronic 283, 285–95
    classification 284, 285
    diagnostic criteria 283
    incidence 283
    non-odontogenic 285
    social and psychological
        impact 284
oropharyngeal airways, and
    anaesthetic-related dental
    injuries 152
oropharyngeal isthmus, sensory
    innervation 79
oropharyngeal suction 185, 243, 245,
    246, 315
orthognathic surgery 241–52
    hypotensive techniques 270,
        271, 272
orthopaedic problems 122
orthopantomogram (OPG) see dental
    panoramic tomogram (DPT)
osteomyelitis 144
osteoradionecrosis 237
osteotomies, postoperative
    management 264
otic ganglion 70
otoplasty (pinnaplasty) 136
outpatient procedures 35, 43, 46, 107,
    123, 231
oversedation 109, 112, 115, 133, 148
oxygen therapy
    for carbon monoxide toxicity
        194–5
    hyperbaric 194, 230, 237
    for oral and maxillofacial patients
        314–15

paclitaxel **232**
paediatric patients
    burns 190, 191, 192

comorbidities 121
consent 34
decreased pulmonary function 199
dental damage during
    anaesthesia 155
general anaesthesia 121
imaging under anaesthetic 264
inhalational sedation 114
limited mouth opening 260
maxillofacial surgery 253–68
non-accidental injury 265
premedication 123–4
preoperative assessment 22
pain
    emotional and psychological factors
        288, 292
    genetic aspects 295
    idiopathic 291–5
    neurovascular 285–90
    odontogenic 284
    postoperative 127, 140, 185, 285
    see also orofacial pain
pain control
    in burn patients 192
    in facial trauma 183, 185
    in head and neck region 218, 234
palatal anterior superior alveolar nerve
    block 94
palatal fistula 258
palate, sensory innervation 79
palliative treatment 230–1, 234
Paracelsus 1
paracetamol
    dose and administration route 127
    in facial trauma 183
    overdose, overlooked 190
    postoperative 201, 218, 219, 244,
        246, 250, 256, 258, 259
    preoperative 275, 277
paranasal sinuses 167
parotid plexus 76
patient assessment
    for conscious sedation 103
    for general anaesthesia 121
patient-controlled analgesia (PCA) 218
patient-controlled sedation (PCS) 112
patients
    anxious see anxiety/phobia
    with learning disabilities 120–2,
        123, 126
    positioning for dental surgery 124
    reassurance during sedation 113
    repositioning 44–5
    uncooperative 126
    see also elderly patients; paediatric
        patients
pectus excavatum 253
peptic ulcer disease 18
percutaneous dilatational
    tracheostomy 55–8
    see also tracheostomy
percutaneous endoscope gastrostomy
    (PEG) tube 233, 234

pericoronitis 284–5
periodontal ligament 168, *169*
periorbital bruising 172
persistent idiopathic facial pain (PIFP)
    293–5
PET scanning 226
Pfeiffer's syndrome see syndromic
    craniofacial abnormalities
pharmacokinetics, in burn patients 201
pharyngeal branches 73
    of the glossopharyngeal nerve 84
    of the vagus nerve 85
pharyngeal pack see throat pack
pharyngoplasty 259
pharynx
    injury 181
    innervation 89
    perforation 159
phenytoin 265
phobia see anxious/phobic patients
phrenic nerve 88
physical examination, preoperative 14
physical status classification (ASA) **12**,
    104, 132
physiological trespass 263
Pierre Robin syndrome 22, **254**, 257
pigmented lesions, removal 140
pilocarpine 236
plaque, and anaesthesia-related injury
    153–4
plastic surgery, history 131
platinum-based chemotherapy agents
    230, **231**
pneumonia, postoperative 316
pneumothorax 191
polysomnography 305
posterior auricular nerve 75
posterior ethmoidal nerve 75
posterior inferior nasal nerve 73
posterior superior alveolar nerve 72
    block 92
posterior superior nasal nerve 73, 81
postherpetic neuralgia 291
postnasal drip 275
postoperative care
    for burn patients 202
    nursing considerations 311–25
    in orthognathic surgery 243
    for paediatric patients 255
postoperative nausea and vomiting
    after otoplasty 136
    ingested blood 135, 136
    in nasal and antral surgery 276, 277
    with nitrous oxide 215
    not affected by throat pack 160
    nursing considerations 312, 323
    in oral surgery 18, 127–8
    in paediatric patients 255, 256
    patient-specific factors 323
    preventing 243–4
post-traumatic neuropathic pain 291
Poswillo report 9, 119

preanaesthetic assessment 211
premedication
    beta-blocker 270
    for day-case anaesthesia 123–4
    in epileptic patients 121
    in nasal/antral surgery 275
    in orthognathic surgery 241–2
    in paediatric patients 22, 253, 265
preoperative assessment
    for cleft lip/palate surgery 257–8
    for dental general anaesthesia 121
    importance 11
    for nasal/antral surgery 275
    for orthognathic surgery 241
    in paediatric patients 253
preoperative investigations 12, **13**
preoperative visit
    ASA guidelines 11
    in hypotensive anaesthesia 271
    in orthognathic surgery 241, 242
    for paediatric patients 22, 253
preprosthetic surgery 247–8
preservatives 133
propofol
    decreased postoperative nausea and
        vomiting 277, 323
    intravenous anaesthesia 184, 215, 244
    intravenous induction 60, 126, 134,
        135, 140, 278
    operator-controlled infusion 112
    in paediatric patients 112, 114
    sedation 39, 107–8
    target-controlled infusion 132
psychiatric disorders
    and orofacial pain 283
    in patients with learning
        disability 122
    in persistent idiopathic facial pain
        (PIFP) 294
psychological illness, severe **105**
psychometric testing 295
psychosocial morbidity 237
pterygo-maxillary buttress 167
pterygopalatine ganglion 71, 72, 73–4
public guardian 34
pulmonary circulation,
    hypotension 271
pulmonary complications,
    perioperative 14
pulmonary embolism 316
pulmonary trauma 177
pulse oximetry
    in burn patients 191, 192, 198, 202
    in conscious sedation 109, 110,
        112, 115
    in hypotensive procedures 272
    overnight 304
    standard care 258, 313
pyramidal fracture 171

radiation caries 236
radiation effects 232–3, 319

radiotherapy
    dose and fractionation 229
    for head and neck cancers 207, 212,
        213, 225–30
    and hypoxia 230
    methods of delivery 227–9
    morbidity 231–3
Ramsay Hunt syndrome 291
recombinant activated protein C 148
regional anaesthesia
    for facial aesthetic procedures
        131, 133
    for mandibular nerve and branches
        94–7
    for maxillary nerve and branches
        92–4
    in nasal and antral surgery 277–8
    in oral and maxillofacial surgery
        91–101
regional analgesia, for donor site
    pain 218
regional nerve blocks **92**
reintubation 44, 184, 218, 219, 249, 315
remifentanil
    analgesia 215, 258
    blood pressure control 134, 215,
        260, 277
    in burn patients 201
    emergence 185
    in head and neck surgery 214, 215,
        218, 222, 260
    infusion 218, 220, 243, 246, 258
    maintenance of anaesthesia 215
    in neonates and infants 256
    rapid recovery 133, 222, 256
    in rhinoplasty 134
    total intravenous anaesthesia 184,
        215, 281
renal circulation, hypotension 270
renal disorders, preoperative
    assessment 20–1
renal failure 318
renal support 147–8
respiratory complications,
    postoperative 314–16
respiratory depression
    benzodiazepines 107
    in conscious sedation 107, 108,
        110, 111
    in intravenous sedation 115
    midazolam 106, 111, 112, 115
    opiates/opioids 108, 112, 126, 185
respiratory disorders
    in patients with learning
        disabilities 122
    preoperative assessment 14
    sleep-related 300–1, 306
respiratory function, assessment and
    monitoring 313
respiratory pattern 304, *305*
respiratory support 147
'responsible minority' defence 28–9
resuscitation equipment 123

reverse carotid flow 99
rhinoplasty 134–5, 280
rhytidectomy 135
Riggs, John 2
right recurrent laryngeal nerve 85
Ring–Adair–Elwyn (RAE) tube 125,
    135, 183, 258, 259, 275–6
risk stratification 11
Robinson, James 3
Rocabado's exercises 292

salbutamol 197
saliva, diminished or absent 154
salivary fistula 320
salivary glands 80, *208*, 220, 265
Second World War, importance for
    anaesthesia 8
sedated patient, monitoring
    110–11, 114
sedation *see* conscious sedation
sepsis 146, 319, 321–2
septic shock 146–8
septoplasty 280
septorhinoplasty 134
sevoflurane 61, 108, 114, 126, 127,
    201, 214
sexual fantasies 116
Sharpey's fibres 168
short ciliary nerves 82–3
short-lasting unilateral neuralgia with
    conjunctival irritation and tearing
    (SUNCT) 289
Simpson, James Young 4
sinonasal tumours 280–1
sinus surgery 280
skin cooling devices 139–40
skin flaps *see* flaps
skin grafts 199–200
skin reaction, in head and neck
    radiotherapy 235
sleep, physiology 299–300
sleep apnoea *see* obstructive sleep
    apnoea
sleep deprivation 302, 303
sleep problems, paediatric studies 306
smoke, toxic compounds 197
smoke inhalation complex 189,
    194, 195
smoking
    cessation 14, 225, 233
    and head and neck cancer 207, 213,
        214, 225, 237
    and radiotherapy 233, 234
    risk factor 14, 15, 144, 154, **155**, 311,
        316, 323
snoring 300, 303, 306
Snow, John 3–5
social factors, in sedation 105, 109
socioeconomic status 121, 144
sodium bicarbonate *see* bicarbonate

solid organ transplant recipients, head and neck cancer 207
solid organ transplantation, preoperative assessment 23
sore throat, associated with throat packs 160
special senses
    alteration 99
    organs 65
speech and language therapists 233
sphenopalatine ganglion, blockade 134
sphenotemporal buttress *173*, *174*
spinal cord ischaemia 272
splanchnic circulation, hypotension 270
stab wounds 180
statins 12–13
statute law 27
steroids
    adverse effects 18, 321
    anti-inflammatory 180, 182
    current medication 13, 14
    in postherpetic neuralgia 291
    postoperative 128, 222, 250
    preoperative 14
    prophylactic 232, 287
    in sepsis 147
    in temporal arteritis 289–90
Stickler's syndrome **257**
stress, in aetiology of pain 288, 292
Sturge–Weber syndrome **254**, 261
stylopharyngeus branch of the glossopharyngeal nerve 84
subglottic tracheal stenosis 199
submandibular ganglion 70–1
submental intubation 62–3, **184**, 242
submentovertex view 169
subperiosteal injection 99
sucralfate 235
suction *see* oropharyngeal suction
suicidal patients, with burns 190
superior alveolar nerves 78
superior cervical ganglion 86–7
superior laryngeal nerve 85
supraclavicular nerves 84
supraglottic devices 35, 42–3, 125, 220–1
supraorbital artery *66*
supraorbital nerve *66*, *67*, 75
supratrochlear artery *66*
supratrochlear nerve *66*, *67*, 75
surgical cricothyroidotomy 49–53
surgical procedures, grading system **12**
surgical tracheostomy 54–5
    see also tracheostomy
sutures, postoperative care 320
suxamethonium 126, 201, 203
swallowing problems 233–4, 315, 322
syncope 100
syndromic craniofacial abnormalities anaesthetic implications 253, 254

associated with cleft palate **257**
and obstructive sleep apnoea 306
surgery 241, 247, 248, 261–2
syringes
    aspirating 99
    computerized 93, *94*
    for dental use 91, **278**
    in liposuction 135
systemic diseases, intraoral manifestations 154, **155**
systemic inflammatory response syndrome (SIRS) 146, 319

target-controlled infusion 112, 133, 214
taste, loss 236
tattoos, removal 140
taxanes 226, 230, **232**
teenagers, psychosocial problems 242
teeth
    anatomy *see* dental anatomy
    deciduous 121, 155
    extraction 124
    identification/nomenclature 151, 167
    inhaled 158, *159*
    innervation 77
    subluxed or avulsed 158
temperature control
    in burn patients 200–1
    during lengthy procedures 262
    in flap perfusion 216
    in orthognathic surgery 243
    postoperative 318–19
temperature monitoring, in burn patients 202
temporal arteritis 289–90
temporal nerve 76
temporomandibular disorders, and orofacial pain 283, 284, 291–3
temporomandibular joint
    ankylosis 260–1
    evaluation 36
    innervation 71
    surgery 249–51
    trauma 175–6
thermal injuries 189–205
    airway damage 195–6
thiopentone 8
throat packs
    in airway surgery 254
    alert label *242*
    in dental abscess patients 147
    in facial surgery 185, 243, 245, 246, 247, 249, 250, 251
    injuries/morbidity associated with 151, 159, 160
    in nasal/antral surgery 275, 276, 277, 279, 280, 281
    in paediatric surgery 254, 258, 259, 262, 264, 265

prevention of PONV 323
ribbon type *127*
safe removal 56, 126, 135, 160
thyroid dysfunction, associated with radiotherapy 237
thyromental distance 37
titanium *see* dental implants
tomotherapy 228–9
tongue
    defects, repair 315
    injuries, anaesthetic related 159
    reduction 265
    sensory innervation 79
    see also macroglossia
tongue tie, division 264
tonsillar branches, of the glossopharyngeal nerve 84
topical anaesthesia
    intraoral 99
    prior to venepuncture 109–10
    see also lidocaine
topical barrier gels 235
total intravenous anaesthesia 134, 135, 214
    see also intravenous anaesthesia
toxicity, in local anaesthesia 100–1
tracheal injuries 178, 180
tracheal tubes 125, 254, 262
tracheostomy
    advantages and disadvantages 53, **184**
    for airway obstruction 60–1
    awake 147, 213
    in burn patients 199
    complications 58–60
    contraindications 53–4
    in critical care 54, 55, 60
    elective 313
    emergency 61–2
    general anaesthesia 61–2
    in head and neck resections 214
    indications 53
    local anaesthesia 61
    and obstructive sleep apnoea 307
    in paediatric patients 255–6, 262
    permanent 59
    techniques 53
    tubes 58–60
    under local anaesthesia 221, 222
tramadol 185, 201, 234, 295
transillumination 41–2
transtracheal block 39
transverse cervical nerve 83–4
trauma
    airway management 46–7
    imaging 169–76
    preoperative evaluation 46
    self-inflicted 100, 127
    see also maxillofacial trauma
Treacher Collins syndrome **254**, **257**, 306
treatment planning, for conscious sedation 105–6

trigeminal nerve (cranial V) 65, 283
trigeminal neuralgia 290–1
trimalar fracture 172
trimetaphan 269
trismus
    after nerve block 99–100
    in facial trauma 183
    in head and neck cancer 220
    infection related 38, 145, 146, 264
    prevention 128
    radiotherapy induced 213, **221**,
        235–6
    in temporomandibular joint
        disorders 250
trochlear nerve (cranial IV) 81–2
tumours *see* head and neck cancer
turbinectomy 280
tympanic nerve 84

undersedation 107, 115
upper respiratory tract, variations 35
urinary catheters, monitoring 202, 318
uvula, vulnerable to injury 159
vagus nerve (cranial X) 84–5
valvular heart disease 17–18, 122
    see also cardiac disorders

varicella zoster virus 291
vascular access 200, 263
vascular injury 178, 180
vascular lesions, laser treatment 141
vascular malformations and
    tumours 261
vasoactive agents, in flap perfusion
    217–18
vasoconstriction 211, 216, 218, 219,
    222, 271, 301, 317, 318
vasoconstrictors 39, 54, 91, 97, 99, 127,
    133, 134, 161, 276–7, 278, 279, 280
vasodilatation 269–70
velocardiofacial syndrome **257**
velopharyngeal insufficiency 258
venous thromboembolism,
    postoperative 316
ventilation
    compromised 313–14
    during sleep 299–300
ventriculoperitoneal shunt 263
videofluoroscopy 233
virus infections 100, 148, 227, 291
vocal cord palsy 212
volume resuscitation 317
    see also fluid resuscitation

Walton series machines 8
warfarin 13
waste gas scavenging 114
Waters view 169
Wells, Horace 2
wounds
    care 319–20
    intraoral 320
    postoperative infection 321–2
wrinkles, treatment 141

xenon scanning 197
xerostomia **213**, 229, 234, 236
xylocaine *see* lidocaine

Young, J.Z. 65

zygoma, fractures 172–4
zygomatic nerve 72, 76
zygomaticofacial nerve 66, 67
zygomatico-maxillary buttress 167
zygomaticotemporal nerve 66, 67